Manual of Acute Hand Injuries

Manual of Acute Hand Injuries

David S. Martin, MD
Plastic and Reconstructive Surgery
Murfreesboro Medical Clinic and Surgicenter
Murfreesboro, Tennessee

E. Dale Collins, MD
Assistant Professor of Plastic and Reconstructive Surgery
Dartmouth-Hitchcock Medical Center
Lebanon, New Hampshire

With 327 illustrations

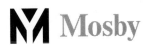 Mosby

St. Louis   Baltimore   Boston   Carlsbad   Chicago   Minneapolis   New York   Philadelphia   Portland
London   Milan   Sydney   Tokyo   Toronto

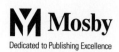
Mosby

Dedicated to Publishing Excellence

A Times Mirror Company

Vice President and Publisher: Anne S. Patterson
Executive Editor: Robert Hurley
Associate Developmental Editor: Marla Sussman
Project Manager: Chris Baumle
Production Editor: Mickie Hall
Designer: Carolyn O'Brien
Manufacturing Manager: William A. Winneberger, Jr.

Printed in the United States of America
Composition by Graphic Composition, Inc.
Printing/binding by R. R. Donnelley & Sons Company

Mosby-Year Book, Inc.
11830 Westline Industrial Drive
St. Louis, Missouri 63146

Library of Congress Cataloging in Publication Data
Manual of acute hand injuries / [edited by] David S. Martin, E. Dale Collins.
    p. cm.
    Includes bibliographical references and index.
    ISBN 0-8151-5861-0
    1. Hand—Wounds and injuries—Surgery—Handbooks, manuals, etc.
I. Martin, David S. (David Scott). II. Collins, E. Dale.
[DNLM: 1. Hand Injuries—therapy—handbooks. 2. Hand—surgery—handbooks. WE 39 M293 1998]
RD559.M276 1998
617.5'75044—dc21
DNLM/DLC
for Library of Congress   97-17955
                                                        CIP

98 99 00 01 02 / 9 8 7 6 5 4 3 2 1

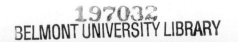

Foreword

The editors, as residents, noted a need for a concise, portable manual for treatment of acute hand injuries. In preparing a manual directed primarily at students, residents, fellows, and young practicing surgeons, the editors have elected to present a proven method of management rather than "cover the waterfront." Faculty of the Division of Plastic Surgery at Washington University, with a particular interest in hand surgery, contributed their experience in many of the chapters. The editors observed and participated in application of these techniques and in evaluating the results. They concluded, from their unbiased observations, that a concise presentation of these methods could be of benefit.

This first edition is a tribute to the indefatigable efforts and intellectual curiosity of the editors—outstanding individuals who epitomize the ideal resident. The manual will be revised at regular intervals by residents, fellows, and staff members working in concert to provide a single volume highlighting the technical advances in hand surgery. It has been an honor to be associated with all involved in its preparation.

Paul M. Weeks, MD, FACS

Preface

Manual of Acute Hand Injuries was designed to be the best friend of both the neophyte and the occasional hand surgeon. Although there are superb references covering all facets of hand injuries by authors of general, orthopedic, and plastic surgical backgrounds, most are burdensomely detailed (and heavy), precluding easy use by some haggard physician evaluating a complicated hand injury in the middle of the night. Most contributors to this book still remember examining a patient and then retreating to an office or call room or trunk of a car where the desired information could be found. Woe be to the physician who, on consulting the reference text, realized that he or she had failed to perform some basic physical examination maneuver, and would therefore have to return to the patient's bedside, complete the proper examination, and again return to consult an encyclopedic text to ascertain how to proceed with treatment. It was the feeling of intense frustration in not having a concise, portable, informative reference that could be used when time was of the essence that led to the writing of this book.

We sought an accessible format that provided the useful details and practical advice often omitted from more distinguished texts. Technique of patient examination, pertinent anatomy, priorities for treatment and their urgency, operative sequence, and the recovery process are emphasized. Repetition of figures and text topics between chapters is intentional; we know the frustration of not knowing where to look to find the desired information. Our intent was to augment the knowledge and confidence of fledgling hand surgeons and those physicians who only occasionally care for patients with upper extremity trauma. It also is designed to assist nurses, physical and occupational therapists, and others who seek to better understand hand injuries.

We had perhaps one of the greatest professional opportunities available: the chance to train as residents and fellows under the tutelage of the plastic surgery faculty of the Washington University School of Medicine in St. Louis. Under the leadership of Dr. Paul M. Weeks, we were provided with a smorgasbord of clinical material, an attitude of intellectual encouragement, and ample opportunity to learn operative skills with a blend of supervision and independence. We are deeply indebted to Dr. Weeks for his dedication and commitment to the teaching of residents and fellows during the course of his exemplary career.

Finally, this book is offered as a special dedication to our late mothers: to Nancy Wallner Martin, an educator with a lifelong zeal for learning and the desire to make learning easy and fun for others, and to Vera Virginia Collins, for a life devoted to the guidance, support, and encouragement of her children.

David S. Martin
E. Dale Collins

Contributor Affiliation List

Thomas J. Francel, MD, FACS
Assistant Professor, Department
  of Surgery
Plastic Surgeon-in-Chief, Barnes-Jewish
  Hospital North
St. Louis, Missouri

Mitchell A. Fremling, MD
Hand Surgery Fellow, Department
  of Orthopedics
Loma Linda University
Loma Linda, California

Louis A. Gilula, MD
Professor of Radiology, Orthopaedic
  Surgery and Plastic Surgery
Washington University School
  of Medicine
Director, Musculoskeletal Section
Barnes-Jewish Hospital
St. Louis, Missouri

Gail N. Groth, OTR, CHT
Occupational Therapist, Milliken Hand
  Rehabilitation Center
Barnes-Jewish Hospital
St. Louis, Missouri

Joan Guccione, OTR, CHT
Occupational Therapist, Milliken Hand
  Rehabilitation Center
Barnes-Jewish Hospital
St. Louis, Missouri

Philip E. Higgs, MD, FACS
Assistant Professor, Washington
  University School of Medicine
Barnes-Jewish Hospital
St. Louis, Missouri

Roger K. Khouri, MD, FACS
Professor, Miami Hand Center
Coral Gables, Florida

Bruce A. Kraemer, MD
Associate Professor, Plastic and
  Reconstructive Surgery
Washington University School
  of Medicine
Director Replantation Service, Director
  BJH Wound Healing Center
Barnes-Jewish Hospital, Barnes-Jewish
  West County Hospital
St. Louis, Missouri

David M. Kupfer, MD
Assistant Clinical Professor of Surgery
University of California, San Diego
Co-Director, California Institute of
  Plastic and Reconstructive Surgery
San Diego, California

Laurent Lantieri, MD
Practicien Hospitalo Universitaire
CHU Henri Mondor, Paris XII
  University
Plastic and Reconstructive Surgery
Hopital Henri Mondor Assisatance
  Puclique des Hopitaux de Paris
Paris, France

Gilbert W. Lee, MD
Assistant Clinical Professor, Division of
  Plastic and Reconstructive Surgery
Department of Orthopaedic Surgery,
  University of California-San Diego
San Diego, California

Susan E. Mackinnon, MD
Professor of Surgery (Plastic and
  Reconstructive)
Chief, Division of Plastic and
  Reconstructive Surgery
Washington University School
  of Medicine
Barnes-Jewish Hospital, St. Louis
  Children's Hospital
St. Louis, Missouri

Kathy A. Mantz, BGS
Nursing Marketing Coordinator, Mosby-
  Year Book, Inc.
St. Louis, Missouri

Viktor M. Metz, MD
Associate Professor of Radiology, Clinic
  for Radiodiagnostic
University Vienna, Austria

S. M. Metz-Schimmerl, MD
Staff Member, Clinic for
  Radiodiagnostic
University Vienna, Austria

Patty Paynter, OTR, CHT
Staff Therapist, Milliken Hand
  Rehabilitation Center
Barnes-Jewish Hospital
St. Louis, Missouri

Erin Casey Phillips, MSOT, OTR/L
Hand Therapist, Milliken Hand
  Rehabilitation Center
Barnes-Jewish Hospital
St. Louis, Missouri

Barbara Sopp, MS, OTR/L, CHT
Staff Occupational Therapist, Milliken
  Hand Rehabilitation Center
Barnes-Jewish Hospital
St. Louis, Missouri

Elizabeth J. Walker, PT
Physical Therapist, Milliken Hand
  Rehabilitation Center
Barnes-Jewish Hospital
St. Louis, Missouri

Greg P. Watchmaker, MD
Children's Hospital
Milwaukee, Wisconsin

Paul M. Weeks, MD, FACS
Professor of Surgery (Plastic and
  Reconstructive)
Washington University School of
  Medicine, Barnes-Jewish Hospital
St. Louis, Missouri

Peter D. Witt, MD, FACS
Assistant Professor of Surgery, Plastic
  and Reconstructive Surgery
Washington University School of
  Medicine
Director, Cleft Lip/Palate, Cleft Palate
  and Craniofacial Deformities Institute
St. Louis Children's Hospital/Barnes-
  Jewish Hospital
St. Louis, Missouri

Mary Beth Wulf, OTR/L, CHT
Occupational Therapist, Loyola
 University Medical Center
Maywood, Illinois

Patty K. Young, MD
Instructor, Plastic and Reconstructive
 Surgery
Washington University School of
 Medicine
Barnes-Jewish Hospital
St. Louis, Missouri

V. Leroy Young, MD
Professor, Plastic and Reconstructive
 Surgery
Washington University School
 of Medicine
Attending Physician, Division of
 Plastic Surgery
Barnes-Jewish Hospital, Barnes-Jewish
 West County Hospital
St. Louis, Missouri

Contents

Manual of Acute Hand Injuries

1

Healing of Specialized Tissues

Gilbert W. Lee, MD
E. Dale Collins, MD
David M. Kupfer, MD
Paul M. Weeks, MD, FACS

The hand is composed of specialized body tissues, which include glabrous skin, bone, tendons, nerves, cartilage, and joints. Adequate treatment of acute hand injuries requires a good working knowledge of the processes by which these specialized tissues heal. Because different tissues heal at different rates, the healing process must be monitored constantly. A thorough understanding of the time, course, and manner in which each tissue heals enables the hand surgeon to incorporate changes into the rehabilitation protocols that will optimize the functional result.

WOUND HEALING: OVERVIEW

The palmar surface of the hand is covered with glabrous, or nonhair bearing, skin. This skin, which is also found on the plantar surface of the feet, heals in a similar manner to skin found elsewhere in the body. Following injury to the skin, the process of epithelization seals the wound, while the processes of fibrous tissue synthesis and remodeling provide wound strength. These wound healing processes are divided into the inflammatory phase, the proliferative phase, and the remodeling phase. When tissue is missing, wound contraction moves tissue edges into closer approximation, so that epithelization and fibrous protein synthesis can occur.

Wound Contraction

It has long been recognized that wounds left open to heal form scars that are much smaller than the original skin defects. The centripetal movement of the raw skin edges, which causes the wound to shrink, is called contraction. The functional and aesthetic result following wound closure by contraction depends on the amount of excess skin that is available to donate to the defect. The face and hands of young people do not have excess skin. Thus, closure of wounds by contraction causes distortion of adjacent structures or loss of joint mobility. Conversely, elderly patients who have much more lax, redundant skin can heal wounds by contraction with little distortion of adjacent structures. If the edges of a hand wound cannot be approximated without holding a joint in flexion or extension, it is certain that wound contraction will result in a flexion or extension contracture, which is the result of dynamic wound contraction.

The process of wound contraction begins approximately 4 days following an injury. During those 4 days, known as the inflammatory phase, the wound amasses the chemicals, cellular components, and energy that will be required to move the skin edges closer together. The process of contraction continues well after the wound edges touch each other, thereby sealing the wound. Myofibroblasts are responsible for the movement of the wound edges. Microscopically, myofibroblasts show the characteristics of fibroblasts and smooth muscle cells, including rough endoplasmic reticulum, microfilament bundles similar to smooth muscle, and abundant microtubules that apparently perform a bracing function. Histochemical studies show that the common contractile protein in smooth muscle cells and myofibroblasts is actin. Experimentally, wound contraction can be inhibited by the application of smooth muscle inhibitors or inhibitors of microtubule formation.

Epithelization

A basic regenerative function of the body is to cover areas denuded of skin with regenerated epidermis. This epithelization is the first sign of wound repair and occurs long before any evidence of connective tissue synthesis. Epithelization is necessary to create a watertight seal for the body. Although this seal protects the body from fluid loss, infection, and particulate contamination, the epidermis offers little strength or structural support to the scar. Thus, a wound that has only a tenuous epithelial barrier is at risk for breakdown. The process of epithelization is rather primitive. It is similar to an embryonic state characterized by rapid cellular proliferation. The regenerating epithelial cells continue to replicate and push forth the wound margins until they are surrounded by dense contact with other epithelial cells and the wound is fully epithelized. This process begins within hours of wound creation. Incised and sutured wounds form an epithelial watertight seal within 24 hours. Early in the process, the epithelium follows the undulations of the wound margin; underlying connective tissue synthesis will eventually push the epithelium into an everted position.

Collagen

Collagen is a protein synthesized by fibroblasts. Type I collagen is the most prevalent type in mature vertebrates. Type II collagen is found in human articular and costal cartilage. Type III collagen, which is found in association with Type I collagen, is most prevalent in tissue undergoing remodeling. It appears to be an important part of those tissues that require an unusual amount of elasticity, such as the aorta, esophagus, and uterus.

Collagen is synthesized within the fibroblasts. A critical step in this synthesis is the hydroxylation of proline and lysine to produce hydroxyproline and hydroxylysine. Hydroxyproline and hydroxylysine are amino acids found only in collagen. After the collagen is synthesized and secreted by the fibroblasts, a procollagen peptidase removes the N-terminal and C-terminal ends of the collagen molecules. This allows the collagen's trihelix structures to interact and bond, forming fibrils and fibers (Fig. 1-1). It is the cross-linking of collagen and the interweaving of the fibers and fibrils that increase the tensile strength of a scar. The collagen within a wound is a dynamic structure that is constantly undergoing remodeling and replacement. After 6 weeks of healing, the amount of collagen in the wound does not increase, but the scar continues to gain strength for at least 2 years. Thus, increases

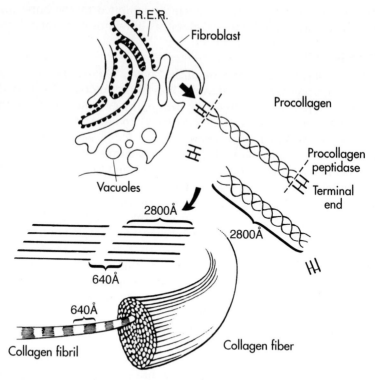

Figure 1-1 Procollagen synthesis occurs within the endoplasmic reticulum of the fibroblast. The C- and N-terminal ends are removed by a procollagenase peptide. The collagen fibrils then bond to form fibrils and fibers.

in cross-linking and the rearrangement of fibers and fibrils must still be occurring.

Summary

The healing of wounds is usually described in terms of two forms: the healing of an incised and sutured wound that is properly coapted (healing by primary intention) and the healing of a wound by contraction and epithelization because tissue has been lost (healing by secondary intention).

Following full-thickness skin loss, elastic skin and muscle forces pull and enlarge the defect. A blood clot forms on the wound surface; it then contracts and dehydrates forming a scab. This scab creates a barrier against further contamination. The first stage of wound healing is called the inflammatory phase. During this phase, an intense inflammatory reaction takes place. There is a huge influx of enzymes, fluid, and protein into the extracellular spaces of the wound. White blood cells accumulate, mast cells release various amines, and thrombi form in peripheral vascular channels.

Approximately 12 hours after the injury, the inflammatory process is well established and epithelial migration—the first clear-cut sign of rebuilding—occurs. In a primary wound, epithelization is complete in 24 to 48 hours. In a secondary wound, migration of cells is rapid initially, but as the line of cells from the wound margin becomes extended and the epithelial probe dwindles to a monolayer, progress becomes slower. As a result, days or even weeks elapse before epithelization is complete. After 4 or 5 days, epithelization is assisted by wound contraction, which moves the wound margins toward the center. After the scab has been removed, there is an intense proliferation of richly perfused capillary loops at the center of the wound. This granulation tissue provides a good barrier against contamination.

Collagen synthesis begins between the second and fourth days, but is not noticeable until the fifth day. Tensile strength in the initial wound is the result of blood vessels growing across the wound, epithelization, and aggregation of globular proteins. Although the strength of the wounds is slight, it is usually adequate by the fifth day to hold the wound edges together without sutures, provided the wound is not under tension. The significant gain in tensile strength begins on approximately the fifth day, when collagen synthesis becomes apparent. Tensile strength measurements usually are recorded beginning on the fifth day. Strength increases rapidly for 17 days, and then slows down for an additional 10 days. The strength of the scar never reaches that of normal skin (Fig. 1-2).

The collagen content of the wound tissue increases rapidly between the sixth and the seventeenth day. It then tapers off over the next three weeks, so that collagen content does not rise after the forty-second day. The gain in strength after the seventeenth day, therefore, is primarily the result of the remodeling of collagen and, hence, is only correlated with total collagen content during the early portion of the healing curve.

BONE REGENERATION
Embryology and Anatomy

Bone is embryologically derived from mesenchymal tissue through endochondral or intramembranous ossification. Endochondral bones are formed from a hyaline cartilage model that becomes partially ossified. Endochondral bones, which include the bones of the limbs, vertebral column, and base of the skull (chondrocranium), retain a cartilaginous portion as articular cartilage and epiphyseal growth plate.

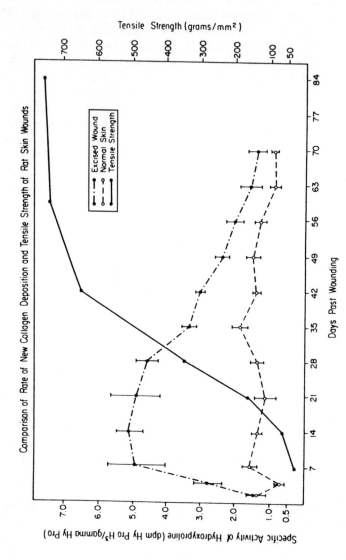

Figure 1-2 Comparison of rate of collagen deposition and tensile strength in healing of rat skin. (From Peacock EE, Cohen IK: *Wound healing.* In McCarthy JR, editor: *Plastic surgery,* Philadelphia, 1990, WB Saunders, p. 174.)

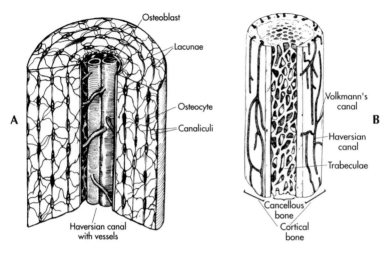

Figure 1-3   **(A)** The osteon, which is the basic unit of cortical growth. **(B)** A wedge of bone, showing the cortical and cancellous components.

Membranous bones develop directly from mesenchymal condensations, without an intermediate cartilage matrix. The cranial vault (neurocranium), facial skeleton, and clavicle are membranous bones. The mandible and the sphenoid, temporal, and occipital bones (chondrocranium) have ossification centers originating from both cartilage and mesenchymal condensations.

The architecture of bone is described morphologically as cortical or cancellous. Cortical bone constitutes the external and internal lamellae of flat bones and the external column of long bones. Cancellous bone is found between the cortical layers of flat bones and in the metaphyseal region of long bones.

The basic unit of cortical bone is the osteon, which consists of the haversian canal with its associated vessels that are surrounded by concentric lamellae of bone in which the osteocytes are embedded. Vessels course through Volkmann canals to anastomose with haversian vessels. This specialized arrangement of cells and vascular elements provides a spatial relationship in which no osteocyte within the matrix lies more than 300 μm from a blood vessel (Fig. 1-3A and B). In remodeling, new haversian systems are formed, as osteoclasts, grouped into a resorbing wedge, resorb older mineralized bone, thereby creating a new tunnel into which vascular elements and osteoblasts migrate and deposit new bony lamellae.

Cancellous bone is structurally characterized by large units of mineralized bone called trabeculae and smaller units called spicules. Osteoblasts reside on the surface of the trabeculae, where they deposit osteoid. Osteocytes are found within lacunae in regions of functional stress where the cross-sectional dimensions of the trabeculae are significantly increased. The axes of the trabeculae are oriented perpendicular to the forces of muscle tension and weight bearing.

Healing of Bone

Bone is a unique tissue in that it is capable of regeneration without formation of a scar. The surgical principles of anatomic reduction, preservation of blood supply, and adequate immobilization promote healing of fractures. The classic histologic observations of fracture healing were made on nonrigidly immobilized fractures. Initially, a hematoma forms at the fracture site due to damaged blood vessels in the periosteum and endosteum. During the subsequent inflammatory phase, there is proliferation of osteogenic cells from the periosteum and endosteum, with gradual replacement of the hematoma by fibrovascular tissue and osteogenic cells. In nondisplaced fractures, endosteal circulation predominates throughout all healing phases. When endosteal circulation is disrupted, periosteal circulation becomes the major blood supply to displaced bone fragments. The overlying soft tissue is also an important source of blood supply to the fractured bone segments, particularly when there is significant periosteal stripping as a result of the trauma. During the initial healing stage, a callus forms at the fracture site consisting of dense fibrous tissue, fibrocartilage, and cartilage. Large caliber vessels, derived from the reunited periosteal and endosteal circulation, penetrate the callus. This rich vascular environment promotes the differentiation of osteogenic cells into osteoblasts that deposit immature woven bone in a random pattern. Osteoclasts also appear, so that ossification and resorption occur concomitantly, gradually transforming the fibrocartilaginous callus into a bony callus. The ultimate healing of the fracture site depends on continued formation of subperiosteal trabeculae that bridge the fracture gap and on remodeling of the cortex.

Cancellous bone heals primarily through formation of an endosteal callus. Cancellous bone heals more rapidly than cortical bone because of its abundant vascularity and the large surface area of endosteal bone. The osteogenic cells lining the trabeculae proliferate and deposit woven bone in the cancellous spaces. The internal endosteal callus gradually remodels so that the axes of the trabeculae become oriented perpendicular to the vectors of force acting on the bone.

Impacted fractures of cancellous bone heal more rapidly than distracted fractures separated by dead space resulting from the juxtaposition of the healing bone units. Further, when fractured segments are accurately aligned and fixed with compression plates, healing proceeds without formation of an internal or external stabilizing callus. In this situation, direct osseous healing occurs rapidly by intracortical remodeling.

Blood supply is the most critical element influencing fracture healing. Soon after a fracture, the blood flow through the adjacent undamaged blood vessel increases; this persists until the fracture is healed. Both periosteal and endosteal circulation also increase by angiogenesis. Within any fracture site, there is death of osteocytes in the cortical and cancellous bone adjacent to the fracture because of disruption of their blood supply. To ensure prompt healing, adequate vascularity to the bone must be preserved. Surgical intervention affects the blood supply to a variable degree depending on the extent of dissection for exposure and the method of fixation. Therefore, operative intervention must be justified by improved anatomic reduction and more stable fixation; periosteal stripping should be kept to a minimum.

Healing of Bone Grafts

There are three biologic mechanisms of bone regeneration after bone transplantation: osteogenesis, osteoconduction, and osteoinduction. Osteogenesis is the formation of new bone by surviving preosteoblasts and osteoblasts within the graft. Healing by this mechanism is more prominent in cancellous bone grafts than in cortical bone grafts, because of the rapid revascularization of the former. A vascularized bone transfer also heals primarily by osteogenesis, as the blood supply to the bone-forming cell is maintained. In contrast, healing by osteoconduction is a prolonged process. The bone graft functions as a nonviable scaffold for the gradual ingrowth of blood vessels and osteoprogenitor cells from the recipient site, with gradual resorption and deposition of new bone. Axhausen referred to this process as creeping substitution. Osteoconduction is the predominant mechanism in healing of cortical grafts. Osteoinduction is the transformation of local host mesenchymal cells into bone-forming cells in the presence of an appropriate inductive stimulus. This process is regulated by insoluble polypeptide morphogens and specific enzymes and enzyme inhibitors. Demineralization of bone prior to implantation is required for osteoinduction to occur.

Healing of Cortical Versus Cancellous Grafts

The healing of autogenous cancellous and cortical bone grafts is essentially the same during the first 2 weeks after transplantation. During the first week, the graft is the focus of an inflammatory response characterized by infiltration of vascular buds into the transplant bed.

Lymphocytes, plasma cells, osteoclasts, and fibrous connective tissue with mononuclear and polynuclear cells, as well as extracellular fluid, surround the graft. By the second week, the inflammatory response subsides with continued fibrovascular proliferation and increasing osteoclastic activity. Within the confines of the graft, osteocytic autolysis proceeds with necrosis of the cellular elements. The necrotic tissue in the haversian canals and marrow spaces is removed by macrophages. The evacuated vascular spaces become filled with primitive mesenchymal tissue. Some peripheral cells remain viable by passive diffusion of nutrients from the surrounding soft tissue.

In the later phases of healing, cancellous and cortical bone grafts can be distinguished by differences in the rate of revascularization, by creeping substitution, and by the completeness of the repair. In cancellous grafts, following the initial inflammatory phase and osteoclastic autolysis, the numerous vascular spaces surrounding the bone are primed for invasion by new blood vessels. Revascularization of cancellous grafts may occur within hours after transplantation through inosculation. However, gradual revascularization of cancellous grafts by host vessel ingrowth into the marrow spaces is usually completed within 2 weeks. In contrast, revascularization of cortical bone grafts occurs more slowly. There is essentially no penetration of a cortical graft by blood vessels during the first week and complete revascularization requires 1 to 2 months or longer. The cortical architecture apparently delays revascularization because the new vessels must follow pre-existing Volkmann and haversian canals from the periphery of the graft into the interior. Delayed vascularization may also be the result of the limited number of vessels available to participate in the process of inosculation.

Concomitant with vascular invasion of a cancellous graft, primitive mesenchymal cells lining the trabeculae differentiate into osteoblasts and deposit a seam of osteoid around the central core of necrotic bone. Thus, repair of a cancellous graft is by initial bone formation. In contrast, cortical graft repair is initiated by osteoclastic activity, with early resorption directed to peripherally located necrotic haversian systems and the interstitial lamellae followed by resorption of the cortical interior. Osteoblasts then appear and begin to deposit osteoid where resorption of the bone has occurred.

In cancellous grafts, the entrapped areas of necrotic bone are gradually resorbed by osteoclasts, and in time, the cancellous graft is completely replaced by viable new bone. In cortical grafts, the initiation of the appositional phase takes place before the necrotic bone has been completely removed. These areas of nonvascularized bone become sealed off from further osteoclastic resorption, leaving the cortical graft as an admixture of necrotic and viable bone.

The mechanical strength of cancellous and cortical grafts is affected by the differences in the healing process. Cancellous grafts initially strengthen as repair is initiated by new bone formation; the mechanical strength then normalizes as the necrotic bone is removed. Cortical grafts weaken to approximately 60% of normal strength for up to several months after grafting because repair is initiated by osteoclastic resorption, which increases the internal porosity of the graft. Thus, cortical grafts require prolonged splinting and activity limitations compared with cancellous grafts.

Periosteum

Onlay bone grafts with intact periosteum seem to revascularize faster, have a greater percentage of osteocyte survival, and maintain volume better than grafts without periosteum. However, studies utilizing radionuclide scanning show that the presence or absence of periosteum has no effect on vascularization of the bone grafts. In clinical practice, it can be difficult to harvest and model the graft while retaining the periosteum. Typically, the periosteum is preserved in the donor site as a guiding envelope for bone healing.

Graft Orientation

Survival of an onlay bone graft is improved when the cortical surface of the graft is placed in contact with overlying soft tissue, and the cancellous surface is placed in contact with the recipient bone.

Stress Loading and Electromagnetic Fields

It is well known that mechanical loading of a bone causes significant increase in its mass. Conversely, bones removed from stress lose mass. Such situations are seen in individuals who are placed in casts or restricted to bedrest. How does bone detect a mechanical load? There are two hypotheses. One is that bone cells can detect a deformation directly; the second is that bone cells can detect a byproduct of deformation, namely, an electromagnetic field (EMF). The second hypothesis is supported by the fact that dry bone produces electrical potentials when it is deformed. These are called stress-generated potentials (SGPs). Observations of SGPs in physiologic bone suggest that if bone cells detect and respond to the naturally occurring SGPs, they may also respond to a signal that is created by an exogenous electromagnetic field. Unfortunately, it is difficult to know what type of exogenous electromagnetic field stimulates bone cells. Although there is little knowledge of the mechanism of action for electromagnetic field stimulation, this technique is occasionally used in instances of fracture nonunion. EMF stimulation is used particularly in cases of scaphoid fracture nonunion, especially when the fracture is near the proximal pole.

ARTICULAR CARTILAGE HEALING
Components and Growth of Cartilage

Cartilage is composed of chondrocytes, matrix, and water. The chondrocytes occupy lacunae in the matrix and are arranged in columns along the lines of stress. The chondrocytes elaborate collagen, elastin, and the protein polysaccharides within the cartilage. The matrix is composed of proteoglycans, complex molecules with a protein core, carbohydrate side chains, and Type II collagen, found almost exclusively in cartilage. Proteoglycans and collagen are polymerized to form a macromolecule that binds water, imparting the characteristic property of viscoelasticity. Water is essential to the nutrition of cartilage, which has no blood or lymphatic vessels. Although oxygen consumption of cartilage is very low, the metabolic activity of individual chondrocytes is similar to that of other tissue cells. Diffusion of nutrients throughout the matrix is facilitated by the shifting of water layers during compression of the cartilage. Immobilization may impair the diffusion of nutrients, causing absorption of the cartilage. The perichondrium is a vascular fibrous capsule that surrounds the cartilage; some of its fibers are in continuity with the collagenous fibrillar network.

Growth of cartilage is both appositional (occurring from the deep layer of perichondrial connective tissue cells) and interstitial (occurring by mitosis of chondrocytes within the cartilage matrix). The perichondrial connective tissue cells secrete matrix elements and become separated from the perichondrium to become intracartilaginous chondrocytes. These chondrocytes undergo mitosis that is followed by secretion of the matrix, causing progressive separation of the cells.

Chondrocytes are not replaced during the life of an individual. Cartilage growth ceases after reaching adulthood, and there is a progressive loss of chondrocytes during an individual's lifetime. Abnormal joint movement leads to premature loss of joint cartilage and subsequently to degenerative arthritis. In contrast to osteoblasts, chondrocytes show little reparative ability, so that following injury, healing is by formation of undifferentiated fibrous tissue.

Properties of Cartilage

There are four types of cartilage based on gross, histologic, and functional differences: morphologic cartilage, fibrocartilage, articular cartilage, and hyaline (elastic) cartilage. Morphologic cartilage has a fixed configuration and is found in such structures as nasal and auricular cartilage. Fibrocartilage is built to withstand large forces and is therefore found in such structures as intervertebral disks and temporomandibular joints. Articular cartilage is adapted to withstand repeated compressive forces and is located in the joints of the extremities. Hyaline cartilage is found primarily at the costochondral junction, where it facilitates expansion of the thoracic cage.

Mature cartilage possesses certain properties that must be considered during surgical manipulation and cartilage transplantation. Viscoelasticity is an intrinsically balanced system of forces and immunologic privilege. Cartilage has memory, that is, it returns to its original position following deformation by an external force. The maintenance of deformation requires less force with time, and if the deformation is continued for several months, the cartilage will remodel to the new shape.

The major constituents of cartilage demonstrate antigenic properties in vitro. Chondrocytes possess transplantation antigens similar to those of other tissues. However, the matrix is only weakly antigenic in vivo. It serves as a protective barrier to the chondrocytes because there are no blood vessels or lymphatics to expose antigenic sites to the host immune system. Thus, a cartilage allograft enjoys relative immunologic privilege. Once a cartilage allograft is carved, some antigen sites become exposed to the host immune system. The outer portion of the allograft may be replaced by fibrous tissue to a degree that may compromise the clinical result.

Cartilage Transplantation

Long-term survival of fresh cartilage autografts has been shown experimentally. Clinical investigators have confirmed that fresh cartilage autografts maintain structure and volume years following transplantation. The presence or absence of perichondrium does not affect graft survival, but less resorption results if the perichondrium is left intact. It is the perichondrium that becomes vascularized after transplantation.

Autogenous cartilage grafts are most commonly used in rhinoplasty, ear construction and reconstruction, and eyelid reconstruction. Their use in hand surgery, however, is quite limited. This because the joints of the hand are difficult to reconstruct with autologous cartilage, and other procedures exist to treat arthritic joints in the hand, such as joint fusion and arthroplasty with autologous tendons or synthetic materials. Perichondrial grafts have been used to reconstruct joints where cartilage has been lost. In these procedures, perichondrium from the costochondral region is transplanted to the joints of the hand to fill in defects where cartilage has been lost. After the perichondrium revascularizes, the transplanted chondrocytes synthesize new cartilage by appositional growth to fill in the defect on the joint surface. Such procedures are most commonly done in the metacarpolphalangeal joints and proximal interphalangeal joints of the hand. Success with perichondrial grafting has been limited to patients under 40 years of age. This may be the result of the loss of reparative capacity in older chondrocytes.

NERVE REGENERATION AND HEALING
Anatomy of the Nerve

To understand the pathophysiology of neural regeneration, one must understand the anatomy of a nerve. A nerve is comprised of many cells or neurons. A neuron has its nucleus in the region of the spinal cord. For the motor neuron, the nucleus is in the anterior horn; for the sensory neuron it is in the dorsal root ganglion. In both cases, the nucleus of the neuron is clearly far removed from any peripheral nerve injury occurring in the hand. Nevertheless, this central site undergoes changes following a transection of the peripheral nerve.

A nerve, such as the median nerve, consists of neurons surrounded by collagen and vessels that comprise an endoneurium. These neurons are then grouped together into fascicles by a multiple layered structure called the perineurium, composed of fibroblast-like cells, and additional collagen and blood vessels. The fascicles have functional characteristics that are determined by maintenance of an internal milieu. The guardian of this internal environment is the blood–nerve barrier, which is regulated by endothelial cells within the perineurium and the endoneurium. Groups of fascicles are separated from each other by an interfascicular epineurium and enclosed by an extrafascicular epineurium. This entire peripheral nerve is then attached to the surrounding tissues by a mesoneurium, through which a segmental extrinsic blood supply can occur. The internal longitudinal blood supply within the nerve is so good that interruption of the extrinsic segmental blood supply may be carried out over considerable lengths without interfering with circulation within the nerve (Fig. 1-4A).

Classification of Nerve Injuries

Injuries to peripheral nerves can occur by means of blunt trauma, traction, burns, lacerations, or injection. Regardless of the mechanism, nerve injuries can be described by a classification system created by Seddon in 1943, expanded by Sunderland in 1951, and modified by Mackinnon and Dellon in 1988 (see Table 1-1). There are six degrees of peripheral nerve injury. Knowledge of the degree to which a nerve is injured aides the physician in determining appropriate treatment for nerve injuries (Fig. 1-4B).

A first-degree injury consists of a localized conduction block on a nerve caused by segmental demyelination of the nerve. Seddon described this as a neuropraxia. Because the nerve axons remain in conti-

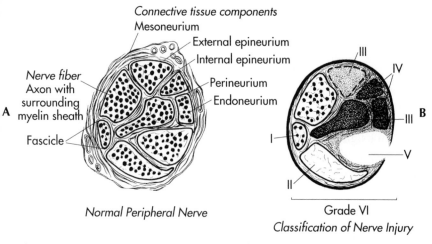

Figure 1-4   (A) Schematic cross-section of normal peripheral nerve. (B) Schematic cross-section of injured peripheral nerve, demonstrating the six degrees of nerve injury.

Table 1-1   Nerve Injury Classification and Relationship of Injury to Recovery

Degree of Injury					
Sunderland Classification	Seddon Classification	Tinel's	Expected Recovery	Rate of Recovery	Surgical Procedure
I	Neuropraxia	−	Complete	Rapid, days to weeks	None
II	Axonotmesis	+	Complete	Slow, (1 in/mo)	None
III		+	Variable	Slow, (1 in/mo)	None or neurolysis
IV		+	None	No recovery	Nerve repair or graft
V	Neurotmesis	+	None	No recovery	Nerve repair or graft
VI*		Varies, depending on combination of injury patterns			

*The neuroma-in-continuity described in Mackinnon and Dellon, *Surgery of the Peripheral Nerve,* 1988.

nuity, no nerve degeneration takes place. Recovery time may vary from minutes to months, depending on the length of time required for the Schwann cells to generate myelin around the demyelinated segment of nerve. Following remyelination, nerve recovery is immediate and complete. If, after a closed injury, full recovery of nerve function occurs within the first 3 months of the injury, the injury is considered to be first degree.

A second-degree injury involves a disruption of the nerve axons without significant injury to the endoneurium or perineurium. Seddon described this second-degree injury as axonotmesis. Distal to the site of the second-degree injury, wallerian degeneration takes place. To repair this level of injury, the proximal nerve must regenerate within the endoneurial sheath all the way to the end target of the nerve. Regeneration occurs at the classic rate of 1 inch/month or 1 mm/day. Because the injury is purely axonal in nature, the basal lamina of the Schwann cells, which makes up the endoneurial tubes, has not been violated. Therefore, regeneration of each axon occurs along its original endoneurial tube, unimpeded by scar tissue. This restores full and original sensory and motor function. Recovery of nerve function occurs after the nerve regenerates to the end organ. Because recovering nerve segments are hyperexcitable, tapping causes an electrical tingling or "crawling ant" sensation that is known as Tinel's sign. Thus, one can follow the progression of nerve recovery by percussing the nerve. The diagnosis of a second-degree injury can only be made after complete recovery from a nerve injury. If the recovery is full, but recovery occurred at the rate of 1 inch/month, with an advancing Tinel's sign present, then the injury is labeled an axonotmesis. If the recovery is incomplete but follows the same time course as an axonotmetic of injury, then it is called a third-degree injury.

A third-degree injury involves disruption of the nerve axons with some degree of intervening scar tissue present within the endoneurium. This type of injury results in an incomplete return of nerve function, since some of the regenerating fibers are blocked by scar tissue and cannot make contact with distal receptors. Because the basal lamina of the Schwann cells is violated, regeneration can result in some mismatching of nerve fibers to inappropriate distal receptors. However, the perineurium remains intact in a third-degree injury, and all regenerating fibers will remain within the involved fascicle. The variation of recovery is broadest in the Sunderland third-degree injury, where it can vary from almost complete recovery to almost no recovery depending on how pure or mixed the fascicle involved is and the degree of endoneurial scarring present.

A fourth-degree injury involves disruption of all of the axons within a nerve, with significant formation of intraneural scarring. This is termed a neuroma in continuity. A Tinel's sign will be present at the level of the injury, but no progression of the Tinel's sign will be noted distal to the injury, because regenerating nerve fibers are blocked by scar tissue. No sensory or motor recovery will occur without surgical intervention. To treat these injuries, excision of the neuroma must be followed by nerve coaptation through primary nerve repair, nerve grafting, or a nerve conduit. A physician generally observes a nerve injury for a period of three months before determining whether or not it is a fourth-degree injury. If after 3 months, no motor or sensory function has returned and no evidence exists of neural regeneration by means of an advancing Tinel's sign, the injury is considered a fourth-degree injury and surgical management is indicated.

A fifth-degree injury is a complete transection of the nerve, also termed a neurotmesis. Fifth-degree injuries are usually easily diagnosed because they occur in association with open wounds. The presence of an open wound and absence of nerve function raises the suspicion of a fifth-degree injury. The open wound should be thoroughly explored to examine the integrity of the nerve and allow for early repair.

The concept of the sixth-degree injury was brought forth by Mackinnon in 1989. A sixth-degree injury is one that combines some or all Sunderland's five degrees of injury. It is this group of injuries that creates the greatest surgical dilemma. A nerve with a six-degree injury may contain fascicles with neuropraxia—some with third-degree injuries, and some with fourth- or fifth-degree injuries. Complete recovery may occur in some fascicles, while none may occur in others. The surgeon is responsible for carefully assessing the preoperative function in each fascicle, or group of fascicles, to be explored. In weighing the pros and cons of nerve exploration, the surgeon should recognize that first-, second- and third-degree injuries offer spontaneous recovery superior to that provided by surgical grafting techniques. Care must be taken, therefore, not to injure those fascicles or normal fascicles while reconstructing the fascicles with fourth- and fifth-degree injuries.

Neural Regeneration

An important concept to grasp is that while nerves of the central nervous system do not regenerate, peripheral nerves do regenerate and therefore can be reconstructed. The ability of a cell to regenerate in the peripheral versus the central nervous system is based on the interactions of that cell with its surrounding connective tissue supporting cell, that is the Schwann cell in the peripheral nervous system versus the astrocyte or oligodendrocyte in the central nervous system.

Following transection of a neuron, the distal axon dies and undergoes a process of wallerian degeneration, first described in 1850. In this process, the remaining Schwann cells remove the axon and myelin debris of the distal neuron by phagocytosis. The only remnant of the axon–Schwann cell relationship will be the remaining Schwann cell nucleus, the cytoplasm, and the basal lamina. This degenerated system has been termed the band of Bunger. Proximally, the same process takes place, but for a variable distance. The nucleus of the injured cell, lying in a central location, will undergo changes varying from cell death to preparation of the cell for regeneration. When the location of the peripheral nerve injury is close to the spinal cord, the degree of loss to the neuron is sufficiently high that the nucleus may die, leaving less than the normal number of nuclei available to carry regeneration of the peripheral nerve to its distal site. The corollary is that the more distal the injury to the peripheral nerve, the fewer the number of central nuclei that will be lost and the greater the number of nerve cells available to regenerate along the peripheral nerve.

Proximal to the nerve transection, if the neuron survives, regenerative changes occur within 24 hours of the injury. At a node of Ranvier proximal to the transection, the axon develops multiple axonal sprouts, each with a growth cone on its end. A single axon may yield as many as 10 or 15 such sprouts; these growth cones actively seek appropriate distal targets to reinnervate. As these sprouts migrate distally, they become ensheathed by a Schwann cell. If this was formerly a myelinated nerve, the Schwann cell will myelinate the axon. If the nerve had been unmyelinated, then the sprouts within the Schwann cell will not develop myelin. This grouping has been termed a regenerating unit by Morris, Hudson, and Weddell.

The regenerating unit is guided distally by a combination of forces, including contact guidance and neurotropism. The growth cone of an axon sprout has an affinity for laminin and Type IV collagen. The basal lamina of a Schwann cell is composed of laminin, fibronectin, and Type IV collagen. Therefore, given a chance, the regenerating axon will travel along the course of basal lamina. The filopodia of the growth cones are electrophilic and seek the cationic region of the laminin. After attaching, there is a contraction of the filopodia's actin polypeptide, which produces axonal elongation. The modulation of this activity appears to occur through the cyclic-adenosine monophosphate (cAMP) system.

In addition to the factors already discussed, chemical mediators in the environment of the wound may also direct the axon sprout to an appropriate distal location. Studies done with the rat have demonstrated that axons will make the appropriate choice of regenerating toward a muscle rather than regenerating toward a tendon in the now classic "Y" forced choice situation. The chemicals within the environment of the regenerating axon that cause the nerve to choose between muscle and tendon are termed neurotrophic factors. These factors are presumed to be locally derived from the distal cut end of the nerve or Schwann cell. This regulation by the target organ is so sufficiently specific that the regenerating motor nerve will choose, as described above, a distal muscle target over a tendon target and, in fact, will choose a specific motor nerve over a sensory nerve as its distal target. The presence of these growth factors may specifically favor sensory rather than motor localization, and this again opens the possibility for future pharmacological modulation of nerve regeneration.

Therefore, in nerve healing, after a nerve division and nerve repair, the axon sprouts multiply the proximal axon count by at least tenfold. This advancing army of axon sprouts may be guided to their distal goal by local mechanical and chemical factors through contact guidance and by neurotrophic factors. These axons travel along, not through, appropriate such structures as the basal lamina, Schwann cells, degenerating nerve fibers, the interfascicular epineurium, and the perineurium. All are driven distally by the central axoplasmic push and pulled distally by neurotrophic or growth factors. The axons regenerate at a rate of 1 mm/day or 1 inch/month. One can follow the progression of neural regeneration by percussing the nerve, with a positive Tinel's sign indicating the level of regeneration. As the neural "front" marches distally, the Tinel's sign advances, representing the leading edge of the axonal sprouts. When the regenerating axons reach the end-targets, differences depend on whether the motor fiber enters a muscle or whether the sensory fiber reaches an appropriate distal sensory receptor. Once the distal connection has occurred, motor nerve to motor end plate or sensory nerve to sensory nerve ending, then appropriate signals are conducted by retrograde axoplasmic transport. A process of maturation now occurs. Classically, the myelinated nerve fiber will undergo an increase in axonal diameter. The thickness of the myelin will also increase in proportion to the diameter of the axon. Once one of the regenerating axons has made an appropriate distal connection, the nucleus withdraws support in some fashion from the remaining axon sprouts. As a result, the majority of the regenerating axons that have not yet reached an appropriate distal target experience a loss of centrally transported building materials and trophic support, and degenerate. This effect is termed pruning. If a given peripheral nerve distal to the repair site is observed over a period of time, the number of nerve fibers present will initially increase. This increase will be sustained over a period of months, determined by the distance between the injury and the distal target. Once regeneration has occurred distally and maturation has begun, the number of nerve fibers at the distal site should diminish to a number approximately equal to that proximal to the site of nerve division.

This general scheme of events is the same for unmyelinated fibers, with the exception that myelin is not formed. It is also the same for the pain and temperature fibers, and sympathetic and parasympathetic nervous system fibers, with the exception that the appropriate end organ, that is, the sweat gland, is reinnervated.

Wound Healing in Nerves

The preceding discussion dealt with neural regeneration at the microscopic level of the axons. That process of neural regeneration takes place in the middle of injury to the macrostructure, the nerve. The nerve is comprised of blood vessels, connective tissue, and neurons. As such, the structure undergoes wound healing just as skin does, with an inflammatory phase, a proliferative phase, and a remodeling phase. Collagen synthesis associated with wound healing can interpose scar tissue between proximal and distal aspects of the transected nerve, thus blocking neural regeneration. Significant tension at the nerve repair site can also cause abnormal scarring, thus blocking satisfactory neural regeneration. Millesi has done the most significant work in this area, demonstrating that a nerve repair under any tension will have more scar tissue at the suture line and will decrease nerve function. Thus, if a nerve repair cannot be carried out without tension, the appropriate treatment is to interpose a conduit between the two ends of the damaged nerve. The purpose of the conduit is to remove this tension and allow neural regeneration to occur across the gap without excess interference from the supporting fibroblasts. Traditionally, the conduit of choice has been the autogenous nerve graft. Alternate strategies for bridging nerve gaps now include the use of veins and synthetic conduits.

The length of a gap across which a nerve will attempt to regenerate has been well worked out in the rat and monkey. A transected nerve will grow in length a mean of 2.5 cm and a maximum of 4 cm searching for an appropriate distal target. Thus, in the absence of direct guidance by a conduit, it appears that the nerve has sufficient ability to reach out over several centimeters searching for an appropriate distal end organ.

Technical Factors

The best results of nerve reconstruction occur in young patients, because neural regeneration is more successful at a younger age. This, however, is clearly outside the ability of the surgeon to control. The next most critical factors are related to scar formation at the repair site. The surgeon can help prevent this by resecting that portion of the nerve which has been damaged. The degree of resection is related to the mechanism of injury, that is, a greater amount of resection is required for an avulsion than for a clean cut. The next critical factor is the amount of tension at the suture line. As emphasized by Millesi, the repair should be as tension free as possible. Resecting even 1 or 2 mm on either side of a clean laceration will give some increased tension. The length of the defect that can be reasonably closed varies with the anatomic location of the injury. For the digital nerve very little gliding or excursion is possible in the nerve, and a nerve defect of even 3 or 4 mm may require a graft to carry out a tension-free reconstruction of the nerve. The median nerve at the wrist, having greater glide and mobility, can tolerate a repair with a defect of 1.5 or 2 cm. Defects of 2 cm or more are clearly under sufficient tension that they cannot be closed without flexing the wrist and widely mobilizing the nerve in the forearm. When the hand is taken out of its fixation postoperatively and the wrist is mobilized, tension develops at the nerve repair site, stimulating scar formation which interferes with nerve function.

Alternatives to autogenous nerve grafting have been discussed in the literature. The use of the bioabsorbable tube and autogenous vein have been described in the rat model, and the bioabsorbable conduit extensively developed in the primate model. The use of the bioabsorbable conduit to bridge nerve defects of less than 3 cm has been successfully applied for the clinical reconstruction of digital nerves, and the technique is now being used by surgeons. In summary, research demonstrates that while a nerve can regenerate across gaps up to 3 cm, the ability to do so is better through a bioabsorbable conduit than through an autogenous vein. Most probably, the autogenous vein lacks sufficient external support resulting in collapse of its lumen, which impedes a certain percentage of the regenerating units from reaching distal target organs. The conduit technique, be it bioabsorbable or autogenous vein, appears to successfully direct proximal axons distally and thereby minimize a painful neuroma formation at the proximal repair site.

Additional technical factors that may be helpful are minimizing the interval between injury and reconstruction. The literature supports the view that sensory recovery is better for nerve repairs at the wrist level if the nerve repair can be carried out less than 3 months, and certainly if less than 6 months, after the nerve injury. However, sufficient reinnervation can occur that reconstruction of a sensory defect is worthwhile no matter how long the interval has been. The end-organ time limitation is different in the motor system since the muscle end-organ, devoid of trophic stimuli from nerve, will undergo interstitial fibrosis and gross atrophy despite the survival of the muscle as a cell. Thus, if muscle cannot be reinnervated by a year, the expectation for functional reinnervation is low.

With a long nerve graft, experimental evidence supports connecting the distal segment of the graft at the time the graft is placed. There is a possibility that scar tissue can occur at the second suture site and therefore impede distal regeneration of the nerve; however, neurotrophic substances may be released distally, collected, and transmitted through the graft. This offers a sufficient possibility to warrant a distal connection at the time of the initial nerve graft. Clinically, if a Tinel's sign does not progress beyond the distal nerve juncture, then a second exploration at the time with resection and second repair of the distal repair site would be appropriate.

The final factor under direct control of the surgeon that may be helpful in achieving the best results for wound healing in a nerve relates to rehabilitation. Traditionally, motor rehabilitation has been emphasized. Sensory reeducation, which entered the armamentarium in the 1970s, has now been demonstrated to improve significantly the results following not only nerve repair but also nerve grafting and nerve reconstruction during digital replants and toe-to-thumb transplants. Early-phase sensory reeducation is begun as soon as neural regeneration is apparent into the distal territory. This not only improves cortical misrepresentation and mislocalization and hypersensitivity, but reorganizes the perception of touch submodalities—that is, movement versus pressure versus vibration. Late-phase reeducation emphasizes object recognition.

TENDON HEALING: TENDON GLIDING AND REPAIR
Functional Anatomy of Tendon Gliding

Tendons transmit muscle action for movement of appropriate joints. For this function to occur most efficiently, the tendons are retained by pulley systems at the wrist and in the digits. Gliding is facilitated by the formation of sheaths that contain a lubricant—synovial fluid. The functional anatomy of these structures will be reviewed prior to considering their reactions to injury and its surgical implications.

The extensor tendons are invested in synovial sheaths located primarily over the radiocarpometacarpal area. These synovial sheaths are enclosed by one dense dorsal retinacular ligament that forms the pulley system for the extensor tendons. There are six synovial extensor sheaths, or compartments, through which all of the extensor tendons to the hand and wrist pass. The tendons of the extensor digitorum communis and the extensor indicis proprius are enclosed in a single synovial sheath that extends 10 to 15 mm proximal to the dorsal retinacular ligament. The synovial sheath of the abductor pollicis longus and the extensor pollicis brevis extends from the intersection of the muscles with the tendons of the radial wrist extensors to the metacarpal phalangeal joint of the thumb. Individual sheaths exist for the extensor digiti quinti, the extensor pollicis longus, and the extensor carpi ulnaris. The extensor carpi radialis longus and brevis share a synovial sheath. The fibro-osseous tunnels of the extensor tendons are limited to the wrist area, with the fibrous portion composed of the dorsal retinacular ligament and the volar surface formed from the ligaments interconnecting the radius, carpal bones, and the metacarpal bones.

The fibro-osseous tunnels of the flexor tendons consist of conduits that begin at the level of the distal palmar crease and extend to the distal phalanx. The posterior wall of each tunnel is formed by the volar plates of the metacarpophalangeal and interphalangeal joints and the periosteum of the intervening phalanges. This tunnel terminates at the insertion of the profundus tendon into the distal phalanx.

The anterior wall consists of a fibrous tissue covering that encircles the flexor tendons and attaches to the lateral edges of the volar plates of the previously mentioned joints and the anterolateral edge of the phalanges. Proximally, the fibers are dense and rigid, forming a pulley system. At the junction of the proximal two thirds with the distal third of the proximal and middle phalanges, the pulley system is evidenced by thickening of the transverse fibers. Over the joint areas the fibers are very thin, and the tunnel is formed primarily from the parietal layer of the synovial membrane.

Synovial sheaths line the fibro-osseous tunnels of all digits. In the index, long, and ring fingers, the synovial sheaths envelope the flexor tendons from a point approximately 10 mm proximal to the proximal border of the deep transverse ligament to the profundus insertion. The thumb and little finger have separate synovial sheaths that extend proximally from the insertion of the profundus through the carpal tunnel and into the distal forearm.

The synovial membranes form a parietal and visceral layer around the flexor tendons, which is most evident within the fibro-osseous tunnels. The parietal synovial layer lines the fibro-osseous portion of the tunnel, while the visceral layer is intimately applied to the tendon surface. The parietal synovial sheath layer is reflected from the fibro-osseous tunnel onto the flexor tendons at the distal insertion of the tendons and again at the proximal extent of the synovial membrane as outlined previously. This forms a closed sac in which the tendons glide. At the proximal reflection, there is an accordion-like fold in the synovial membrane that allows unimpeded excursion of the flexor tendons. After reflection of the parietal synovial membrane onto the tendon, it is termed the visceral synovium. At the level of the sublimis tendon decussation, the visceral synovium of the profundus tendon is reflected volarward, forming a thin process to join the sublimis at the proximal

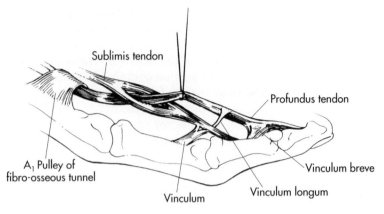

Figure 1-5   Segmental nutrient vessels within the vincular system of the flexor tendons.

extent of its decussation. Blood vessels penetrate the vinculum breve of the sublimis and extend through the vinculum longum of the profundus tendon to supply that tendon (Fig. 1-5). Occasionally, the vinculum longum of the profundus arises at the midpoint of the proximal phalanx and can be detected externally as a lateral weakness in the fibro-osseous tunnel through which the vascular system penetrates to gain access to the long vinculum. In such instances, the vinculum longum can measure 1.5 inches in length.

As a result of these arrangements, the blood supply of the flexor profundus within the digital sheath is derived from three sources: the proximal palmar vessels, the vinculum longum, and the bony tendinous insertion (vinculum breve). The sublimis tendon derives its blood supply from the proximal palmar vessels and its vinculum breve. Studies have shown that the proximal portion of the profundus is less well perfused than the distal portion. This distal portion is perfused primarily through the vinculum breve, while the proximal portion is perfused primarily by palmar vessels. The vinculum longum alone can not maintain the normal levels of perfusion in any portion of the profundus tendon. This implies that laceration of the profundus tendon at the level of the vinculum longum (dividing the latter) leaves the free ends of the tendons adequately nourished by the remaining proximal and distal vascular sources. The importance of these observations will be emphasized when discussing healing within the sheath.

Tendon gliding is facilitated by the physical arrangement of the structures immediately surrounding the tendon. The paratenon is a loose areolar tissue containing long, elastic fibers running between the tendon and the surrounding tissues. As the tendon glides, the curled, elastic fibers straighten out to permit an unimpeded excursion. All tendons have some form of mesotenon or mesentery. In the fibro-osseous tunnels, the mesotenon is represented by the vinculum longum and the vinculum breve. Outside the synovial sheath, where the tendon lies in its paratenon, a mesotenon is traversed by the vascular supply of the tendon.

Response of Tendons to Injury

Most studies of tendon healing have been concerned with healing within the synovial sheaths located in fibro-osseous tunnels. Of course, the same synovial reaction to injury would be expected in the synovial sheaths that extend around the flexor tendons into the forearm. Consequently, the primary difference in the digit is the presence of the rigid nonyielding fibro-osseous tunnel that encircles the tendons. Therefore, any discussion of tendon healing in the digit must deal with the reaction to injury by the individual structures and with the interaction among the individual structures when one is injured—that is, the effects of trauma to the perisheath area, the fibro-osseous tunnel and underlying parietal synovium, and the visceral synovium and tendon. The role of the endotenon and tendon cell, as well as the role of the vinculum, must also be considered.

Trauma to the perisheath structures that does not violate the parietal or visceral synovium has no adverse effects on tendon gliding. Even when the anterior aspect of the fibro-osseous tunnel (including parietal synovium) is excised, a new sheath forms with the development of only light filmy adhesions between the underlying tendon and the new sheath. It should be emphasized that the visceral synovium was not violated. However, when the parietal and visceral synovium are lacerated—that is, laceration of the sheath and the tendon at the same level—the stage is set for rigid scar formation between the cut tendon ends and the free edge of the fibro-osseous tunnel. If the free end of the tendon retracts into an area of intact parietal synovium, the tendon end rounds off and no adhesions are formed with the lateral walls. The need for violation of both visceral and parietal synovium to produce adhesion formation is evidenced by simple placement of a fine wire suture into an intact digital flexor tendon. This causes a significant tendinous and peritendinous reaction.

Because the scar that forms in the fibro-osseous tunnel can be so dense as to completely restrict tendon gliding, one must be concerned with how the reacting cells (fibroblasts) arrive at the site of the injury. Observations on the derivation of the fibroblasts in tendon healing have resulted in basically three theories concerning their origin. One proposes that the tendon ends provide the fibroblasts responsible for repair; a second suggests that the peritendinous tissues provide the initial fibroblastic ingrowth, followed later by the appearance of fibroblasts from the free tendon ends; and the third proposes that only the peritendinous tissue can provide the fibroblasts necessary for tendon healing.

Extensive studies of tendon ends displaced from the site of sheath laceration support the concept that the connective tissue cells comprising a tendon are capable of producing immature cells. After tendon injury, the cells within the epitenon and endotenon react earliest and account for the largest amount of proliferating tissue. The more differentiated and specialized connective tissue cells in the tendon bundles react later. This is based on the observation that soon after an injury proliferation of the epitenon (visceral synovium) covers the end of the tendon and that only after 2 to 3 weeks does cellularity develop between the bundles within the tendon. This observation, coupled with the observation that maintenance of the integrity of either the visceral or parietal synovium minimizes adhesion formation, has practical clinical implications.

Tendon Healing

Lindsay, Matthews, Potenze, Peacock, Furlow, and others have studied the mechanism of tendon healing extensively. More recently, the studies of Manske, Gelberman, Mass, and others have greatly increased our understanding of this process. It is now generally agreed that flexor tendons possess an intrinsic capacity to heal themselves by diffusion, without depending on extratendinous cells or surrounding adhesions. Lundborg showed that in rabbits flexor tendons deprived of their blood supply can heal without adhesion formation. He removed flexor profundus tendons from the sheaths of rabbit toes, cut them in half, sutured them together, and placed them in a rabbit's knee in the suprapatellar pouch. The tendons were analyzed macroscopically and microscopically at periods ranging from 1 to 6 weeks. Healing without adhesion formation took place, and Lundborg concluded that flexor tendons did possess an intrinsic capacity for healing with nutrients supplied by diffusion from the synovial fluid. Potenza and Herte and others, however, disagreed with this conclusion, believing that cells from the synovium actually seeded onto the surface of the tendons to heal them. More recently, Manske, Gelberman, Mass, and others have used various animal models to show that flexor tendons do have an intrinsic capacity for healing. They placed cut segments of flexor tendons in tissue culture media and demonstrated the presence of a healing process by light and electron microscopy. It has also been shown that there is neovascularization present within the sheath of healing flexor tendons, which suggests that vascular perfusion plays a role in the healing of intrasynovial tendinous connective tissue. The presence of an intact vincular system does improve the results of flexor tendon repair in Zone II.

Even though the exact process of tendon healing is not completely understood, it is now known that flexor tendons do possess an intrinsic capacity to heal themselves. Whether or not adhesion formation from the surrounding soft tissues is an integral part of the repair process is questionable. Recent evidence suggests that it is not necessary.

During the past several years, Gelberman and his associates have carefully evaluated the healing processes of flexor tendons with in vivo and in vitro studies. They compared repaired flexor tendons that were totally immobilized to tendons treated with varying degrees of protected passive mobilization. The tensile strength and gliding function were consistently greater in the mobilized tendons. In the immobilized tendons, adhesions surrounding the repair site attached it to the sheath. In contrast, the mobilized tendons had a smooth gliding surface and good healing, showing that adhesions are not necessary for healing at the repair site. In their in vitro studies, Gelberman and his associates extensively reviewed the cellular mechanism of repair, demonstrating phagocytosis of debris by epitenon cells and collagen synthesis by endotenon cysts. These studies provided the first experimental evidence that early, controlled, passive mobilization of repaired flexor tendons within the digital sheath could be beneficial. Their recent studies indicate that increasing the duration and frequency of protected passive mobilization following flexor tendon repair can have a beneficial effect on the tensile strength of the healing flexor tendon, and ultimately improve tendon function. Current studies are underway with the use of a continuous passive motion machine.

Despite the intense efforts of these and other authors, many questions remain. What, then, is the nutritional pathway for the flexor tendon within the digital sheath? How does the severed tendon heal in the sheath? If diffusion from the synovial fluid is a more effective nutritional pathway than perfusion, should the digital flexor sheath be repaired or reconstructed at the time of tendon repair? How should early protected passive mobilization be carried out following tendon repair? Should one use elastic band traction with a palmar pulley or a continuous passive motion machine on an intermittent basis? Unfortunately, the answers to many of these questions requires additional research. Until such research provides definitive answers, treatment plans for flexor tendon injuries should be formulated based largely on clinical results and experience.

Development of Gliding Function

As noted earlier, scar between tendon ends undergoes reorganization so that the nonpurposefully oriented fibrils and fibers disappear. If gliding function is to occur, scar along the longitudinal surface of the tendon must undergo a remodeling process that is quite different from that exhibited between the tendon ends. For adhesions to permit satisfactory gliding function, a loose arrangement of the collagen bundles must exist to permit longitudinal gliding. Failure to glide appears to be related to the quantitative and qualitative characteristics of the adhesions surrounding the repair. Large quantities of scar, as occurs after infection, can restrict motion. Scar induced by dense fibrous structures (that is, the periosteum or the bone or palmar fascia) is slow to undergo satisfactory remodeling and may completely inhibit tendon gliding.

Adhesion formation is a normal part of tendon healing, but minimizing such adhesions is essential for tendon gliding. Many surgical techniques are predicated on the goal of adhesion prevention. Even a minimal gain in motion correlates with favorable changes in the physical properties of the dense connective tissue around the repair site. Why secondary remodeling of newly synthesized connective tissue in the healing tendon wound should produce different physical characteristics in portions of the same scar is unknown. The scar between the tendon ends becomes oriented along the long axis of the tendon and exhibits marked gain in tensile strength. The scar between the tendon and surrounding structures must become loose and filmy for gliding function to be regained. Possibly, the newly synthesized connective tissue remodels in response to inductive influences of the tissue with which it is in intimate contact.

Many physicians have asked, why not wrap the tendon in a foreign material that completely prevents adhesion formation? Unfortunately, experimental use of tendon wrapping has been shown to noticeably delay tendon healing. The observation that free tendon grafts completely encircled with a foreign material undergo necrosis has often been cited to support the need for peritendinous cells or synovial fluid to participate in healing. This observation leads to the conclusion that any mechanical procedure designed to prevent adhesion formation would impair tendon healing so severely as to render the methods unfeasible.

Biochemical Control of Adhesion Formation

The biosynthesis and degradation pathways of collagen—the primary component of scar—have been elucidated. Biochemical agents have been identified that can modify collagen synthesis and organization, thereby quantitatively and qualitatively altering scar formation. Reduction in synthesis can be obtained by altering the synthesis of ribonucleic acid (RNA) or by disrupting the orderly incorporation of amino acids into polypeptide chains. The conversion of proline-rich procollagen to tropocollagen may be interrupted by alteration of any of the five parameters necessary for proline hydroxylation. The chelating of iron, the absence of molecular oxygen, the blockage of alpha ketoglutarate, the absence of proline hydroxylase, and—most widely recognized—the lack of ascorbic acid, all interfere with the hydroxylation of proline and the normal production of mature collagen. After tropocollagen is released from the fibroblast cell, collagen assembly and intermolecular binding may be inhibited and thereby yield collagen with physical properties that are unsuitable for functions requiring great tensile strength. The most widely discussed agents that interfere with collagen organization are the lathyrogens. These agents—of which β-aminopropionitrate (BAPN) is the best known—interfere with the formation of aldehyde groups needed to form inter- and intramolecular cross-links as the collagen matures. Becuase the ultimate functional result of a tendon repair graft is determined by the qualitative characteristics of the collagen deposited in response to wounding, qualitative control of the scar could be beneficial. β-aminopropionitriate acts on newly synthesized collagen, while having very little effect on mature collagen. Yet most mature collagen is subject to degradation by collagenase and remodeling by the deposition of nascent collagen. The most dramatic effects of a lathyrogen are on bone, vascular structures, and healing wounds. The effect on bone results in marked deformity of the animal. Collagen turnover in the major vessels of an animal treated with lathyrogens leads to the deposition of collagen of minimal tensile strength; thus aneurysm formation is frequent. The healing wound of the lathyritic animal contracts normally, but does not gain significant tensile strength. Peacock reports that alteration in the inter- and intramolecular bonds of nascent collagen around a tendon repair can be produced without damage to other tissues. After a primary tendon repair in chickens had been performed, a secondary procedure—tenolysis—was performed, and the animals were given BAPN. The work required to produce longitudinal tendon motion was significantly less in the treated group. The difficulty of transferring these observations to humans is obvious. Above all, the control values for the development of tendon gliding in man are not known. Some patients produce favorable scar and develop gliding very rapidly, while others develop unfavorable scar and gliding is delayed or never develops adequately. Of course, many patients' reactions fall between these two extremes. Because the lathyrogens have a systemic effect, the results of administration could be disastrous. Biochemical control of scar formation has not been localized to the site in question, and certainly clinical use is not feasible at this time.

Operative Control of Adhesion Formation

Development of operative methods for controlling or producing favorable scar formation requires recognition of the biological characteristics of the tissues that predispose to the development of unfavorable scar in a wound. A healing wound promotes formation of tissues necessary for repair or for regeneration of the injured structures. For example, the fracture callus incites the production of extremely dense periosteal-like tissue. The presence of a repaired tendon within the immediate area of the fracture callus results in the formation of extremely dense scar between the fracture callus and the healing tendon. Similarly, lacerations or avulsions of the periosteum produce dense unfavorable periosteum and surrounding structures.

The dermis, palmar fascia, volar plates, and fibro-osseous tunnels (including the periosteum) are composed of dense interlacing bundles of collagen organized into rigid nonyielding structures. Each of these structures produces scar that is unfavorable for tendon gliding. The dense fibrous tissue of the palmar fascia is attached to the overlying palmar skin by multiple septa that extend into the dermis. In addition, fibrous attachments of the palmar fascia extend vertically to the metacarpals. These attachments produce a rigid, nonyielding, immobile palmar fascia, and tendon injuries in the palm of necessity injure them. If repaired and left unattended, dense adhesions will develop between the repaired tendon and the palmar fascia. Since the palmar fascia is immobile, tendon gliding would be restricted. Therefore, overlying fascia should be excised to expose the tendon repair to the subcutaneous fat and muscle—structures that cause much less severe scar formation.

Similarly, healing fractures produce callus formation, which results in dense adhesions between the bone and the adjacent structures. Remember that a phalangeal fracture that produces tears in the posterior wall of the fibro-osseous tunnel predisposes one toward scar formation around the flexor tendons during the period of immobilization. Adhesions between the periosteum and flexor tendons can "check-rein" the interphalangeal joint, resulting in eventual fibrosis of the joint. Consequently, when physicians see a phalangeal fracture, they should be concerned with more than simply a fractured bone. The periosteum of the fibro-osseous tunnel has been violated; the fracture edge has impinged or impaled the flexor tendons; and probably there are associated tears of the anterior portion of the fibro-osseous tunnel. The extensor tendon apparatus often is involved to a lesser degree. Yet, direct closed injury can cause intense periosteal reaction that incorporates the intact extensor apparatus into the resulting callus. During immobilization, the joints become stiff in extension by the check-reining effect of the scar on the extensor apparatus. Therefore, early range of motion exercises are instituted with hand fractures as soon as is allowed by appropriate fracture management to preserve tendon gliding and prevent joint contractures.

Finally, consider further the avulsing injury over the dorsum of the hand, which eliminates all skin and subcutaneous tissues and lacerates the extensor tendons. The presence of dense dermis, such as a skin graft applied immediately to the bone and tendon, will preclude subsequent tendon movement throughout the area because of the nature of the adhesions formed between the dermis, the bone, and the tendon. To reconstruct this defect, remember that there are two basic tissues within the hand that are predisposed to favorable scar formation: subcutaneous tissue/fat and synovial sheaths. Therefore, soft tissue defects with exposed tendons (devoid of paratenon) should be covered with vascularized subcutaneous tissue, which allows for tendon gliding. Such transfers of vascularized tissue are known as flaps. Because fatty tissues do not incite a significant fibroblastic response, wound coverage with flaps results in minimal scarring between the recipient site and the flap, which allows for maximal tendon gliding. Flaps do not induce dense fibrous tissue formation, except around their periphery where the dermis of the flap abuts the dermis of the recipient site. As a result, use of a flap limits the area of unfavorable scar tissue formation to the periphery of the flap. In cases where the tendons are destroyed and soft tissue coverage is suboptimal, polymeric silicone rods are inserted in the subcutaneous tissue for approximately 2 months. During this time, a pseudosynovial sheath forms around the silastic rods. At a second stage, tendon grafts can be passed through the new sheaths with better subsequent gliding than had the grafts been placed primarily in the subcutaneous tissue.

SUMMARY

Failure to appreciate the significance of scar formation in the injured hand can result in impaired tendon gliding, joint motion, nerve regeneration, and skin compliance. Tissues of the hand respond to injury and surgery (which is controlled injury) in virtually the same manner. Following injury or surgical intervention, the wound healing processes outlined in this chapter come into play and the reparative process begins. The characteristics of the resulting scar determines the eventual functional outcome. Scar formation and degradation occur simultaneously, providing a remodeling of both favorable and unfavorable scar and hopefully functional reorganization. Through this remodeling and reorganization, unfavorable scar may be converted to favorable scar.

Unfavorable scar interferes with all phases of restorative hand surgery—tendon gliding, joint motion, nerve regeneration, fracture healing, and skin compliance. Interference with tendon gliding results from the persistence of unfavorable scar adhesions. It may interfere with motion by limiting intracapsular and extracapsular movements associated with normal joint movement. Nerve regeneration is inhibited by interposition of new scar between the nerve ends, thereby impairing the return of nerve function. Fractures can result in scarring of surrounding and subcutaneous tissue structures, thereby causing joint stiffness. Finally, scarring in the skin can interfere with joint motion and tendon gliding, either directly or by producing contractures across flexion creases. In the case of the repaired flexor tendon, the scar that forms between the coapted tendon ends undergoes remodeling to yield a rigid scar (certainly favorable for the transmission of the unmodified muscle action to the digits). Yet, the same scar forms adhesions with the structures in juxtaposition to the tendon. This scar must undergo a totally different remodeling process to yield supple adhesions that will permit tendon gliding. Consequently, there are many wound environments produced by a single injury, for example, between the tendon ends, between the tendon and its milieu, between the bone ends, between bone and tendon, between the nerve ends. Each injured structure induces the formation of scar which may be either favorable or unfavorable. Postoperative modification of favorable and unfavorable scar is required to achieve optimal function in the injured part. The postoperative rehabilitation of the injured hand requires a team effort, with the surgeon and therapist working in concert to prevent excessive scar formation and to modify the normal scar that has already formed.

SELECTED REFERENCES

Axhausen G: Ueber den histologischen vorgang bei der transplantation vongelenkenden. *Arch Klin Chir* 99:1, 1912.

Barbul A: Immune aspects of wound repair, *Clin Plast Surg* 17(3):433-441, 1990.

Brennwald J: Bone healing in the hand, *Clin Orthop* 214:7-10, 1987.

Dellon AL: Wound healing in the nerve, *Clin Plast Surg* 17(3):545-570, 1990.

Fitzsimmons RJ, Baylink DJ: Growth factors and electromagnetic fields in bone, *Clin Plast Surg* 21(3):401-406, 1994.

Gelberman RH, Khabie V, Cahill CJ: The revascularization of healing flexor tendons in the digital sheath: a vascular injection study in dogs. *J Bone Joint Surg* 73(A):868-881, 1991.

Gelberman RH, Siegel DB et al: Healing of digital flexor tendons: importance of the interval from injury to repair, *J Bone Joint Surg* 73(A):66-75, 1991.

Mackinnon SE, Dellon AL: *Anatomy and physiology of the peripheral nerve.* In *Surgery of the peripheral nerve,* New York, 1988, Thieme, pp. 1-34.

Madden JW, Peacock EE: Studies on the biology of collagen during wound healing. I: Rate of collagen synthesis and deposition in cutaneous wounds of the rat, *Surgery* 64:288, 1968.

Manske PR: Flexor tendon healing, *J Hand Surg* 13B:237-245, 1988.

Manske PR, Lester PA: Flexor tendon nutrition, *Hand Clin* 1(1):13-24, 1985.

Millesi H, Berger A, Meisl G: Experimental study of healing of transected peripheral nerves. *Chir Plast (Berlin)* 1:174, 1972.

Morris J, Hudson A, Weddell G: A study of degeneration and regeneration in the divided rat sciatic nerve based on electron microscopy. A Zellforsch Mikrosk Anat 124:76. 1972.

Motoki DS, Mulliken JB: The healing of bone and cartilage, *Clin Plast Surg* 17(3):527-544, 1990.

Peacock EE: *Wound healing and wound care.* In Schwartz SI, editor: *Principles of surgery,* ed 5, New York, 1989, McGraw-Hill, pp. 307-330.

Peacock EE, Cohen IK: *Wound healing.* In McCarthy JG, editor: *Plastic surgery.* Philadelphia, 1990, WB Saunders, pp. 161-185.

Seddon HJ: Three types of nerve injury, *Brain* 66:237, 1943.

Seradge H, Kutz JA, Kleinert HE, Lister GD, Wolff TW, Atasey E: Perichondrial resurfacing arthroplasty in the hand, *J Hand Surg* 9A: 880-886, 1984.

Sunderland S: A classification of peripheral nerve injuries producing loss of function, *Brain* 784:491, 1951.

Weeks PM, Wray RC: *The biological basis for management.* In Weeks P, Wray CR, editors: Management of acute hand injuries: a biological approach. St. Louis, 1973, CV Mosby, pp. 3-104.

2

Evaluation of Hand Injuries

Mitchell A. Fremling, MD
Thomas Francel, MD, FACS
Paul M. Weeks, MD, FACS

CONTROL OF BLEEDING
    Direct Pressure and Elevation
    Pressure Dressing
    Tourniquet

LISTEN
    Injury
    Occupation/Social
    Hand-Dominance
    Previous Medical History

LOOK
    Posturing
    Viability
    Sweating

ASSESSMENT
    Vascular
    Nerve
    Muscle/Tendon
    Bones/Ligaments/Joints
    Skin and Specialized Structures

ANESTHESIA IN THE
EMERGENCY DEPARTMENT
    Local and Regional Anesthesia
        in the Emergency Room
    Anesthesia in the Operating
        Room

CARE AFTER INITIAL
EVALUATION
    General Care
    Amputated Parts

OPERATING ROOM

SELECTED REFERENCES

The initial evaluation of a hand injury is very important, as the ultimate outcome is often determined by the initial care provided. Complications or misdiagnoses may lead to serious disabilities. A stepwise progression of examination is important because once certain points in the evaluation and treatment have been reached (i.e., the administration of anesthesia, pain medication), it may be difficult—if not impossible—to return to an earlier step of the evaluation process. This is especially true if other injuries are present. The development of an evaluation strategy following the listen, look, assess, and stress method ensures a complete evaluation for all types of hand injuries.

CONTROL OF BLEEDING

Although bleeding from upper extremity injuries may be profuse, blind clamping or ligation of bleeding vessels is strongly discouraged because it may result in inadvertent injury to adjacent nerves and tendons. Most small vessels will stop bleeding with pressure and elevation alone; large caliber vessels (i.e. digital, radial, and ulnar arteries) should not be clamped or ligated in the emergency department, as this may complicate subsequent repair.

Direct Pressure and Elevation

Immediate control of bleeding can usually be obtained by direct pressure. Using gloves, place several surgical sponges directly over the wound and apply firm pressure while the extremity is elevated. In the badly fractured hand, care must be taken not to cause further injury as pressure is applied. Pressure may be released periodically to assess the status of hemostasis. If an extended period of direct pressure and elevation fail to stop the bleeding, then evaluation in the operating room is indicated.

Pressure Dressing

During patient transport or evaluation of other injuries, a pressure dressing may be employed as a substitute for direct pressure. Intermittently, status of the extremity and the pressure dressing should be evaluated to ensure that it is adequately controlling blood loss and not functioning as a tourniquet. Frequent reevaluation of the dressing status is essential. Bleeding will often resume when the dressing is removed for evaluation. Patients should never be discharged from the emergency department with a pressure dressing in place.

Tourniquet

A tourniquet may be used to control bleeding for a brief period of time to halt otherwise uncontrollable bleeding or to limit bleeding during examination or surgical procedures. However, a tourniquet does render the extremity distal to it ischemic and therefore should not be used injudiciously. In addition to its ischemic effects, tourniquets may directly induce nerve damage. The risk of nerve injury is directly proportional to the magnitude of pressure and the duration of application. Wider tourniquets are less likely to result in a nerve injury.

Arm Tourniquet

In the emergency department, cast padding and a blood pressure cuff may be used on the upper arm as a tourniquet. If not contraindicated, the arm may be exsanguinated with elevation and/or an elastic wrap before inflation of the cuff to allow better visualization of the wound. This is done by firmly wrapping the hand and arm with the elastic wrap in a distal to proximal direction. The blood pressure cuff is then inflated to 200 to 300 mmHg. This pressure may be safely maintained for up to 2 hours to control bleeding, but as a result of ischemia-induced pain, most conscious patients will only tolerate this for 10 to 20 minutes without pharmacologic manipulation, such as regional or general anesthesia. Another important consideration is that use of the tourniquet in the emergency department may limit the period of time that it can be safely used in the operating room during a second tourniquet run. As a result, use of a full upper extremity tourniquet in the emergency department is generally limited to a brief period of time, either as a means of evaluation or as a means of obtaining rapid control of severe bleeding until a pressure dressing can be fabricated or the patient transported to the operating room.

Finger Tourniquet

After a complete evaluation, finger tourniquets may be applied to allow visualization during minor surgical procedures that are performed in the emergency department. Following digital blockade (see sec. on Anesthesia in the Emergency Department), the patient will tolerate a finger tourniquet for a significantly longer period of time than an arm tourniquet. The finger may be exsanguinated with elevation and/or direct pressure. A tourniquet may be applied using a 1/2-inch penrose drain or the finger of a surgical glove using a small surgical clamp with the handle directed proximally. Alternatively, the cut finger from a glove of the appropriate size may be rolled down the finger to simultaneously exsanguinate and act as a tourniquet.

Documentation

The time at which a tourniquet is placed should be carefully noted, and the duration monitored so as not to exceed 2 hours of tourniquet time. The use of a tourniquet and its duration should be documented in the patient's medical record. Again, improper use of a tourniquet may result in serious injury. It should be used only when no other acceptable alternative is available, and every step should be taken to ensure that its use is as brief as possible.

LISTEN

Most patients arrive in the emergency department with a bandage in place and bleeding already under control. In this situation, obtain as much of the history as possible before removing the dressing, because removal of the dressing is often painful for the patient and may cause bleeding to begin again.

Injury

The mechanism of the injury should be elucidated. In crush-type injuries, estimate the forces applied and the duration of exposure. If machinery was involved, obtain specific details regarding the type of machinery and the mechanism of action. In hyperextension or fracture injuries, the patient should estimate the direction and degree of maximum extension or angulation. If the skin is broken by penetrating trauma, estimate depth of penetration. If the skin was exposed to heat, acid, or other caustic agents, duration of exposure and details of initial treatment at the scene are especially important.

Occupation/Social

Knowledge of the patient's occupation and hobbies are essential for determining the goals in treatment of hand injuries. For example, the primary goal in a concert pianist may be to restore fine manual dexterity, while the goal in a heavy laborer may be to restore power grip. The patient's occupation and social situation may also dictate the practicality of such goals. Some patients may be unwilling or unable to make the time commitment necessary for postoperative recovery and the rehabilitation of a finger replantation following traumatic amputation. In these patients, a revision amputation may better suit their needs.

Hand Dominance

The medical team should also note which hand is dominant in the patient.

Previous Medical History

To assess the patient's ability to undergo potentially lengthy operative procedures and to provide appropriate care for the patient postoperatively, obtain a thorough medical history that includes a list of medications and allergies.

LOOK

The first step of the physical examination should be a visual assessment of the patient's injuries. Documentation should be meticulous, as the initial emergency department evaluation is often an extremely important source of comparison in later examinations. The use of diagrammatic representations is strongly encouraged. In immature or obtunded patients, visual inspection combined with palpation and radiographic examination may be the only means of evaluation available.

Posturing

A great deal can be learned from the position the hand assumes at rest. Abnormal angulation of bones and/or joints should be noted. In

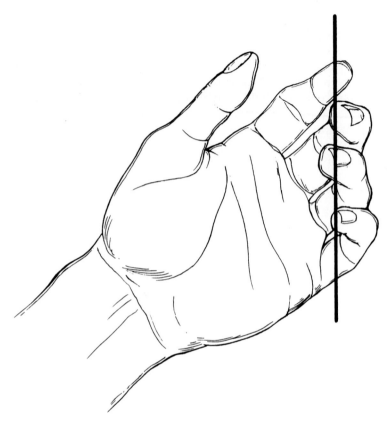

Figure 2-1   With intact flexor tendons, the fingers assume a partially flexed position that creates a cascade from the index through the little finger. A break in the smooth cascade of these digits may indicate a flexor tendon laceration.

the uninjured supine hand, the fingers cascade smoothly when at rest. A broken cascade of the fingers when the hand assumes a supine position often indicates tendon injury (Fig. 2-1).

Viability

The condition of the soft tissues should be noted and injuries documented diagrammatically. Areas of questionable viability should be noted for more extensive evaluation.

Sweating

The presence or absence of sweating in all or portions of the hand may provide important clues to the status of the innervation of the hand. Normal skin should be slightly moist. Nerve disruption with loss of sympathetic tone results in drying of the skin within the distribution of the affected nerve.

ASSESSMENT

Once the initial visual inspection is completed, systematic evaluation of the hand should begin. Again, emphasis is placed on careful documentation of all systems, including normal findings.

Vascular

Anatomy

   Arteries

     (Fig. 2-2)

     SUBCLAVIAN ARTERY

      The right subclavian artery arises from the brachiocephalic artery; the left subclavian artery takes off directly from the aorta. Distal to this level, the arterial anatomy of the arms is symmetric in most individuals.

     AXILLARY ARTERY

      After passing beneath the clavicle and reaching the distal edge of the first rib, the subclavian artery becomes the axillary artery. After giving off a number of branches to the scapula, shoulder, and lateral chest wall, the axillary artery becomes the brachial artery at the distal edge of the teres major muscle.

     THE BRACHIAL ARTERY

      The brachial artery travels down the medial aspect of the arm through the biceps, brachialis, and the triceps muscles, giving off the deep brachial (profunda brachii) artery along with superior and inferior ulnar collateral arteries. In the cubital fossa, the brachial artery lies deep to the bicipital aponeurosis, superficial to the brachialis muscle, and medial to the biceps brachii tendon. Just distal to the elbow, it divides to form the radial artery and the ulnar artery. Occlusion or laceration of the artery proximal to this division will usually render the distal extremity ischemic. However, division of either the radial or ulnar divisions of the artery individually is usually well tolerated because of collateral flow from the remaining artery.

     THE RADIAL ARTERY

      The radial artery crosses the biceps brachii tendon, gives off several radial recurrent branches, and then travels down the radial aspect of the proximal forearm deep to the brachioradialis muscle. It becomes superficial again at the junction of the middle and distal third of the forearm, as the brachioradialis becomes tendonous. At the distal forearm, the radial artery is easily palpa-

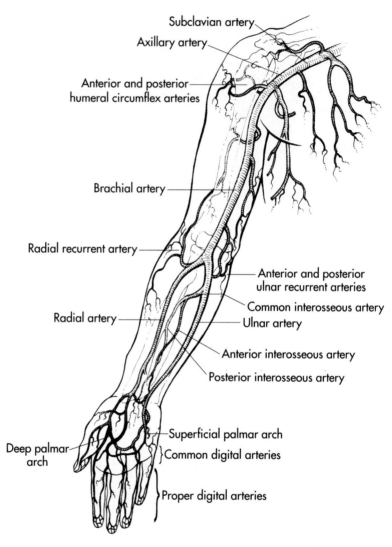

Figure 2-2   The arterial anatomy of the upper extremity.

ble between the flexor carpi radialis tendon and the brachioradialis tendon. Several centimeters proximal to the distal wrist crease it gives off a superficial palmar branch. This provides the smaller radial contribution to the superficial palmar arch. The radial artery proper travels deep to the abductor pollicis longus and extensor pollicis brevis tendons; it becomes palpable again in the anatomic snuff box (formed by the extensor pollicis longus and brevis tendons). At the base of the first metacarpal, it passes between the two heads of the first dorsal interosseous muscle and provides the larger radial contribution to the deep palmar arch.

THE ULNAR ARTERY

The ulnar artery gives off recurrent branches and the common interosseous artery in the proximal forearm. The common interosseous artery bifurcates almost immediately to form the anterior and posterior interosseous arteries, which travel along their respective surfaces of the interosseous membrane between the radius and ulna. The ulnar artery travels down the forearm deep to the flexor carpi ulnaris muscle. In the distal forearm, it is joined by the ulnar nerve, which lies just ulnar to the artery. The artery enters the hand, through Guyon's canal, between the pisiform bone and the hook of the hamate. Here it gives off the deep palmar branch of the ulnar artery that provides the lesser ulnar contribution to the deep palmar arch. The ulnar artery proper continues superficially to form the superficial palmar arch.

PALMAR ARCHES

The superficial palmar arch travels just deep to the palmar aponeurosis. It gives off the proper digital artery to the ulnar side of the little finger and the common digital arteries to the ring, long, and index fingers. The common digital arteries travel between the flexor tendons. Just proximal to the web spaces, they divide to form the proper digital arteries of the radial side of the little finger, both sides of the ring and long fingers, and the ulnar side of the index finger. The deep palmar arch travels in a plane between the flexor tendons and the palmar interosseous muscles. The deep arch gives off the common digital artery to the thumb (princeps pollicis artery) and the proper digital artery to the radial aspect of the index finger. It also gives off palmar metacarpal arteries. These arteries anastomose with the common digital arteries just prior to their bifurcation into the proper digital arteries.

THE PROPER DIGITAL ARTERIES

The proper digital arteries travel along the lateral aspect of each digit accompanied by the digital nerves and veins. Just distal to the distal interphalangeal joint the digital artery divides into multiple branches.

Veins

(Fig. 2-3) Venous drainage of the hand is much more variable than the arterial supply. In addition to the venae commitantes, which travel with the named arteries, there are multiple superficial veins. Thus a dual system of venous drainage exists. As a result of

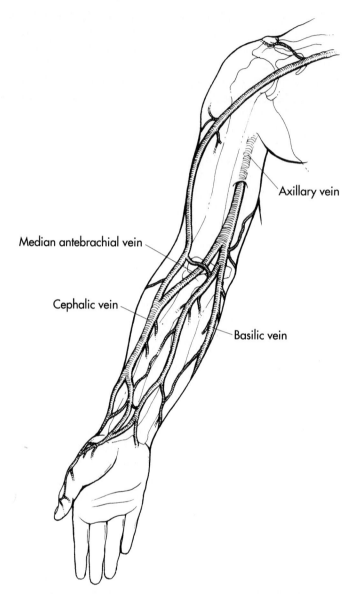

Figure 2-3   The venous anatomy of the upper extremity.

this redundancy, nearly complete amputation is required for total interruption of venous outflow. The superficial veins form an anastomotic network in the dorsum of the hand. They coalesce along the radial aspect of the forearm to form the cephalic vein and the ulnar aspect to form the basilic vein. Just distal to the cubital fossa, the cephalic vein branches to give rise to the median antebrachial vein, which crosses the cubital fossa to anastamose with the basilic vein just below the medial epicondyle. The superficial veins join the deep brachial veins in the axillary region to form the axillary vein.

Examination

Visual inspection

In most settings, perfusion of the digits is easily determined by assessing the color, temperature, and capillary refill. In some situations, however, the determination of perfusion may be quite difficult. Color and temperature are most useful when unaffected digits can be used for comparative purposes; if all the digits of the injured hand are affected, use the digits of the uninjured hand for comparison. A relatively cool and pale digit is problematic for arterial insufficiency. Capillary refill is determined by squeezing the fingertip or by the application of focal pressure using a blunt probe. If refill after blanching is slow (greater than 2 seconds) and/or incomplete, then arterial insufficiency is suspected. Extremely brisk capillary refill combined with dark blue coloration suggests venous insufficiency. It is important to note that some degree of capillary refill may occur even in an amputated digit because of redistribution of stagnant blood. Therefore, capillary refill must be interpreted as a relative rather than an all-or-nothing phenomenon. If the perfusion status of a digit is still indeterminate after this visual inspection, it may be appropriate to further assess blood flow by puncturing the fingertip with a sterile 20-gauge needle. This should be performed only if the patient is insensate in the area to be tested; this is not uncommon in patients with a digit that is almost completely amputated. The return of briskly flowing, bright-red blood following puncture excludes the diagnosis of arterial insufficiency. Slowly flowing, dark venous blood or no blood return at all suggest arterial insufficiency. Copious amounts of dark blood suggest venous insufficiency. If available, a doppler probe may prove invaluable in determining the vascular status of a digit if an arterial signal distal to the level of injury can be obtained.

Allen test

Occlusion or severance of both the radial and ulnar artery in combination should be easily determined on the basis of the injury pattern, bleeding, and the marked decrease in blood flow to all of the digits of the affected hand (some blood flow may reach the hand through the interosseous arteries if they remain intact). Division or occlusion of a single artery may be somewhat more difficult to determine, as bleeding will frequently stop with extended direct pressure and the remaining patent vessel may provide adequate blood flow to the hand. In this situation the Allen test (Fig. 2-4) is employed to

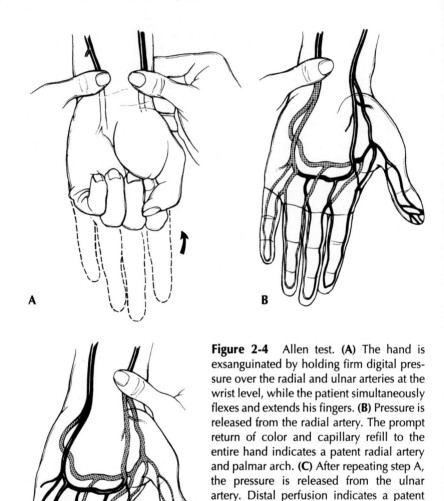

A

B

C

Figure 2-4   Allen test. **(A)** The hand is exsanguinated by holding firm digital pressure over the radial and ulnar arteries at the wrist level, while the patient simultaneously flexes and extends his fingers. **(B)** Pressure is released from the radial artery. The prompt return of color and capillary refill to the entire hand indicates a patent radial artery and palmar arch. **(C)** After repeating step A, the pressure is released from the ulnar artery. Distal perfusion indicates a patent ulnar artery.

determine the patency of both vessels. In this test, both the radial and ulnar artery are firmly compressed at the wrist. The hand is exsanguinated by elevation and by the patient opening and closing his/her hand (if not contraindicated by other injuries) (Fig. 2-4*A*). The radial artery is released while pressure is maintained over the ulnar artery; if the palm and all five digits fill with blood, then the radial artery is patent with good collateral blood flow into the ulnar artery system (Fig. 2-4*B*). The entire test is then repeated for the ulnar artery (Fig. 2-4*C*). Normal filling time for either artery should be fewer than 5 seconds under normal conditions.

Doppler probes

Doppler probes may be helpful in this vascular evaluation, but interpretation may be difficult if collateral blood flow from the intact artery results in retrograde flow through the distal portion of the severed artery. Alternate occlusion by pressure over the arteries may help to distinguish direct flow from collateral flow.

Nerve
Anatomy

Three major nerves—the median, ulnar, and radial—supply both motor and sensory innervation to the hand and forearm (Fig. 2-5). Two other nerves—the lateral antebrachial cutaneous and medial antebrachial cutaneous—supply most of the remaining sensory innervation to the forearm.

The median nerve (Fig. 2-6)

The median nerve is formed in the axilla by a coalescence of branches from the lateral and the medial cords of the brachial plexus, with contributions from C5, C6, C7, C8, and T1. The me-

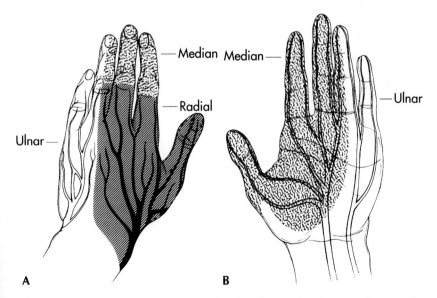

A   B

Figure 2-5   The sensory innervation of the hand. Note that there may be considerable overlap of the territories and considerable variation between individuals.

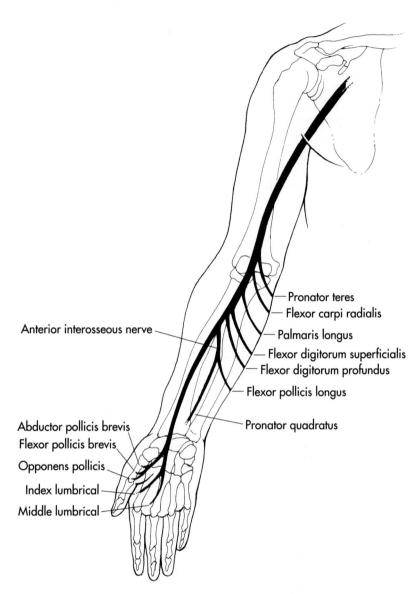

Figure 2-6   The median nerve motor innervation in the hand and forearm. Note that the anterior interosseous nerve typically innervates the radial half of the flexor digitorum profundus, the flexor pollicis longus, and the pronator quadratus.

dian nerve travels down the anteromedial aspect of the arm deep to the biceps muscle adjacent to the brachial artery. It continues across the elbow into the forearm superficial to the brachialis muscle in the central portion of the arm. At the elbow, the median nerve lies medial to the brachial artery, which in turn lies medial to the biceps tendon (TAN: tendon–artery–nerve). The median nerve passes deep to the lacertus fibrosus and enters the forearm between the superficial and deep heads of the pronator teres muscle. After passing through the pronator teres, the median nerve passes deep to the flexor digitorum superficialis under the flexor digitorum superficialis (FDS) arch. At approximately this level, the median nerve gives off the anterior interosseous nerve, which travels along the anterior surface of the interosseous membrane in the interval between the flexor pollicis longus and the flexor digitorum profundus. The anterior interosseous nerve provides motor input to the radial half of the flexor digitorum profundus, the flexor pollicis longus, and the pronator quadratus. After passing beneath the FDS arch, the median nerve travels down the forearm in the plane between the flexor digitorum superficialis and flexor digitorum profundus to the most distal portion of the forearm. At that point, it becomes more superficial among the tendons of these muscles. At the wrist, the median nerve lies just deep to and between the flexor carpi radialis and palmaris longus tendons (if present). In the distal forearm, the median nerve gives off a superficial branch, the palmar cutaneous branch of the median nerve, which provides sensation to the proximal palm of the hand. In its superficial location in the distal wrist, the palmar cutaneous branch is highly susceptible to injury, and untreated divisions frequently result in painful neuromas. The median nerve then passes through the carpal tunnel accompanied by the flexor tendons to the fingers. Somewhat variably at this level, the median nerve gives off the recurrent motor branch to the thenar eminence. The motor branch characteristically follows a recurrent course from distal to proximal to innervate the abductor pollicis brevis, the opponens pollicis, and the superficial head of the flexor pollicis brevis. Immediately on leaving the carpal tunnel, the median nerve divides into three common palmar digital nerves. The first divides proximally to supply the proper palmar digital nerves to the thumb and the radial aspect of the index finger. The second and third divide more distally and give branches to the ulnar aspect of the index finger, the radial and ulnar aspects of the long finger, and radial aspect of the ring finger. In the fingers, the digital nerves are located just palmar to and central to the digital arteries. Clearly defined neurovascular bundles may be identified to a level distal to the distal interphalangeal joints.

The radial nerve (Fig. 2-7)

The radial nerve is formed in the axilla from the posterior cord of the brachial plexus with contributions from C4 to T1. The nerve passes medial-to-lateral deep to the triceps along the posterior aspect of the middle third of the humerus, accompanied by the profunda brachii artery. Fractures of the humerus at this level can result in injury to the radial nerve. This produces a transient or, less commonly, permanent nerve palsy. In the spiral groove, the radial nerve gives off the posterior antebrachial cutaneous nerve, which provides sensation to the dorsal forearm. Distal to the spiral groove, the radial nerve pierces the lateral intermuscular septum at the junction of the middle and distal thirds of the humerus and passes across the elbow anterior to the lateral epicondyle between the brachialis and brachioradialis muscles. Deep to the brachioradialis muscle, the radial nerve gives off motor branches to the brachioradialis and extensor carpi radialis muscles, and then divides to form the superficial sensory branch radial nerve and the deep radial (posterior interosseous) nerve. The superficial radial nerve continues along the undersurface of the brachioradialis muscle into the distal forearm (accompanied by the radial artery in the middle third of the forearm). It exits from under the brachioradialis at approximately the musculotendonous junction at the distal third of the forearm and passes dorsally over the wrist. At that point, it divides into multiple branches that provide sensation to the radial side of the dorsum of the hand and fingers to approximately the level of the proximal interphalangeal joints (Fig. 2-5*A*). The radial nerve and its branches are very superficial in this location, and therefore very susceptible to trauma. Untreated divisions at the wrist often lead to painful neuroma formation. In the proximal forearm, the posterior interosseous branch of the radial nerve gives off motor branches to the extensor carpi radialis brevis and the supinator. It then passes deep into the forearm between the superficial and deep heads of the supinator muscle. After passing through the supinator, branches are given to the extensor digitorum communi, extensor digiti minimi, extensor carpi ulnaris, extensor pollicis longus and brevis, abductor pollicis longus, and the extensor indicis proprius. The terminal branches of the posterior interosseous nerve provide deep sensation to the dorsum of the carpus.

The ulnar nerve (Fig. 2-8)

The ulnar nerve is formed in the axilla from the medial cord of the brachial plexus with contributions from C8 to T1. It runs down

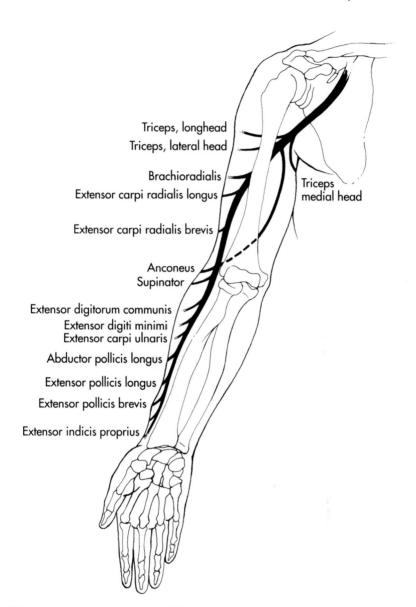

Figure 2-7   Muscles innervated by the radial nerve. After passing through the spiral groove, the radial nerve also gives off motor branches to the lateral half of the brachialis muscle (not shown here).

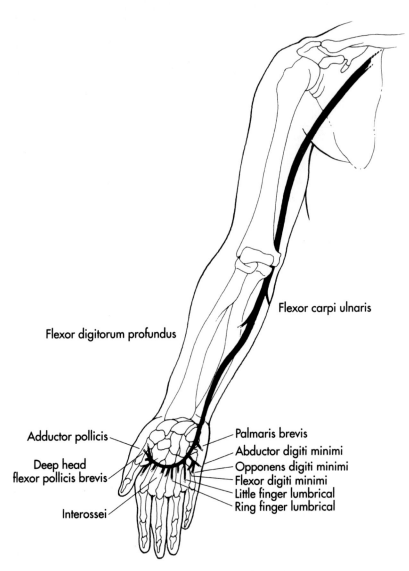

Figure 2-8 Motor innervation of the ulnar nerve.

the medial aspect of the arm piercing the medial intermuscular septum dorsally at the midarm; it then continues distally between the septum and the triceps muscle, accompanied by the superior ulnar collateral artery. The nerve passes into the forearm via the cubital tunnel, whose entrance is formed by the medial epicondyle and the olecranon. Within the tunnel, the nerve passes between the two heads of the flexor carpi ulnaris. It then continues along the undersurface of this muscle down to the distal wrist. Proximally, the nerve gives off motor branches to the flexor carpi ulnaris and to the ulnar half of the flexor digitorum profundus. Proximal to the wrist (~8 to 10 cm), the nerve gives off a dorsal sensory branch that passes dorsally from under the flexor carpi ulnaris. It then divides to provide sensory branches to the ulnar dorsum of the hand and the dorsum of the ring and little finger out to the level of the proximal interphalangeal joints (Fig. 2-5*A*). In the distal forearm, the ulnar nerve gives off a palmar sensory branch that gives sensation to the ulnar surface of the palm. The ulnar nerve is joined by the ulnar artery in the midforearm. At the distal wrist, the ulnar artery and nerve lie side by side beneath the tendon of the flexor carpi ulnaris, with the ulnar artery radial to the nerve. Both artery and nerve pass into the hand through Guyon's canal between the pisiform and hook of the hamate. Within the canal, the nerve divides into superficial and deep branches. The superficial branch supplies motor innervation to the palmaris brevis muscle and sensation to the hypothenar eminence. It then divides into digital branches, with a proper digital nerve to the ulnar aspect of the little finger and a common digital nerve, which divides into proper digital nerves, to the radial aspect of the little finger and the ulnar half of the ring finger (Fig. 2-5*B*). The deep branch of the ulnar nerve accompanies the deep branch of the ulnar artery. Together they pass between the abductor digiti minimi and the flexor digiti minimi brevis, and then pass through the opponens digiti minimi muscle. The deep branch of the ulnar artery continues in a plane dorsal to the flexor tendons. The deep palmar arch and the deep branch of the ulnar nerve follows along with it, giving motor branches to the small and ring finger lumbricals, all of the interossei, adductor pollicis, and the deep head of the flexor pollicis brevis.

The lateral antebrachial cutaneous nerve

The musculocutaneous nerve is a continuation of the lateral cord of the brachial plexus and receives contributions from C4 to C6. This nerve provides motor input to the flexors of the arm, but does not provide any motor input distal to the elbow. It does however, continue distally into the forearm as the lateral antebrachial cutaneous nerve, which provides sensation to the radial aspect of the forearm. In the proximal forearm, the nerve runs with the cephalic vein along the medial aspect of the brachioradialis muscle. Typically two or more branches of the nerve separate distally into the anterior and posterior branches. Distally, there may be significant overlap of the sensory territories of the lateral antebrachial cutaneous nerve and the radial sensory nerve.

The medial antebrachial cutaneous nerve

The medial antebrachial cutaneous nerve arises directly from the medial cord of the brachial plexus. It runs down the medial aspect of the upper arm adjacent to the basilic vein. In the forearm, it gives off both anterior and posterior branches and provides sensation to the ulnar aspect of the forearm.

Examination

Sensory evaluation

A sensory evaluation should be performed in a systematic fashion, based on the patient's injuries and subjective complaints. Sensory examination should always be completed prior to the administration of a local anesthetic, sedation, or potent narcotic pain medication.

TWO-POINT DISCRIMINATION

The simplest and most reliable means of sensory examination of the hand is the measurement of two-point discrimination. We employ the "Disk-criminator®," a commercially available device for measurement of two-point discrimination, but the two ends of a bent paper clip will suffice if such a device is not readily available. Needles or other potentially painful instruments are discouraged during the initial evaluation, as they will make it difficult for the patient to concentrate and frequently result in poor cooperation during further evaluation. Two-point discrimination can be performed as a static or as a moving exam, with the points passed proximally to distally across the pulp of the finger being tested. Of the two, moving two-point discrimination is more consistently reproducible. This test should be performed with the patient in a relaxed, relatively painless, position. Ideally the hand should rest on a firm, flat surface to prevent motion of the fingers as pressure is applied. If the injury prevents placing the patient's hand on a flat surface, support each digit individually as it is tested. Perform the test with the patient's eyes closed, so that the patient's responses will not be altered by visual input. Testing should proceed from widely spaced prongs (8 mm or more) to progressively narrower prongs. Patient responses should be limited to "one," "two," or "I don't know." The recorded value should be the lowest value at which the patient can consistently distinguish two points. Abnormal values in the digits are greater than 6 mm for static two-point discrimination and greater than 4 mm for moving two-point discrimination. Typically, a complete sensory examination usually requires only a few minutes. As a general rule, a complete evaluation of the injured extremity should be performed. The evaluation of uninjured regions of the extremity provides useful information for comparison purposes and may result in the detection of unsuspected damage. The results of this exam must be carefully recorded to serve as the basis for comparisons in subsequent serial assessment.

Thus, two-point discrimination testing provides significant insight into the status of the sensory innervation of the hand. However, if a significant laceration has occurred, our policy is to surgically explore those patients who complain of persistent numbness when touched lightly in the appropriate anatomic distribution. This policy applies even if the "two-point discrimination" test results are normal. Overlapping patterns of innervation may sometimes produce a normal two-point discrimination, even if a nerve is partially or completely lacerated. In small children or obtunded patients, who are unable to comply with formal sensory testing, surgical exploration of a potentially lacerated nerve may be necessary to exclude a diagnosis of injury.

INTERPRETATION

Interpretation of the sensory examination depends on the mechanism of injury and the findings from the rest of the evaluation. The implications of sensory loss following a crush injury or fracture are significantly different from the implications of sensory loss following a laceration. Sensory loss following a proximal crush injury or fracture may indicate that there is ongoing pressure on the nerve. As a result, consideration should be given to emergent surgical decompression of the appropriate region. Alternatively, sensory loss following a laceration with perfusion intact may indicate nerve division and the need for either immediate or delayed surgical exploration and repair in the operating room. Temporary impairment of the nerve may occur following any injury in which the nerve is mechanically traumatized (neuropraxia or axonotemesis). If nerve division or ongoing compression can be excluded, management of this type of injury is usually expectant, because in many instances recovery will proceed without intervention.

SERIAL EXAMINATIONS

In crush injuries or fractures with relatively mild sensory deficits, serial sensory examinations may be useful in differentiating a neuropraxia from an ongoing compression neuropathy. Progressive worsening of the sensory examination following this type of injury is an ominous sign. In such instances, emergent surgical decompression may prevent permanent nerve damage. Compression of the nerves may occur in isolation (e.g., carpal tunnel syndrome) or as part of a compartment syndrome (see sec. on

Assessment—Muscle/Tendon). A compression neuropathy may occur anywhere along the length of a nerve that is subjected to increased ambient pressures. Crush injuries, blunt trauma, burns, or fractures all may produce swelling that can result in a compression neuropathy. If the diagnosis is made early, surgical release is curative. Failure to make the diagnosis or a delay in therapy may result in permanent nerve injury. Further discussion of the pathophysiology and management of nerve injuries is outlined in Chapter 6.

Motor evaluation

Motor evaluation is outlined below. in the discussion of muscle/tendon examination (see sec. on Assessment—Muscle/Tendon). Loss of function in specific muscles or muscle groups may be correlated with sensory examination to determine the degree and level of nerve injury.

Muscle/Tendon

Anatomy

The antebrachial fascia envelops the musculature of the forearm; septae penetrate between the individual muscles and divide the arm into flexor and extensor compartments.

The extrinsic flexor muscles

These muscles of the forearm may be divided into superficial, intermediate, and deep groups.

The superficial flexor group originates from the medial epicondyle of the humerus and constitutes the primary flexors of the wrist. It includes the pronator teres (a pronator of the forearm), flexor carpi radialis, palmaris longus (present in 80% of forearms), and flexor carpi ulnaris (Fig. 2-9).

The intermediate flexor group consists of the flexor digitorum superficialis muscles. These muscles originate from the medial epicondyle, proximal ulna, and proximal radius. They give rise to four tendons that pass through the carpal tunnel in the palm and insert at the base of the middle phalanges of the index, long, ring, and little fingers. They also act to flex the fingers at the proximal interphalangeal joints.

The deep flexor group consists of the flexor digitorum profundus and the flexor pollicis longus (Fig. 2-10). The flexor digitorum profundus arises from the proximal ulna and interosseous membrane. It gives rise to four tendons that pass through the carpal tunnel, then pass through the superficialis tendons from dorsal to palmar under the A1 pulley, and insert at the bases of the distal phalanges of the index, long, ring, and little fingers. They act to flex the distal

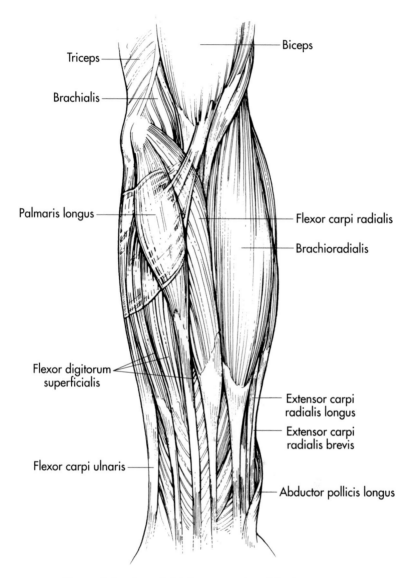

Figure 2-9   Superficial flexor muscles of the forearm.

interphalangeal joints of these digits. The flexor pollicis longus originates at the midradius and interosseous membrane, passes through
the carpal tunnel, inserts at the base of the distal phalanx of the
thumb, and acts to flex the interphalangeal joint of the thumb.

The action of the extrinsic finger flexors depends on a series of

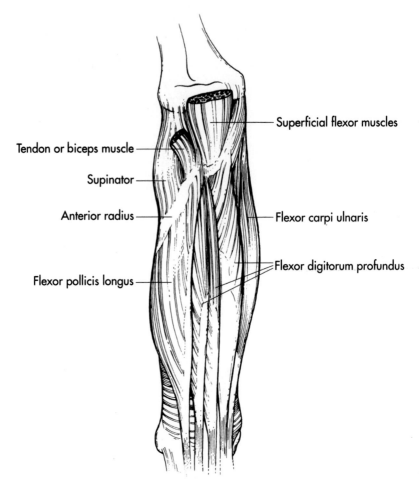

Superficial flexor muscles

Tendon or biceps muscle

Supinator

Anterior radius

Flexor carpi ulnaris

Flexor digitorum profundus

Flexor pollicis longus

Figure 2-10   Deep flexor muscles of the forearm.

pulleys located along the volar aspects of the digits. In addition to the transverse carpal ligament, these pulleys prevent bowstringing of the tendons and allow their action across the interphalangeal joints. The most important of these are the second and fourth annular pulleys of the index, long, ring, and little fingers (Fig. 2-11). In the thumb, the oblique pulley is the most important for preventing bowstringing (Fig. 2-12).

The extrinsic extensor muscles

These muscles of the forearm may also be divided into superficial and deep groups.

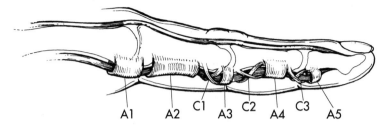

Figure 2-11   Flexor tendon pulley mechanism of the fingers.

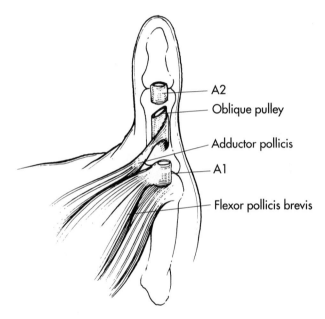

A2

Oblique pulley

Adductor pollicis

A1

Flexor pollicis brevis

Figure 2-12   Flexor tendon pulley mechanism of the thumb.

The muscles of the superficial extensor group arise from the lateral supracondylar ridge, the lateral epicondyle, and proximal radius. They consist of the brachioradialis, the extensor carpi radialis longus and brevis, extensor digitorum communis, extensor digiti minimi, and extensor carpi ulnaris (Fig. 2-13).

The muscles of the deep extensor group arise from the midradius, interosseous membrane, and ulna. They consist of the supinator (which supinates the forearm), the abductor pollicis longus, extensor pollicis brevis, extensor pollicis longus, and extensor indicis proprius (Fig. 2-14).

The extensor tendons' actions depend on six extensor retinacula

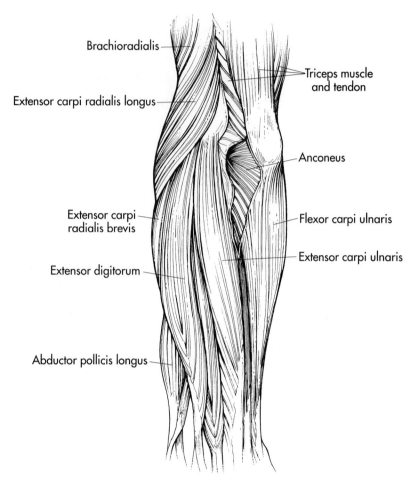

Figure 2-13 Extensor muscles of the hand and wrist.

located along the dorsum of the wrist (Fig. 2-15). The first contains the abductor pollicis longus and extensor pollicis brevis tendons; the second the extensor carpi radialis longus and brevis tendons; the third the extensor pollicis longus tendon; the fourth the extensor indicis proprius and digitorum communi tendons; the fifth the extensor digiti quinti proprius tendon; and the sixth the extensor carpi ulnaris tendon.

Fascia

The antebrachial fascia of the forearm continues distally into the palm. Centrally, the deep fascia forms the palmar aponeurosis that

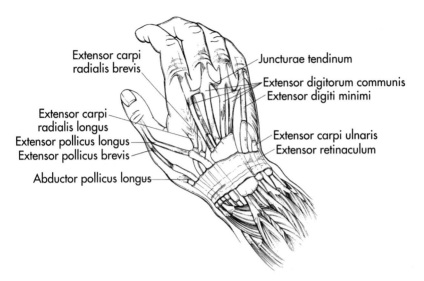

Figure 2-14 Extensor tendons of the hand and wrist.

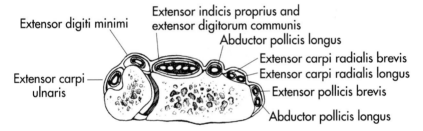

Figure 2-15 Compartments of the extensor retinaculum.

creates a thick protective layer over the relatively superficial tendons, arteries, and nerves in the palm. The deep fascial layer also envelops the thenar and hypothenar muscles, forming the thenar and the hypothenar compartments.

Intrinsic muscles of the hand

The muscles in the thenar compartment are the abductor pollicis brevis, the opponens pollicis, the flexor pollicis, and the adductor pollicis. These muscles abduct, oppose, flex, and adduct the thumb at the level of the carpometacarpal joint.

The muscles of the hypothenar compartment are the abductor digiti minimi, the flexor digiti minimi brevis, and the opponens digiti minimi (quinti). These muscles abduct, flex, and oppose the little finger at its metacarpal-phalangeal joint.

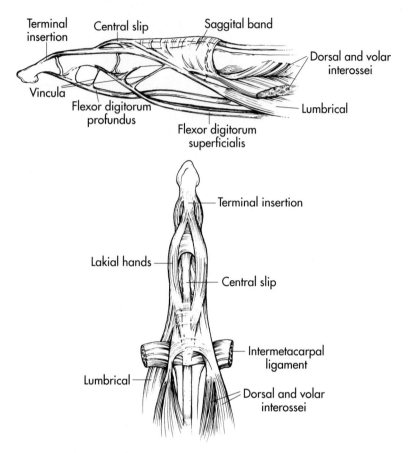

Terminal insertion

Central slip

Saggital band

Dorsal and volar interossei

Vincula

Flexor digitorum profundus

Lumbrical

Flexor digitorum superficialis

Terminal insertion

Lakial hands

Central slip

Intermetacarpal ligament

Lumbrical

Dorsal and volar interossei

Figure 2-16   Extensor mechanism of the finger.

The dorsal and palmar interosseous muscles lie between the metacarpals and function in a complex manner to allow adduction and abduction of the digits at the level of the metacarpal–phalangeal joints, flexion at the metacarpal–phalangeal joints, and extension at the interphalangeal joints. The extrinsic extensors, the interossei, and the lumbricals (along with the extrinsic flexors) interact to produce various degrees of extension at the metacarpal phalangeal (MP), proximal interphalangeal (PIP), and distal interphalangeal (DIP) joints of the fingers. The extrinsic extensors exert more force at the MP joint level, while the intrinsic extensors exert more force at the PIP and DIP joints. Distal to the MP joint level, the tendons of the extrinsic and intrinsic extensors merge to form the extensor hood of the finger (Fig. 2-16).

The lumbricals arise from the flexor digitorum profundus tendons in the palm and contribute to flexion at the metacarpal–phalangeal joint and extension at the interphalangeal joints.

Examination

The examination may be directed in part by the nature and location of the patient's injuries (i.e., for a volar wrist laceration attention would be directed toward testing flexion). However, it is possible to have tendon interruption without laceration. This may be the result of the sharp edges of a fracture (e.g., distal radial fractures and extensor pollicis longus rupture) or avulsion of the tendon from its insertion site (e.g., a mallet finger resulting from disinsertion of the extensor tendon from the distal phalanx; similarly the flexor digitorum profundus may also be avulsed from its distal insertion site). In addition, etiologies other than division or avulsion, including vascular or nerve injuries, may result in loss of function. Thus, in all but the simplest of injuries it is advisable to perform a complete examination of muscles and tendons of the forearm and hand. When performed in a systematic fashion, such an examination may be completed in a matter of minutes. In patients with associated injuries, the administration of pain medications or local anesthesia (following complete neurologic examination) may sometimes improve patient compliance with tendon evaluation.

Extrinsic flexors

To test the function of the flexor pollicis longus, ask the patient to flex the tip of the thumb. Then, assess the flexion strength at the IP joint of the thumb against resistance. The flexor digitorum profundus for each digit should be tested individually by stabilizing the PIP joint in extension and asking the patient to flex the tip of the finger (Fig. 2-17). Isolated testing of the flexor digitorum superficialis tendons to the individual fingers is possible because the flexor digitorum profundus tendons arise from a common muscle belly. Thus, by holding all of the fingers not being tested in full extension, the action of the flexor digitorum profundus on the finger being tested is eliminated. Flexion across the proximal interphalangeal joint, while the other fingers are held flat against the table in full extension, indicates an intact flexor digitorum superficialis tendon (Fig. 2-18). In some patients, the muscle belly to the flexor digitorum profundus tendon of the index finger may function independently, making examination of the flexor digitorum superficialis tendon to the index finger difficult. In a small percentage of patients, the superficialis tendon to the little finger may be absent as a normal anatomic variant. The flexor carpi ulnaris, palmaris longus, and flexor carpi radialis can be tested by asking the patient to flex his or her wrist and manually palpating each of these tendons. The pal-

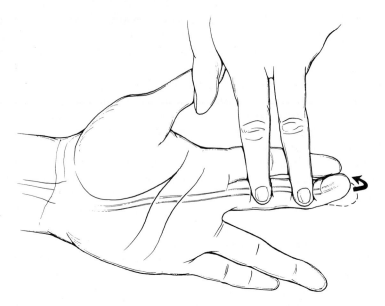

Figure 2-17   The flexor digitorum profundus is tested by holding the proximal interphalangeal joint in extension and asking the patient to flex the finger.

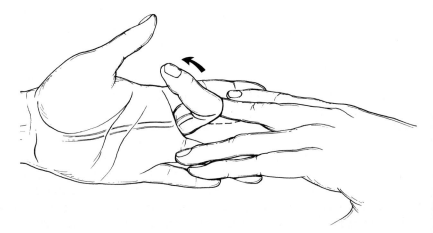

Figure 2-18   The flexor digitorum superficialis is tested by holding all fingers not being tested in full extension and asking the patient to bend the finger.

maris longus may be made more prominent by having the patient actively oppose his/her thumb to his/her little finger while flexing his/her wrist. (The palmaris longus tendon is absent in approximately 15 to 20% of people).

Extrinsic extensors

The tendons of the first compartment—the abductor pollicis longus and extensor pollicis brevis—are tested by asking the patient to maximally abduct the thumb and manually palpating each tendon. Similarly, the tendons of the second compartment—the extensors carpi radialis longus and brevis—can also be tested by palpation when the patient is asked to make a fist and then actively extend the wrist against resistance. The tendon of the third compartment—the extensor pollicis longus—is tested by having the patient place his/her hand flat on the table and then having the patient lift only the thumb. The tendons of the fourth compartment—the extensor indicis proprius and the extensor digitorum communi—are tested by having the patient actively extend (straighten) his/her fingers at the MP joint level. Function of the extensor indicis proprius is ascertained by having the patient extend the index finger with all of the other fingers in full flexion (thus eliminating the action of the EDC on the index finger). Likewise, the tendon of the fifth compartment—the extensor digiti minimi—is also tested by having the patient make a fist with all of the other fingers and then actively extend the little finger. The extensor carpi ulnaris may be palpated dorsally just distal to the ulnar head by having the patient actively extend and ulnarly deviate the hand at the wrist.

While these tests indicate dysfunction of the extrinsic flexors and extensors to the hand, they fail to distinguish between neurologic, muscular, or tendonous etiologies. Frequently, the pathology may be distinguished on the basis of history and visual inspection alone (for example, failure of the flexor tendons associated with a laceration at the distal wrist crease is almost certainly the result of tendon transection, while failure associated with a laceration at the level of the midhumerus is most likely the result of a median nerve injury). However, this may not always be the case. In patients who are neurologically impaired as the result of central or peripheral nervous system injuries, the status of the tendons may still be assessed by observation of resting posture and by evaluation of the tenodesis effect. With the wrist in a neutral position, the fingers will typically assume a resting cascade with progressive flexion moving from radial to ulnar. A break in this normally smooth cascade (i.e., one or more of the fingers lays in full extension breaking the cascade) indicates tendon disruption. The tendon status may be further assessed by passively flexing and extending the wrist. When the wrist is flexed, tone is increased in the finger extensors. This results in passive extension of the fingers (Fig. 2-19A). With passive extension of the wrist, tone is increased in the flexor tendons. This results in flexion of the fingers (Fig. 2-19B). This tenodesis effect will not occur if the tendon is not in continuity.

Intrinsic muscles

The thenar muscles—the flexor pollicis brevis, opponens pollicis, and abductor pollicis brevis—are tested as a group by having the patient bring the thumb and little finger into opposition, so that the nails are parallel. They can also be tested by having the patient lay the hand on the table palm up and then bring the thumb up to form a 90-degree angle with the palm. Simultaneously, the examiner actively palpates the thenar musculature. The adductor pollicis is tested individually by having the patient hold a piece of paper between the thumb and the radial aspect of the proximal phalanx of the index finger. If the adductor is nonfunctioning, the patient will need to compensate by using the flexor pollicis longus resulting in flexion at the IP joint (Froment's sign). The hypothenar muscles—the abductor digiti minimi, flexor digiti minimi, and opponens digiti minimi—are tested as a group by having the patient abduct the little finger and palpating the muscle group. Interosseous function can be tested by having the patient spread the fingers apart with and without resistance. It may also be tested by having the patient place the hand flat on the table palm down, hyperextend the middle finger, and then alternately radially and ulnarly deviate the finger. The patient may also be asked to "cross" the fingers.

Extensor hood

Extensor hood injuries may be deceptive in their initial appearance. As a result, partial lacerations and avulsions may go unrecognized. Without proper management they may lead to serious deformity of the involved digit. Pain over the distal interphalangeal joint, with or without an avulsion fragment visible on an X-ray, may represent an avulsion of the terminal slip of the extensor mechanism from the distal phalanx. Pain and swelling may mask the inability of the patient to fully extend at this joint. Left untreated, this type of injury will progress to a mallet finger deformity, with a flexion contracture at the DIP joint level. Pain and swelling over the PIP joint level following trauma may represent an avulsion of the central slip of the extensor mechanism. Initial evaluation may fail to reveal an extension deficit because of the actions of the lateral bands of the extensor mechanism. However, if left untreated, this disruption of the extensor mechanism may lead to volar displacement of the

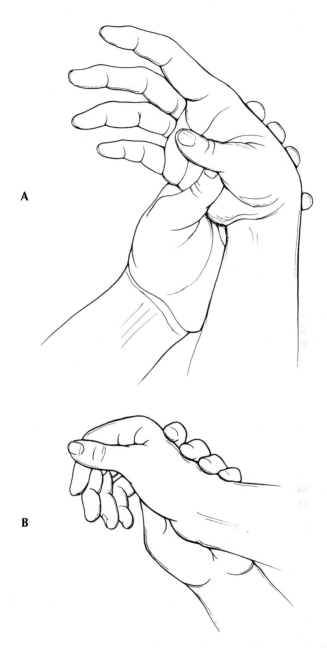

Figure 2-19   The status of the tendons may be assessed by passively flexing and extending the wrist. **(A)** When the extensor tendons are intact, passive flexion of the wrist results in extension of the fingers. **(B)** When the flexor tendons are intact, passive extension of the wrist results in flexion of the fingers.

lateral bands, with the resultant characteristic Boutonniere deformity (flexion contracture at the PIP joint and fixed extension at the DIP joint). Similarly, seemingly superficial lacerations of the dorsum of the finger may produce lacerations of the extensor hood. This can also result in complex deformities of the fingers if left untreated. Therefore, careful inspection of wounds in this location is indicated, with subsequent anatomic repair of any defects encountered. In closed injuries, if the diagnosis of possible extensor injury remains in question at the time of the initial evaluation, a follow-up examination within seven days is indicated. After several days have elapsed, pain and swelling will diminish and a more thorough examination will be possible. Conservative (closed) treatment of these avulsion-type injuries of the extensor mechanism is usually effective even if instituted several weeks after the initial injury.

A Compartment Syndrome

A compartment syndrome is an elevation of pressure within a confined space (or compartment), so that circulation is compromised to the structures within it.

Pathophysiology

In the hand and forearm, the space is defined by the enveloping antebrachial fascia and its septations, which travel through the various muscles and muscle groups. Within these confined compartments, swelling as a result of bleeding and/or edema can lead to an elevation of intracompartmental pressure. Progressive elevation of pressure results in progressive impairment of perfusion to the structures contained within the compartment. It is possible to have a compartment syndrome that involves isolated compartments, such as the volar or dorsal compartments of the forearm, or a syndrome that involves the entire arm. A variety of insults, including crush-type injuries, fractures, prolonged ischemia, burns, and envenomation, may produce an elevation of intracompartmental pressures and lead to compartment syndrome. Any insult that produces swelling may cause this syndrome. With early diagnosis, compartment syndrome may be effectively treated; if diagnosis is delayed even a few hours, the patient may be left with a permanently functionless limb! Therefore, it is essential that the examiner maintain a high index of suspicion regarding the presence of a possible compartment syndrome and be able to recognize the signs of this syndrome so that surgical decompression may be performed prior to the development of irreversible injury.

Diagnosis

The signs of compartment syndrome are pain that is disproportionate to the injury, palpably swollen compartments, pain on passive or active stretching of the involved muscle(s), decreased strength in the involved muscle compartment, hypesthesia or anesthesia in the sensory distribution of the nerve in the involved compartment, and loss of distal pulses. These signs may occur individually or in combination; the presence of *any* of these signs in the traumatized upper extremity should prompt an immediate investigation for possible compartment syndrome. Diagnosis may be made entirely on clinical grounds.

Measurement of compartment pressures

In the unconscious, uncooperative, or pediatric patient, or in patients with equivocal exams, direct measurement of intracompartmental pressures may be necessary. Several commercial devices are available for measuring compartment pressures. Monitors designed for measuring central venous pressure or arterial blood pressure may be converted for measuring intracompartmental pressures by attaching the tubing to an 18-gauge needle, which is then inserted into the compartment. If one of these devices is not available, the "Method of Whitesides" may be employed by using equipment that is available in most emergency departments (Fig. 2-20). In this technique, a three-way stopcock is connected through intravenous tubing to a mercury manometer, a 20 cc syringe (filled with air), and an 18-gauge needle. The stopcock must be of the type that will allow all three ports to be open simultaneously. The 18-gauge needle is inserted into a bottle of bacteriostatic saline, and the saline is aspirated to fill one-half of the tubing between the needle and the stopcock. The stopcock is then closed to the needle so that the saline will not be lost, and the needle is inserted using sterile technique into the compartment to be tested. The stopcock is then opened to all three tubes, and the plunger of the 20 cc syringe is slowly depressed until the saline column in the tube is seen to move (this may be best appreciated by monitoring the air–saline interface). At this point, the pressure reading on the mercury manometer reflects the compartment pressure. A minimal amount of saline should be injected so as to not contribute to further increases in the compartment pressure.

Management

In normotensive patients a compartment pressure greater than 30 mmHg is considered pathologic. Extensive decompression should be performed in the operating room as soon as possible. Although measurement of compartment pressures may be a useful adjunct to the clinical examination, immediate surgical decompression is indicated whenever compartment syndrome is suspected even in the face of apparently normal pressure measurements. The conse-

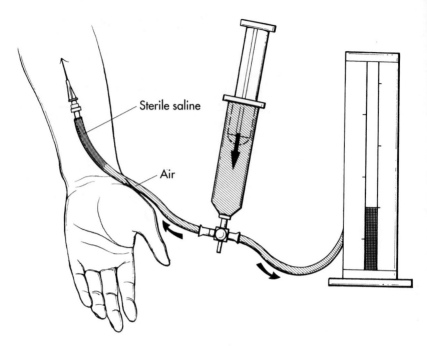

Figure 2-20 The Method of Whiteside. The plunger is depressed until the air fluid interface is seen to advance. The pressure is simultaneously read from the manometer.

quences of a potentially unnecessary compartment release are minor when compared with the devastating results of an unreleased compartment syndrome.

Bones/Ligaments/Joints
Anatomy
The bones of the hand and wrist are illustrated in Fig. 2-21.
Wrist
The radius articulates with the ulna at the radioulnar joint; the convex head of the ulna is seated in the concave sigmoid notch of the radius. The primary stabilizer of this joint is the triangular fibrocartilage, which originates from the dorsoulnar corner of the distal radius and inserts at the base of the ulnar styloid. Strong fibers travel over the dorsal and volar surface of the ulnar head, as well as its distal surface, securing the radius to the ulna throughout a wide range of motion (pronation and supination). There are two rows of carpal bones. The proximal row articulates with the radius and ulna at the scaphoid and lunate fossae. This articulation is stabilized by

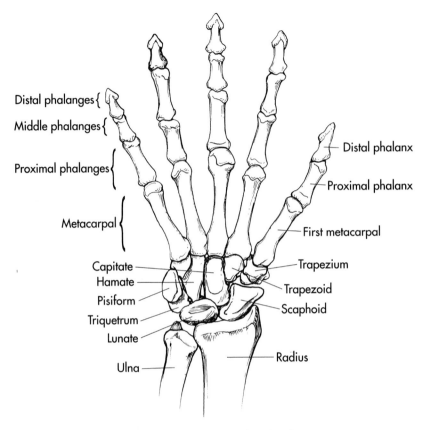

Figure 2-21   Bones of the hand and wrist.

strong volar (extrinsic) ligaments, primarily the radioscaphocapitate, the radiolunate, and the radioscapholunate ligaments (Fig. 2-22). The articulations between the carpal bones are also stabilized by strong volar (intrinsic) ligaments, most significantly the scaphoid–lunate, lunate–triquetrum, and the deltoid (or V) ligaments.

The carpometacarpal (CMC)
    CMC articulation of the thumb metacarpal with the trapezium has two degrees of freedom and is stabilized by five discrete ligaments: the posterior intermetacarpal ligament, the posterior oblique carpometacarpal (dorsal) ligament, the radial carpometacarpal ligament, the anterior intermetacarpal ligament, and the anterior oblique carpometacarpal (ulnar) ligament. Of these, the strongest and most important is the anterior oblique ligament, which resists hyperextension and radial subluxation of the joint.

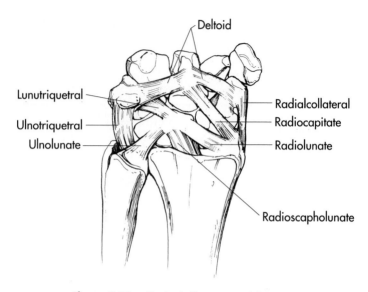

Figure 2-22   Extrinsic ligaments of the wrist.

Strong dorsal and volar carpometacarpal and intermetacarpal ligaments support the carpometacarpal joints of the other metacarpals. These strong ligaments, a significantly limited range of motion, and the support of the adjacent metacarpals and surrounding intrinsic musculature make dislocations of these joints very uncommon.

The metacarpophalangeal joints (MCP)

The MCP joints are condyloid, with two degrees of freedom. The joints are stabilized by strong collateral ligaments laterally and the volar plate palmarly. Accessory collateral (metacarpal glenoidal) ligaments provide additional support interconnecting the metacarpal head with the volar plate. Further support is provided by the volar intermetacarpal ligaments and the surrounding tendons and muscles that cross the joint.

The interphalangeal joints

The interphalangeal joints are hinge joints, with only one degree of freedom permitting flexion and extension. These joints are also supported by collateral ligaments, a volar plate, and the tendons that cross the joint. The collateral ligaments consist of a true portion spanning the joint and a more volar fan-shaped accessory portion that connects the proximal phalangeal head to the volar plate.

Evaluation

Although evaluation of bony and ligamentous injuries of the hand and wrist relies heavily on radiographic evaluation, a thorough physical examination remains essential both as a diagnostic tool and as a means by which radiographic examination may be directed. In a sensate hand, acute fractures and ligamentous tears are always associated with tenderness to palpation directly over the site of the injury. Thus, evaluation for bony and ligamentous injuries should include gentle palpation of the entire hand and gentle passive and active range of motion of all joints. Information obtained from the initial examination should be shared with the radiologist and technician before obtaining radiographs, so that special views may be obtained as needed.

Fractures

Standard radiographs of the hand may not be sufficient to evaluate fractures that are nondisplaced or minimally displaced or fractures that are not profiled in a standard series.

SCAPHOID FRACTURES

This is especially important for nondisplaced scaphoid fractures, which may be very difficult to diagnose radiographically in the acute setting. A patient with significant pain to palpation over the anatomic snuff box (between the extensor pollicis longus and brevis tendons, just distal to the radial styloid) following trauma should be managed as a scaphoid fracture even in the absence of radiographic evidence on plain film. Repeat the radiographs in 7 to 14 days or perform another type of radiological evaluation (e.g., bone scan or CT) to make or exclude the diagnosis.

METACARPAL AND PHALANGEAL FRACTURES

Another setting in which radiographs alone are not sufficient to determine therapy are fractures of the metacarpals and phalanges. Although plain radiographs provide useful information in the evaluation of these injuries, they are frequently unable to adequately assess subtle rotational malalignments. Rotational alignment is evaluated by having the patient gently make a fist and assessing for scissoring or overlap of the involved digit(s). In addition, in the Boxer's fracture (i.e., fracture of the small finger metacarpal neck with apex dorsal angulation) or in dorsally angulated fractures of the other metacarpals, the degree of extensor lag may be assessed by having the patient fully extend the fingers either with or without anesthesia. The degree of extensor lag and rotational malalignment supplement the radiographic evaluation in determining the course of therapy.

Ligament injuries

Physical examination also compliments radiological examination in the evaluation of ligamentous injuries of the hand.

LUNOTRIQUETRAL TEARS

Patients with acute traumatic lunotriquetral dissociation, with disruption of the lunotriquetral ligament, will typically have a dorsiflexion type injury to the wrist and will complain of pain over the ulnar aspect of the wrist. A physical examination will reveal pain in response to palpation directly over the lunotriquetral joint. In the lunotriquetral ballottement test, described by Reagan, the examiner stabilizes the lunate with the thumb and index finger of one hand, while the triquetrum and pisiform are alternately displaced dorsally and palmarly with the other hand. A positive result elicits pain, crepitus, and excessive laxity.

SCAPHOLUNATE TEARS

Patients with traumatic scapholunate dissociation will also typically have a dorsiflexion type of injury. However, the pain in scapholunate dissociation is radially located and may be localized by palpation directly over the scapholunate joint. Watson has described the "scaphoid shift test" for evaluation of scapholunate dissociation. In this test, the examiner's four fingers of the same hand as that to be examined are placed dorsally over the radius. The thumb is used to exert pressure palmarly over the distal pole of the scaphoid. The examiner's other hand is then used to move the wrist from ulnar to radial deviation. Palpable dorsal displacement of the scaphoid will occur with this maneuver in the case of scapholunate dissociation. Comparison with the uninjured hand is important. Considerable experience with this test may be required before the examiner becomes proficient in its application.

GAMEKEEPER'S THUMB

Although gentle palpation and range of motion may be safely performed in most settings, it is sometimes prudent to obtain plain films of the hand before more aggressive manipulations. One example of this is acute ulnar collateral injuries of the MP joint of the thumb (Gamekeeper's thumb or Skier's thumb). These injuries are produced by forced radial deviation of the thumb, which produces a partial or complete tear of the ulnar collateral ligament or an avulsion at its insertion into the phalanx at the interphalangeal joint. Therapy is determined by the severity of the injury, which in turn is determined by the instability of the joint on physical exam under local anesthesia. However, this form of stress testing may complicate the injury by interposing the adductor aponeurosis between the proximal portion of the torn ligament and its distal site of insertion (Fig. 2-23). This prevents healing of the injury without surgical intervention. If plain films are obtained before stress testing and an avulsion fracture is found, therapy may be based on the position of the thumb and the displacement of the fracture fragment. This makes stress testing, and its inherent risks, unnecessary. In the absence of an

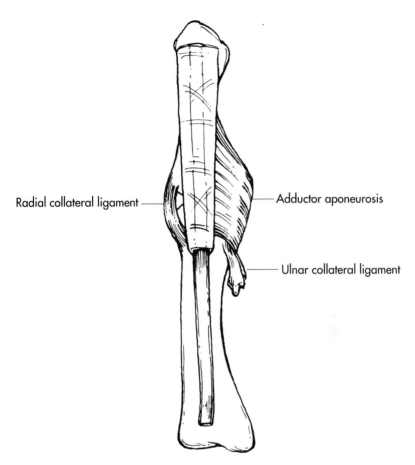

Radial collateral ligament

Adductor aponeurosis

Ulnar collateral ligament

Figure 2-23   Stener's lesion. Following disruption of the ulnar collateral ligament of the MP joint of the thumb, the adductor aponeurosis may become interposed (between the ligament and the proximal phalanx) preventing healing of the ligament.

avulsion fracture or a painful palpable lump over the ulnar aspect of the joint (Stener's lesion), the examiner must weigh the risks and benefits of stress testing. If testing is performed, it should be in both full extension and 30 degrees of flexion. Testing in flexion provides more direct information regarding the ulnar ligament, because the ligament is under maximal tension in this position. Laxity of 30 degrees more than the contralateral thumb MP joint is considered diagnostic of a complete rupture of the collateral ligament.

Neurologic impairment

As already discussed, all fractures should be evaluated for possible compression neuropathy and/or compartment syndrome. More severe fractures may also require serial examinations in the hospital to monitor the patient for the development of a compression neuropathy or compartment syndrome.

Skin and Specialized Structures

Anatomy

The skin of the hand and forearm is remarkably specialized in its form and function. The glabrous skin of the palm and fingers is thick and tethered with an irregular surface and a high density of sensory receptors. By comparison, the skin on the dorsum of the hand and the forearm is relatively thin and mobile. The nailbed complex plays an important role in fine grasp and in providing additional support for the fingertip (Fig. 2-24). The nailbed complex is referred to as the perionychium. The distal skin of the complex is the hyponychium; the thin layer of skin overlying the most proximal portion of the nail plate is the eponychium. The pocket beneath the eponychium from which the nail plate arises is known as the nail fold. The nailbed is divided into the distal sterile matrix and proximal germinal matrix by a visible

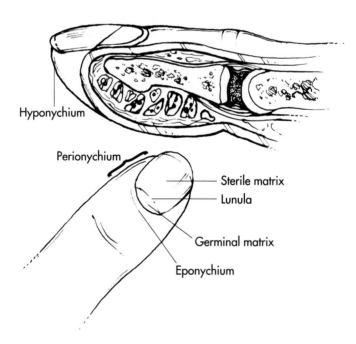

Figure 2-24 The fingertip and nail complex.

moon-shaped crescent called the lunula. Damage to the sterile matrix with irregular healing will result in an abnormally shaped nail, while damage to the germinal matrix may interrupt growth of the nail and result in an abnormally shaped nail. Because the nailbed is extremely thin between the nail plate and the distal phalanx, it is susceptible to lacerations either from tears or deformation of the nail plate or from fractures of the distal phalanx.

Evaluation

Lacerations

In addition to evaluating the underlying structures, all lacerations should be evaluated for the viability of adjacent tissues, the adequacy of soft tissue coverage, and the presence of any foreign bodies. The viability may be assessed by visual inspection of the damage, by checking for capillary refill, and by checking the skin edges for bleeding. Any nonviable tissue will need debridement before closure or coverage of the wound. Adequacy of soft tissue coverage may be assessed by manually coapting the skin edges and assessing the tension across the closure by palpation and visual inspection. The skin should pull together with minimal tension; when closed, the tissues should remain pink and capillary refill must remain within a normal range. If closure with minimal tension is not possible, another form of coverage will be necessary. One of the greatest problems for physicians in the emergency department is retained foreign bodies. With this in mind, it is essential to not only perform a thorough evaluation for foreign bodies in all lacerations, but also to carefully document this evaluation in the patient's medical record. A number of foreign bodies are radioopaque and may be seen on plain films. These include metal, rock, and a variety of glasses. Wood is not usually visible on plain radiographs. If the history suggests the presence of a potentially radioopaque foreign body, radiographs should be obtained. Special views may be necessary to prevent the underlying skeleton from obscuring the foreign body. It is essential to remove any foreign materials from the skin surface or overlying dressings before obtaining radiographs. Plain films alone are not sufficient to rule out the presence of a foreign body, and all lacerations should be visually inspected, manually explored with gentle probing, and thoroughly irrigated prior to closure.

Nailbed injuries

Unrepaired lacerations of the nailbed may result in nail deformity. Therefore, the most important question to answer when evaluating nailbed injuries is whether there is a nailbed laceration that requires repair. In some settings, there will be a tear in the nail plate or the nail plate will be avulsed; this will allow direct visual inspection of the nailbed. However, in most settings, there will be no tear or only a slight tear in the nail plate, and it may then become necessary to remove the nail plate in order to assess the nailbed. It has been suggested that all subungal hematomas above a certain size be explored by removing the nail plate, but our practice is to include other factors in making this decision. The mechanism of injury, the severity of associated injuries, the condition of the nail plate, and the presence or absence of an underlying fracture should all be considered. A displaced fracture of the distal phalanx directly under the nailbed greatly increases the likelihood of a significant nailbed laceration, while the absence of a fracture and an intact nail plate make a significant tear less likely. If a nailbed laceration is suspected, the nail plate should be removed using a blunt-tipped scissors or an elevator under finger block anesthesia. If the nail plate is removed for evaluation, it should be replaced following repair of the nailbed to prevent scar tissue formation between the eponychium and the nailbed, to act as a biologic splint, and to reduce pain. Lacerations of the nailbed should be repaired with fine suture under magnification. In patients with smaller subungal hematomas, in which a significant nailbed tear is thought to be unlikely, decompression of the hematoma by making a hole in the nail plate with a 19-gauge needle or, more preferably, an ophthalmic cautery will greatly decrease patient discomfort.

Thermal burns

The hands are more susceptible to damage from burns than any other area of the body, because their position of function makes them more likely to be exposed to intense heat. Further, their distal perfusion makes them more susceptible to vascular compromise. Because of the number of joints involved and the heavy reliance on flexibility and motion, serious burns may result in devastating loss of function. Fortunately, the hand is afforded some protection by the extremely thick glabrous skin along its palmar surface, which makes the palm more burn resistant than thinner skin elsewhere on the body. Unfortunately, the dorsal skin of the hand is relatively thin, and it is not uncommon to have a full thickness burn or a poorly managed partial thickness burn in this area render a hand functionless.

Evaluation of hand burns is similar to the evaluation of burns elsewhere in the body, and initial management is based primarily on visual inspection, assessment of tissue perfusion, and sensory evaluation. Although blistering on the palmar surface may make this evaluation difficult, blisters in this location are usually not debrided during the initial evaluation unless they are already ruptured or are so extensive that rupture is inevitable. Some authors advocate repeated aspiration of the contents of blisters on the palmar surface of the hand using a needle syringe and sterile technique. Because the skin on the dorsal surface of the hand is much thinner and blisters in this location are more likely to rupture, large blisters in this location may be routinely debrided during initial inspection. Small blisters should be left intact. Moist, red or pink, sensate skin indicate a partial-thickness injury, whereas, dry, white or charred, insensate skin is indicative of a full-thickness injury. The perfusion status of each digit must be carefully checked, as swelling in combination with circumferential burns may result in serious vascular compromise. In these instances, it may be necessary to perform escharotomies in order to salvage the hand or its digits.

Because thermal burns involving the hand will require frequent reevaluation, debridement, dressing changes, and physical therapy, hospitalization is often indicated. Silver sulfidiazene or another topical antimicrobial should be applied after completion of the initial inspection. Dressings must allow for swelling, full range of motion of the digits, and frequent inspection of perfusion status. In burns involving the entire hand, it may be more practical to leave the hand without a formal dressing and instead rely on frequent applications of silver sulfidiazene combined with saline-moistened gauze or a loose-fitting plastic bag to maintain a moist environment.

Chemical burns

The initial first aid for chemical burns is frequently given in the field. With the exceptions of elemental sodium, potassium, or lithium, such treatment consists of removal of the offending agent followed by immediate and copious irrigation with water. If irrigation was not performed or was felt to be inadequate, this should be repeated immediately upon arrival at the emergency department. A few common agents require specific therapies.

ACID AND BASES

Neutralization of acids with basic solutions and bases with acidic solution should not be performed, as neutralization typically produces an exothermic response that increases the damage to the tissues. In mild alkali burns, skin pH has been shown to return to normal only after one hour of shower lavage. Thus for acid or alkaline burns, a minimum of one to two hours of water lavage is recommended. Acids cause tissue damage by cellular dehydration, destruction of cellular membranes, and liquefaction necrosis. This action tends to be rapid. However, if the offending agent is not removed, damage may continue for as long as 24 hours. Alkali burns cause tissue destruction by combining with tissue elements to form fatty soaps. These reactions may continue for days. Therefore as a general rule, acids cause more immediate damage, while bases cause more delayed and extensive soft tissue damage. This should be taken into consideration in determining the level of postburn monitoring following a chemical exposure.

HYDROFLUORIC ACID

The initial therapy for hydrofluoric acid burns is removal of the offending agent and any overlying clothing, followed by immediate and copious irrigation. Following irrigation, topical application of calcium gel may be used to inactivate the free fluoride ions. The gel should be massaged into the tissues for 30 minutes, with subsequent reapplications based on the recurrence of pain and the severity of the burn. In more severe burns with obvious tissue damage and severe pain not relieved by topical calcium gel application, subcutaneous infiltration of 10% calcium gluconate solution 0.5 ml per cm^2 has been shown to relieve pain and decrease tissue damage. In very severe burns, intraarterial injections of calcium have been used, but this technique has been associated with a relatively high-complication rate and is not recommended. All patients with significant hydrofluoric acid burns should have their serum calcium and magnesium levels checked and should be monitored for systemic signs and symptoms of hypocalcemia and hypomagnesemia.

PHOSPHORUS BURNS

Phosphorus burns should also be treated with copious irrigation; residual particles may be identified by washing briefly with 1% copper sulfate to form black cupric phosphide to aid in direct removal.

ELEMENTAL SODIUM

Elemental sodium is one of the few chemical agents that should not be treated with water lavage. Elemental sodium combines with water to form NaOH, producing heat and even explosions. Treatment consists of covering the agent with oil, followed by direct removal/excision.

POISON CONTROL

Poison control information is an excellent resource in the management of chemical exposures and is easily accessed by phone or computer from most emergency departments.

Injection injuries

Injection injuries with high-pressure paint guns or similar devices may produce extensive soft tissue injury that requires surgical exploration, irrigation, and debridement in the operating room. Initial visual inspection may only reveal a small break in the skin at the injection site, but injection injuries with high-pressure spray guns frequently propagate throughout the soft tissues of the hand and even into the forearm. The location of pain and soft-tissue swelling is useful in determining the extent of the injection. Many paints possess some degree of radioopacity and plain films may also be useful. Unfortunately, the caustic and recalcitrant nature of these substances frequently leads to significant soft tissue damage. Early surgical exploration with irrigation and debridement of the affected tissues is indicated.

Frostbite

When an extremity is exposed to cold for a prolonged period of time, ice crystal formation may occur within the tissues; this condition is commonly referred to as frostbite. The severity of the tissue damage depends on a variety of factors, including temperature, wind chill, protective clothing, contact with water or cold objects, and the patient's internal temperature, and may range from mild superficial blistering to complete loss of the extremity. Initial evaluation of the acutely frostbitten hand reveals firm pale tissue. Ice crystal formation usually develops from distal to proximal and superficial to deep, so that the tips of the fingers are most frequently affected. However, it is usually not possible to accurately predict the extent of the damage at the initial evaluation. If thawing has already occurred, the entire hand may appear pink and swollen and the patient may complain of severe pain. With more severe injuries, blistering will usually develop over the next 48 hours. Subsequently, skin necrosis occurs with demarcation between viable and nonviable tissues and, in severe cases, mummification of entire digits. Initial treatment depends on the timing of the patient's initial presentation. If the patient arrives with a frozen hand, it should be rapidly thawed in warm (38-42°C) water. Thawing may be extremely painful and may require sedation as well as an analgesia. Multiple pharmacologic therapies have been suggested to limit tissue loss because of frostbite. Aspirin, nonsteroidal antiinflammatories (NSAIIDs), steroids, topical aloe vera, and a variety of other agents have been used in an attempt to inhibit the inflammatory response and vasoconstricting mediators. Intravenous dextran has been used in an attempt to inhibit platelet aggregation. Direct vasodilators, such as intraarterial reserpine, have also been used. Unfortunately, clinical trials with these agents have not been very encouraging. There is *no* role for early surgical debridement in cases of frostbite. Once the hand has been thawed, care is primarily directed toward protecting the injured tissues from any mechanical damage that might contribute to further tissue loss. Large bulky dressings, with or without such topical antibiotics as silver sulfidiazene, are applied, and the patient is then serially monitored over several days for the development of necrotic tissues. This may be done as an outpatient for minor cases of frostbite or in the hospital for more severe cases. Once clearly demarcated, necrotic tissues should be debrided in order to limit the spread of infection.

Envenomation

Hands are a common site of envenomation. A wide variety of snakes, spiders, scorpions, and insects are capable of envenomation. Hand surgeons and emergency department physicians should familiarize themselves with the species endemic to their geographic location.

SPIDER BITE

Although a variety of spiders endemic to the United States produce local effects with envenomation, the Brown Recluse Spider (*Loxosceles* sp.) is the only common spider capable of producing serious tissue damage and even loss of limb. Although other spiders such as black widows, funnel spiders, and tarantulas may inflict serious bites, local wound management is usually relatively uncomplicated and is typically overshadowed by the potential for serious and even life-threatening systemic toxicity. Local wounds produced by these and other common spiders usually respond well to conservative measures. Unfortunately, this is not true of the brown recluse spider whose venom contains phospholipases and lipases capable of producing widespread local-tissue necrosis.

The brown recluse spider typically lives in dry, dark, quiet areas, such as attics or wood piles. The spider has a delicate body habitus, is tan or brown, and possesses a characteristic violin-shaped marking on its dorsal surface. The initial bite is typically only mildly painful and the initial lesion red, edematous, or blanched. Later, this lesion may evolve a characteristic blue–grey halo. Over the following hours to weeks subsequent tissue breakdown may occur depending on the severity and location of the envenomation. Blebs and an irregularly bordered purpuric lesion typically precede the necrosis, which takes the form of a large eschar. In severe envenomations—and especially in infants and small children—systemic toxicity may occur. In rare instances, this may even lead to death.

Multiple treatments have been advocated for the management of local-tissue necrosis, including steroids, heparin, dextran, antihistamines, hyperbaric oxygen, and early surgical excision. Review of the literature provides little objective support for any of these modalities. Dapsone, a therapy originally developed for the treatment of leprosy, has shown some ability to limit the severity of the tissue destruction. Unfortunately, this drug has the potential for serious side effects, including chemical hepatitis, hemolysis, methemoglobinemia, and leukopenia, and therefore should probably be reserved for rapidly progressive, severe bites in adult patients. Adult doses of 50 to 500 mg/d, divided twice daily have been used. Colchicine 1.2 mg followed by 0.6 mg every 2 hours for 2 days and then every 4 hours for 2 additional days may be added. Complete blood counts and methemoglobin levels should be monitored. Although an antivenin has been developed, it is not available for routine clinical use at the present time.

Several weeks should elapse before embarking on definitive surgical debridement and reconstruction. This will allow the lesion to fully demarcate. The results of early surgical intervention have been found to be inferior to delayed debridement and reconstruction.

SNAKE BITE

The initial evaluation of a snake bite in the emergency department should include an attempt to identify the snake responsible for the bite. There are two families of venomous snakes endemic to the United States: the pit vipers (*Crotalidae*), including rattlesnakes, copperheads, and cottonmouths (water mocassins), and the coral snake (*Elapidae*). The coral snake has short fangs and injects its victims with a neurotoxin through a chewing motion. It is brightly colored with red, yellow, and black stripes. It can be distinguished from similar nonpoisonous snakes by the saying: "Red next to yellow can kill a fellow . . . red next to black, venom lack." Although potentially serious, coral snake bites are relatively uncommon.

Pit viper bites account for the majority of poisonous snake bites in the United States. There is considerable variability in the markings of the pit vipers, even among members of the same species. General features of a pit viper that may help distinguish it from nonpoisonous species include a triangular-shaped head rather than a rounded head, elliptical pupils rather than round pupils, the presence of paired heat-sensing pits anterior to the eyes, and a single row of subcaudal plates below the anal plate instead of the double row seen in nonpoisonous snakes. In addition, species-specific markings and, in the case of the rattlesnake, the presence of a rattle will help to distinguish a pit viper from a nonpoisonous snake. If the snake was captured or killed, it should be taken to the emergency department for specific identification. Care should be taken when handling a killed snake as envenomation may still occur following death.

When the snake or a description of the snake are not available, examination of the bite marks may help to distinguish a poisonous from a nonpoisonous bite. Nonvenomous snakes lack fangs and characteristically produce four rows of scratches with their upper teeth and two rows with their lower teeth. This is in contrast to the paired puncture marks of the pit vipers. *Determination of envenomation.* Envenomation does not always occur with a pit viper bite. Factors affecting envenomation include the specific species of snake, age of the snake, seasonal variations, and the depth and duration of the bite. Because treatment of pit viper bites is not benign, envenomation should be documented before instituting specific therapy. Typically, pain, erythema, and edema surrounding the fang marks that progresses and spreads proximally are present within 30 minutes of an envenomation. If these signs and symptoms have not occurred within 4 hours, a significant pit viper envenomation almost certainly has not occurred.

Pathophysiology. The effects of envenomation can be broadly categorized as local and systemic. Local effects may produce pathology in two ways: direct tissue toxicity and decreased tissue perfusion secondary to swelling. Although direct tissue toxicity may affect the tissues throughout the limb, actual tissue loss related to envenomation is usually limited to the area immediately surrounding the fang marks. This tissue loss may progress over many days and produce an ulcerated lesion that is slow to heal. If this occurs, loss of tissue perfusion secondary to swelling will usually take place within the first 24 to 48 hours. If left untreated, single or multiple compartment syndromes may have devastating effects that result in loss of limb function or complete loss of the limb.

Management.   As coral snake bites are less common and the systemic effects far outweigh the local effects, discussion of management will be directed toward pit viper bites only. Animal studies have indicated that the classic field treatment of incision and aspiration of venom from the bite site may decrease the severity of the envenomation, but only if it is performed immediately. In these studies, aspiration after 15 minutes had little or no effect. Additionally, incision by nonexperienced personnel has been associated with significant morbidity. Therefore, this therapy should probably be reserved for documented pit viper bites, within 15 minutes of the bite, and only be performed by experienced individuals. It should be noted that wide excision of the bite site as a means of removing the venom is still advocated by some authors, and this therapy should be differentiated from simple incision and suction in terms of timing and application.

Transport.   When possible, patients should be kept calm and be transported as quickly as possible to an emergency facility. Although time is of the essence, death from pit viper bites is relatively rare. When it occurs, it usually takes place at least several hours after the initial envenomation. The bite site should be kept level with the heart. A very light tourniquet placed proximal to the bite decreasing lymphatic flow without decreasing venous or arterial blood flow may be of benefit in limiting the spread of the venom. Ice or icepacks placed directly on the bite site are associated with increased tissue necrosis and should not be used.

Evaluation. If it has been determined that the patient has suffered an envenomation, laboratory studies including CBC, creatinine, electrolytes, liver function tests, prothrombin time, partial thromboplastin time, thrombin time, fibrinogen, type and crossmatch, and urinalysis should be obtained. A baseline electrocardiogram should be obtained. A large bore intravenous line should be established. Serial vital signs and continuous cardiac monitoring should be followed. Tetanus prophalaxis, if appropriate, should be administered. The circumference of the limb should be measured and recorded at the same level every 15 to 30 minutes.

Antivenin. Antivenin plays a role in the management of both systemic and local toxicity of snake venom. It is derived from the serum of horses hyperimmunized with *Crotalidae* snake venom. Because its use is associated with a significant risk for anaphylactic reactions and delayed serum sickness, its administration should be limited to patients with significant envenomation. Efficacy at decreasing local toxicity is proportionate to the amount of antivenin administered and the speed with which it can be administered. This creates a paradoxical situation in that delay of administration allows the clinician to more accurately assess the severity of the envenomation, but decreases his/her ability to treat the envenomation with antivenin. Before the administration of antivenin, skin testing should be performed to check for anaphylaxis. At a distant site, inject subcutaneously 0.02 cc of saline diluted serum. The weal should be observed for 10 minutes for signs of erythema, itching, or hives. A syringe of 1:1000 epinepherine should be kept available to treat reactions. If the patient passes this test, 0.2 to 0.5 cc of antivenin may be administered slowly by intravenous infusion. Again, monitor carefully for signs of anaphylaxis. Despite these precautions, the patient may still develop an anaphylactic reaction to antivenin administration. Therefore, administration should be performed in an emergency room or intensive care unit that is equipped to deal with an anaphylactic reaction. Although not well documented, premedication with parenteral antihistamine and 0.25 mg of epinephrine subcutaneously (less for children) probably decreases the incidence of anaphylactic reaction and lessens the severity of such reactions when they do occur. This protocol should probably be used even in the absence of a positive skin test. Dilution of the antivenin allows more controlled administration and may decrease the severity of anaphylactic reactions by allowing early recognition of the reaction and discontinuance of administration. Because antivenin is more effective if it is administered early, patients should be given antivenin as soon as it becomes apparent that they have suffered a serious envenomation. Initial dosing should be proportionate to the suspected severity of the envenomation, with subsequent dosing based on continued progression of local manifestations (especially edema) and systemic manifestations. Typical doses range between 10 and 100 cc, but higher doses may be appropriate in severe envenomations.

Fasciotomy.   Whether or not antivenin is administered, patients with envenomation should be monitored hourly for at least 24 hours for the development of compartment syndrome. Evaluation of compartment syndromes is discussed in Vascular—Muscle/Tendon Section. If a compartment syndrome is suspected, a fasciotomy must be performed immediately to prevent permanent disability.

Animal bites

Because of their potential for producing infection, even seemingly trivial animal bites may produce serious disability to the hand. The risk for infection depends on the animal responsible for the bite, the size and severity of the breaks in the skin, the location of the bite, the force of the bite (and thus the degree of crush and tissue destruction), the patient's immune status, and the initial care for the bite. Initial care consists of immediate and copious irrigation either with a syringe and blunt-tip needle or pulse lavage with one of a variety of commercially available irrigation systems. The timing of the irrigation is critical; irrigation within an hour of the bite has the potential to remove nearly all of the saliva and potentially infectious organisms. After the first hour, irrigation becomes less and less effective. Therefore, no time should be wasted in initiating irrigation as soon as the patient arrives in the emergency department. Sharp debridement can also be utilized to decrease the risk for infection and should be utilized in large wounds with significant contamination and devitalized tissues. Suturing and closure of wounds has the potential for creating a dead space and subsequent abscess formation. In general, puncture wounds, small wounds in noncosmetic locations, wounds in which treatment has been delayed, and wound with significant surrounding soft tissue trauma should not be closed. Closure may be considered in larger wounds, in which there is minimal tissue crush and in which copious irrigation was performed shortly after the bite occurred. Monofilament, nonabsorbable nylon sutures should be used for closure. Partial wound closure or closure with drains left in place may be used in marginal wounds. Aggressive irrigation, debridement, and the liberal use of drains in the operating room may be necessary in large wounds that have exposed bone, joints, and/or tendons. In larger wounds that are not closed primarily, delayed primary closure may be possible after several days of dressing changes. The routine use of antibiotics in acute bite injuries is somewhat controversial. Opponents cite no definite decrease in the infection rate when antibiotics are used acutely combined and the risk of developing resistant strains of bacteria. However, because of the high risk for the development of infection in bite wounds of the hand, one should have a low threshold for administering antibiotics either acutely or at the first sign of infection. Once infection develops, treatment should include hospitalization for intravenous antibiotics, immobilization, elevation, and surgical drainage and debridement of abscess or devitalized tissues.

DOG BITES

Dog bites range from small puncture wounds to skin tears to severe crush injuries. Treatment has already been outlined in this chapter.

CAT BITES

Cat bites frequently consist of a series of benign-appearing puncture marks in the hand that are difficult to irrigate effectively. Cat saliva characteristically contains Pasteurella multocida that may produce a rapidly progressive, painful cellulitis. Early administration of penicillin may prevent this infection. Once it has developed, hospitalization for intravenous penicillin, immobilization, and elevation are indicated. Occasionally surgical intervention is necessary.

HUMAN BITES

Human bites frequently result when one potential patient strikes another potential patient in the mouth with a clenched fist. A tooth may break through the skin and pass through the tendon of the fist into underlying bone or joint. Patients with this characteristic injury may deny this mechanism because of fear of legal repercussions. The depth of the wound can be assessed by having the patient clench the fist; if the hand is only examined with the fingers extended, the break in the underlying tendon and joint capsule may be missed.

Human saliva contains a variety of organisms with the potential for producing serious infections. Streptococcus viradans and staphylococcus aureus are among the most common causes of infection, but a wide variety of anaerobic organisms may also be present in patients with poor oral hygiene. In reliable patients who are seen early and have skin-only involvement, copious irrigation followed by a course of oral antibiotics and dressing changes combined with frequent follow-up visits in the outpatient setting may be indicated. If the bite may have entered the joint or if infection has already occurred, surgical irrigation and debridement, followed by intravenous antibiotics, immobilization, and elevation are indicated.

Infections

When a patient arrives in the emergency room in a delayed state of trauma, complicating infections must be considered.

CELLULITIS

Cellulitis is characterized by warmth and erythema surrounding a break in the skin. The skin is usually tender to the touch and may be swollen or indurated, but should not feel fluctuant with a collection of fluid beneath the skin surface (this would suggest an abscess). The patient may be febrile and may have an elevated white count. Streptococcus is a frequent pathogen in nonbite wounds. In less severe infections, outpatient treatment with oral antibiotics is effective against gram positive cocci. Immobilization, elevation, and follow-up within 24 to 48 hours is appropriate. In more severe infections or in compromised patients, such as diabetics, hospitalization with intravenous antibiotics is indicated.

ABSCESS

Abscess formation may occur anywhere in the hand, but assumes a characteristic pattern of spread based on its location. On the dorsum of the hand, the overlying skin is mobile. This allows the infection to travel in a subcutaneous plane. On the volar surface and in the fingertips, the skin is thick and tethered, which limits the spread of the abscess. Infections that develop around the soft tissue fold of the fingernail are referred to as paronychia. A felon is an abscess that occurs deep within the distal pulp of a finger or thumb. Pyogenic flexor tenosynovitis may occur when infection develops within the confined space of the flexor tendon sheath. Abscesses in the palm characteristically develop in the web spaces between the fingers, in the thenar space deep to the thenar muscles, or in the midpalmar space deep to the flexor tendons.

Dorsal abscesses are easily diagnosed because the thin skin overlying the pus allows direct palpation of the fluctuant mass;

palmar abscesses are much more difficult to diagnose because the thick and teethered overlying skin makes it difficult to palpate the abscess. Focal areas of pain and swelling in the palm following penetrating trauma should raise the clinician's suspicion for a possible abscess. Not infrequently, the patient will undergo an unsuccessful course of antibiotic therapy before the diagnosis of a palmar abscess is made.

Infection of the flexor sheath or pyogenic flexor tenosynovitis is characteristically associated with Kanavel's four signs: a flexed position of the finger, symmetric enlargement of the entire finger (sausage digit), marked tenderness to palpation but only directly over the tendon sheath, and severe pain upon passive extension of the digit.

Unlike cellulitis, which typically responds rapidly to appropriate antibiotic therapy, abscesses do not resolve until the collection of pus (bacteria, white cells, fluid, and debris) is drained. The location and size of the abscess dictate the surgical approach. Small abscesses, such as felons and paronychial abscesses, may be drained in the emergency department under digital block if appropriate equipment is available. Larger and more proximal abscesses should be drained in the operating room under regional or general anesthesia. Small stab incisions may allow the abscess to decompress, but are no substitute for widely incising and thoroughly irrigating the abscess. There is no role for a conservative approach in managing abscesses; such an approach will only prolong the patient's infection and in the long run result in greater morbidity. All abscesses must be completely opened, thoroughly irrigated, and the wound left open for subsequent dressing changes.

ANESTHESIA IN THE EMERGENCY DEPARTMENT
Local and Regional Anesthesia in the Emergency Room

The administration of local anesthetic is used in the emergency department for stress testing, reduction of displaced fractures and dislocated joints, and repair of lacerations.

Anesthetic Agents

Lidocaine is currently the most commonly used local anesthetic in most emergency centers. Plain 1% or 2% lidocaine is preferred as cases of vasospasm, with loss of digit attributed to the use of epinephrine with local anesthetic, have been reported. The discomfort of infiltration may be lessened by decreasing the acidity of the lidocaine (bicarbonate added), using a small gauge needle (25-30 gauge), and slow administration of the agent to lessen the discomfort of tissue distention. The acidity of lidocaine is reduced by adding 1 ml of sodium bicarbonate (1 mEq/ml) to each 10 ml of local anesthetic, to give a final concentration of 0.1 mEq/ml.

Anesthetic Administration

If anesthesia is necessary, the decision to administer a local or regional anesthetic should be based on the location and severity of the injury.

Local administration

Local administration is most useful for the management or exploration of lacerations in the forearm and small lacerations of the dorsal hand and palm.

Hematoma block

Local administration of anesthetic agent directly into a fracture site before reduction is referred to as a hematoma block. A larger-gauge needle is used in this type of infiltration. The needle is inserted directly into the fracture site while gently aspirating. When blood return from the fracture hematoma is noted, the anesthetic is injected. This form of anesthesia is most useful for fractures of the metacarpals and the distal radius.

Digital block

Digital block is useful in the management of lacerations, nailbed injuries, fractures, and dislocations of the fingers. A true ring block, with infiltration of anesthetic agent distal to the MCP joint, may result in obstruction of blood flow by elevation of local tissue pressure. Insertion of the needle at the interdigital web space, with infiltration in the region of the digital nerve 0.5 cm proximally, averts this problem (Fig. 2-25). Branches of the radial or ulnar nerve may be blocked by raising a thin weal in the skin dorsally over the MCP. A total of 3 to 5 ccs of 1% lidocaine is usually sufficient to block a single digit. Alternately, Chiu's intrathecal technique, in which a 25-gauge needle is inserted directly into the flexor sheath in the midline of the digit at the level of the A1 pulley (using sterile technique), may be used. The needle typically enters the tendon substance and is then gently withdrawn. Simultaneously, gentle pressure is applied on the syringe. As the potential space between the tendon and the sheath is reached, the anesthetic rapidly infuses. Digital pressure is held at the base of the A1 pulley during and for 30 seconds after the infusion. The anesthetic exits the sheath proximally to provide a block of the common and proper digital nerves and also dissects dorsally from the sheath to block the dorsal sensory branches as well. This technique uses 3 cc of plain 1 or 2% lidocaine, allows digital block with a single needle stick, and involves almost no risk of direct nerve injury. This technique provides reliable anesthesia for the entire digit distal to the level of the MCP. In cases where

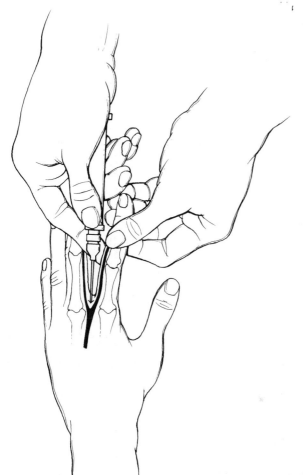

Figure 2-25   Digital block of the finger is performed by insertion of the needle into the interdigital web space and infiltration 5 mm proximally along the palmar surface. This is performed on both sides of the digit. A dorsal weal at the level of the MP joint is performed to block dorsal or ulnar branches.

postprocedure monitoring of sensation will not be necessary, a long-acting local anesthetic, such as bupivicaine, may be mixed with the lidocaine to give prolonged relief. This may be particularly appropriate for cases in which a digital tourniquet is applied, because the vasodilatory response following release of the tourniquet may rapidly reverse the digital block and result in a rapid return of painful sensation to the digit.

Median nerve block

The median nerve may be blocked at the wrist if a larger area of anesthesia is required. At this level, the median nerve lies just radial and dorsal to the palmaris longus deep to the antebrachial fascia (Fig. 2-26). A 1½-inch small (25-27) gauge needle is inserted approximately 1 cm proximal to the distal wrist crease between the palmaris longus and the flexor carpi radialis. (If the palmaris longus is absent, the needle is directed just ulnar to the flexor carpi radialis.) When blocking large nerves, it has sometimes been recommended that the needle be inserted until paresthesias are elicited prior to infiltration of lidocaine. We feel that this is a dangerous practice, because injection of local anesthetic agent directly into the nerve may result in permanent nerve damage. Therefore, we recommend instructing the patient before performing a block of one of the larger nerves of the need to inform the operator of any sensations of paresthesia or "electric shock" feelings radiating into the distribution of the nerve. If this response is produced, the needle should be withdrawn and redirected prior to infiltration. Typically 5 cc of lidocaine are infiltrated in the vicinity of the nerve. Because of the larger diameter of the nerve, it will take 10 minutes or longer for the anesthetic to take full effect.

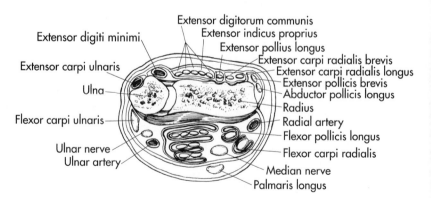

Figure 2-26   Location of the median and ulnar nerves in the distal forearm.

Ulnar nerve block

The ulnar nerve may also be blocked at the wrist. At this level, the nerve is located between the flexor carpi ulnaris and the ulnar artery (Fig. 2-26). Infiltration is performed by inserting the needle beneath the radial edge of the flexor carpi ulnaris. A small-gauge needle should be used and gentle aspiration performed prior to infiltration. If the ulnar artery is inadvertently punctured, the needle should be withdrawn and direct pressure applied for 5 to 10 minutes. The dorsal sensory branch of the ulnar nerve may be blocked by raising a weal dorsally over the ulnar half of the wrist.

Radial nerve block

The dorsal sensory branches of the radial nerve may also be blocked by raising a subcutaneous weal over the dorsum of the wrist just distal to the radial styloid, extending from just lateral to the radial artery to the midpoint of the dorsum of the wrist.

Anesthesia in the Operating Room

Exam under Anesthesia in the Operating Room

Using a local or regional anesthetic, it is often possible to perform an adequate examination of most potentially nonoperative conditions in the emergency department. However, in uncooperative patients, pediatric patients, or in patients with multiple injuries, examination in the operating room may be more informative and less stressful for both physician and patient.

Procedures under Anesthesia in the Operating Room

In some instances, the patient may be taken to the operating room because it is not technically possible to perform a planned procedure in the emergency department because of inadequate supplies, facility, or personnel. In these instances, it may be appropriate to perform the procedure using one or more of the techniques of administration already discussed. However, in some instances, anesthesia in the operating room is indicated. These include procedures requiring anesthesia of the entire upper extremity, either because of the extent of the injury or because a tourniquet will be required to create a bloodless field for a period beyond 10 to 15 minutes. In such cases, either a Bier block with administration of anesthetic into the venous system distal to an inflated tourniquet, an axillary block with administration of a regional blockade at the level of the axillary artery, or a brachial plexus block performed at a more proximal level may be administered by qualified personnel. The choice of block depends on the nature of the injury and the time requirements for the planned procedures. Although it is technically possible for the surgeon to administer these blocks, administration by an anesthesiologist allows the surgeon to focus entirely on the surgical procedure, while the anesthesiologist assumes responsibility for the block, sedation, and patient monitoring.

CARE AFTER INITIAL EVALUATION
General Care

The care of specific injuries is discussed in later chapters. If care is to be delayed, then apply a dressing that provides comfort and stability. It is *never* permissible to leave a compression-type dressing on an unattended patient. A standard dressing consists of a nonadherent layer (especially if there are multiple lacerations or abrasions and the dressing is to be left in place for longer than a few hours), a bulky layer consisting of gauze fluffs or wraps, plaster supporting the injured part(s), and finally an outer layer consisting of further gauze wrap, Coban®, and/or ACE® wrap. If prolonged immobilization is likely, then the MCPs should be splinted in flexion and the PIPs and DIPs in extension to minimize stiffness. In this position, the collateral ligaments of these joints are maximally stretched, thereby preventing shortening of the ligaments during the period of immobilization. Again, it is crucial that the dressing has adequate bulk and the outer wrapping be applied loosely. In significant injuries, the hand will likely swell significantly during the following 24 to 48 hours, converting a snug dressing into a tourniquet. Unless severely injured, the fingertips should be exposed so that circulation and sensation may be easily monitored. The frequency and the setting for such evaluation depends on the type and severity of injury and ranges from care in the outpatient setting to hourly monitoring by skilled nurses and physicians in the hospital. Almost irrespective of the injury, elevation for the ensuing 48 hours is beneficial in limiting swelling, bleeding, and bruising.

Amputated Parts

The care of amputated parts deserves special mention. With proper care and cooling, some amputated digits may be replanted up to 24 hours after the initial injury; unfortunately, some parts may be unintentionally destroyed within a matter of minutes when cooling is employed improperly. Because amputated parts lack circulation, they are more susceptible to rapid cooling and the formation of ice crystals in the tissues (frostbite) than nonamputated parts. Therefore, amputated parts should never be placed directly on ice. Following inspection, the amputated part should be wrapped in a saline-soaked (normal saline or ringer's lactate) sterile gauze. This is then placed in a plastic bag, which is placed in an ice slurry. If there is a prolonged delay, the part should be reinspected periodically to make sure that it is being kept cool but not freezing. If the part and patient are to be transported to another facility, it is essential to control the patient's bleeding prior to transport. This can usually be accomplished with a snug dressing and elevation. It is possible for a patient to exsanguinate from an amputation—bleeding must be controlled prior to transport!

OPERATING ROOM

The determination of whether or when to take a patient to the operating room depends on a multitude of variables, and the development of an elaborate criterion is beyond the scope of this chapter. However, several simple principles may be of assistance. Immediate operative evaluation/therapy is always indicated in possible compartment syndromes, vascular injuries resulting in possible loss of perfusion, acute nerve compression syndromes secondary to trauma, and grossly contaminated open wounds (especially those with associated fractures and open joints). Additionally, immediate operative intervention is often indicated for multiple tendon lacerations, nerve lacerations, or multiple fractures. It may be possible to perform an adequate irrigation of an open fracture of a digit in the emergency department when the bone is well exposed, tissue damage is minor, and contamination is minimal, but in the absence of proper equipment or in a patient who is unwilling or unable to comply with this procedure in the emergency department, immediate irrigation and debridement in the operating room are indicated. More proximal open fractures require irrigation and debridement in the operating room. In infants, preschool children, and obtunded or neurologically compromised adult patients, it is often necessary to evaluate potential nerve lacerations in the operating room as it is frequently not possible to perform an adequate sensory exam in these patients. All complete flexor tendon lacerations should probably be repaired in the operating room unless the emergency department has highly specialized equipment. Given their more superficial location, it may be possible to perform uncomplicated extensor tendon repairs in the emergency department. With regard to isolated digital nerve or flexor tendon injuries, it is likely that the results of primary (immediate) versus delayed primary (within a week) repairs are equivalent. Therefore, if there are factors which make an immediate trip to the operating room suboptimal (intoxication, associated injuries, medical problems, etc.), it may be prudent to copiously irrigate the wound, perform a primary closure of the skin, and then return within seven days to perform a repair of the lacerated tendon or nerve in the operating room.

Although a trip to the operating room may seem to significantly increase the time and cost of caring for the patient's injuries, the cost of inadequate initial care of hand injuries can be enormous. Thus, it is essential for the surgeon to recognize situations in which management in the operating room is likely to improve the patient's outcome and to employ this option whenever such situations arise.

SELECTED REFERENCES

Agur AM: *Atlas of anatomy,* ed 9, Baltimore, 1991, Williams & Wilkins.

Allen C: Arachnid envenomations, *Emer Med Clin North Am* 10(2): 269-298, 1992.

April EW: *Anatomy,* Media, PA, 1984, Harwal.

Bentivegna PE, Deane LM: Chemical burns of the upper extremity, *Hand Clin* 6(2): 253-259, 1990.

Bergman RA, Afifi AK, Jew JY, et al.: *Atlas of human anatomy in cross section,* Baltimore, 1991, Urban & Schwarzenberg.

Clemente CD: *Gray's anatomy,* ed 13, Philadelphia, 1985, Lea & Febiger.

Frederick HA, Carter PR, Littler JW: Injection injuries to the median and ulnar nerves at the wrist, *J Hand Surg* 17A: 645-647, 1992.

Fremling MA, Mackinnon SE: Injection injury to the median nerve, *Ann Plast Surg* 37(5): 561-566, 1996.

Gold BS, Barish RA: Venomous snakebites: current concepts in diagnosis, treatment, and management, *Emerg Clin North Am* 10(2): 249-267, 1992.

Gold BS, Wingert WA: Snake venom poisoning in the United States: a review of therapeutic practice, *South Med J* 87(6): 579-589, 1994.

Green DP, editor: *Operative hand surgery,* ed 3, New York, 1993, Churchill Livingstone.

Idler RS, Manktelow RT, Lucas G, et al.: *The hand,* ed 3, New York, 1990, Churchill Livingstone.

Kirkpatrick JJ, Enion DS, Burd DA: Hydrofluoric acid burns: a review, *Burns* 21(7): 483-493, 1995.

Mackinnon SE, Dellon AL: *Surgery of the peripheral nerve,* New York, 1988, Thieme.

May JW, Littler JW, editors: *Plastic surgery,* vol 7-8, Philadelphia, 1990, WB Saunders.

McKay W, Morris R, Mushlin P: Sodium bicorbonate attenuates pain on skin infiltration with lidocaine, with or without epinephrine, *Anesth Analg* 66: 572-574, 1987.

Meals RA, Seeger LL: *An Atlas of forearm and hand cross-sectional anatomy,* New York, 1991, Churchill Livingstone.

Moore KL: *Clinically oriented anatomy,* ed 2, Baltimore, 1985, Williams & Wilkins.

Simon RR, Brenner BE: *Emergency procedure and techniques,* 2nd ed., Baltimore, 1987, Williams & Wilkins.

Snyder CC: Animal bite wounds, *Hand Clin* 5(4): 571-590, 1989

Sutherland SK: Antivenom use in Australia: premedication, adverse reactions and the use of venom detection kits, *Med J Aust* 157: 734-739, 1992.

Young VL, Pin P: The Brown Recluse Spider bite, *Ann Plast Surg* 20(5): 447-452, 1988.

3

Imaging Evaluation of the Hand and Wrist

Viktor M. Metz, MD
S. M. Metz-Schimmerl, MD
Louis A. Gilula, MD

Injuries to the wrist and hand often result in subtle clinical and radiological findings that necessitate a careful evaluation of the bones, cartilages, ligaments and joint capsule for an appropriate diagnosis to be reached. Different imaging techniques have been established for better evaluation of what is normal or abnormal on the distal forearm, wrist and hand. Available tools for the radiologist include standard radiographs in different routine and detailed views, bone scan, arthrography, computed tomography (CT), and magnetic resonance imaging (MRI). The standard radiograph remains the most valuable and readily available imaging technique. It should be used as an initial approach to wrist and hand trauma. However advanced imaging techniques can add significant information about bone, cartilage, and soft tissues disorders that affect the hand and wrist and may influence treatment. This chapter defines and illustrates the advantages and disadvantages of the most common imaging techniques.

RADIOGRAPHY
Routine Roentgenographic Survey

For a routine roentgenographic survey of the wrist and hand, a minimal of four views centered for the wrist and three views for the hand, are recommended. These views should include posteroanterior (PA), lateral, and oblique projections. For the wrist, a fourth view—the PA view with ulnar deviation—is recommended. For examinations of the wrist, the central beam should be over the capitate head; for examinations of the hand, it should be over the midportion of the third metacarpal.

For the PA view of the hand or wrist, the hand is placed flat on the cassette to profile the carpometacarpal joints in the neutral position. The axis of the third metacarpal should be colinear with the axis of the radius (Fig. 3-1). The neutral position (without any ulnar or radial deviation) is of major importance because under normal conditions, the scaphoid foreshortens and assumes the configuration of a signet ring, (Fig. 3-2) with radial deviation or palmar flexion, and elongates with ulnar deviation or dorsal flexion. A signet ring sign, however, seen on a true neutral PA view suggests a pathologic condition seen in patients with rotatory subluxation of the scaphoid (RSS). Therefore a PA radiogram, performed in radial deviation which foreshortens the scaphoid, may lead to a misdiagnosis. In addition, for the PA view of the wrist, the humerus should be abducted 90 degrees from the chest wall so that the elbow is at the same level as the shoulder and flexed 90 degrees.

For the oblique (semipronation) view (Fig. 3-3), the hand is rotated 45 degrees off the cassette and the fingers held straight (positioned on a step sponge) to obtain the interphalangeal and metacarpophalangeal joints in true profile. In this view, the trapeziotrapezoid and the trapezioscaphoid joints are profiled and parallel, providing an additional view of the head of the capitate.

The lateral view (Fig. 3-4) is performed by further rotation of the hand into a radioulnar projection. For this projection the humerus is adducted against the chest wall with the elbow flexed 90 degrees. For evaluation of the hand, the fingers must be spread to avoid overlapping. For examination of the wrist, it is important to keep the wrist and fingers straight (without any flexion or extension) for optimal evaluation of carpal alignment. Recognition of an acceptable lateral wrist position can be made when the ventral cortex of the pisiform is midway

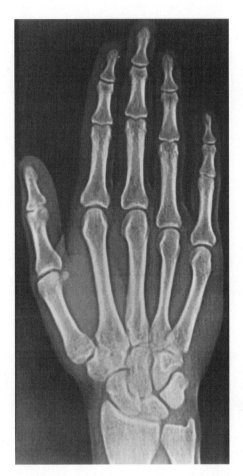

Figure 3-1   Posteroanterior radiographic view of the hand. The hand (not the wrist) is placed flat on the cassette in the neutral position, with the axis of the third metacarpal colinear with the axis of the radius.

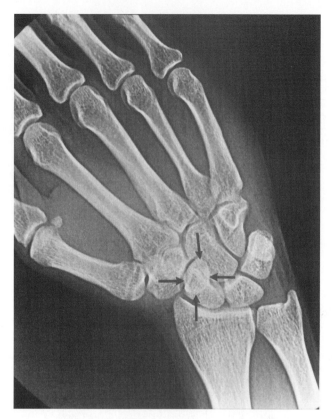

Figure 3-2 Posteroanterior radiograph of the hand in radial deviation. The scaphoid foreshortens in radial deviation under normal conditions and takes the configuration of a signet ring. The entire bone looks like a ring with a stone (arrows) in the center of the ring.

between the ventral surfaces of the distal pole of the scaphoid and the head of the capitate, which is the SPC (scapho-piso-capitate) relationship.

Special Views

Other views may be necessary to investigate specific problems in various sites of the wrist and hand. Because the distal articular surface of the radius is angled ventrally, the radiocarpal joint is not in profile in a routine PA view (Fig. 3-1). To better profile the radiocarpal joint (Fig. 3-5), the central beam must be angled 10 to 20 degrees toward the elbow, or the wrist must be draped over an angle sponge with the central beam directed vertically through the joint.

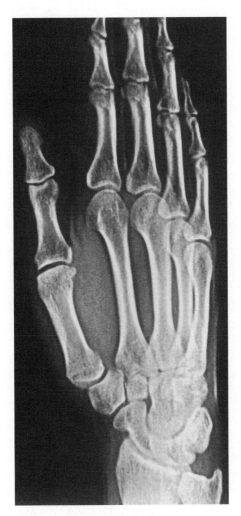

Figure 3-3   Oblique view of the hand. The hand is rotated 45 degrees off the cassette with the fingers held straight, providing oblique views of all bones. This view also provides depiction of the trapeziotrapezoidal, the scaphotrapezio-trapezoidal, the metacarpophalangeal, and interphalangeal joints in true profile.

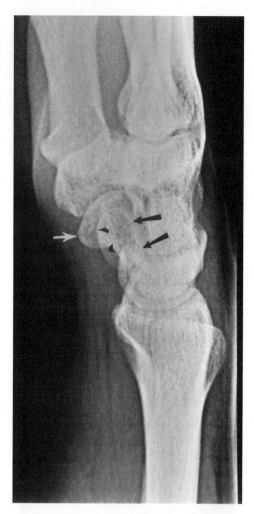

Figure 3-4   For the lateral view, the wrist is rotated further into a radioulnar projection. For evaluation of carpal alignment, it is important to keep the wrist and fingers straight without any flexion or extension. A good lateral of the carpus is recognized when the ventral surface of the pisiform (arrowheads) lies between the distal pole of the scaphoid (white arrow) and the ventral cortex of the capitate head (black arrows).

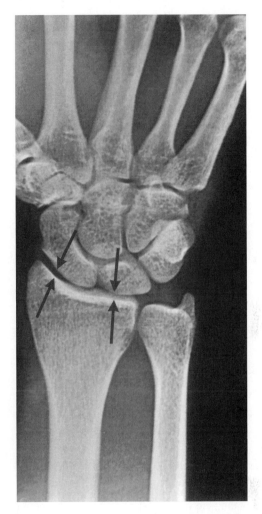

Figure 3-5   The radiocarpal joint is clearly recognized by looking at parallel articulating cortices (arrows). For a better profile of the radiocarpal joint specifically, the central beam can be angled 10 to 20 degrees towards the elbow.

To better profile the carpal scaphoid (Fig. 3-6), the wrist is initially placed in the routine PA view and then ulnarly deviated as far as possible. The central beam is angled 20 degrees toward the elbow. The film in this position demonstrates the scaphoid, free of the distortion caused by its normal volar tilt when the wrist is in the neutral position.

Radiographic evaluation of the carpal tunnel (Fig. 3-7) is commonly performed by placing the forearm flat on the cassette and maximally

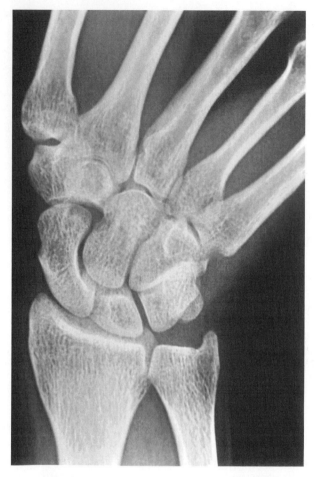

Figure 3-6 Posteroanterior view in ulnar deviation allows better profile of the scaphoid by elongating the scaphoid than exists with the normal volar tilt of the scaphoid when the wrist is placed in neutral position. The scaphoid waist can be elongated more by adding angulation of the tube 20 degrees toward the elbow.

dorsiflexing the hand by means of the patient's opposite hand or a strap. The central beam is directed toward the cup of the palm at about a 15 degree angle. This view can also be obtained by placing the fingers on the cassette and moving the forearm forward to extend the wrist. The degree of the central beam angulation depends on the amount of wrist hyperextension. The carpal tunnel view demonstrates an axial view of the hook of hamate, the pisiform and the volar margin of the

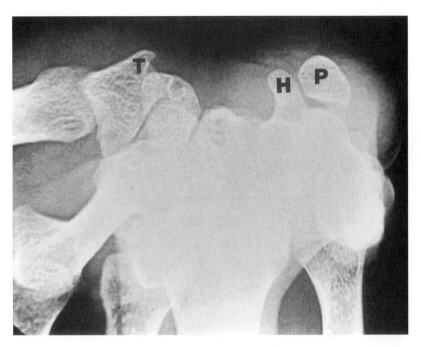

Figure 3-7   Radiograph of the carpal tunnel demonstrates an axial view of the hook of hamate (H), the ventral tubercule of the trapezium (T), and the pisiform bone (P).

trapezium. Optimal depiction of the pisiform bone and a profile of the pisiotriquetral joint can also be achieved in an AP semisupinated oblique position, in which the wrist is supinated 30 degrees from the lateral position.

The second through fifth digits normally are well depicted on the routine PA and oblique views (Figs. 3-1, 3-2). Anteriorposterior (AP) views profile slightly different portions of the carpometacarpal, the metacarpophalangeal, and the interphalangeal joints, and may be of additional value for depiction of occult fractures or erosions. For the lateral projection of an individual digit, which should always be obtained when evaluating a digit, it may be necessary to overpronate the hand, place the index or long finger against the cassette, and keep the other digits out of the field to prevent superimposition (Fig. 3-8). For true frontal and lateral projections of the thumb, which is depicted in an oblique view on routine PA radiographs, it may be necessary to overpronate the forearm and hand to position the dorsum of the

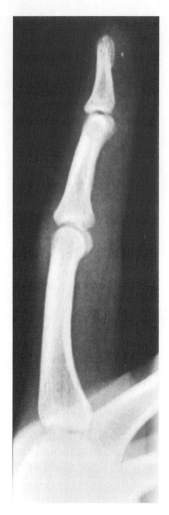

Figure 3-8   Lateral radiograph of the second digit. The hand is overpronated, and the radial side of the second digit is placed against the cassette.

thumb in contact with the cassette surface (Fig. 3-9). The true lateral projection of the thumb can be obtained by overpronating the hand and placing the radial surface of the thumb on the cassette.

Fluoroscopic spot films should be performed when detailed carpal views fail to demonstrate an abnormality in a clinically suspicious area. Instability series under spot filming or videotaping should be performed if there is any clinical or plain film suspicion of carpal ligament

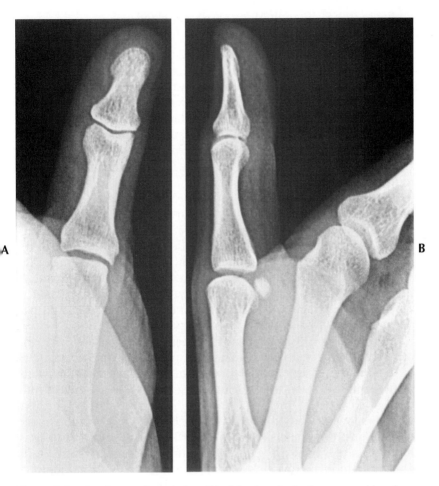

Figure 3-9   For the true frontal view **(A)** of the thumb, the forearm and hand are overpronated and the dorsum of the thumb is placed on the cassette. The true lateral radiograph **(B)** of the thumb is obtained by overpronating the hand and placing the radial side of the thumb on the cassette.

disorders. Such a full instability series includes bilateral PA views in neutral, radial and ulnar deviation, a semipronated oblique view, lateral views in neutral, full flexion and extension and radial and ulnar deviation, CLIP wrist maneuvers, 30 degrees off lateral view to profile the pisotriquetral joint, and AP clenched fist views with the wrist in neutral, ulnar, and radial deviation. Views are obtained of both wrists. A tailored wrist instability series has been described by Truong, Mann, and Gilula.

Radiographic Evaluation of the Wrist and Hand

Soft Tissue Evaluation

Soft tissue evaluation is often underestimated, but its recognition may be the key for correct diagnosis in trauma of the wrist and hand. Good film quality is required to demonstrate the soft tissues clearly, without diminishing the bony details. Proper exposure allows evaluation of the skin, subcutaneous fat, and the soft tissues of the tendons, capsules, and muscles, while still penetrating the bony structures sufficiently. Several superficial and deep fat planes on the PA and lateral radiogram have been described that are useful in evaluation of trauma radiographs of the wrist and hand.

The pronator quadratus fat pad (Fig. 3-10) is located between the pronator quadratus muscle and the volar flexor tendon sheaths. It is constantly visible as a straight or concave lucency on the lateral radiograph. Displacement of this fat pad is associated with fractures of the distal radius or ulna and with radiocarpal dislocation. Swelling of the pronator quadratus fat pad in the absence of an obvious fracture of the distal radius or ulna is an indirect sign for a fracture. Especially in a Salter I or II fracture of the distal radius, alteration of the fat pad may be the only radiographic abnormality.

The dorsal skin-subcutaneous fat zones of the forearm, wrist, and hand are superficial fat planes that form three compartments at regions of the forearm, wrist, and hand, and can be evaluated on the lateral plane (Fig. 3-10). Dorsal forearm swelling occurs in two thirds of fractures of all forearm fractures. When both dorsal forearm and dorsal wrist swelling can be visualized, it may be the result of (a) a radial fracture involving the distal articular surface of the radius, (b) a fracture of a carpal bone associated with a distal forearm fracture, or (c) a dislocation of the distal radioulnar joint, the radiocarpal joint, or intercarpal joints. Dorsal wrist swelling often occurs in fractures or dislocations of the carpal bones, but may also be observed in patients without fractures. However, if significant dorsal wrist swelling is present, a fracture should be searched for diligently. Dorsal hand swelling is strongly associated with fractures of the metacarpals II to V. Combinations of dorsal wrist and hand swelling after trauma occur in cases of (a) carpometacarpal dislocation, (b) proximal intraarticular fracture of one or more metacarpals II to V, or (c) combinations of metacarpal and carpal fractures.

The scaphoid fat pad, seen on the PA view (Fig. 3-11), lies between the radial collateral ligament and the tendon of the abductor pollicis longus muscle and courses from the radial styloid to the trapezium. Because fractures of the scaphoid may be extremely subtle, attention should always be directed to the scaphoid fat pad. An ulnar deviated

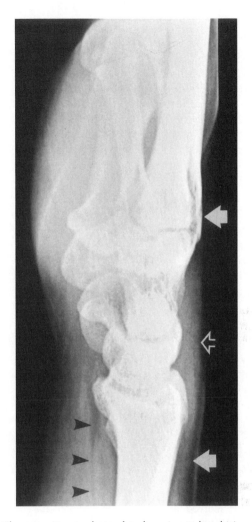

Figure 3-10   The pronator quadratus fat plane (arrowheads) is superficial to the pronator quadratus muscle. The dorsal skin-subcutaneous fat zones (arrows) are well defined on the lateral radiograph dorsal to the metacarpals, the wrist, and dorsal forearm. The normal fat stripe over the wrist (open arrow) is concave to horizontal over the carpal bones.

PA view may be an additional projection for observing the swelling of the scaphoid fat pad, because this position accentuates the fat pad and allows its contour to be visualized in its entire extension. Swelling, displacement, or obliteration of this fat pad occurs in one third of all carpal fractures and is usually associated with scaphoid fractures.

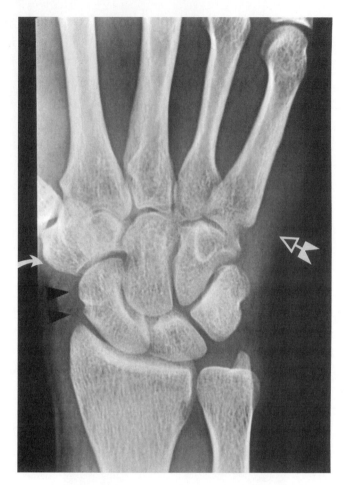

Figure 3-11   On a posteroanterior radiograph, the scaphoid fat pad (arrowheads), the thenar (curved arrow), and the hypothenar (open arrow) skin-subcutaneous fat planes are commonly seen. When they are displaced or obscured, they may be used as landmarks for evaluation of occult fractures underlying the abnormal fat plane.

However, the scaphoid fat pad may also be altered in cases of fractures of the radial styloid, other radial fractures with an intraarticular component, and in fractures of the trapezium.

Swelling of the thenar skin-subcutaneous fat plane (Fig. 3-11) are associated with fractures of the first metacarpal, sometimes with fractures of the proximal first phalanx, and rarely with fractures of the trapezium.

Hypothenar swelling may occur in cases with fractures of metacarpals II to V and in patients with hamate fractures (Fig. 3-11).

Metacarpophalangeal joint swelling may be indicative of a fracture at that region. Injuries at the metacarpophalangeal joints lead to a focal swelling over the joint and involve only the more distal parts of the dorsal hand soft tissues. Swelling at the interphalangeal joints may also be an indicator for a fracture. The swelling at that region tends to be more tubular and unilateral swelling around an interphalangeal joint may be an indirect sign of rupture of the collateral ligament.

Soft Tissue-Evaluation of the Hand

Alignment deformities, which may result from ruptured tendons or ligaments, can be detected or suspected on routine radiograms.

The "mallet finger" deformity is suspected when a distal phalanx is maintained in palmar flexion as a result of rupture of an extensor tendon to the distal phalanx. This abnormality may be diagnosed only on the lateral view, because the distal phalanx of a mallet finger can be extended passively on a PA view (Fig. 3-12).

Another deformity that results from rupture of a extensor tendon is the "button hole" deformity. In this condition, the extensor tendon is ruptured from its attachment to the dorsal base of the middle phalanx or there is a rupture of the central slip that keeps the tendon over the dorsal midline of the proximal interphalangeal joint. In this deformity, the finger is flexed at the proximal interphalangeal joint and extended at the distal interphalangeal joint (Fig. 3-13).

Rupture of the *flexor tendons* may be without roentgenographic signs or may cause slight dorsal subluxation at the distal or proximal interphalangeal joints. A ventral bone fragment may be avulsed from the base of the distal phalanx and may remain in anatomic position or may be retracted and displaced ventral to the diaphysis or even the base of the middle phalanx.

If eccentric swelling at one side of an interphalangeal joint can be detected in a patient, it is suggestive of a collateral ligament injury. Disruption of the ulnar collateral ligament of the first metacarpophalangeal joint, which is often accompanied by a fracture of the base of the proximal phalanx, is known as the Gamekeeper's thumb (Fig. 3-14). Routine dorsovolar PA and oblique views commonly are sufficient to demonstrate a possible associated fracture. However abduction stress views of the thumb may need to be performed in some patients for evaluation of the collateral ligament. An increase to more than 30 degrees in the angle between the first metacarpal and the proximal phalanx is characteristic of abnormality of this ligament. Comparison views with the opposite side can be very helpful in detecting normal variations. It is very important not to perform such stress

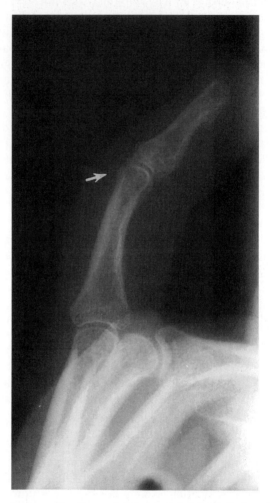

Figure 3-12   In the mallet finger, deformity of the distal phalanx is maintained in palmar flexion because of the rupture of the extensor tendon to the distal phalanx. This condition may be overlooked on the PA view and may be diagnosed only on the lateral view. Swelling is present dorsal to the middle phalanx and DIP joint. A small avulsion fracture (arrow) from the base of the distal phalanx indicates extensor tendon injury.

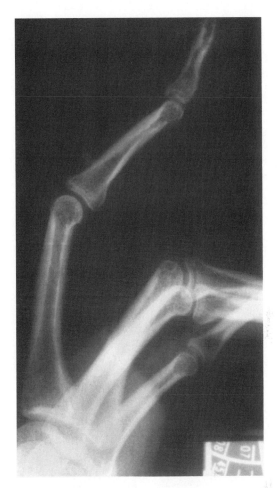

Figure 3-13   Lateral radiograph shows a "button hole" or boutonnière deformity of the long finger. In this condition, the finger is flexed at the proximal interphalangeal joint and extended at the distal interphalangeal joint.

views when an avulsion fracture is present at the joint to be stressed, because stress can flip the bone fragment into the joint or trap the fragment under soft tissue, thereby changing a nonsurgical to a surgical treatment.

Analysis of the Osseous Structures

After careful examination of the soft tissues, the osseous elements should be evaluated for evidence of fractures, joint space width, parallelism of the joint spaces, alignment, and any other abnormality. Understanding what is normal and using some basic principles will lead to a correct diagnosis.

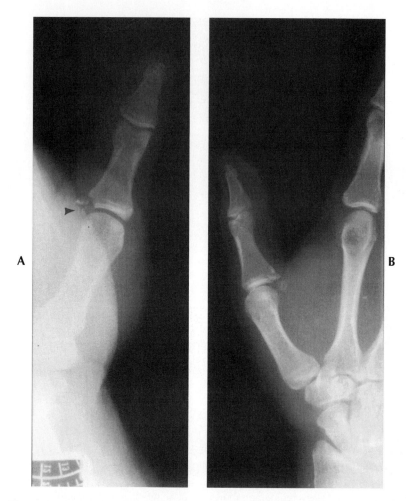

Figure 3-14   Gamekeepers thumb. Comminuted intraarticular fracture involves the ulnar aspect of the base of the proximal phalanx on frontal **(A)** and obliqued lateral **(B)** views. A smaller second fracture fragment is located proximal (arrow).

Under normal conditions, the radiocarpal, intercarpal, and carpometacarpal joint space widths are 2 mm or less and may decrease from proximal to distal. However, accurate measurement of a joint space width is only possible if the joint space in question is in true profile and measurement is performed at the joint's midportion between parallel articulating cortices. If a joint space is not in profile on standard or detailed radiographs and there is any clinical or radiological suspicion of an abnormality, fluoroscopic controlled views should be performed. Sometimes, in healthy individuals, joint space width may be slightly

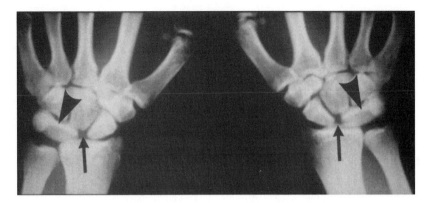

Figure 3-15   Posteroanterior view of both wrists shows bilateral lunotriquetral osseous coalitions (arrowheads) with bilateral widened scapholunate joint spaces (arrows) that can be normal variants.

wider than 2 mm, but they should be of symmetric width. A comparison with the contralateral side should be performed in any unclear case to exclude normal variants. When a joint space is 4 mm wide or more, it is considered abnormal and indicates ligamentous defects. A narrow lunotriquetral or even an "abnormal" wide scapholunate joint space can be a normal variant in patients with carpal lunotriquetral coalition (Fig. 3-15).

As in any other area of the body, the concept of parallelism of articulating joint surfaces helps to differentiate normal from abnormal bone alignment. This concept, however, can only be used when the joint in question is in true profile. On the correctly performed routine PA view (Fig. 3-1), parallelism exists between the radius, scaphoid, and lunate bones; between the bones of the proximal and distal carpal rows; at the intercarpal joints of the proximal and distal carpal rows; between the distal carpal bones and the metacarpals; and between the metacarpophalangeal and interphalangeal joints. Occasionally, joints may be parallel but not of symmetric width with respect to other joints of the wrist and hand. This condition can occur when there is articular fluid spreading articular surfaces, when there is a tear of the capsule, or even when there is a subluxation or dislocation and the bone ends still project parallel on the PA view.

Under normal conditions, the articular surfaces between the bones mentioned above on a true PA view do not overlap. Overlapping of articular surfaces between those bones indicates subluxation or dislocation. Between the trapezium, the trapezoid and the base of the first metacarpal parallelism on the PA view is not recognizable because the articulating surfaces of those bones are not profiled in this view.

Three normal smooth carpal arcs have been described that can be observed in the PA or AP view (Fig. 3-16*A*). Break (stepoff) of any of these arcs may indicate ligamentous/bony abnormality at the site of the broken arc (Fig. 3-16*B*). Arc I joins the main convex curvatures of the proximal surfaces of the proximal carpal row. Arc II can be drawn joining the concave distal curvatures of the proximal carpal row. Arc III outlines the proximal major convexities of the capitate and hamate. However, with radial and ulnar deviation, a small stepoff may be seen at the site of the lunotriquetral joint, with the triquetrum moving distally and proximally with respect to the lunate which is considered a normal variant. Similar, but less pronounced, displacement may occur at the scapholunate joint between radial and ulnar deviation. Another congenital variation is that sometimes the triquetrum is smaller than the lunate in its proximal–distal dimension. In this condition, a stepoff of Arc I may be seen at the lunotriquetral joint; however Arc II is still smooth.

Normal Angles and Measurements

Understanding normal carpal anatomy on the lateral wrist radiograph is essential to correctly interpret carpal alignment. The key structures for correct identification of normal or abnormal carpal alignment are the capitate, lunate, scaphoid, and radius (Fig. 3-17). The capitate, which is rigidly fixed in the base of the third metacarpal bone, is centered with its rounded head to the distal concavity of the lunate. The lunate rests in the concavity of the distal radius. The axes of these three bones average within 10 degrees of coaxial in most cases and are coaxial in only 11% of cases. The axis of the capitate (Fig. 3-17) can be defined by drawing a line from the midportion of the capitate head to the superimposed midportion of the bases of the metacarpals II to V. The lunate axis (Fig. 3-17) can be drawn by joining the distal volar and dorsal portions (poles) of the lunate with one line and drawing a second line perpendicular to the first line. The axis of the scaphoid (Fig. 3-17) can be determined by drawing a straight line touching or tangent to the distal and proximal ventral poles of the scaphoid. Finally, the radius axis is defined by a line that runs through the middle of the diaphysis of the radius. For evaluation of possible carpal malalignment (ligament instability), two angles should be measured: the scapholunate and the capitolunate angles. Under normal conditions, the scapholunate angle (Fig. 3-17) is between 30 and 60 degrees; it is questionably abnormal between 60 and 80 degrees, and it is definitely abnormal at more than 80 degrees or less than 30 degrees. However these measurements are only reliable if the wrist is examined in a true lateral and neutral position, without any flexion or extension

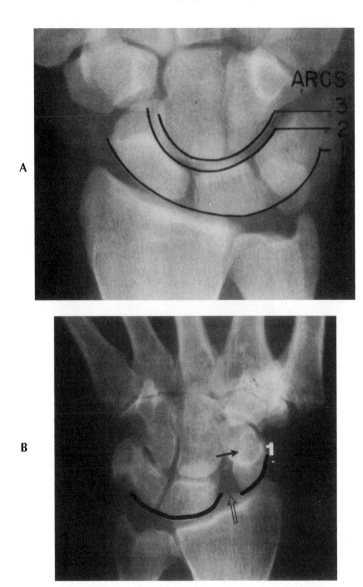

Figure 3-16   Neutral posteroanterior view of the wrist. **(A)** Three normal carpal arcs can be found: Arc 1 joins the outer proximal convexities of the scaphoid, lunate, and triquetral bone; Arc 2 joins the distal concavities of these same three carpal bones; Arc 3 joins the proximal convexities of the capitate and hamate bones. **(B)** Neutral posteroanterior view of the wrist demonstrates a broken Arc 1 because of rupture of the scapholunate ligament indicated by a scapholunate diastasis (open arrow). The scaphoid is somewhat foreshortened (rotated) and takes the configuration of a signet ring (arrow). (Reprinted with permission from Gilula LA: Carpal injuries: analytic approach and case exercises. *AJR* 133:503-517, 1979.)

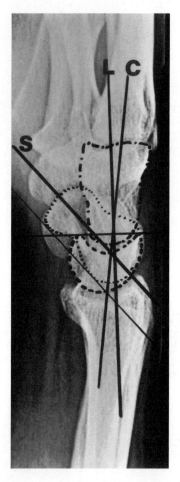

Figure 3-17   Method for determination of the carpal axes on the lateral radiograph (see text). S = scaphoid axis; C = capitate axis; L = lunate axis; dots outline the scaphoid; dashes outline the lunate; dots and dashes outline the capitate.

and ulnar or radial deviation. The capitolunate angle (Fig. 3-17) is normal at less than 30 degrees and abnormal when more than 30 degrees.

On the PA and lateral radiographs, four radiographic measurements are of importance for treatment and radiological follow-up after distal radius fractures. Radial angulation (or inclination) is the angle created between a line drawn along the distal radial articular surface on the PA view and a line drawn perpendicular to the long axis of the radius. This angle should be between 16 and 28 degrees (mean:20 degrees)

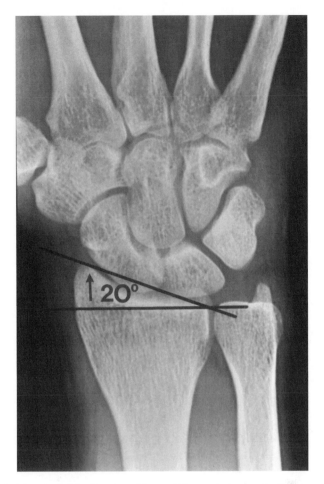

Figure 3-18   Radial inclination. The radial angulation or inclination is determined by drawing one line joining the distal articular surface of the radius and another line perpendicular to the long axis of the radius. The mean angle is 20 degrees (range 16-28 degrees).

(Fig. 3-18). Prominent loss of this angle indicates a radial fracture with impaction or overlap of fragments in most cases. The palmar tilt (or palmar slope) of the distal radius is measured on the lateral view as the angle between the distal articular surface of the radius and a line drawn perpendicular to the long axis of the radius (Fig. 3-19). This angle is normally between 0 and 20 degrees. The radial length, measured on the PA radiograph (Fig. 3-20), relates the length of the radius to the ulna. It is defined by the distance between two perpendicular

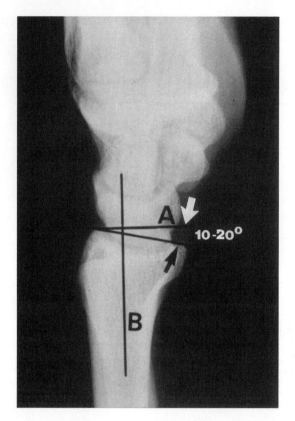

Figure 3-19   Palmar tilt. The palmar tilt is the angle between a line drawn perpendicular to the long axis of the radius (B) and a line joining the distal articular surface of the radius (A). Normally this angle is between 0 and 20 degrees.

lines to the long axis of the radius, one joining the tip of the radial styloid process and the other the surface of the ulnar head. Normally the radial length is 10 to 18 mm (mean:11-12 mm). The radial shift (or radial width), measured on PA view (Fig. 3-21), is defined as the distance between the longitudinal axis through the center of the radius and the most radial point of the radial styloid process. Both the injured and the uninjured wrists should be measured and compared to verify abnormalities; comparison with an opposite normal wrist is helpful in excluding normal variants. In addition, knowing what is normal in an individual patient can make any reconstructive or restorative surgery more satisfactory for both surgeon and patient.

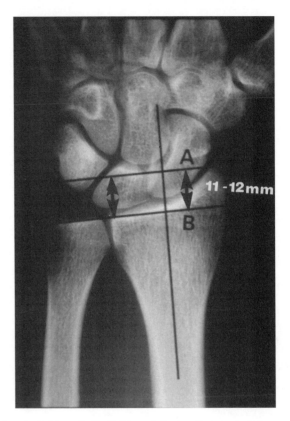

Figure 3-20   Radial length. Radial length is the distance between a line drawn perpendicular to the axis of the radius (B) and a line parallel to line B that joins the tip of the radial styloid process. Radial length is 10 to 18 mm (mean is 11-12 mm).

Carpal Ligament Instabilities

Carpal instabilities are conditions that may occur after interruption of the extrinsic and/or intrinsic carpal ligaments. Two types of carpal instabilities can be differentiated: static and dynamic. Static instabilities are constantly present and can be diagnosed on routine PA and lateral radiographic views. Dynamic instabilities are not constantly present; they need stress or motion to produce them. The latter may be diagnosed only by using special stress views or by the instability series mentioned earlier in this chapter. Carpal instabilities may be without clinical symptoms and may even occur as normal variants.

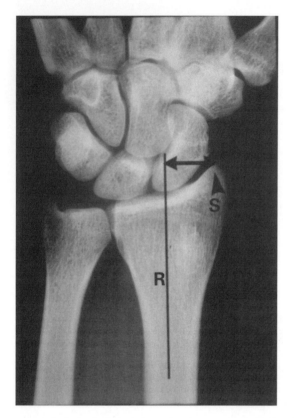

Figure 3-21   Radial shift. Radial shift is the distance (doubleheaded arrow) between the long axis through the center of the radius (R) and the most radial point of the radial styloid process (S).

Therefore, in any case with suspected instability of the wrist, radiological examination of the contralateral wrist should be performed to exclude the possibility of a normal variant. In other cases, carpal instability may progress to further disruption, leading to severe loss of wrist function and advanced degenerative joint disease. Six static carpal ligament instabilities have been described: dorsiflexion instability or dorsal intercalated segmental instability (DISI), palmar flexion instability or volar intercalated segmental instability (VISI), ulnar translocation, dorsal and palmar carpal subluxation, and rotatory subluxation of the scaphoid (RSS), or so-called scapholunate dissociation. One of the most important radiographic keys for detection of static carpal instability is to identify the position of the lunate.

Dorsiflexion instability (DISI) (Fig. 3-22) is a condition in which

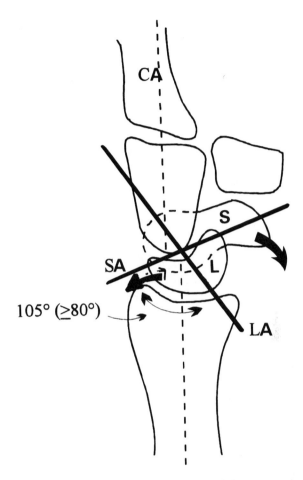

Figure 3-22   Schematic drawing of dorsiflexion instability (DISI). The scapholunate angle, which is normally between 30 and 60 degrees, increases to more than 60 degrees (an increase of this angle between 60 and 80 degrees is questionably abnormal; an angle of more than 80 degrees is definitely abnormal). The capitolunate angle remains normal or may also be increased. With DISI, the scaphoid (S) rotates volarly (larger thick arrow) and the lunate (L) tilts dorsally (thick arrow). Here the scapholunate angle is 105°. SA = scaphoid axis; LA = lunate axis; and CA = capitate axis.

the distal articular surface of the lunate tilts too far dorsally. The scaphoid bone may keep its normal position or, more commonly, tilt ventrally more than normal. This leads to an increased scapholunate angle of more than 60 degrees; this angle becomes definitely abnormal when it reaches more than 80 degrees. The capitolunate angle is nor-

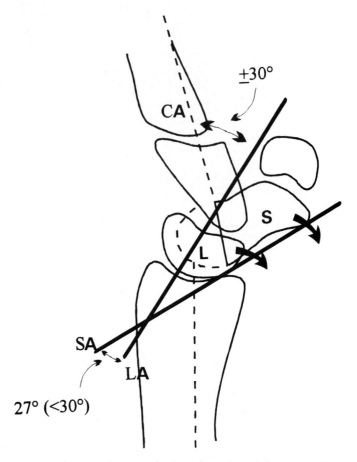

Figure 3-23   Schematic drawing of palmar flexion instability (VISI). The scapholunate angle is less than 30 degrees, or the capitolunate angle is more than 30 degrees, or both angles are increased. With VISI the scaphoid (S) rotates volarly (thick arrow) and the lunate (L) tilts volarly too (thick arrow). SA = scaphoid axis; LA = lunate axis; and CA = capitate axis.

mally 0 to 30 degrees; it may remain normal or may increase to more than 30 degrees.

In palmar flexion instability (VISI) (Fig. 3-23), the distal articular surface of the lunate faces too far palmarly. In this condition, the lunate and the scaphoid are flexed palmarly, leading to a scapholunate angle that may be 30 degrees or less. The capitolunate angle may be increased to more than 30 degrees.

When VISI or DISI is suspected and one or both of the scapholunate or the capitolunate angles show abnormalities, two additional lat-

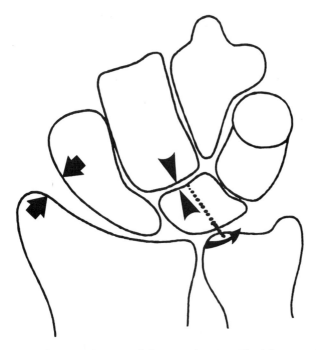

Figure 3-24   Schematic drawing of ulnar translocation. The joint space between the radial styloid and the scaphoid (between arrows) is wider than the other joint spaces of the wrist (between arrowheads). In addition more than one half of the proximal articular surface of the lunate is ulnar to the radius (curved arrow). This should be evaluated in the position in which the third metacarpal axis is collinear with the long axis of the radius.

eral views—in maximal extension and flexion—should be performed of both wrists. These additional views show if there is normal or abnormal motion between the carpal bones on flexion and extension. Normally, during wrist flexion, the lunate axis should flex with respect to the radius axis, and the capitate axis should flex with respect to the lunate axis. Similarly, during wrist extension, the axis of the lunate should extend with respect to the radius axis, and the capitate axis should extend with respect to the lunate axis. Abnormal intercarpal motion (lack of these findings on flexion and extension) is consistent with carpal ligament instability and supports the diagnosis of VISI and DISI. Because abnormal intercarpal alignment and motion may be found in some asymptomatic persons, comparison views of the opposite wrist should be obtained to exclude possible normal variants.

Ulnar translocation or translation (displacement) is a condition in which the carpus has merely subluxed ulnarly. Type I (Fig. 3-24) de-

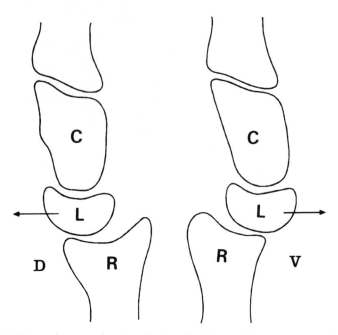

Figure 3-25 Schematic drawing of a lateral radiograph demonstrates palmar (P) and dorsal (D) dislocation of all the carpal bones. The drawing on the left represents an old dorsally impacted distal radius fracture. C = capitate; L = lunate; and R = radius.

scribes the condition in which the entire carpus is subluxed ulnarly. It can be diagnosed on the neutral PA view when the space between the radial styloid and scaphoid is wider than the width of other intercarpal joints and/or when more than one half of the proximal articular surface of the lunate is ulnar to the radius. Type II exists when there is a marked scapholunate diastasis, the scaphoid remains in the scaphoid fossa of the distal radius, and the remainder of the carpus is translated ulnarly.

In dorsal or palmar subluxation (Fig. 3-25), all the carpal bones are displaced dorsal or palmar to the midplane of the distal radius, as seen on the lateral view. Dorsal subluxation usually follows an old Colles' fracture and palmar carpal subluxation may be associated with a chip fracture off the ventral surface of the radius. Both conditions, dorsal and palmar subluxation, result from severe abnormalities of the radiocarpal ligaments. Palmar carpal subluxation is very uncommon and often has an associated ulnar carpal subluxation.

Rotatory subluxation of the scaphoid or scapholunate dissociation is the condition in which the scaphoid is abnormally aligned within the scaphoid fossa. It can be diagnosed when the scapholunate joint space is 4 mm or wider (Fig. 3-16*B*). This increase in the width of the scapholunate joint space (Terry Thomas sign) indicates a rupture of the scapholunate interosseous ligament (scapholunate dissociation). If there are additional abnormal radiocarpal ligaments, the scaphoid tilts ventrally and the term "rotatory subluxation" of the scaphoid is applicable. If the scaphoid tilts ventrally, it foreshortens and has a "signet ring" shape on the neutral PA radiograph because of overlapping edges of the scaphoid (Fig. 3-16*B*). Abnormal scaphoid foreshortening is supported when the radioscaphoid angle on the lateral view is less than 110 degrees (the scapholunate angle may increase while the capitolunate angle remains normal). As mentioned earlier in this chapter, scaphoid foreshortening can be produced in any patient if the wrist is in radial deviation. For that reason, foreshortening of the scaphoid on a PA view without other correlative findings for abnormal scaphoid position cannot reliably be called rotatory subluxation. In addition, when evaluating the width of the scapholunate joint space, it is important to measure the width of this joint at its midportion because the proximal edges of the scaphoid and lunate are rounded and measurement along its proximal margins will produce a falsely abnormal width. In isolated rotatory subluxation of the scaphoid, only the ligaments around the scaphoid are abnormal; the other radiocarpal ligaments are still intact. Only the scaphoid has abnormal motion, and the lunate has some or all of its normal motion resulting from its other normal ligamentous attachments. Therefore the flexion and extension lateral views show normal lunate motion in isolated rotatory subluxation. However, rotatory subluxation of the scaphoid may progress to DISI (occasionally VISI) over time.

Carpal Fractures and Dislocations

Carpal dislocations can be divided into two gross types, lunate and perilunate, with or without associated fractures. The normal anatomic position is identified by the distal radial articular surface, the lunate, and the capitate. Generally, on the lateral view, whichever bone is centered over the radius, whether it is the lunate or the capitate, is the bone that is considered in regular anatomic position. In lunate dislocation (Fig. 3-26) the lunate is displaced ventrally or dorsally away from the radius, and the head of the capitate is centered over the radius (ventral or dorsal lunate dislocation respectively). By contrast, in perilunate dislocation the lunate stays in anatomic position to the radius, and the capitate head is displaced ventrally or dorsally with respect to the radius (ventral or dorsal perilunate dislocation). If there is an additional fracture of a carpal bone, the term "trans" indicates which

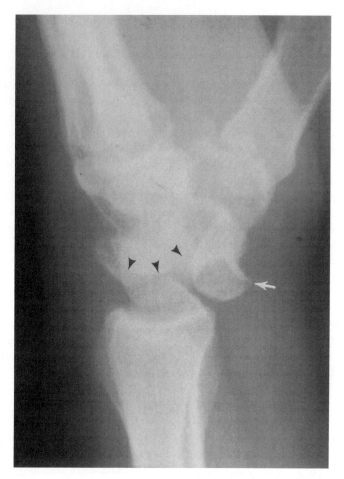

Figure 3-26   Ventral lunate dislocation. The lunate (arrow) is dislocated ventrally out of the distal concavity of the radius. The head of the capitate (arrowheads) is centered over the midshaft of the radius.

bone is fractured (e.g., a fracture of the scaphoid and dorsal dislocation of the capitate and its attached carpal bones would be referred to as transscaphoid dorsal perilunate dislocation). The term "midcarpal dislocation" can be used when there is a dislocation between the capitate and the lunate with other carpal bones and neither the lunate nor the capitate is centered over the distal radius (Fig. 3-27). In rare cases, a carpal fracture dislocation separates the carpometacarpal axes in the sagittal plane (Fig. 3-28). These dislocations are called "axial fracture dislocations." In those cases, the fractured bone is again named first

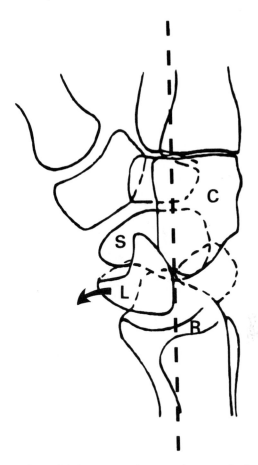

Figure 3-27   Midcarpal dislocation. Schematic drawing of a lateral radiograph demonstrates the condition of a midcarpal dislocation. The lunate (L) is displaced ventrally; the head of the capitate (C) is displaced dorsally. The midpoint axis of the radius passes between the lunate and the capitate. Therefore neither the capitate nor the lunate centers over the radius (R). S = scaphoid. (Reprinted with permission from Gilula LA: Carpal injuries: analytic approach and case exercises. *AJR* 133:503-517, 1979.)

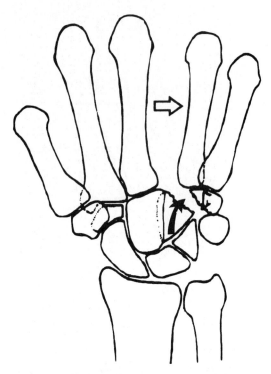

Figure 3-28 Schematic drawing of a transhamate peripisiform axial–ulnar dislocation. The carpal fracture dislocation separates the carpometacarpal axes ulnarly (open arrow). The fractured bone is the hamate (curved arrow).

by using the term "trans" and then adding the site of carpal joint separation (e.g., transhamate, peripisiform axial fracture dislocation) (Fig. 3-28).

SCINTIGRAPHY (RADIONUCLIDE BONE IMAGING, RNBI)

RNBI is an extremely sensitive (but with low specificity) imaging modality for evaluation of subtle wrist and hand injury. This technique is very valuable for detecting or excluding osseous, osteochondral, and some soft tissue abnormalities. RNBI is used especially in patients following acute trauma with significant clinical symptoms and in whom standard radiographs fail to demonstrate a definite lesion. It is also used in patients in whom the presence of a fracture is suspected, even though the symptoms are not completely typical. Scintigraphy is also very useful to localize an abnormality in subacute or chronic situations with persistent clinical symptoms but normal radiographs.

For RNBI, technetium-99m is usually coupled to phosphate compounds, such as methylene diphosphonate. The use of three-phase radionuclide scintigraphy provides information faster than the usual 2 to 3 hours required for bone images. Phase I (= radionuclide angiography), which is obtained during the first 1 to 2 minutes after injection of the radionuclide, provides valuable blood flow information. Phase II (= blood pool images), which is obtained at approximately 5 minutes after injection, and Phase III (= delayed bone images), which is obtained 2 to 3 hours later, are useful in detecting abnormalities of soft tissue and cartilage or bone, respectively. The bone scan must be sufficiently detailed to examine both wrists in dorsal, ventral, lateral, and oblique views to enable localization of any increased bone turnover in a specific site of the wrist and hand.

In most fractures of the distal radius, wrist, and hand, standard radiographs usually define the presence of a fracture. In some cases, however, when radiographs have been normal but the patients have symptoms or in patients with suspected bone, cartilaginous, or ligamentous abnormalities of the wrist and hand after trauma, RNBI may be very helpful in detecting abnormalities. In areas of intense, focal tracer uptake, an occult fracture must be excluded with additional, more detailed roentgenograms in different planes or with other imaging techniques such as CT or MRI. Mildly increased focal tracer accumulation suggests a ligamentous or cartilaginous abnormality or an osseous or osteochondral area of lesser activity. The lack of focal tracer accumulation on delayed images is useful in excluding osseous involvement.

The use of the three-phase bone scan technique allows determination of the age of a fracture as well as fracture healing when radiograms are inconclusive. In the acute phase after trauma (2-4 weeks), all three phases of bone scan are positive. On delayed pool images, the fracture site shows very intense tracer uptake with unsharp margins. In the subacute stage (4-12 weeks), the radionuclide angiography becomes normal; the blood pool images as well as the delayed pool images stay positive and become more focal with respect to the fracture line. In the chronic phase, radionuclide angiography and blood pool images are normal, and the activity on the delayed pool images slowly decreases over a period of 3 to 8 months.

RNBI may be helpful for evaluation of posttraumatic bone pain and delayed fracture healing and fracture nonunion. In cases with bone bruise, radionuclide angiography usually is normal. Blood pool images and delayed images show minimal to moderate increased tracer uptake. Patients with reactive nonunion of the fracture usually have normal radionuclide angiography. On the blood pool images, they have a variable increase of activity ranging from normal to 2+ increase and focal increased tracer uptake from 1+ to 3+ on delayed images. By using a single RNBI examination, differential diagnosis between delayed union and reactive nonunion may be impossible. However, if the blood pool images are normal and the amount of activity associated with the delayed images is minimal, the lesion is more likely to be in an end stage of healing. If typical patterns of fracture nonunion can be demonstrated on radiographs, RNBI may be helpful for evaluation of the degree of nonspecific stress change taking place (degree of activity on delayed images) and the amount of synovial-type inflammation present (degree of activity on blood pool images).

RNBI is also used for diagnosis of reflex sympathetic dystrophy (RSD), a condition that is not uncommon after distal radius fractures or fractures of carpal bones. A specific scintigraphic pattern for RSD has been established with a sensitivity and specificity of 96% and 97%, respectively, on delayed bone images that show diffusely increased activity involving predominantly the juxtaarticular zones of bones of the wrist and hand. Three-phase scintigraphy is a valuable method, especially for diagnosing the early stages of RSD, which are often not detected on conventional radiograph, and for the follow-up assessment of therapeutic regimes. However bone scintigraphy by itself is not diagnostic and must be correlated with clinical findings to make a diagnosis of RSD.

Another condition in which RNBI may be useful is evaluation of posttraumatic avascular necrosis (AVN) of carpal bones or carpal bone fracture fragments. Early detection of AVN is of major importance for treatment and prognosis. RNBI is superior to radiographs for early detection of AVN, but has a very low sensitivity. The sensitivity of magnetic resonance imaging (MRI) for detection of AVN is similar, or even higher than RNBI, but MRI is much more specific and should therefore be used as the imaging modality of choice in such cases.

ARTHROGRAPHY
Wrist Arthrography

When a patient's history, plain films, and instability series suggest a ligamentous or cartilaginous abnormality, arthrography may be helpful in identifying those defects.

Normal Arthrogram

The wrist consists of several synovial lined major and minor compartments that usually do not communicate. The major compartments are the radiocarpal compartment (RCC), the distal radioulnar compartment (DRUC), and the midcarpal compartment (MCC). Minor compartments are the first carpometacarpal compartment of the thumb (I CMC), the pisotriquetral compartment, and the common carpometacarpal and intermetacarpal compartments.

The RCC (Fig. 3-29A) is bordered proximally by the distal radial articular cartilage and the triangular fibrocartilage complex (TFCC). (The triangular fibrocartilage, or the TFC, is the cartilaginous structure that extends from the ulnar aspect of the radius to send out attaching fibers to the base of the ulnar styloid. The triangular fibrocartilage complex, or TFCC, is the TFC plus its surrounding soft tissue attachments to the adjacent anatomic structures.) Distally the RCC is bordered by the cartilaginous surfaces of the bones of the proximal carpal row and the interosseous ligaments between these bones. Three normal recesses of the RCC can be seen constantly: the prestyloid, the ventral radial, and the dorsal carpal. The DRUC (Fig. 3-29B) outlines the proximal surface of the TFCC, which extends a variable distance from its radial attachment on the distal radius to the base of the ulnar styloid, outlining the articulation between them. Contrast outlines the articular cartilage of the ulnar head. The midcarpal compartment extends between the proximal and distal carpal rows (Fig. 3-29C). Normally there is no communication between the MCC and RCC or between the RCC and the DRUC.

Technique

Arthrography is best performed by utilizing fluoroscopic control and frequent spot filming with the patient prone on the fluoroscopy table, the arm raised above the head, the elbow extended, and the wrist prone. Under sterile precautions, a 2:1 mixture of dilute water-soluble contrast to 1% lidocaine is used. Ulnar access to the midcarpal joint is obtained at the junction of the lunate, triquetrum, capitate, and hamate, or the needle is introduced radially over the distal scaphoid next to the capitate just proximal to the trapezoid. For distal radioulnar joint arthrography, the needle is introduced into the joint a few millimeters proximal to the distal surface of the ulna along the midportion of the distal radioulnar articulation. Access to the radiocarpal joint is through the radioscaphoid region, if the site of the pain is ulnar. If the patient's pain is radial sided, the needle can be placed in the region from the radiolunate joint, or ulnar, to the lunotriquetral joint along the proximal edge of the triquetrum. Needle placement is always away from the symptomatic site in the midcarpal and radiocarpal joints, so that local contrast extravasation will not be confused with pathology. The joints are fully distended with contrast until the patient has mild discomfort. After full distension of the joints the needle is removed and the wrist is observed fluoroscopically under exercise. Exercising the wrist in several positions may open a small communicating defect that may not be apparent otherwise. For a "complete" arthrographic study of the wrist designed to show the maximal number of abnormal communicating and noncommunicating defects, the MCC, the DRUC, and the RCC should be injected. To see if a defect on the symptomatic

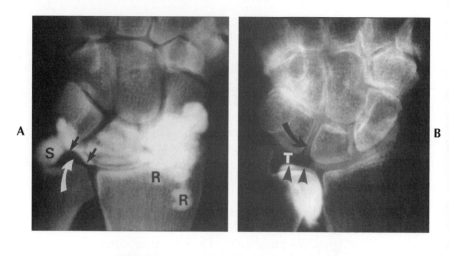

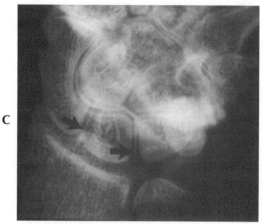

Figure 3-29   Normal wrist arthrography. **(A)** Radiocarpal arthrogram. S = prestyloid recess; R = ventral radial recesses; curved arrow = triangular fibrocartilage; and small arrows = distal surface of the triangular fibrocartilage. **(B)** Arthrogram of the distal radioulnar joint. Arrowheads = proximal surface of the triangular fibrocartilage and T = triangular fibrocartilage as a radiolucent band. There is residual contrast after midcarpal arthrography (curved arrow). **(C)** Midcarpal arthrography. Contrast extends between the proximal and distal carpal rows and contrast outlines the distal surface of the scapholunate and lunotriquetral ligaments (just proximal to tips of arrows).

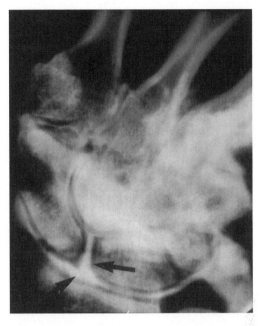

Figure 3-30   Radiocarpal arthrography demonstrates a communication from the radiocarpal compartment to the midcarpal compartment because of a defect of the scapholunate ligament (arrows). The scapholunate joint is abnormally wide.

side is also present on the asymptomatic side, injection of the same compartment in the opposite wrist may be of value.

Abnormal Arthrogram

The most common sites of abnormal intercompartmental communications resulting from ligamentous tears or defects are the scapholunate and the lunotriquetral ligaments (with or without abnormal widening or malalignment of the scapholunate [Fig. 3-30] and lunotriquetral joints) and the TFC. Traumatic TFC defects are classified according to the location of the lesion. Class IA lesions are small communicating perforations of the horizontal portion of the TFC located 2 to 3 mm ulnar to the radial attachment of the TFC and are seen on either or both radiocarpal and distal radioulnar joint injections (Fig. 3-31). Class IB lesions are avulsions of the TFCC from its insertion into the distal ulna (with/without fracture of the ulna styloid). In this condition, radiocarpal arthrography may or may not reveal an abnormality depending on whether this is a communicating defect (Fig. 3-32). However, distal radioulnar arthrography will detect contrast leakage into the ulnar soft tissue attachment of the TFC. Type IC lesions

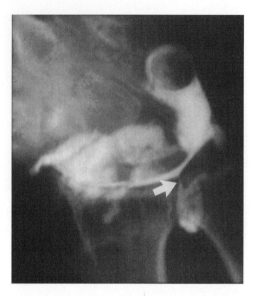

Figure 3-31 Radiocarpal arthrography. A small communication to the distal radioulnar compartment near the radial attachment of the TFC is demonstrated. (arrow).

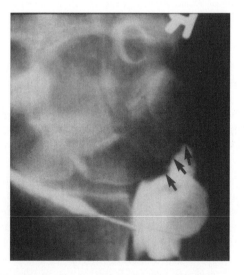

Figure 3-32 Distal radioulnar arthrography demonstrates contrast surrounding the proximal attachments of the TFCC at the ulnar styloid (arrows), indicating a peripheral detachment of the TFCC. Because there is no communication to the radiocarpal compartment, this abnormality would be overlooked by performing only radiocarpal wrist arthrography.

are avulsions of the TFCC from its distal attachment to the lunate or triquetrum. On arthrography, a capsular leak may occur on either radiocarpal or even midcarpal injection, depending on the location of the torn tissue. Class ID lesions are complete avulsions of the TFCC from its attachment to the radius and can be seen with either radiocarpal or distal radioulnar joint injections.

In general, ligamentous, cartilaginous, or capsular defects may be communicating or complete (through and through) and are usually seen on both adjacent compartments that are injected (bidirectional communication). A communicating defect may also occur in a "one-way valve" behavior (unidirectional communication) and can therefore be overlooked by injecting only one compartment. A ligamentous or cartilaginous defect may also occur as a noncommunicating or incomplete defect (not through and through or not communicating between two adjacent compartments) and can therefore be detected only by injecting both adjacent wrist compartments. For example, a noncommunicating defect of the TFC or a proximal avulsion of the TFCC from the base of the ulnar styloid can be seen only with DRU arthrography and not with RC arthrography (Fig. 3-32). In addition, patients may have more than one abnormality in different compartments that would be missed by using single compartment arthrography alone.

Current Status of Wrist Arthrography

The clinical significance of some arthrographic findings is difficult to access. As known from the literature, there is often poor correlation between symptom sites or sides and abnormalities detected on arthrography. The reason for the poor correlation for arthrographic abnormalities is uncertain, but ligamentous and triangular fibrocartilage defects increase in number with age. Therefore asymptomatic defects must exist. Abnormalities detected on arthrography must always be carefully correlated with clinical and physical examinations. Perhaps the use of bilateral wrist arthrography to detect asymmetric defects may show asymmetric defects that may have better correlation with symptom sites.

Arthrography of the Fingers and Thumb

The most common indications for finger arthrography are to demonstrate acute injuries of the capsule and collateral ligaments of the finger, tendon derangements, and defects of the volar plate of the metacarpophalangeal joints. Arthrography should be performed acutely because the joint capsule usually (but not always) seals spontaneously in less than one week. The most frequent finger joint evaluated by arthrography is the metacarpophalangeal joint of the thumb. Arthrography is used to diagnose disruption of the ulnar collateral ligament in patients in whom clinical examination or stress radiography results are equivocal. Arthrography technique is also helpful to inject steroid into a joint when it is important to verify that the steroid has been placed intraarticularly.

Technique

For arthrography of the metacarpophalangeal and interphalangeal joints, the hand is placed palm down on the fluoroscopic table with the fingers slightly flexed. Under fluoroscopic control and sterile precautions, a needle is inserted into the joint of interest from a dorsolateral or dorsomedial approach, adjacent to the extensor tendons. The needle should be placed away from the site of probable pathology. In this technique, 1 to 1.5 ml of dilute contrast medium for the metacarpophalangeal joint and 0.5 to 1ml for the interphalangeal joints are injected under fluoroscopic control and spot filming. The needle is then removed. Posteroanterior, lateral, and oblique views should be obtained after the procedure.

Normal Arthrogram

Under normal conditions, contrast medium in the metacarpophalangeal or interphalangeal joints passes in a curvilinear fashion between the adjacent proximal and distal cartilaginous surfaces of the metacarpophalangeal and interphalangeal joints. The joint capsules are smooth, with proximal and distal recesses at the radial, ulnar, dorsal, and ventral aspects of the articulations. The proximal recesses, especially of the metacarpophalangeal joint of the thumb, are commonly larger than the distal recesses; they are also larger dorsal than ventral. At the metacarpophalangeal joint of the thumb, the proximal recesses can measure up to 20 mm in length, whereas the distal recesses are usually not longer than 5 mm (Fig. 3-33). Slight indentations seen on the posteroanterior radiograph at the joint line are produced by collateral ligaments. The volar plate produces an indentation on the palmar surface of this capsule as seen on the lateral view (Fig. 3-33). Normally there is no extravasation of contrast outside the joint capsule, except along the needle track.

Abnormal Arthrogram

Following an acute or subacute tear of the collateral ligaments (Fig. 3-34) or the capsule, contrast extravasates into the soft tissues. Such extravasation may be helpful to evaluate ligamentous injuries of the ulnar aspect of the metacarpophalangeal articulation of the thumb. In these patients, radial directed stress shows damage to the ulnar collateral ligament, joint capsule, and volar plate. However, as mentioned earlier in this chapter, such extravasation is seen most commonly in the acute or subacute phase. After the acute phase has passed, the joint capsule may become fibrosed and close the defect. In late cases, the joint capsule along the ulnar side of the first metacarpophalangeal

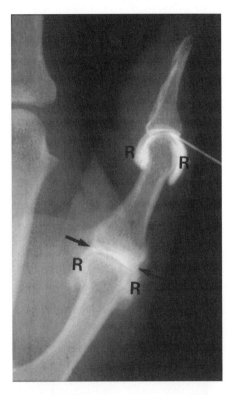

Figure 3-33   Normal arthrography of the metacarpophalangeal joint and the interphalangeal joint of the thumb. The joint capsules are smooth, and there are proximal and distal, radial and ulnar, and volar and dorsal recesses (R). The arrows demonstrate the indentations caused by the soft tissues at the joint. Ventrally is the volar plate.

joint may become irregular and bulging, suggesting a diagnosis of collateral ligament tear. Another lesion that may be diagnosed with arthrography is the Stener lesion of the thumb. In this lesion the proximal portion of the torn ulnocarpal collateral ligament is folded back and trapped by the aponeurosis of the adductor pollicis muscle. It appears on arthrography as a filling defect on the ulnar side of the joint capsule. Injuries of the volar plate can be diagnosed on arthrography as extravasations of contrast material ventrally, occasionally with additional filling of the adjacent tendon sheaths.

COMPUTED TOMOGRAPHY (CT)

The main advantages of CT are improved contrast resolution and planar representation of the carpal bones without the superimposition of anatomic structures inherent in radiography. Another advantage of

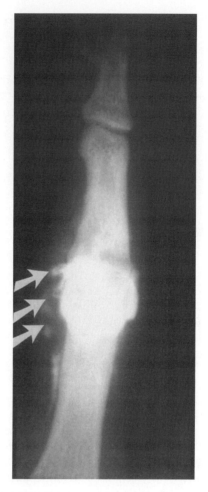

Figure 3-34   Abnormal arthrogram of the proximal interphalangeal joint. Contrast extravasates into the soft tissues due to collateral ligament rupture (arrows).

CT is that primary images in different planes (e.g., axial, coronal, and sagittal) can be obtained. Furthermore, spiral-CT technique allows multiplanar reconstructions in any desired plane and high-quality, three-dimensional reconstructions by a single examination. In the majority of cases of wrist fractures, the routine radiographic examination is satisfactory to solve radiographically demonstrable clinical problems. In selected cases however, CT examination of the wrist can be diagnostically very useful. Indications for wrist CT include valuation of the distal radioulnar joint and distal articular surface of the radius, evaluation of complex or occult carpal fractures, and assessment of fracture healing and postsurgical alterations. In such cases, CT may add significant information when compared to conventional radiography.

Diagnosis of distal radioulnar subluxation or dislocation can be made on a true lateral radiograph. However, it may be difficult to obtain a true lateral radiograph because pain in an acutely injured wrist and casting or inconsistent positioning by the technologist may be a limiting factor. Positioning the wrist as little as 10 degrees off lateral makes the lateral radiograph completely unreliable in the assessment of distal radioulnar joint congruity (Fig. 3-35*A* and *B*). In addition, the ulna may be subluxed only in certain positions, and the dorsally prominent ulna may be a normal variant. Comparison with the opposite wrist in true lateral position may be helpful. CT is the technique of choice for corroborating distal radioulnar subluxation or dislocation. For diagnosis of distal radioulnar congruity by using CT, axial, 2 mm thick, contiguous sections should be performed through the distal radioulnar joints. Initially the hands are placed prone on the table and the thumbs side by side with the distal radioulnar joints at the same level for symmetry. Two lines are drawn on these images: one through the dorsal border of the distal radius at the sigmoid notch and Lister's tubercle; the second through the palmar border of the distal radius at the level of the sigmoid notch (Fig. 3-36). Articulation of the distal radioulnar joint is considered normal if the ulnar head lies between these two lines. Additional axial CT scans must be performed in a position of supination and an additional pronation (or some other position that is painful for the patient) in hopes of finding the subluxation in the painful position. This is done to avoid picturing a dynamic subluxation that is reduced during CT scanning. Other authors cited poor experience with these criteria and introduced the epicenter and congruity methods as being more accurate for diagnosis of distal radioulnar incongruity.

Another indication for CT is to demonstrate the occult fracture of the distal radius suspected on the basis of physical examination findings and focally positive RNBI when plain films are normal. For preoperative evaluation of the size and position of fragments in complex comminuted distal radius fractures and exact evaluation of the distal articular surface of the radius, CT is superior to conventional radiographs. For CT examination of distal radius fractures, imaging in two planes (axial and sagittal or axial and coronal) with thin sections is usually sufficient. The axial plane is useful to show the configuration of the fracture patterns involving the distal articular surface of the radius and shows the degree of diastasis of radioscaphoid and radiolu-

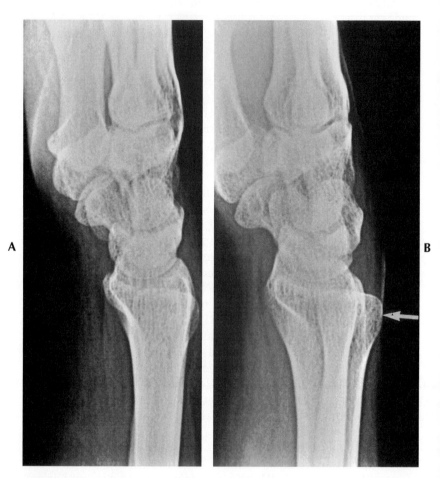

Figure 3-35 True lateral radiograph of a healthy wrist **(A).** There is no evidence of subluxation of the distal radioulnar joint. The same wrist which is performed slightly off lateral **(B)** may lead to a misdiagnosis of dorsal subluxation of the distal radioulnar joint (arrow).

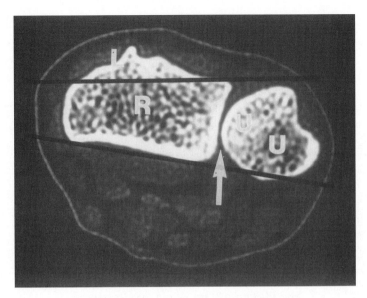

Figure 3-36   Axial CT scan at the level of the sigmoid notch (arrow) and Lister's tubercle (L). Two lines, one drawn through the dorsal border of the radius and the other through the palmar border of the radius, are shown. Under normal conditions, the ulna should lie between these two lines. A tiny amount of the ulna projects palmar to the palmar line. This is normal.

nate fossae fragments, incongruity of the distal radioulnar joint, and volar and dorsal cortical comminution of the radius. Sagittal and coronal planes are useful for depiction of congruity and angulation of radiocarpal joint surfaces, the degree of dorsal and volar surface comminution, and elevation or depression of distal radial articular surface fracture fragments (Figure 3.37*A* and *B*). Recognition of fracture fragment size and position is of importance when deciding whether to operate and, sometimes, which approach may be most beneficial. Central pylon-type fracture depression may be undetectable on conventional radiographs.

Fractures of the carpal bones, especially fractures of the scaphoid and the hook of hamate, sometimes are difficult to diagnose on conventional radiographs and may be overlooked. Therefore, injuries to patients with negative radiographs but definite, focal clinical symptoms (especially tenderness) or hot spots over the carpal bones, should be further investigated by using CT or MRI. Fracture complications can only be avoided by early detection. Fractures of the scaphoid waist are slow healing and may be associated with nonunion and/or avascular necrosis of the proximal fracture fragment. It is extremely important to determine as early as possible whether or not fracture alignment has

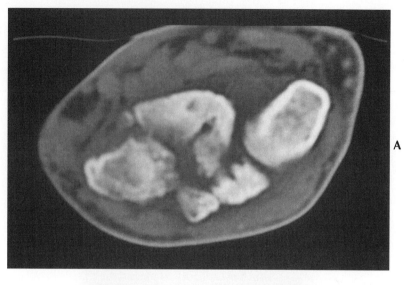

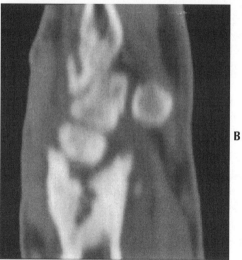

Figure 3-37 Axial CT **(A)** scan through the distal radius demonstrates severe comminuted intraarticular fracture of the distal radius. CT excellently demonstrates the number of fracture fragments and the amount of fracture fragment displacement. Multiplanar reconstructions of this axial scan shown in (A) and sagittal plane **(B)** adds further information about the amount of fracture depression or presence or absence of intraarticular fracture fragments that may be difficult to detect on conventional radiographs. Here the lunate lies proximal between the displaced large ventral and dorsal distal radius fracture fragments.

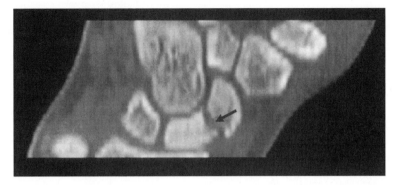

Figure 3-38   Coronal reconstruction of an axial CT scan in a patient with scaphoid fracture (arrow). Coronal CT allows excellent evaluation of radioulnar offset between scaphoid fracture fragments. When direct coronal CT scans are obtained, reconstructions will not be necessary.

the potential for anatomic healing. Our preferred way to image the scaphoid by CT is to use two planes, the oblique sagittal (the long axis of the scaphoid is parallel to the scan plane) and the coronal. The long sagittal axis of the scaphoid provides information about palmar or dorsal angulation and displacement of fracture fragments. This is the best view to demonstrate dorsal gapping of fracture fragments at the fracture site. The coronal plane (Fig. 3-38) provides assessment of radioulnar offset between the proximal and distal fracture fragments. Most fractures of the hook of the hamate are located at its base (oriented in the coronal plane) and therefore are often difficult to detect on routine radiographs. As with the scaphoid, complications of nonunion and necrosis of untreated fractures of the hamate may occur. Fractures of the hook of the hamate are well shown with the axial CT projection as a linear gap transversing its base. An additional examination in the sagittal plane allows detection of craniocaudal shift or angulation of the hook. Fractures of other carpal bones may be surveyed effectively with the coronal plane, as the entire carpus can be examined with relatively few thin sections. However, depending on the plane of the fracture, a second CT plane may be necessary. If a spiral-CT unit is available, the wrist can be examined rapidly in whatever plane is desired (if the patient can position the wrist in the desired position) with thin sections (1 mm). Because of the ability of this technique to obtain multiplanar reconstructions in any desired plane, additional planes can be reconstructed later.

Evaluation of the distal radius and wrist following treatment of radius or wrist fractures can be difficult with plain films or even with conventional tomography because of artifacts from casting material or metal implants or the inability to obtain proper positioning. CT has advantages over conventional radiographs and conventional tomography in assessing fusions because CT avoids overlapping bone surfaces seen on radiographs and blur seen on conventional tomography. CT is very sensitive in detecting subtle calcification or areas of bone formation. Therefore CT provides an excellent means to evaluate posttreatment success and fracture healing. CT is a very reliable method to determine carpal fracture nonunions, bone graft incorporation, and osseous fusion. However, exact positioning of the forearm and wrist and a careful selection of the scan planes is mandatory to obtain a good quality CT exam.

CT has advantages over plain radiography and conventional tomography in assessment of treatment planning, fracture healing, and postoperative followup. However, because of its higher costs, CT should be reserved for cases in which plain radiographs are insufficient to make diagnoses or treatment decisions or in which a significant discrepancy exists between plain radiographs and clinical symptoms.

MAGNETIC RESONANCE IMAGING (MRI)

Because of the improvement in MR techniques and the development of dedicated surface coils, MRI has provided an important, new, noninvasive approach for examination of the wrist. Compared with all other imaging modalities, this method allows simultaneous and direct visualization of bone, cartilage, and soft tissue. Although MRI cannot be used as the imaging technique of choice for evaluating the acute injured wrist and hand, it provides a powerful new diagnostic tool. MRI is presently used in the evaluation of trauma-related injuries, such as carpal ligamentous disruptions, triangular fibrocartilage complex (TFCC) disruptions, distal radioulnar joint instability, occult fractures of the distal radius and carpal bones, median nerve compression, rupture of flexor and extensor tendons, reflex sympathetic dystrophy, and avascular necrosis of carpal bones.

Because of the complex anatomy and the small size of the wrist, MR imaging currently is best performed with a high, field-strength magnet (1.5T). However lesser quality MRI may also be performed with a lower field magnet of 0.5, when dedicated wrist surface coils are available. The wrist should be examined in the neutral position, with the axis of the radius and the third metacarpal colinear and without flexion or extension. This will maintain consistent alignment of the carpus. The hand should be properly fixed to avoid motion artifacts. Dedicated wrist surface coils should be used to provide optimal signal-to-noise ratio and uniform signal intensity throughout the image field of view. For routine examination commonly T1-weighted SE sequences and 3D-GRE sequences are performed to allow accurate diagnoses. Selection of the imaging plane depends on the clinical question.

During the last few years, much attention has been given to evaluating abnormalities of the TFC and the ligaments of the wrist with MRI. It is the only imaging modality that allows direct topographic visualization of the TFC and the intrinsic and extrinsic carpal ligaments. The most important structures for wrist stability are the scapholunate and the lunotriquetral intrinsic ligaments (Fig. 3-39*A*), the TFC (Fig. 3-39*A*), and the volar and dorsal extrinsic carpal ligaments (Fig. 3-39*B*). Recent studies have found MRI to be very accurate in delineating TFC perforations (communicating defects), perforations of the interosseous ligaments of the proximal carpal row, and perforations of the extrinsic ligaments. However, for accurate evaluation of structures that are less than 1 to 2 mm thick, thin MR sections (1 mm or less) have to be performed. It is important to know that degenerative changes of the TFC and carpal ligaments can be the cause of perforations and can be found even in the second and third decades of life. On MR images, degenerative defects may have appearances and signal intensities similar to those of posttraumatic perforations. Therefore, it may be difficult to decide whether these changes are posttraumatic or the result of age-related degeneration. Synovial fluid collection in the DRUC and MCC is reported as more common in patients with traumatic than degenerative perforations of the TFC and scapholunate and lunotriquetral ligaments; it may therefore be an indirect sign for traumatic tears. However, small amounts of fluid may also exist in normal persons. Abnormalities of the carpal ligaments and the TFC detected on MRI must be carefully correlated with clinical findings and symptoms.

As discussed earlier in this chapter, diagnosis of subluxation or dislocation of the distal radioulnar joint may be difficult, or even impossible, on plain films. Compared with CT, MRI has the additional advantage of simultaneous identification of the radioulnar ligaments and the TFC. It also allows more accurate characterization of associated effusion in the distal radioulnar joint, which may be a secondary sign of ligament and TFC pathology.

MRI has also proved to be a very important diagnostic tool in evaluating occult fractures and posttraumatic necrosis or necrosis of a fracture fragment (Fig. 3-40) of carpal bones. Compared with plain radiography and sometimes even with scintigraphy, MRI may be more sensitive in detecting early osteonecrosis. Because MR findings depend on the death of fat cells, which takes from 2 to 5 days, avascular necrosis may be seen as early as 5 days after trauma. Evaluation of fracture

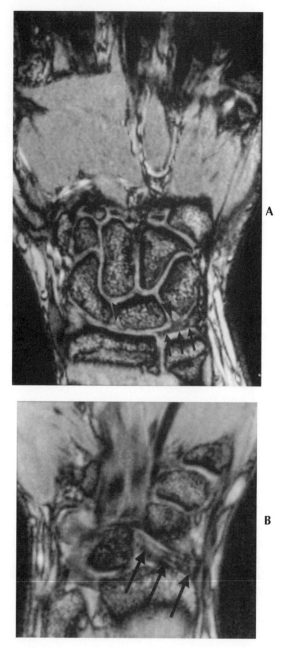

Figure 3-39 **(A)** Coronal GRE MRI of a healthy wrist. MRI allows direct and simultaneous depiction of bones and soft tissues of the wrist. The scapholunate and lunotriquetral intrinsic ligaments of the proximal carpal row (arrowheads), the TFC (arrows), and even the extrinsic carpal ligaments, such as the radioscaphocapitate ligament **(B)** can be depicted by using MRI.

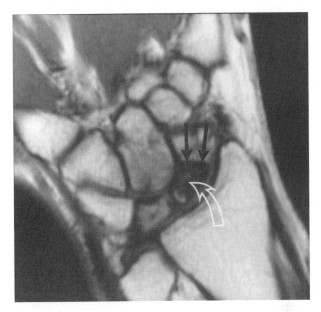

Figure 3-40   Coronal T1 weighted MRI of the wrist demonstrates fracture of the scaphoid waist (arrows). The proximal fracture fragment has a very low signal intensity indicating abnormality in this marrow space (open arrow). Additional MRI sequences are necessary to separate this from healing reaction, avascular necrosis or even marrow edema.

healing or follow-up after bone graft incorporation are other conditions in which MRI may be superior to other imaging techniques, particularly if medullary continuity of adjacent bones is questioned. When the status of bone union with apposing cortical surfaces is questioned, thin-section CT may be more valuable than MRI. Therefore, a very early diagnosis of bone bridging, which is imperative for a successful treatment, can be made by using CT. However, if gadolinium is used, MRI may be able to give additional information about possible revascularity between bone fragments that is not possible with other imaging techniques, with the exception of radionuclide imaging, which is not as specific as MRI.

As for related injuries of flexor or extensor tendons and injuries to the median nerve, which are possible complications in distal radius fractures or complex carpal fractures, MRI can be a helpful diagnostic imaging modality. Similar evaluation of carpal tunnel disease after malunions of distal radius fractures can be performed successfully with MRI.

Reflex symphathetic dystrophy (RSD) is a common complication associated with distal radius fractures or fractures of the carpal bones.

MRI has been reported as a helpful imaging technique in diagnosis and follow-up of RSD. A coexistence of signal intensity changes of soft tissue and bone marrow because of edema, which seem to be typical features in patients with RSD, has been described. In addition, MRI potentially allows detection of the different stages of RSD, which affects therapeutic procedures. Bone scintigraphy has also been claimed to be valuable in making the diagnosis of RSD when all three phases of a bone scan are abnormal. However, making the diagnosis of RSD without clinical correlation is fraught with problems, as it is not uncommon to have changes on bone scintigraphy suggesting RSD that are completely incompatible with this diagnosis clinically.

ULTRASONOGRAPHY

Ultrasonography has been used successfully for many conditions of the hand and wrist. It has been more commonly used in Europe than the United States because of the less frequent availability of CT and MRI scanners, especially in their early development. Gradually, with continual improvement of ultrasound, musculoskeletal ultrasound has been increasingly used in the United States. Ultrasound has the advantage of examining structures during active motion, or in "real time," a situation that is not possible with any other technique except fluoroscopy. However, ultrasound provides detail of soft tissues, a feature not possible with fluoroscopy. The use of ultrasound is highly machine and operator dependent, and this technique may be best developed with ultrasonographer and referring physician working together. Ultrasonography may be very helpful in evaluating the internal character of tendons, as well as their functional and anatomic characteristics, the status of many ligaments, cartilage, and osseous surfaces, and characteristics of soft tissue masses. With thoughtful development of this technique by the referring physician and ultrasonographer, many valuable uses of ultrasonography in the hand and wrist can be identified. However, effective ultrasonography of the musculoskeletal system can be developed best in each institution by someone interested in this area. Merely requesting such an exam may not produce worthwhile answers.

SUMMARY

Imaging of the hand and wrist is an important part of evaluation of the patient with clinical symptomatology related to this part of the body. Knowledge about the use of the many different imaging techniques available today is necessary to provide expeditious evaluation and satisfactory treatment of patients. Working together, imagers and physicians can provide worthwhile approaches to dealing with patients, especially those in whom the precise diagnosis is not obvious. This chapter provides some information that can serve as a basis from which focused evaluations of patients can be developed.

SELECTED REFERENCES

Bowers WH, Hurst LC: Gamekeeper's thumb: evaluation by arthrography and stress roentgenography. *J Bone Joint Surg* 59A:519, 1977.

Brody GA, Stoller DW: *The wrist and hand.* In Stoller DW, editor: *Magnetic resonance imaging in orthopaedics and sports medicine,* ed 1, Philadelphia, 1993, Lippincott.

Bush CH, Gillespy T, Dell PC: High-resolution CT of the wrist: initial experience with scaphoid disorders and surgical fusions. *AJR* 149:757, 1987.

Cone RO, Szabo R, Resnick D, et al.: Computed tomography of the normal radio-ulnar joints. *Invest Radiol* 18:541, 1983.

Curtis DJ, Downey EF Jr., Brower AC, et al.: Importance of soft-tissue evaluation in hand and wrist trauma: statistical evaluation. *AJR* 142:781, 1984.

Ganel A, Engel J, Oster Z, et al.: Bone scanning in the assessment of fractures of the scaphoid. *J Hand Surg* 4:540, 1979.

Gilula LA: Carpal injuries: analytic approach and case exercises. *AJR* 133:503, 1979.

Gilula LA, Totty WG, Weeks PM: Wrist arthrography: the value of fluoroscopic spot viewing. *Radiology* 146:555, 1983.

Gilula LA, Weeks PM: Post-traumatic ligamentous instabilities of the wrist. *Radiology* 129:641, 1978.

Gold RH: *Arthrography of the wrist.* In Arndt RD, Horns JW, Gold RH, editors: *Clinical arthrography,* ed 1, Baltimore, 1985, Williams & Wilkins.

Golimbu CN: *Wrist.* In Frioozina HF, Golimbu CN, Rafii M, et al., editors: *MRI and CT of the musculoskeletal system,* ed 1, St. Louis, 1992, Mosby Year Book.

Hardy DH, Totty WG, Reinus WR, et al.: Posterioanterior wrist radiography: importance of arm positioning. *J Hand Surg* [Am] 12:504, 1987.

Hindman BW, Kulik WJ, Lee G, et al.: Occult fractures of the carpals and metacarpals: demonstration by CT. *AJR* 153:529, 1989.

Höglund M, Tordai P. *Ultrasound.* In Gilula LA, editor: *Imaging of the wrist and hand.* Philadelphia, 1995, WB Saunders.

Holder LE: *Radionucleide bone imaging in surgical problems of the hand.* In Gilula LA, editor: *The traumatized hand and wrist,* ed 1, Philadelphia, 1992, WB Saunders.

Kellerhouse LE, Reicher MA: *Osteonecrosis and fractures of the wrist.* In Reicher MA, Kellerhouse LE, editors: *MRI of the wrist and hand.* New York, 1990, Raven, p. 107.

Kraemer BA, Gilula LA: *Metacarpal fractures and dislocations.* In Gilula LA, editor: *The traumatized hand and wrist,* ed 1, Philadelphia, 1992, WB Saunders.

Levinsohn EM, Palmer AK: Arthrography of the traumatized wrist. Correlation with radiography and carpal instability series. *Radiology* 146:647, 1983.

Manaster BJ: The clinical efficacy of triple-injection wrist arthrography. *Radiology* 178:267, 1991.

Mann FA, Wilson AJ, Gilula LA: Radiographic evaluation of the wrist: what does the hand surgeon want to know? *Radiology* 184:15, 1992.

Mauer AH: Nuclear medicine in evaluation of the hand and wrist. *Hand Clin* 7:183, 1991.

Metz VM, Mann FA, Gilula LA: Three compartment wrist arthrography: correlation of pain site with location of uni- and bidirectional communications. *AJR* 160:819, 1993.

Metz VM, Mann FA, Gilula LA: Lack of correlation between site of wrist pain and location of noncommunicating defects shown by three compartment wrist arthrography. *AJR* 160:1239, 1993.

Mikic Z: Age related changes in the triangular fibrocartilage of the wrist. *J Anat* 126:367, 1978.

Mino DE, Palmer AK, Levinsohn EM: The role of radiography and computerized tomography in the diagnosis of incongruity of the distal radio-ulnar joint. A prospective study. *J Hand Surg* [Am] 8:30, 1983.

Palmer AK: Triangular fibrocartilage lesions: a classification. *J Hand Surg [Am]* 14:594, 1989.

Resnick D: *Arthrography and tenography of the hand and wrist.* In Dalinka MK, editor: *Arthrography,* ed 1, New York, 1980, Springer Verlag.

Sartoris DJ, Resnick D: *Plain film radiography: routine and specialized techniques and projections.* In Resnick D, Niwayama G, editors: *Diagnosis of bone and joint disorders,* ed 2. Philadelphia, 1988, WB Saunders.

Schimmerl S, Schurawitzki H, Imhof H, et al.: Morbus Sudeck- MRT als neues diagnostisches Verfahren. *RFortschr Röntgenstr* 154:601, 1991.

Stewart NR, Gilula LA: CT of the wrist: a tailored approach. *Radiology* 183:13, 1992.

Taleisnik J, *Radiographic examination of the wrist.* In J Taleisnik, editor: *The wrist.* ed 1, New York, 1985, Churchill Livingstone.

Totterman SM, Miller R, Wasserman B, et al.: Intrinsic and extrinsic carpal ligaments: evaluation by three-dimensional Fourier transform MR imaging. *AJR* 160:117, 1993.

Totty WG, Gilula LA: *Imaging of the hand and wrist.* In Gilula LA, editor: *The traumatized hand and wrist,* ed 1, Philadelphia, 1992, WB Saunders.

Truong NP, Mann FA, Gilula LA, Kang SW: Wrist instability series: increased yield with clinical-radiologic screening criteria. *Radiology* 192:481, 1994.

Wilson AJ, Gilula LA, Mann FA: Unidirectional joint communication in wrist arthrography: an evaluation of 250 cases. *AJR* 157:105, 1991.

4

Skin and Soft Tissue Injury of the Upper Extremity

Thomas J. Francel, MD, FACS

The skin and soft tissue are essential components for useful functioning of the upper extremity. Even "insignificant" injuries to the skin and/or poor soft tissues may dramatically impair upper extremity function. There is no excess skin on the extremities; therefore, small skin defects may require more extensive surgical intervention than initially anticipated. Scar formation after complete wound healing may limit the excursion of the motor units or involve cutaneous nerves, which can lead to a painful extremity. Loss of soft tissue may leave vital structures exposed (e.g., nerves, arteries, tendons), resulting in injury to these structures because of desiccation. The closure and healing of skin and soft tissue of the upper extremity should be addressed early and correctly.

The skin of the upper extremity is characterized by a high density of sense organs. Quickly adapting fiber receptors (i.e., Pacinian and Meissner's corpuscles) sense touch and vibration. These are tested by moving two-point discrimination and object identification. Slowly adapting receptors (i.e., the Merkel cell complex) sense constant touch and pressure. This is tested by static two-point discrimination. Many sensory receptors are present at the base of the hair follicles on the dorsum of the hand and forearm. There are marked differences between the palmar and dorsal skin of the hand. The palmar skin cushions the forces generated during gripping. The thinner dorsal skin permits more movement and allows for venous and lymphatic vessel distension to improve drainage of the hand.

Another interesting anatomic variation between the palmar and dorsal skin involves the blood supply. The nourishing arteries and venous system are axial on the dorsum of the hand, but tend to be more vertically oriented on the palm. Therefore, a short palmar flap may be devascularized by a shear injury, whereas a much longer dorsal flap will tolerate extensive undermining and survive intact. Reconstructive surgeons utilize this difference by employing random dorsal skin flaps for soft tissue coverage. Palmar based skin flaps require direct neurovascular pedicles (e.g., the Moberg advancement flap) for viable transfers.

There are some very specialized soft tissue structures within the upper extremity. The septa in the fingertip pulp distribute shear forces and pressure, and are similar to the plantar surface of the foot. Pulp stability is required in the fingertip to endure the pinch mechanism, as well as the extreme shearing that occurs when you place your fingertip onto the surface of an object and push. The palmar skin has many vertical septa to the palmar fascia. This allows for the best functional grip and keeps the skin tense over the object that is held. The nails and the nailbed of the fingers also are very specialized. The nails protect the delicate fingertip pad, contribute to sensation, and enhance the ability to pick up fine objects. Nails support the fingertip pad beyond the end of the distal bony phalanx. A deformed nail also is very noticeable from the cosmetic viewpoint.

In discussing soft tissue injuries, it is essential to point out that the underlying structural support for the soft tissue of the upper extremity is the bone. Many aspects of bone reduction and healing need to be addressed to obtain the best possible soft tissue reconstruction of an upper extremity injury. This supportive scaffolding needs to be replaced correctly to allow better draping of the soft tissue and skin. An early bone deformity followed by secondarily soft tissue contracture is very difficult to correct at a later time. Therefore, correct bone reduction and healing should be addressed early in the patient care plan.

Soft tissue reconstruction must address blood supply, tendons, muscles, and nerves. These structures are all located within the soft tissue of the extremity and must be reconstructed individually to obtain the best functional result. The upper extremity blood supply from the elbow distally is redundant (radial and ulnar). Therefore, an injury isolated to a single vessel may not require repair unless evidence exists of vascular compromise to the distal structures. Smooth tendon excursion allows for very precise movements of the hand. This is facilitated by an overlying synovium that allows for easy gliding and a pulley system that directs the forces of flexion. The muscles of the upper extremity include the intrinsic muscles of the hand and the larger extrinsic muscles of the forearm. Function and coordination of the individual motor tendons and nerves is important. The nerves of the upper extremity continue distally through the soft tissues to end in sense organs at the skin level. They also contribute fine motor control required for good upper extremity function. The nerves tend to accompany the vessels and therefore, any type of injury to vessels or nerves is particularly significant because an injury to either probably means an injury to both.

Aesthetic outcome also is important in soft tissue reconstruction. This may require replacing damaged skin, with a consideration for dermal thickness and sensory organs. The reconstructive surgeon must consider the thickness of the tissue used for reconstruction because many areas of the upper extremity are extremely thin. Adding bulky replacement tissue would be very unsightly, and the available donor sites are limited.

The first three sections of this chapter address the initial evaluation and treatment of acute and chronic injuries. They concentrate on emergency room treatments and the initial hospitalization. The last section is dedicated to more complicated reconstructions that should be done by an experienced hand surgeon. These include skin grafts and the multiple flaps that are available for soft tissue replacement.

EVALUATION OF WOUNDS

Early during the evaluation of a hand injury, the patient must be examined completely to exclude other injuries. This includes life-threatening injuries that would take precedence over the upper extremity injury. In following the protocols of Acute Trauma Life Support, an injury that is life threatening needs to be treated before consideration is given to limb-threatening injuries. It often is impossible to directly address the extremity injury while the patient is being resuscitated for other major organ injuries.

History and Physical Examination

Personal History

Employment and hand dominance are the most important information that can be obtained from the patient early in the evaluation. These should be listed in the first section of the History and Physical (i.e.; "a right-hand dominant 34-year-old carpenter . . ."). This important information will communicate to the treating physician the implications of the patients' injury. An injury to a dominant hand of a carpenter will be more functionally significant than an injury to a dominant hand in a person who is employed in a management position. Also, injuries to nondominant hands tend to be overcome more easily by the patient than injuries to the dominant hand.

Mechanism of Injury

The history of the injury itself is important in determining future treatment. The initial evaluation should include the time of the injury, as well as conditions since the time of the injury. A good example would be a sharp fingertip amputation that occurred approximately 2 hours ago, in which the part has been kept cooled since the initial accident. The position of the digits in the hand at the time of injury is important to document. A tendon injury that occurs when a patient is grasping a sharp object will be at a different level than an injury that occurs if a patient falls with an open hand onto a piece of glass. If the fingers are flexed at the time of injury, the tendon laceration occurs distal to the entrance wound on the skin. This type of injury requires more extensive soft tissue exposure to adequately repair. More limited excursions of the extensor tendons and the fibrous connections between them makes position at the time of injury less important for dorsal injuries.

The mechanism of injury also is an important determinant in predicting severity and guiding treatment. In general, quick sharp injuries fare better than those resulting from tearing or crushing. A crush injury subjects the surrounding tissues to periods of ischemia and extremes of pressure. Crush injuries often require more extensive debridement and are more likely to damage multiple functional components of the upper extremity. An important factor in considering the mechanism of injury is the degree of energy dissipated into the soft tissues. A low-velocity injury, such as a fall, will have very minimal energy transferred into the surrounding tissues. As a result, an early reconstruction may be performed. In contrast, a very high-energy injury may involve structural damage that is not initially apparent. A good example of this is a forearm fracture caused by a crush mechanism. Often the initial debridement does not reveal the full extent of the injury. A second or third exploration and debridement is required to remove all of the devitalized structures. Premature reconstruction following a high-energy crush injury will be hampered by subsequent complications and will achieve a less desirable functional result.

Environmental Contamination

The contamination of the wound also should be ascertained during the initial history. A sharp laceration by a kitchen knife is different than a sharp laceration in a factory. The degree of contamination of the wound may dictate therapeutic interventions, such as leaving a contaminated wound open to allow some "cleaning" of the wound before definitive closure. A good example is a laceration over the metacarpal heads on the dorsum of the hand. This occurs most commonly when a patient's fist encounters a tooth when striking someone's mouth. This laceration should not be closed, because the incidence of septic joint after this type of injury is very high. Rather, it should be left open and the area irrigated. This subject will be addressed further when individual complex penetrating injuries are discussed.

Of utmost importance in all injuries is the tetanus immunization of the patient. In previously immunized patients with a clean wound and an immunization less than 10 years previously, no injection is needed. If it is a dirty wound with an immunization more than 5 years old, then often a toxoid injection is given. In patients who have not been immunized previously and who have a clean wound, a toxoid injection regimen is started. In patients who have not been immunized previously and who have a contaminated, dirty wound, a toxoid injection regimen is started, and 50 units of human tetanus immunoglobulin is given (Table 4-1). All of these patients require early follow-up to evaluate their wounds within a few days after injury.

Physical Examination

After a patient's tetanus status is confirmed, the patient's history is obtained and the mechanism of the injury is learned, the patient should be examined as described in Chapter 2. A stepwise progressive examination is important because the structures must be evaluated in

Table 4-1   Tetanus Immunization Guideline ·

Previously immunized patient	
Clean wound, immunization <10 yr ago	No injection needed
Dirty wound, immunization >5 yr ago	Toxoid injection
Patient not previously immunized	
Clean wound	Toxoid injection
Dirty wound	Toxoid injection and 50 units of human tetanus immune globulin (HTIG)

a particular order; it often is difficult to turn back. Frequently, before the hand surgeon arrives, multiple examiners have elicited a painful response from the patient. Therefore, the final examination is limited by secondary pain or the patient's anticipation of pain. Therefore, the initial examination is very important, as are consecutive follow-up examinations by the same examiner. The physical examiner needs to observe the posturing of the hand, as well as the viability of the tissues. A vascular examination is required of all patients, and nerve testing should be done to exclude sensory and motor nerve damage. The nerve deficits should be diagrammed to better portray the extent of the injury. If tendons are injured, the examination should include testing of the superficialis as well as the profundus tendons. The forearm muscles need to be examined, along with the intrinsic muscles in the hand.

Examination of the combative, comatose, or young patient can be difficult. Examining the posture of the hand probably is the most important test in evaluating the extent of tendon injuries. Compression of the forearm musculature also will allow the tendons to move; an absence of movement can be used to determine the extent of tendon injury. This method of examination is particularly effective with children because it avoids any type of pressure or pain at the area of injury. The presence (or lack) of sweating is an excellent test for distinguishing nerve injuries in an otherwise unreliable patient, such as a child, because it does not illicit the painful response associated with pin-prick testing.

Antibiotic Therapy

After examination of the patient and the extent of the injuries, it is appropriate to decide whether antibiotics should be started. The degree of contamination needs to be considered before exposing the patient to the risk of antibiotics. These risks include anaphylaxis, development of resistant organisms, and a superinfection with fungus. If a vital structure is exposed, some type of antibiotic coverage should be initiated. Injury to poorly vascularized tissue, including bone cortex and tendons, and the presence of marginally viable soft tissues also suggest the need for antibiotic coverage. In patients who have open fractures associated with soft tissue injuries, antibiotic coverage has been shown to decrease the risk of osteomyelitis.

Appropriate initial antibiotic therapy includes giving the patient an initial dose of an intravenous first-generation cephalosporin, followed by oral antibiotic therapy. If the patient has a penicillin allergy or an allergy to cephalosporins, then another appropriate antibiotic may be selected. In certain instances, it is more appropriate to initiate broader coverage that may include better gram-negative coverage or anaerobic coverage. This is especially important after farm equipment injuries, where contamination is heavy as a result of exposure to many gram-negative organisms and anaerobic bacteria. Patients with diabetes also tend to have mixed flora infections, including gram-negative organisms.

Radiographic Evaluation

After the examination is completed, X-rays are obtained. Remove all jewelry on the hand before taking X-rays because the jewelry may obscure some bony injuries. Also, the patients should remove all jewelry before swelling, because jewelry may serve as a constrictor and thereby compromise the vascularity of the extremity. The appropriate X-rays to be obtained will be covered in more detail in Chapter 3.

TREATMENT OF ACUTE INJURIES

Preparation

Control of Bleeding

A tourniquet may be necessary to control bleeding during repair of the injury and should be in place before the preparation of the skin. The longest time that a tourniquet may be inflated is approximately 2 hours. After 2 hours, there is significant soft tissue injury secondary to ischemia and injury to the tissues directly beneath the tourniquet. Before 2 hours, the patient may have a significant amount of ischemic pain, which could be an indication that injury may be in progress. A tourniquet should only be used to control obvious bleeding; it should be released to repair the injury. With the combination of a tourniquet and a pressure dressing, hemostasis should be obtained. If this cannot be accomplished, the patient should be taken immediately to the operating room.

Lighting

Adequate lighting is a requirement. An adjustable mobile light is the most practical one for use in the emergency room. The physician repairing the injury should be as comfortable as possible and should have a chair available so that these repairs are not done while the patient is standing.

Skin Preparation

The fibroblasts in the wound are as sensitive as bacteria to destruction after exposure to most antiseptic solutions. This includes betadine and hydrogen peroxide. For this reason, it is more appropriate to use betadine on the surrounding skin that is intact to decrease colonization in the area and use sterile saline to irrigate the open wound to remove as much contamination as possible. This may be delivered by a syringe and an angiocath. In the severely contaminated wound, a very dilute betadine solution may be most appropriate.

Repair and Closure

Equipment Setup

Uncomplicated lacerations often are closed in the emergency room. The most important thing is preparation before initiating closure of these wounds. A Mayo stand should be set up, with the sterile equipment placed on it. A tourniquet may be necessary to control bleeding during the repair and should be in place before preparation of the skin. An additional light stand may be necessary to give cross-lighting and prevent shadows within the operative field. Magnification equipment should be available. It often is required to visualize the vital structures deep to the skin and to allow precise placement of sutures. This should all be set up before preparation of the sterile field. Sterile drapes are used to keep the operative field sterile. A wide sterile field is required so that the ends of the sutures, as well as the instruments, are always on the sterile field. This is especially important between the Mayo stand and the sterile field, where the tails of the suture often may drag across the contaminated skin or clothing (Fig. 4-1).

Local Anesthesia

The local anesthetic employed when treating an upper extremity injury should not contain epinephrine/adrenaline. This is especially true if a finger or a hand block is being performed, because epinephrine constricts the arteries within the area and may lead to ischemia of the digit/hand. In all upper extremity work, a solution of plain lidocaine or marcaine is recommended for local anesthesia. Under appropriate supervision, IV Regional Anesthesia (Bier Block) also may be employed in the emergency room, but individuals using this method of local anesthesia need to be experienced with the technique as well as proper management of potential complications.

Uncomplicated Lacerations

Closure of an uncomplicated laceration is best done with loose, simple, monofilament permanent sutures. These sutures have the least

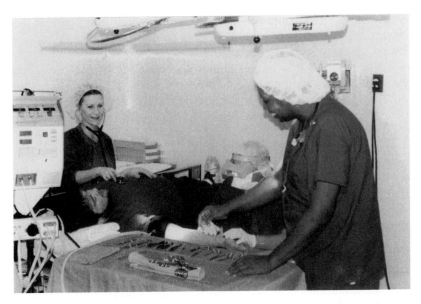

Figure 4-1   A mock set-up in the emergency rooms shows an almost ideal situation. The treating physician has a magnifying apparatus on his head. Such an apparatus should easily be available. Also note that the patient has a tourniquet in place in case extra bleeding is encountered, and all the instruments are well within reach of both the surgeon and the assistant. A different assistant is caring for the patient. Also note that adequate lighting is available.

amount of tissue reaction, as well as the least amount of tissue trauma with passage of the suture material. The use of permanent sutures also encourages follow-up, which should be done in the office of a hand specialist.

The closure of uncomplicated lacerations should be free of any tension. Because the extremities have very little extra skin, a tight closure indicates a more extensive injury with skin loss or significant edema and is likely to result in more complications if closed primarily. This includes the development of infection and tissue necrosis at the areas that were sutured together under tension. In this case, it is more important to leave the wound open and allow dressing changes than to further compromise the surrounding tissues, especially in a very strategic location. A tight closure of a wound may extend the tissue damage and cause local necrosis, which can lead to a much more difficult problem than was present before the initiation of treatment. Usually an uncomplicated closure does not require placement of any deep sutures. If deep suturing is required, then a second examination should be performed to make sure that the function of the extremity is intact. Sometimes there is a laceration of the muscle bellies, and the function will be normal. If this is the case, the fascia over the muscle belly may be closed, but this is not necessary.

Follow-up of "uncomplicated lacerations" is mandatory. Frequently, injuries that were not noticed initially will become obvious on the second or third day postinjury. This includes partial lacerations of tendons, neuropraxias, and devitalized tissue. If there is any question at the time of closure, the patient should be reevaluated within 48 hours. This could be done as a follow-up in the emergency room, outpatient clinic, or the office of a hand specialist. The patient should have a minimum of one follow-up with the hand specialist to ensure that all the deep structures are functioning adequately. This may be done at the time of the initial suture removal, approximately 5 to 10 days after the injury, as dictated by location.

Complex Penetrating Injuries

Angiography

The evaluation of the deep vital structures is important with complex penetrating injuries. The initial evaluation is particularly significant because a patient will be less likely to cooperate fully during subsequent examinations. The integrity of arterial perfusion to the upper extremity needs to be documented. This may require an immediate arteriogram if there are no pulses or if the viability of the extremity is questionable. This may be performed in the radiology department, but some surgeons have advocated urgent exploration and intraoperative arteriogram because, in all probability, some type of an operative procedure will be required to revascularize the limb. The ischemic time of the extremity may be reduced if the patient does not have to go first to radiology and then to the operating room. This is a controversial issue, and the decision should be guided by an experienced hand surgeon.

Treatment

Once the integrity of the vital structures is confirmed, treatment of the injury itself may be started. Initially, the viability of the soft tissue needs to be evaluated, and the contamination of the wound mechanically addressed. After adequate anesthesia is obtained in the injured area, irrigation of the soft tissues is performed. This is most commonly done with sterile saline through a syringe and an angiocath. This develops enough pressure to adequately cleanse all but the dirtiest wounds. If the wound is large and heavily contaminated, then a mechanical irrigation device in the operating room is required. To determine the viability of soft tissue, rub the edge of the skin or muscle with a sponge.

If there is bleeding of any type from the dermis of the skin or the underlying muscle, the tissue should be considered viable until it is allowed to demarcate. At this time, it is very important to remove all foreign bodies (e.g., gravel) from a wound. Leaving debris will only encourage infection and may lead to traumatic tattooing of the area. This may be very difficult to correct at a later time. Traumatic tattooing is more easily prevented than it is treated.

If the patient is a poor anesthetic risk because of general health problems, other injuries, intoxication, or a full stomach, this may be performed in the emergency room. The wound may then be loosely closed with two or three sutures to prevent retraction of the skin, and the patient should be admitted to the hospital for continued intravenous antibiotics. At that time, the hand consultant should schedule a "second look" operation to be performed the following day when the patient is stable. At the very least, these wounds should be cleaned and closed loosely, and the hand placed in a functional splint to improve the comfort of the patient and prevent further injury with motion. The patient should be admitted and the hand elevated to allow adequate drainage, control edema, and prevent vascular compromise.

Stab Injuries

Stab injuries usually have entrance wounds that appear "insignificant" enough to be closed in the emergency room. These cases require an intensive, exact physical examination to determine the function of the extremity. Every nerve and tendon of the hand needs to be examined comprehensively, not just the structures around the entrance wound. The depth and direction of penetration is not apparent by looking and superficially examining the entrance wound. A very "insignificant" entrance wound at the wrist may have lacerated all of the tendons, nerves, and arteries at that level if the sharpened edge is pointed dorsally. Conversely, a large entrance wound may have minimal deeper injury if the sharpened edge is pointed volar to cut the skin, but the dull edge pushes the vital structures deeper and out of the path of harm. In general, the structures injured by a sharp mechanism may be repaired acutely because the energy dissipated into the surrounding tissues is minimal, and rarely is further tissue necrosis a problem over the following days.

Gunshot Wounds

Compared with stab injuries, only under very unusual circumstances should a gunshot wound be treated in the emergency room and the patient released. This is because the energy dissipated as a bullet transverses the soft tissue is proportional to the caliber and the speed of the projectile. This should be determined from the initial history given by the patient. A low-velocity shotgun injury may mimic a high-velocity, low-caliber rifle injury because the total energy transferred to the soft tissue may be equal. Surprisingly, tendons and nerves frequently are spared transection unless they are directly hit. Blood vessels and muscles also can be injured by a shock wave as a bullet pierces the soft tissue. These structures may respond with spasm and necrosis. Similarly, diffuse nerve damage can occur despite being structurally intact. Therefore, the extent of soft tissue injury is not appreciated initially and only becomes apparent over the ensuing days. Hospitalization, antibiotics, and operating room debridement usually are required after a gunshot wound to the upper extremity.

Bites

There is significant morbidity associated with bites of the upper extremity. As a general rule, these patients need a thorough examination, radiographs to rule out chip fractures or tooth fragments, extensive irrigation, and hospitalization with elevation, splinting, and intravenous antibiotics. Deviation from this rule may be considered in a compliant patient without deep involvement, who can be further examined within 24 hours, but this approach should be recommended cautiously. Tetanus immunization needs to be confirmed. Uniformly good results are seen in patients who seek care immediately after injury and receive the appropriate treatment.

Mammalian bites

Human bites of the hand should never be overlooked or downplayed because of the severe complications that can result if appropriate therapy is not instituted rapidly. These wounds are considered contaminated puncture wounds, with increased risk of tetanus and deep tissue involvement. Proper antibiotic treatment covers *Streptococcus, Staphylococcus,* and other aerobic oral organisms. Eikenella corrodens is an anaerobic gram-negative rod that exhibits synergism with *Streptococcus, Staphylococcus* aureus, bacteroides, and other gram-negative organisms. The morbidity in instances in which medical care is delayed is more severe. Penicillin and/or amoxicillin derivatives are recommended as initial therapy, with the addition of clindamycin and gentamycin if improvement is not rapidly apparent.

Special caution should be exercised with clenched-fist injuries. An examiner needs to be suspicious of any laceration over the dorsal aspect of the metacarpophalangeal joint, and this injury needs to be treated as a human bite until proven otherwise. The fist striking a mouth drives the tooth and its bacteria into the metacarpophalangeal joint, often through the extensor tendon (Fig. 4-2). When the fist is opened, the laceration of the tendon retracts proximally

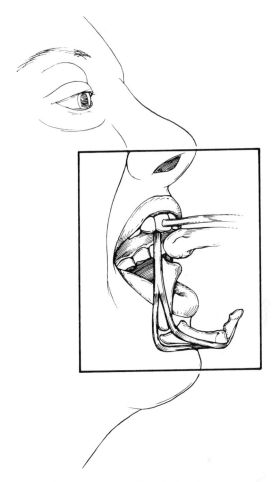

Figure 4-2   Clenched fist injuries usually involve the extensor tendon and may perforate through the dorsal capsule of the metacarpal phalangeal joint, exposing the joint to bacteria inoculum.

and seals over the puncture wound of the metacarpophalangeal joint capsule. Besides septic joint complications, the infection may spread with the extensor tendon to involve the lumbricals, interosseous muscles, and eventually the forearm. Early and aggressive operating room exploration and treatment will prevent septic arthritis, tenosynovitis, myositis, and osteomyelitis. A negative exploration in a high-risk patient more than outweighs the high morbidity if neglected.

Nonhuman mammalian bites deserve some special considerations. Antibiotics to cover domestic mammalian oral flora should appropriately treat alpha hemolytic streptococcus (dogs) and *Pasteurella* (cats). All wildlife species should be considered rabid after an unprovoked attack, and animal control authorities should be notified. The animal should be captured, killed, and analyzed. Domestic animals need to be quarantined and observed for 10 days. Previously immunized patients at significant risk require only two doses of human diploid cell vaccine (HDCV). Human rabies immune globulin (HRIG) is used with five to six doses of HDCV as the primary immunization after exposure. The vaccine may be stopped if the animal is determined by observation of brain tissue analysis to have been nonrabid. Local treatments for nonhuman mammalian bites include irrigation, debridement of nonviable tissue, dressings, and delayed closure. Appropriate dressings may consist of saline wet-to-dry dressings for active debridement, saline wet-to-wet over vital structures, or silver sulfadiazine in grossly contaminated wounds to decrease bacterial counts. Secondary repairs of tendons and nerves are performed after the wound has healed.

Nonmammalian bite

ENVENOMATION

Envenomation injuries usually are the result of nonmammalian bites. As a general principle, poisonous bites by nonmammals are painful compared with bites by nonpoisonous animals. Envenomation injuries in the United States are seldom mortal, although some have been associated with great soft tissue morbidity (i.e., bites from a brown recluse spider). Approximately 15 deaths per year occur from snakebites, mostly in the southern United States during the summer months.

URGENT CARE

Immediate care of reptilian bites includes placement of a lymphatic obstructing tourniquet, if it can be applied within 30 minutes of the injury. In conjunction with elevation of the extremity at the level of the heart, a *properly* placed tourniquet has been shown to decrease the spread of venom. Conditions of a properly placed tourniquet include allowing arterial inflow and intermittent venous outflow as well as the ability to get the victim to immediate care. Often in the field, a tourniquet is placed too tightly without the ability to get the victim to the emergency room for definitive care before ischemia develops in the soft tissues (especially the more sensitive muscle and nerve tissues). This greatly increases the morbidity of the affected limb. An incision into the subcutaneous tissue at the site of envenomation and suction may be helpful if the victim can be treated within 30 minutes after the envenomation injury. For obvious reasons, the person performing suction should be free of breaks in the oral mucosa. This is one of the rare hand injuries for which ice should *not* be applied. Studies show that cooling the extremity potentiates the local necrotic effect of the snake venom. Laboratory tests done immediately on admission should include a complete blood count, coagulation studies, electrolytes, blood sugar, renal function tests, urine analysis, and a type and crossmatch. The complete blood count and platelet count should be tracked several times a day for the first few days, and all urine samples should be tested for myoglobin.

ANTIVENOM

Once the victim arrives in the emergency department, antivenom should be initiated for significant injuries. Briefly, the envenomation therapy consists of continuous intravenous drip of North American Coral snake antivenom for eastern coral snakes (without evidence of fang marks) and polyvalent antivenom for all other pit viper snake bites (with fang marks present). Some surgeons have recommended full-thickness excision of the skin and subcutaneous tissue for severe envenomation injuries to decrease and/or remove the toxic load to the victim. This is difficult to perform within time constraints of venom spread and requires delayed reconstruction.

COMPLICATIONS

If the venom has spread significantly into the hand or forearm, edema and necrosis may contribute to elevated pressures within the compartments. Intracompartmental pressures of the interosseous, thenar, carpal tunnel, and forearm fascial compartments must be recorded for any question or compartment syndrome. Pressures greater than 30 mmHg require release of the constricting fascia. If pressures cannot be recorded and paraesthesias are present, a release is mandated. Prompt treatment of increased compartment pressures should not be delayed even if measurements are inconclusive, particularly when clinical findings strongly suggest impending compartment syndrome.

Spider bites

Significant spider bites usually are attributed to the Black Widow or Brown Recluse spiders. The Black Widow spider (distinguished by the red hourglass on the black body) envenomation actually causes little local soft tissue injury. Systemic signs of envenomation require antispasmodics (diazepam and methocarbamol), narcotics, and calcium gluconate.

The Brown Recluse spider (brown fiddle on a brown body) bite, in contrast, causes severe soft tissue necrosis. Classically, the patient does not remember the initial injury, but recently was working in a previously undisturbed area (e.g., attic, basement, garden, or woodshed). During the ensuing 24 to 48 hours, the patient starts to have severe pain and erythema at the envenomation site. This is when they usually come to the emergency room. Some physicians recommend early excision of envenomated areas to decrease subsequent necrosis, although on a practical level, this area is difficult to determine initially. It may be more prudent to delay excision until after the definitive degree of necrosis has been established. Oral dapsone frequently is recommended to reduce ongoing inflammation, followed by late excision of the most severely damaged soft tissue. Skin grafting frequently is required to reconstruct the soft tissue defect.

Injection Injuries

Injection injuries with paint or petroleum products are associated with high morbidity. Patients demonstrate an apparently minor skin disruption, with rapid progression toward a hand-extremity-threatening emergency requiring aggressive surgical interventions. A key to timely recognition is pursuing the history of the injury. This includes the force of the injection as well as the material involved. If the pressure is low, the material may not be injected deeply. However, a high-pressure gun may inject material following planes into the hand, through the carpal tunnel, and proximally into the forearm. It is crucial to not let a minor entrance wound lull the examiner into believing that the deep tissues and planes have not been violated because significant tissue damage and digital loss can ensue. The physical examination should document the entrance wound, neurovascular status of the extremity and digits, and active range of motion. Circumferential measurements should be made and reviewed. Compartment pressure measurements may be indicated. X-rays may delineate the extent of the injury if the material is radiopaque and can be visualized within the planes of dissection.

Because the injection of air or water is less injurious to the tissue, surrounding soft tissue damage is not as great. Air and water, even if injected under high pressure along tissue planes, are less toxic to the tissues than paint or petroleum, and the tissue response is less severe. Therefore, edema and swelling are less, and tissues may not be compromised. Elevation and close observation are indicated. If the limb shows progressive edema and compartment signs (i.e., impaired vascularity, increasing pain or tenderness, or decreasing sensation), immediate surgical intervention is required.

In contrast to air and water injections, the high-pressure injection of paint or petroleum products (e.g., grease) requires immediate surgical attention. Paint and petroleum products result in more local tissue inflammation than air or water, and therefore, the injury progresses rapidly. These products start a vicious pathway of (1) local tissue injury, (2) inflammation, (3) edema and compression within fascial compartments, and (4) vascular and neurologic compromise. Rapid intervention is mandatory to prevent further compression of vital structures and improve the opportunity to salvage the limb. Operative decompression requires excision of the entrance site and release of all involved fascial planes. This includes the digits (midaxial release is preferred by the author), palm, and carpal tunnel. If required, this should extend to releasing the forearm compartments. This also should include the interosseous muscle compartments. All nonviable tissue and foreign material should be removed carefully, as prolonged contact with paint or grease will increase tissue damage. All open wounds should then be irrigated copiously with antibiotic solution under pulsatile pressure. The skin of larger wounds may be loosely closed over Penrose drains. If there is any question as to the viability of the tissue of these wounds, they should be left open and a "second look" operation planned within 24 hours. The extremity is loosely dressed and splinted.

Postoperative treatment includes elevation and intravenous antibiotics for broad-spectrum coverage. The wounds must be inspected frequently to determine whether there is ongoing injury and necrosis. Often, additional operative explorations are needed to further debride nonviable tissues. Hand therapy for active and passive range of motion should be started soon after establishing control of the infection. Most significant injection injuries develop functional loss, and early therapy may minimize the deficit. Wounds are closed secondarily according to principles outlined later in this chapter.

Reconstruction

An early consultation with an experienced hand surgeon is imperative whenever a complex penetrating injury to the hand occurs. This is especially true after gunshot wounds, bites, envenomations, and injection injuries because these injuries result in extensive soft tissue destruction and exposure of vital structures. Changing an acute, complex injury into a chronic wound should be avoided. This will be addressed further in the section on neglected wounds later in this chapter. Briefly, if a wound is allowed to become chronic in nature, function is compromised. This occurs because of (1) the scarring of tissue beds required for gliding and (2) the further debridement of involved tissues to obtain fresh tissue for primary healing. Soft tissue defects need to be filled early with healthy, well-vascularized tissue to achieve primary healing. Early reconstruction may be required to maintain function.

BURNS

Stabilization

Physiologic stabilization of the patient is of utmost importance after arrival at the hospital if the hand burn is associated with a greater than 20% total body surface area burn. This includes the basic "ABCs" of resuscitation. The airway is stabilized, including placement of an endotracheal tube if there is evidence of upper airway compromise (e.g., hoarseness, soot, history of smoke inhalation at the burn site); intravenous access is established by at least two large peripheral lines; and fluid resuscitation is started. Physiologic monitoring is begun, including use of a urinary catheter, cardiac monitoring, peripheral oxygen saturation, and a gastric decompression tube to monitor gastrointestinal function and prevent stress ulcerations. More extensive burns may require a Swan–Ganz monitor or an indwelling arterial catheter. After patient stabilization, the depth and area of the burn are assessed (rule of nines, Lund–Browder chart). Fluid resuscitation is then tailored to a formula [Parkland formula (lactated ringers solution at 4 ml/kg per percent burn) or hypertonic saline at the Parkland rate]. Half of this fluid resuscitation is given during the first 8 hours after the burn. Fluid administration is tailored appropriately based on physiologic monitoring of vital signs, urine output, sensorium, and so on. Emergency procedures to correct a threatened life or limb need to be performed early in patient care. These include a cricothyroidotomy or tracheostomy, escharotomies, fasciotomies, or debridement of necrotic muscle compartments. Tetanus prophylaxis must be addressed. Electrical and chemical burns will be addressed individually later in this chapter.

Thermal Burns of the Hand

Minor Burns

Burns of the hand need to be treated correctly to prevent severe deformities and loss of function. Minor burns, which frequently are seen in the emergency room, include cooking burns, barbecue burns, and hot water accidents. First- and second-degree burns are treated with local topical therapy, and patients are released with analgesia. Local therapy includes topical antibiotics (usually sulfadiazine) changed twice a day, nonadherent impregnated gauze, and elevation of the extremity. These patients require a follow-up visit within 48 hours to check that there is no streptococcal infection and that wound healing is progressing satisfactorily. Penicillin is indicated if the burn is erythematous and very tender, with signs of a local infectious process. A follow-up examination should check for edema and make sure that the digits and hands are not compromised vascularly. Minor first- and second-degree burns usually heal with minimal sequelae.

Deep Dermal Burns

In contrast, any third-degree burn to the hand requires hospitalization and a team approach, including stabilization, if needed, a hand surgeon, and a hand therapist. It is better to err on the conservative side, encouraging hospitalization to prevent the conversion of a partial-thickness to full-thickness burn because of inadequate care and subsequent infection.

Dorsal hand burns

The most common third-degree burns occur in conjunction with other burns, usually on the dorsum of the hand as the victim clutches his hand in the fetal position at the time of the burn. Obviously, in this position, the skin most frequently injured extends from the proximal interphalangeal (PIP) joint to the wrist. Unfortunately, this also is the thinnest skin on the hand and burns in this area frequently extend through the dermis to involve the tendons, joint capsule, and metacarpal bone (fourth degree). Deep dermal burns of the dorsum of the hand frequently result in severe hypertrophic scarring and restricted motion. Therefore, if it does not appear that the burned skin will heal in 3 weeks, the burn is aggressively excised early and soft tissue coverage is achieved by one of several methods.

Volar hand burns

Isolated palm burns are rare and occur because the patient either has grasped a hot object or has fallen onto an outstretched hand into a fire, furnace, or oven. Because the dermis of the palm skin is thick, full-thickness burns are rare. When they do occur, they usually are the result of prolonged contact. The grasping hand cannot release the object because of an adhesion that develops between the burned skin and the hot object. This same mechanism occurs with cold injuries. Palmar skin usually reepithelializes quickly, but if it appears that it will not heal within 3 weeks, aggressive debridement and full-thickness skin grafting has been recommended.

Escharotomies

Burn resuscitation requires large amounts of fluid to maintain perfusion to vital organs. The increased permeability of the capillaries to crystalloid tends to result in significant edema and swelling throughout the body. If this occurs in conjunction with a circumferential burn eschar on the extremity, it induces a tourniquet effect and may com-

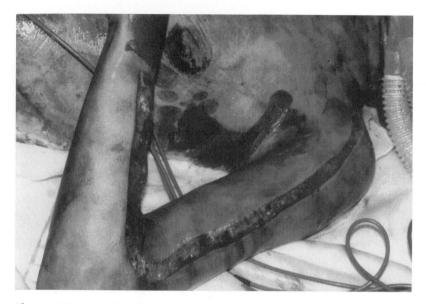

Figure 4-3   Lateral escharotomies of an elderly patient after a circumferential burn that has compromised the blood flow to the left hand.

promise the vital structures of the extremity. It is imperative that the examiner consider this and when detected, correct it promptly with escharotomies. Palpable pulses at the wrist conform blood flow to this level, but Doppler ultrasound examinations are necessary to confirm flow in the palmar arch, and the individual digits. If at any time during resuscitation these Doppler signals become absent, or diminished, intervention is mandated. Treatment modalities include correcting hypovolemia, relaxing secondary peripheral vascular constriction, and release of eschar restriction. Reduction of sensation also is an important indicator that the limb may be compromised, but this can be confusing if the burns are deep and involve sensory receptors, or if the burns are electrical with direct nerve damage. Intracompartmental pressures greater than 30 mmHg also are an indication for aggressive surgical decompression. Adequate escharotomies may be performed at the bedside with electrocautery, good lighting, and hemostats (Fig. 4-3). An eschar is insensitive and therefore, local injection usually is not necessary. In general, a release of a constricting eschar of the upper extremity starts proximally in the lateral arm, crosses the elbow along the lateral flexion crease, continues to the radial aspect of the wrist flexion crease, and extends along the radial aspect of the thenar muscles onto the radial aspect of the thumb (Fig. 4-4). If pulses do not return after

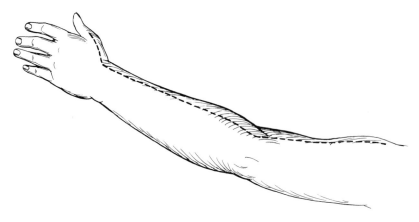

Figure 4-4   Medial escharotomies, as outlined, should continue down the arm and into the hand.

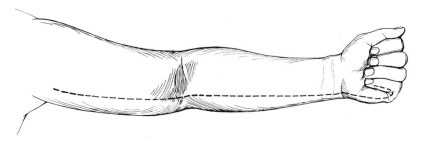

Figure 4-5   Lateral escharotomies continue down across the elbow and along the ulnar aspect of the hand and little finger.

this procedure, a medial escharotomy should be performed. A medial escharotomy starts in the axilla, crosses the elbow above the medial epicondyle, and can extend distally to the ulnar aspect of the little finger (Fig. 4-5). Interosseous releases are accomplished through vertical incisions on the dorsum of the hand between the metacarpals. The carpal tunnel also should be released to avoid acute compression and median nerve injury. Digital escharotomies are performed via ulnar midaxial incisions dorsal to neurovascular bundles. If the escharotomies are performed adequately, the Doppler signals should immediately improve. The escharotomies are then covered with topical antibiotics and loosely dressed without circumferential bandages. The skin of the carpal tunnel is loosely closed with two or three nylon sutures to avoid desiccation of the median nerve. The extremity is then elevated to control edema.

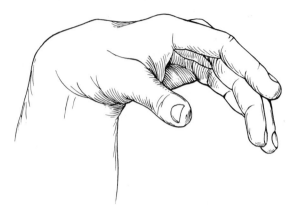

Figure 4-6   The injured patient often will hold the hand in a flexed position at the wrist, with the fingers extended. This decreases the lymphatic outflow and causes marked dorsal swelling and hyperextension of the metacarpal phalangeal joints.

Splinting and Therapy

When the extremity is injured, the hand resorts to the "wounded paw" position (Fig. 4-6), which is characterized by flexion of the wrist, extension of the metacarpophalangeal joints, and flexion of the interphalangeal joints. This position increases edema and swelling over the dorsum of the hand and fingers, which further compromises the hand. To prevent this deformity, place the hand in a splint within 24 hours of the burn. The splint should maintain the wrist in approximately 20° of extension, the metacarpophalangeal joints in approximately 45° of flexion, and the interphalangeal joints in approximately 10° of flexion. The thumb needs to be placed in abduction to prevent thumb web contracture (Fig. 4-7). Active motion against rubberband traction may be initiated to keep the joints supple. Severe passive flexion should be avoided to prevent rupture of the extensor tendons, which may be injured in a full-thickness dorsal skin burn. In deep burns involving the metacarpophalangeal joint capsules, most physicians advocate K-wire stabilization of the metacarpophalangeal joint at approximately 80° of flexion. This also has the advantage of placing the metacarpophalangeal joint in a position that assures adequate dorsal skin coverage. This permits full metacarpophalangeal flexion.

Surgical Treatment

Early Excision and Grafting

Deep dermal burns will not heal in 3 weeks because of damage to the dermal elements. Treatment of these burns requires excision and

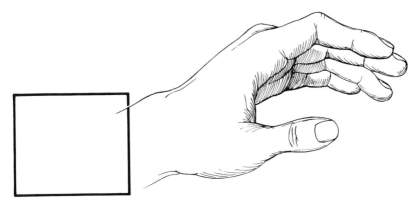

Figure 4-7   When in doubt, the safest splinting position of the hand is in the position of function. This places the wrist at 30°, the metacarpal phalangeals at 60°, the PIP joints at 10°, and the DIP joints at 5°.

grafting. Excision of the burn is best performed by tangential excision with a guarded knife or dermatome. The wound/eschar is excised in layers until punctate dermal bleeding is visible. This indicates viable remaining tissue. With deeper burns, full-thickness excision of the burn eschar is performed in the adventitial plane above the dorsal veins and peritenon of the extensor tendons. These two methods leave a viable bed for split-thickness skin grafting. Deeper burns require distant nonburn soft tissue transfers by pedicle or free microvascular transfer to replace adequate tissue for future tendon grafting. Care must be taken to prevent web contractures or burn syndactyly deformities because these are very difficult to correct secondarily. It is crucial that ample healthy soft tissue in the area is provided to allow for later reconstruction.

Full-thickness burns to the palm and volar aspects of the digits are unusually rare because of the thick dermis in these areas. If they do occur and it is obvious that they will not heal in approximately 3 weeks, excision and full-thickness skin grafting has been advocated.

The hand should be immobilized during skin graft adherence, and then an aggressive range of motion should be started to maintain pliable joint skin.

Secondary Burn Deformities and Reconstruction

Anticipation and prevention will reduce the need for secondary reconstructive procedures. This includes adequate therapy to maintain joint motion, prevention of hypertrophic scarring by aggressive excision and grafting, and placing thicker grafts on the areas where there is significant motion (metacarpophalangeal joints or proximal interphalangeal joints). The patient needs to be counseled that the time to full recovery is extended. Individual aspects need to be addressed in the correct order. A patient may wonder why the reconstructive surgeon is concentrating on repairing the soft tissue when the tendons and nerves have not been addressed. Reestablishing soft, pliable tissue is necessary before tendon or nerve grafts can be placed because the grafts will not function without a well-vascularized bed from which to obtain nourishment. Also, scar contractures limit the range of motion, and the joint must have motion before force can be applied across the joint by tendons for motion. The timing of reconstructive procedures also is important. Bilateral procedures probably should not be performed simultaneously. As much as possible, the procedures should be accomplished before the patient is discharged, so the patient can work closely with hospital support staff.

A few specific points of reconstruction need to be addressed. The tissue used (i.e., skin grafts, abdominal flaps, groin flap, free microtransfers) depends on the surgeon; excellent results have been realized using a variety of techniques. The contracted skin underestimates the size of the full defect, which is often much larger than anticipated. Therefore, flaps must be large enough to cover the joint without tension as it progresses through the range of motion. The palmar skin is rarely excised because even damaged skin has a significantly higher number of sensory receptors than transferred soft tissue. The palmar scar is released over the flexion crease by incision, and the defect is covered with soft tissue. Correction of the dorsal hooding, traumatic burn syndactyly, and first web adduction contractures usually require local flaps, if available, as well as skin grafting.

Electrical Burns

Initial Evaluation

The hand is most frequently the entrance site in electrical injuries, which travel under the skin to the forearm and more proximal regions. The entrance site usually is small, but the injury extends through the tissue supplying the least resistance (i.e., muscle and nerve). Another frequent area of localized skin injury is the elbow. During most injuries, the elbow is slightly flexed. As a result, the electricity can arc across the flexion crease, causing extensive skin injury. There often are associated thermal burns if clothing catches fire and the victim loses consciousness. Circumferential burn eschars are common because the unconscious victim cannot extinguish the flames. X-rays also should be taken to search for fractures from cationic contractions of the muscles against joints secondary to the electrical voltage. Peripheral nerves have a high potential for recovery, and nerve release should be performed early to prevent secondary compression disorders. This is especially prudent because sensation testing is an unreliable indicator after electrical injury. Cardiac monitoring often is necessary because of associated arrhythmias.

Treatment

In electrical injuries, muscle necrosis must be excluded by checking the urine for myoglobin and hemoglobin, because such injuries can lead to loss of limb and renal failure. The use of mannitol and bicarbonate to alkalinize the urine will promote rapid diuresis. The extremity must be elevated and vascular status closely monitored by Doppler pulses and compartment pressures. Extensive muscle necrosis causes marked swelling within the fascial planes, and full-extremity fasciotomies frequently are required. The full extent of muscle necrosis is not realized at the initial debridements, and multiple "second-look" operations often are required. The clinical picture of muscle twitching, normal muscle color, and bleeding help to determine viability and may be enhanced by the intraoperative addition of intravenous fluorescein to assist in establishing lines of demarcation. The wounds are left open and dressed with topical physiologic dressings. Topical antibiotics are used on the associated thermal burns. Secondary wound closure by skin grafting usually is accomplished, although soft tissue transfers may be necessary.

Chemical Burns

The depth of chemical burns is related directly to the length of contact with the offending agent. These agents may induce damage long after the initial contact by progressing into the dermis. Extensive chemical burns require physiologic stabilization. The initial stabilization includes immediate irrigation of the burned skin with copious amount of saline to remove or dilute the offending agent. Some antidotes or neutralizers have been described (Table 4-2), but if these are

Table 4-2   Treatment of Common Chemical Burns

Agent	Common Use	Treatment
Phenols	Disinfectant and laboratory material	Ethyl alcohol or polyethylene glycol
Hydrofluric acid	Glass etching	Subcutaneous calcium injections
Lime	Soil alkalizer and mechanical removal	Water irrigation
White phosphorous	An incendiary	1% copper sulphate irrigation

not readily available, saline or water irrigation is good initial therapy. Like envenomation injuries, some physicians have advocated early, urgent excision of the involved skin and dermis to remove the agent, followed by a secondary skin grafting.

FROSTBITE
Risk Factors

A number of factors contribute to tissue damage after cold temperature insult. These include environmental, anatomic, and preexisting medical conditions (Table 4-3). As with thermal injuries, cold injuries also exhibit a spectrum of tissue damage. A first-degree injury is termed frostnip. The skin is blanched and slightly numb; rapid rewarming reverses this cold injury. If rewarming is not instituted, the cold injury may progress until it involves the dermis, subcutaneous tissue, and deeper structures. Chilblains and trench foot usually occur from prolonged exposures to cold and wet conditions. The temperatures that cause these injuries range from 30° to 50°F and there tends to be chronic irreversible damage to the tissues.

Tissue Injury

Etiology

True frostbite develops with prolonged exposure of tissues to low temperatures and the formation of ice crystals within the cells and tissue. The length of time required for tissue damage depends on the associated wind chill. As a point of reference, tissue exposed to 0°F and a 10-mph wind would freeze in approximately *1 hour,* but with 0°F and a 40-mph wind, the tissues would freeze in *10 minutes.*

Table 4-3   Factors Contributing to Depth of Cold Injury

Environmental	Anatomical	Preexisting Conditions
Temperature	Fingers, toes	Previous frostbite
Duration of exposure	Nose, ears	Smoking history
Wind velocity	Cheek	Peripheral vascular disease
Inadequate clothing	Heels wrist	Diabetes
Immobilization Moisture	Shin, forearm	Malnutrition
Contact with ice or metal		Lack of acclimatization (<6 weeks)
Constricting clothing		Altered mental status (alcoholism, drug use, psychiatric illness, etc.)

Mechanism of Tissue Damage

Cold exposure initially produces vasospasm and vasoconstriction. Secondary arterial–venous communications open to transfer the core body heat to the periphery. If the core body heat cannot be maintained, this response reverses to conserve core body heat at the expense of the extremity. The mechanism of injury in true frostbite involves direct tissue damage to the cells, with the formation of ice crystals. This occurs initially in the interstitium and plasma. Ice crystals in the interstitium establish a hyperosmolar environment that results in cellular dehydration and electrolyte imbalance. The crystals themselves will cause mechanical destruction of the cell wall. Plasma ice crystals cause hemoconcentration and increased viscosity. There also is direct endothelial damage that produces sludging and stasis within the vessels. Increased sympathetic tone also produces vasoconstriction and shunting.

Classification

Frostbite has been described traditionally as first, second, third, or fourth degree. This has been replaced by the more useful clinical classifications of superficial and deep injury. This scheme is superior because differences in the depth of an injury often are difficult to determine initially, and they really do not influence the outcome as predictably as with thermal burns. A superficial frostbite, which involves the skin only, results in minimal debridement and skin loss. It is characterized by (1) supple soft tissues, (2) pain with rewarming, (3) reactive hyperemia with warming, and (4) development of clear, watery blisters. The skin ultimately heals, resulting in tissues that may be more sensitive to future cold injury. Deep frostbite, however, involves all levels of injury to deeper structures. This may include muscle, tendon, nerve, vessels, and bone. A deep frostbite is characterized by (1) thick, firm skin and subcutaneous tissue, (2) anesthesia after rewarming, (3) lack of reactive hyperemia with warming, and (4) development of purple/red blisters. The tissue has a blue/gray discoloration that remains after warming and progresses over the next few days to dark, dry gangrene. At different areas there will be variations in the depth of the injury, which can be determined only with time and healing.

Management

Systemic

It is important not to immediately concentrate on the affected extremities and thereby overlook precipitating causes (e.g., seizures, head injuries, stroke, and so on). Initially, core body temperature should be restored by the application of blankets, warming devices, and warm intravenous fluid. A complete history and physical examination should then be taken to determine the risk factors and exclude life-threatening situations. Tetanus toxoid is required if not up to date. Some physicians have recommended systemic heparinization, low molecular weight dextran, or antifibrinolytic agents to reverse intracapillary sludging or prevent the extension of clots. Regional sympathectomy also has been attempted to decrease vasospasm and thereby, theoretically, decrease tissue damage. Other more moderate groups have recommended aspirin to prevent platelet sludging and ibuprofen to counter the effects of thromboxane and prostaglandins released from the blister fluid.

Local Care for Acute Injuries

Acute

The first step is thawing the frozen extremity. This should only be done in the emergency room before hospitalization because thawing and refreezing have severe consequences that can result in tissue loss. In the worst case scenario, the digits are rewarmed rapidly in the emergency room, the patient is allowed to depart, and the digits refreeze on the way home. Rapid rewarming is accomplished by completely immersing the extremity in a warm-water bath (40-44°F) for approximately 20 to 40 minutes. For this purpose, a whirlpool bath is ideal. The digits will become very painful, and the rewarming procedure is continued until there is flushing of the digits. The extremity is then elevated and placed into splints. It is "dressed" open to avoid constricting bandages. Local applications of aloe vera on intact blisters has been shown to interfere with thromboxane released by the injured skin. If the blisters rupture, they are dressed with sulfadiazine cream (Silvadene 1%). Antibiotics are started if there are any signs of infection, and whirlpool treatments continue twice a day to facilitate debridement and help ease the motion of the joints. Early and aggressive physical therapy is mandatory to avoid joint stiffness and wound contracture. Intrinsic plus splinting is necessary as the intrinsic muscles appear more sensitive to cold injury. Surgery for release of the intrinsic muscles rarely is indicated.

Surgical treatment

Premature surgical debridement is inappropriate. It may take as long as 2 to 3 months for the digits to demarcate fully. Often the amount of soft tissue that is viable at 2 months is greater than would have been predicted during the initial hospitalization. The only exception to this rule is the presence of an uncontrolled infection where an open guillotine amputation is indicated. When clear demarcation occurs, an amputation is completed and maximal functional length is preserved. Three-phase bone scans may show slight radioactivity, and this tissue should be considered viable. The amputation stumps are (1) primarily closed, (2) allowed to granulate and covered by the application of split-thickness skin grafts, (3) treated with local tissue flaps, if available, or (4) treated with distal flaps, either pedicle or microtransfer. Aggressive physical therapy needs to continue through the period of surgical intervention. If not, the patient may end up with a healed, but functionless extremity.

Frostbite in Children

Complex skeletal abnormalities may be seen after a growing hand suffers a cold injury, particularly injury to vulnerable chondrocytes in the cartilaginous growth plate. This causes premature closure of the phalangeal epiphyses. Epiphyseal closure occurs approximately 6 to 12 months after the cold injury, and not surprisingly, affects the distal joints to the greatest degree. The final outcome is shortening of the digits, marked skin redundancy, thick and poorly contoured nails, distal interphalangeal joint radial deviations (especially little finger), and joint laxity. These changes are common and do not appear to correlate with the initial soft tissue injury suffered. For an unspecified reason, the duplicating chondrocytes appear more sensitive than even the skin that has been exposed directly to the cold injury. Functionally, the children perform well, and only rarely is an arthrodesis or angular osteotomy required in adulthood.

CRUSH INJURIES
Etiology

Crush injuries are induced by blunt trauma and vary greatly in severity from minor bruising to loss of the limb. The amount of tissue damage is directly proportional to the force and time of the injury. Hitting a thumb with a hammer is an instantaneous force usually well tolerated by the soft tissues and bone. That same thumb, if crushed and stuck in a press, will suffer much greater tissue injury and may require amputation.

Serious crush injuries of the hand and forearm are severely mutilating and are covered later in Chapter 10. In these cases, the mechanism and length of tissue crushing must be documented. An instantaneous injury is tolerated much better by the soft tissues than a prolonged compression in which the extremity is extracted from the machinery with great difficulty. A crush injury may induce systemic sequelae, as well as local tissue destruction similar to electrical burn injuries.

Physiologic Stabilization

Resuscitation

The basic "ABCs" of resuscitation must be followed. Intravenous access must be established and a liberal amount of fluid given. Monitoring should be initiated and may include cardiac monitoring, peripheral oxygen saturation, and urinary catheter. Fluid intake needs to be adjusted according to the physiologic parameter. This fluid requirement may be much more than initially anticipated.

Systemic Injuries

After a crush injury, muscles release myoglobin, potassium, and creatinine phosphokinase (CPK) systemically. The myoglobin is released by the mechanism of rhabdomyolysis, especially after more than 4 hours of muscle ischemia. Blood studies must be performed to check these values. The quantitative results also may help to determine the extent of muscle injury. Serial blood examinations may show continuing muscle necrosis, which should be addressed surgically. The urine must also be checked for the presence of myoglobin. In these crush injuries, the kidneys are at risk for damage from myoglobin precipitation in the renal tubules as well as hypotension. Adequate rehydration is very important to avoid decreasing the blood flow to the kidneys. Rapid diuresis should be promoted by mannitol infusion. Secondary to this diuresis, rapid fluid replacement must be maintained. Bicarbonate should be added to resuscitation fluids to alkalinize the urine to promote passage of myoglobin through the renal tubule. All of these steps should be initiated early in the treatment plan to prevent kidney failure and the subsequent need for dialysis.

Acute Compartment Syndrome

Acute compartment syndrome occurs when the pressure within a confined space increases, thereby compromising the neurovascular function. The causes of acute compartment syndrome may be decreased enclosed space (tight fascial closures, traction), increased internal pressure (bleeding, increased capillary pressure or filtration), or externally applied pressure (casts, lying on extremity).

Pathogenesis

Pathophysiology

When local tissue pressure is elevated, the veins are compromised, thereby increasing the venous pressure. If venous pressure is increased, the gradient between the arterial and venous systems is decreased. This subsequently decreases the local blood flow to the tissues encased within the compartment. As oxygenation, nutrient, and waste perfusion is lowered, the metabolic demands of the local tissues are not met. This results in loss of function and, ultimately, muscle ischemia and necrosis. A lower arterial pressure (hypotension, arterial occlusion) may severely limit the arterial inflow. As a result, a lower compartment pressure will be measured. Therefore if the patient has a systolic pressure of less than 100 mmHg, compartment pressures may be elevated at < 20 mmHg and release is indicated.

Result if untreated

The end result of ischemic muscle loss and nerve injury is known as a Volkmann ischemic contracture. The upper extremity loses ulnar and median nerve function and sensation. The extremity is fixed in pronation with hyperextension of the metacarpophalangeal joints and flexion of the interphalangeal joints. Often, this contracture results in an amputation because the limb is insensate and functionless.

Prevention

Because acute compartment syndrome is a devastating complication, early steps should be taken for its prevention. These include (1) maintaining blood pressure and limb profusion, (2) removing tight dressings, especially circumferential Ace wraps or elastocrepe bandages, (3) bivalving and extremity cast including the underlying bandages, and (4) keeping the limb at heart level to maintain arterial venous gradient.

Clinical Findings

Signs and symptoms

Because the failure to diagnose and treat acute compartment syndrome is so devastating, the examiner should constantly consider it in every extremity injury. The signs and symptoms usually involve problems with peripheral circulation and sensation. Muscle and nerve ischemia is characterized by severe pain. If these clinical signs are nonconclusive, then tissue pressure must be measured. The differential diagnosis includes arterial occlusion or nerve injuries (Table 4-4).

Peripheral circulation measurements

The measurement of peripheral circulation is a poor indicator of injury within the fascial compartments, because peripheral pulses and capillary filling usually are intact until late in the process. For distal pulses to be obliterated, the pressure within the compartment

Table 4-4   Differential Diagnosis of Compartment Syndrome vs Other Etiology

	Arterial	Venous	Compartment Syndrome	Nerve Injury
Pain	✓		✓	
Paresis	✓	✓	✓	✓
Pulseless	✓		Late	
Paresthesia	✓	✓	✓	✓
Palor	✓		Late	
↑ Pressure			✓	

must be elevated to a level greater than the systolic blood pressure. This is rare and occurs late in the process, typically when surgical intervention does not halt tissue necrosis.

Pain

The pain associated with ischemia appears out of proportion to that expected for the apparent injuries. The pain typically is progressive, persistent, and not relieved by immobilization or narcotics.

Passive stretching

Pain is evident with muscle stretching by passive motion of the fingers, especially with forced extension (volar compartment) or flexion (dorsal compartment). The brachioradialis and the extensor carpi radialis are tested with wrist flexion. Interosseous testing is performed by abduction and adduction of the fingers with the metacarpophalangeal joints in extension and the interphalangeal joints flexed. The thenar muscles are tested by passive stretching of the muscles. The stress pain is present in almost all cases of increased compartment pressure and is a reliable sign. Unfortunately, pain may be absent because of nerve ischemia or proximal nerve injury, or because the patient is obtunded or intoxicated.

Paresis

The progressive weakness associated with paresis usually is a late sign of worsening muscle viability and also may be the result of proximal direct nerve injury.

Paraesthesias

The progression of paraesthesias is indicated by careful initial and subsequent sensory examinations. Most compartments are transversed by sensory nerves with distal distributions, and diminished sensation is indicative of ongoing nerve ischemia. Nerve function is a sensitive indicator of nerve damage and should be tested by sensation (normal, diminished, absent) and sensibility (two-point discrimination, pin prick).

Palpation

Palpation of the compartments during the acute stage will confirm an edematous muscle with a firm, tense, and tender compartment.

Objective Testing and Measurement of Compartment Pressures

Clinical findings alone often are enough to indicate the necessity for exploration and complete fasciotomies to release the fascial compartments. In some patients, the diagnosis of elevated compartment pressures may not be evident, but still cannot be excluded. Objective measurements in these cases may be imperative—or at least prudent—particularly if clinical signs and symptoms are confusing or if there are coexisting vascular and peripheral nerve injuries, other major

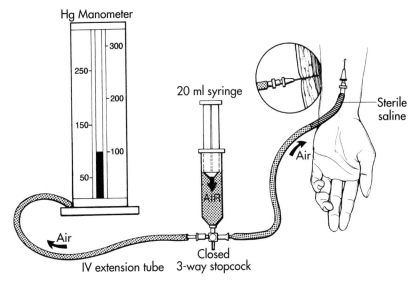

Figure 4-8   The Whiteside infusion technique to measure compartment syndrome is shown. The lined area within the intravenous tubing is sterile saline, and the dotted area is air. The needle should be placed well within the muscle compartment to gain a correct compartment pressure reading.

organs have been traumatized, or the patient is unresponsive or uncooperative.

Whiteside infusion technique

This technique is based on measuring the air pressure required to inject saline into the fascial compartment. The set-up is shown in Fig. 4-8. A 20-ml syringe is attached to a three-way stopcock. One intravenous extension tube is attached to the stopcock in a mercury manometer. Another intravenous extension tube is attached to the last port of the stopcock in a sterile 18-gauge needle. Saline is then aspirated through the needle and should fill approximately one half of the extension tube. The stopcock to this extension tube is then closed to prevent the loss of saline when the needle is removed. The needle is then inserted into a muscle belly. The stopcock is open to all three ports, and gradually the plunger of the syringe is depressed. When the pressure of the plunger exceeds to compartmental pressure, the saline will begin to enter the compartment and move along the intravenous tubing. When this occurs, the pressure registered by the mercury manometer is recorded.

There are reported difficulties with the infusion technique. The results are less reproducible than other techniques and it cannot continuously monitor compartmental pressure because repeat needlesticks would be required at 1- to 2-hour intervals. In addition, mercury manometer readings may not be accurate for less than 15 mm or more than 100 mm. Finally, the needle may be plugged by muscle tissue when it is advanced into the muscle belly.

Wick catheter/slit catheter technique

Both of these catheters increase the surface area for recording pressures (Fig. 4-9). They also prevent tissue obstruction of the recording orifice and allow for continuous monitoring through a saline-equilibrated tube, without the need to flush or use continuous infusion. These techniques also use a standard blood pressure transducer, which is more reproducible and accurate if correctly equilibrated than the mercury manometer.

Both catheters are introduced through a 14-gauge needle cannula, which is introduced approximately 2 to 3 cm into the muscle. The catheters are then threaded through the cannula, and the needle is removed. In this fashion, they remain in contact with the muscle compartment and may be used for continuous monitoring.

Companies manufacturing these catheters determined that a malfunction of these catheters increased the risk to the patient. For legal reasons, these catheters are no longer produced commercially and must be fashioned individually.

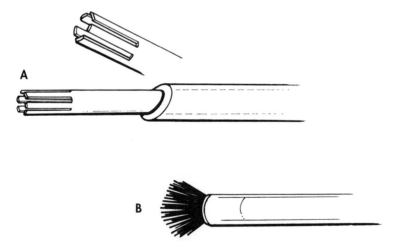

Figure 4-9 Two catheters that appear to be better than the needle catheter and do not occlude as readily are the slit catheter **(A)** and the wick catheter **(B).** These need to be fabricated by the surgeon.

Pressure Threshold for Fasciotomy

The pressure recommendations for fasciotomies vary with the differing techniques used for measurement. The Whiteside infusion technique recommends that fasciotomy be performed when the tissue pressure rises to within 10 to 30 mmHg of the diastolic pressure of the patient. The Wick catheter technique has supported release of the compartment if the pressures are approximately 45 mmHg.

Because fairly straightforward decompression techniques prevent disastrous consequences, we recommend fasciotomies for intracompartmental pressures greater than 30 mmHg in the volar and dorsal compartments and 15 mmHg in the interosseous nerve compartments. These guidelines assume that the patient is normotensive. This also is especially important when you consider the time of compression; if greater than 8 hours, it may indicate more severe muscle necrosis. If the patient is hypotensive with low perfusion to the muscle compartment, then a fasciotomy should be considered when pressures reach 20 to 25 mmHg.

A fasciotomy should be performed whenever the magnitude of the injury or clinical findings suggests increasing compartment pressures, even if measured intracompartmental pressures do not reveal any problem.

Treatment

The treatment for acute compartment syndrome is immediate surgical decompression of the compartments involved. Once elevated, compartmental pressures are documented or clinical findings prove consistent with ischemia to the muscle of the forearm or hand, the patient should be taken urgently for decompression. Conservative therapy, except for increasing perfusion by raising the blood pressure, is of no benefit once the diagnosis is established. Whether the skin needs to be incised to release the compartments underneath is controversial. In these conditions, I have found that the skin often is compromised because of the underlying pressure. As a result, full-skin incision with fasciotomy is recommended. This also offers the opportunity to directly assess the state of the underlying muscle.

The location of the skin incision locations depend on the physician, but a few principles should be maintained. For example, damage to cutaneous nerves and veins should be avoided if possible. The median and ulnar nerves should be released as they pass through their distal tunnels to prevent subsequent scarring around the nerves and acute compression syndromes. The flexion creases should be maintained by avoiding straight-line incisions across them. Every attempt should be made to ensure that the vital structures (peripheral nerves and arteries) are covered at the completion of the fasciotomy by readvancing the skin flaps. This will avoid desiccation and further injury to the structures.

Our preferred skin incisions are shown in Fig. 4-10*A-C*. Note the decompression of the dorsal, as well as the interosseous, compartments. The fingers are released by the placement of a midaxial incision in the finger, with extension at a 45 degree angle at the most proxi-

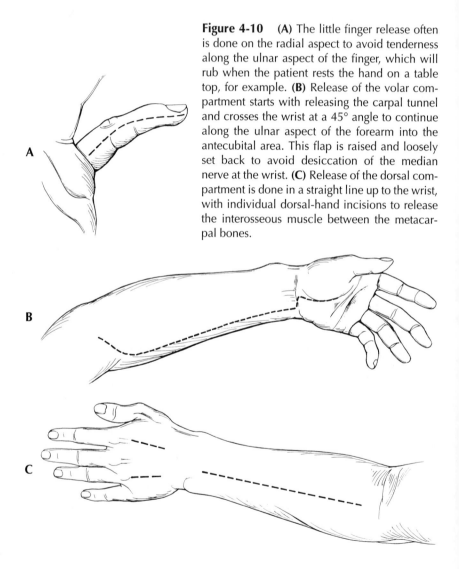

Figure 4-10   (A) The little finger release often is done on the radial aspect to avoid tenderness along the ulnar aspect of the finger, which will rub when the patient rests the hand on a table top, for example. (B) Release of the volar compartment starts with releasing the carpal tunnel and crosses the wrist at a 45° angle to continue along the ulnar aspect of the forearm into the antecubital area. This flap is raised and loosely set back to avoid desiccation of the median nerve at the wrist. (C) Release of the dorsal compartment is done in a straight line up to the wrist, with individual dorsal-hand incisions to release the interosseous muscle between the metacarpal bones.

mal flexion crease. Care must be taken not to injure the neurovascular bundler at that level. The finger release includes incisions through Cleland's ligament around the neurovascular bundle, continuing volar to the flexor tendons to release the opposite Cleland's ligament and the transrectinacular ligaments. These incisions are straight because fewer veins and cutaneous nerves are damaged in this release.

Once the skin has been opened, the volar forearm flap is raised and each muscle compartment inspected. Next, the fascial compartments are opened, and an episiotomy is performed of any muscle that appears ischemic. The incision across the wrist is closed loosely to cover the median nerve, as well as the ulnar nerve and artery. The remaining skin incision is left open to allow continued decompression. Most of these incisions can be closed in approximately 5 to 10 days. On rare occasions, skin grafting is needed for areas of skin loss. In general, the scars are hypertrophic because of the tension and tissue anoxia at the time of the initial injury. Subsequent revisions usually are unnecessary, although serial excision of skin-grafted areas may be done.

FINGERTIP INJURIES
Mechanism

Fingertip injuries probably are the most common hand injuries seen in the emergency room because the fingers (particularly the middle and long fingers) and the nails are the most distal aspects of the hand. The most common mechanisms of injury are closing doors, crushing between two objects, and tool and equipment injuries. Because these injuries are so common, treating physicians should be knowledgeable about the great range of injuries incurred. This section deals only with blunt injuries that do not involve the initial loss of soft tissue. A later section (Wound Coverage Options) deals specifically with soft tissue loss in fingertip injuries. Sometimes crush injuries may lead to soft tissue loss; if this occurs, the reader is referred to a later section on soft tissue coverage for fingertips.

Bone Injuries

Approximately 50% of fingertip crush injuries are associated with fractures. In general, these injuries involve the distal tufts of the phalanx and only need to be stabilized externally by a stack splint or an aluminum finger splint on both the volar and dorsal surfaces. This protects the finger from further injury and stabilizes the bone fragments. If the fracture is proximal to the "waist" of the distal phalanx or involves the articular surface, then more aggressive intervention should be considered. If the fracture heals as a nonunion, the distal finger may lack the stability needed for pinching or pushing, and arthritis in the joint may be debilitating. K-wire screw fixation may be indicated in these circumstances, but this is a controversial approach because the healed soft tissue may be enough to stabilize the distal finger. A Herbert screw also has been used with success.

Nailbed Injuries

Function of the Nail

The nail stabilizes the soft tissue distal to the bony phalanx. It contributes to sensation and assists a person in picking up small objects. An irregular nail is a very objectionable deformity, especially in a woman. Care must be taken to correctly repair nailbed injuries to obtain an optimal result.

Anatomy and Growth of the Nail

Anatomy

The nail plate is made of onychia and is very similar to keratin from the skin. It arises from the germinal matrix proximally and grows distally above the sterile matrix (Fig. 4-11*A*). The nail plate is attached intimately to the nailbed through longitudinal ribs and furrows. The surrounding soft tissue includes the epionychium proximally, the perionychium surrounding the lateral aspects, and the hyponychium distal to the attachment of the nail plate to the nailbed. The lunula is a white area of the nail plate distal to the epionychium, which is not fully cornified and is much softer than the distal nail plate. The blood supply is from the dorsal branches of the volar digital arteries, and the innervation arises from the common digital nerves.

Growth

The nail grows approximately 0.1 mm per day and, therefore, it takes approximately 100 days to grow to full length. After removal of the nail, there is an initial delay of approximately 1 month before the new nail "grows out." Therefore, it may take 4 to 6 months for nail growth to be completed, and up to 1 year for the new nail to be fully mature.

Pathology of Nail Bed Injuries

The etiology of most nailbed injuries involves a crushing mechanism. If a sharp object strikes a finger with enough force to penetrate the nail plate and injure the nailbed, it commonly will continue through the phalanx and amputate the fingertip. For amputation injuries, see the section on wound coverage options. Most commonly, the fingertip is compressed between two hard objects (Fig. 4-11*B*). The compression of the fingertip causes the nail, which is a convex structure, to buckle. This buckling drives the hard nail plate into the nailbed

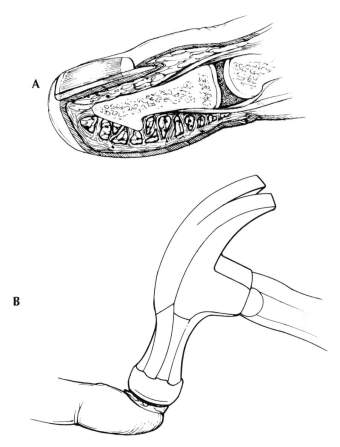

Figure 4-11   **(A)** The anatomy of the nail is very complex. The germinal matrix and the sterile matrix are underneath the nail itself. The eponychial fold needs to be preserved, if at all possible, to avoid scarring in the area. **(B)** Most nailbed injuries occur because of a crush injury, as seen in this injury caused by a direct blow from a hammer.

toward the firm, bony phalanx. It is the soft tissue (i.e., the nailbed), located between these two firm surfaces, that absorbs the energy. If it is a low-energy force, a single laceration is seen where the nail has buckled. A higher-energy blow dissipates more energy and causes stellate lacerations of the nailbed. A high-energy injury frequently shatters the distal bony tuft and explodes the sterile matrix of the nail into many fragments. These lacerations of the nailbed need to be repaired accurately to prevent subsequent nail deformities.

IRREGULARITIES IN NAIL GROWTH

The essential elements of nail growth are the germinal matrix, nailbed, and the supporting bony scaffold. Each of these elements must heal satisfactorily to prevent irregular nail growth. An unrepaired injury to the germinal matrix will result in either no nail regrowth or a soft, immature nail. If the nailbed is not repaired, a scar will result, and a new nail will not adhere to the scar or to the nailbed distal to the scar. If there is a significant loss of bony support for the distal soft tissues, the new nail will follow the drooping nailbed and result in a hooked nail (the so-called parrot beak deformity). To prevent these irregularities, the following techniques are recommended. Bony stabilization technique depends on the level of fracture. If it is a distal tuft comminuted fracture, as are most injuries, external stabilization is adequate. If the fracture occurs at the waist of the phalanx, internal fixation with K-wires should be considered. If this fixation is not precise, more damage may be done to new nail growth. Because the periosteum is in close contact with the nailbed, small irregularities in bone reduction will result in nailbed deformity and subsequent nail nonadherence. If an adequate reduction cannot be obtained, it may be best to use the old nail as an external splint to maintain the nailbed and the phalanx. The bone will then remodel underneath the old nail. Interarticular fractures involving more than 25% of the cartilage surface should be fixated to maintain articular integrity and reduce late occurrence of osteoarthritis.

Subungual Hematoma

Etiology

The most common minor injury of the nailbed is a subungual hematoma. Because the nailbed is located between the buckled nail and the phalanx, its ability to absorb energy is minimal. Even a low-impact injury is enough to cause disruption of the nailbed vessels, with bleeding under the nail plate. This hematoma separates the nail plate from the nailbed. Subsequent scarring of the nailbed will cause nail plate deformity. In addition, the pressure under the nail plate to tamponade the bleeding often causes significant pain.

Treatment

As a general rule, if less than 25% of the nail plate has been elevated by a hematoma with pain, then drainage alone is indicated. Local anesthesia rarely is necessary. The preferred method of drainage is to puncture the nail plate until the hematoma and pain are relieved. The defect in the nail can be small, but must stay open to prevent reaccumulation of the hematoma, which can occur with premature closure. A scalpel opening is insufficient and may penetrate the nail plate to injure the nailbed. The best method to drain a subungual hematoma is with the an ophthalmologic cautery or a heated paper clip. When the tip of either instrument is red hot, place it on the nail plate directly over the hematoma. The nail plate (which is itself insensate) will burn and evaporate as the heated tip penetrates. There will be an immediate flush of blood, and the cautery tip is cooled instantly. Further penetration of the tip should not occur, and injury to the nailbed is rare. Because the nail plate has evaporated and is not simply pushed aside by a scalpel, the drainage holes should be permanent and "grow out" as the nail plate continues to be pushed distally by the germinal matrix. This allows for continued drainage over the next few days until the nail plate can again reattach to the matrix of the nailbed. Antibiotic ointments, a dressing, and a protective splint are the basic follow-up treatments. The patient should have almost immediate relief from the throbbing pain caused by the blood tamponade under the nail. If this does not occur, the hematoma has not been drained adequately.

Injury to Germinal Matrix

Treatment

If the injury penetrates the germinal matrix, the nailbed needs to be closely reapproximated using fine, chromic, catgut sutures. To ensure accurate approximation, the sutures need to be placed precisely with the help of magnification equipment. Even the smallest distortion will be noticeable as a new nail grows. If there is a loss of germinal matrix in a situation where the closure would be under tension, some physicians advocate lateral relaxing incisions in the proximal eponychial folds. Patients tolerate lateral defects better than central nail deformities. The skin of the nail wall is then sutured using 6-0 nylon suture. The nail fold must be maintained approximately 2 to 3 weeks before the new nail starts to grow. This is performed by replacing the old nail. If this is not available or is damaged beyond use, then replacement with either Silastic sheath or nonadherent gauze is recommended.

If this fold is not maintained by a spacer, the dorsal roof will scar down to the ventral floor. The scarring will make it difficult for the new nail to grow, and it will grow deformed. This is easy to prevent, but almost impossible to correct secondarily.

Nailbed Lacerations

Nail Plate Removal

It is difficult to decide when to remove an "intact" nail to fix a nailbed laceration. Generally, if more than 25% of the nail is undermined by a hematoma, the nail should be removed and the nailbed explored and repaired.

Preparation for Repair

Finger block with 1% lidocaine is performed. Care must be taken to ensure that both digital nerves and the dorsal innervation has been anesthetized successfully. While waiting for the block to "set up" (approximately 10-15 minutes), the Mayo stand, instruments, and suture (6-0 chromic, 6-0 nylon) are prepared. The finger is prepared with Betadine, and sterile drapes are placed. The blood in the finger may be exsanguinated by the use of a 1-inch Penrose drain. The Penrose is wrapped distally to proximally to remove the blood. At the most proximal wrap, a clamp is placed to maintain pressure and the Penrose drain is unwrapped distally to proximally. *Careful:* a 1-inch Penrose drain is the smallest that should be used because anything smaller places excessive pressure over a small area and may injure vessels and nerves.

Nailbed Repair

Nail plate removal

The nail is removed, with the patient under anesthesia, by slipping a small clamp, Iris scissors, or periosteal elevator beneath the nail plate from the perionychial fold to perionychial fold and under the epionychium. After this is performed adequately, the nail should be removed gently to avoid further injury by tearing the nailbed.

Repair of the nailbed

Once the nail is removed, inspect the nailbed (Fig. 4-12). Obvious nonviable tissue should be removed, but this should be done very conservatively. The nailbed is attached to the periosteum, and simple advancement of the tissues cannot be performed easily. The accurate approximation of the nailbed should be performed using magnification equipment and a fine, chromic suture on a round needle (Fig. 4-13). Small flaps are sutured to allow the nail to rest flat on the matrix once the repair is performed. A special note should be made about nailbed avulsions. If one occurs proximally, it should be sutured back into position under the nail fold. If tissue is missing on inspection of the nailbed after injury, it still may be attached to the nail itself. It should be removed carefully and sutured into the defect as a free graft. This is done using chromic catgut sutures with precise placement of the suture and only three knots.

Replacement of the nail plate

The next step is to clean the nail. Often, a portion of the proximal soft nail is trimmed so that the nail can be inserted more easily back into the nail fold (Fig. 4-14). To allow for drainage of blood, the nail is perforated at a site not directly over the repair. It is then

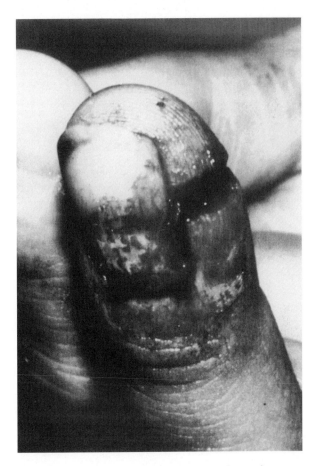

Figure 4-12   A normal mechanism of fingertip injuries is a burst injury secondary to a crush. All that is seen is the laceration along the ulnar aspect of the finger. Care must be taken to examine the nailbed if complete repair is to be achieved.

sutured along the eponychial folds away from the bony phalanx. Some physicians suture the nail distally, but if an undrained hematoma should develop, the proximal nail will elevate out of the nail fold to drain the hematoma. This often is not discovered until the first dressing change, which occurs days after some early adhesion has formed between the dorsal roof and the germinal matrix. After experiencing this a few times, we prefer to suture laterally, after placing the drain hole. If the nail is not available, then Silastic sheet, nonadherent gauze, or even the foil from the suture package may be used to keep the nail fold open.

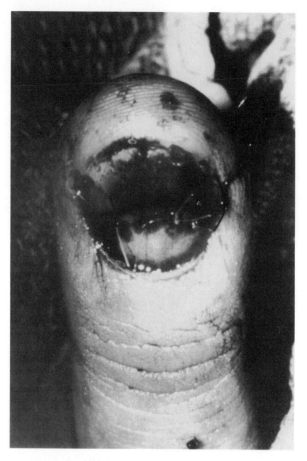

Figure 4-13 The nailbed has been removed and repair of the nailbed laceration has been performed using absorbable sutures.

Dressing and splint

The final step is to dress the finger with nonadherent 2 × 2 inch gauze dressings and tube gauze. A Stax or aluminum splint is then placed over the fingertip to avoid further trauma. At this time, consider placing a Marcaine block in the same manner as the initial finger block. The area is already anesthetized, and the injection should not be painful. This should give the patient approximately 8 hours of pain relief and will make further pain control easier. The arm should be placed in a sling, the hand elevated, and an appointment made with a hand surgeon for a follow-up in 3 to 5 days.

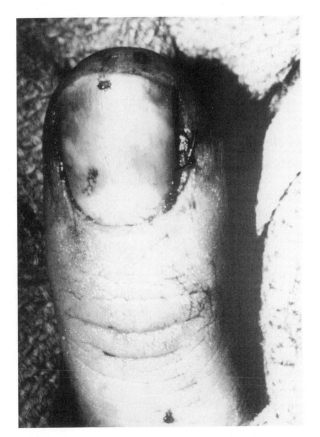

Figure 4-14   The nail plate has been replaced in the eponychial fold to allow growth of the new nail plate from the germinal matrix.

SOFT TISSUE INFECTIONS
Etiology

Infections of the upper extremity are not uncommon. Infections may occur after injuries that initially are thought to be minor. This occurs because the hand often is injured while performing a task in a "dirty environment." Even if the initial injury is clean, the tissues may be exposed subsequently to a contaminated environment. This can lead to inflammation, edema, increased skin tension, and abscess formation. If progressive treatment is not initiated, this may lead to functional losses and even amputation. In compromised patients (i.e., diabetics, transplant patients) this may even lead to death. Although staphylococcal infections occur most frequently, almost all bacterial, fungal, and viral organisms have been cultured from hand infections.

Most infections are contained within the skin and soft tissues. Sometimes these can progress to the deep spaces of the hand (palmar and thenar) and forearm. Treatment of "early" cellulitis may prevent further extension of the infecting organisms to form abscesses in the deep spaces or around the tendons.

History and Physical Examination

Previous Medical History

Care must be taken to identify diabetics and other immunocompromised patients because infections spread rapidly in these patients. "Infections" in persons with a history of gout are difficult to diagnose adequately because the erythema of an acute gouty attack may closely resemble bacterial cellulitis.

Duration

The duration of symptoms might be a useful factor in determining the location and aggressiveness of the offending organisms. Streptococcal and anaerobic infections spread rapidly—in a matter of hours—whereas staphylococcal and pseudomonas infections need time to become established. Acute cellulitis and flexor tenosynovitis usually become established within 24 hours. Deeper infection (peronychiae, felons, deep space) develop in 2 to 5 days.

Occupation

Farm equipment injuries result in the most serious tissue contamination, including gram-negative organisms. Persons who handle fish are prone to mycobacterial infections. Dentists are prone to viral infections (herpetic whitlow) and gardeners have a higher percentage of fungal (sporotrichosis) infections than the general population. Children are prone to oropharangeal bacteria infections in the form of paronychia. The same is true for nail biters and people with short manicures.

Examination

A special note should be made of hand positioning because this may be helpful in detecting deeper infections. The lymphatics of the hand drain through the dorsal surface. Therefore, the dorsum of the hand often is swollen even though this is not the location of the infection. Careful documentation of ascending lymphangitis should be completed. The involvement of axillary lymph nodes and deltopectoral nodes represents a more severe infection.

Laboratory Data

Laboratory testing should include a complete blood count with differential, serum glucose, uric acid (if appropriate), and gram stain and cultures of purulent exudate, if present. Some physicians recommend the injection of saline and aspiration of the soft tissue at the leading edge of the cellulitis, but I have not found this to be particularly helpful. X-ray examination should be undertaken if there is a possibility of a foreign body or if there is significant swelling of the finger or hand.

Initial Management of Acute Infections

REST

As soon as a patient arrives with a possible hand infection, the following treatment program should be started immediately:

R—rest

E—elevation

S—splinting and immobilization (position of function with wrist in 20° of extension, metacarpophalangeal joints in 45° of flexion, and interphalangeal joints in 10° of flexion)

T—tetanus status

S—staphylococcal coverage

This should be adequate to reverse progression of any early superficial infections in an immunocompetent patient.

Drainage

Deeper, more severe infections require hospitalization, intravenous antibiotics, and hydrotherapy to stimulate blood flow. Incision and drainage is required if an abscess has developed. This may be performed without local anesthesia if the skin is attenuated sufficiently at the area of pointing. Otherwise, local blocks or general anesthesia may be required. Cultures should be taken of all drained material to determine specific antibacterial therapy.

Antibacterial Therapy

Initial

The most common organism is gram positive, which should be adequately treated by nafcillin or first-generation cephalosporin. In communities with high penicillin and cephalosporin resistance, vancomycin therapy may be justified in serious infection. If an improvement by clinical examination is not apparent within 24 hours, broader coverage is required to include gram-negative organisms and anaerobic bacteria. This may include the addition of clindamycin and gentamycin until a specific organism can be identified.

Immunocompromised patient

Initial antibiotic coverage for patients who have diabetes or are otherwise immunocompromised should be of a sufficiently broad spectrum to cover mixed organisms, including anaerobic bacteria. The morbidity associated with hand infections in this patient population is severe and needs to be treated aggressively by an experienced hand surgeon. Hospitalization usually is required.

Ambulatory antibiotics

A patient with established cellulitis of the hand frequently will ask not to be hospitalized and will request another therapeutic option. This decision should be met with some reluctance on the part of the hand surgeon. However, we have successfully treated patients with "ambulatory" antibiotics. This requires successful drainage of an established infection (perionychia or felon), no systemic signs of spread (afebrile and a normal leukocyte count and differential), the ability to permanently mark the erythematous area for further evaluations, proximity of the patient's residence to the hospital, and a very compliant, motivated nonimmunocompromised patient who will return for evaluation and intravenous antibiotics every 6 to 8 hours. Any deviation from these requirements is a contraindication for this treatment modality.

Specific infections

Paronychia

Early. An acute paronychia is the most common infection of the hand, accounting for approximately 30 to 40% of all cases. It affects the skin and soft tissues that surround the periphery of the nail plate. The most common causes include a deformed nail, a "hang nail," nail biting, inappropriate manicures, and/or a penetrating injury. Appropriate medical treatment consists of an antibiotic that is effective against *staphylococcus aureus* (the most common causative agent), warm soaks, elevation, and immobilization. Often, progression of the infection can be halted with early effective treatment.

Late. Without appropriate treatment, the infection may spread to involve the eponychium—even to the eponychium on the other side (the so-called "run around" infection). Pain, swelling, and erythema are associated with suppuration and fluctuants. Once the infection is localized, it should be drained. Incisions for adequate drainage must avoid the germinal epithelium to prevent a chronic nail deformity. The author's preferred incision is a linear incision at the fluctuant point. Often, if the skin is thin, the skin may be removed to allow for long-term drainage. Double linear incisions are done for "run around" infections. If a subungual abscess develops, the nail must be removed—or, at least, the lateral third excised.

Adequate drainage must be maintained by unroofing or packing the wound. If there is associated erythema, antibiotics should be maintained. Daily soaks should continue to promote drainage and increase local blood flow. The patient must follow-up with a visit to a hand specialist in the next few days.

FELON

Etiology. A felon is an infection of the distal pulp space of a digit. It is the second most common type of hand infection (approximately 25% of cases). The most common cause is a penetrating injury, including finger-stick blood testing. The initial symptoms usually include cellulitis and pain. During the next 48 hours, if the infection is not controlled, the distal pulp becomes tense, extremely tender, swollen, and shows signs of early skin necrosis.

Anatomy. The severe, rapid, painful progression of a fingertip infection is unique because of the anatomy of the pulp space. The palmar skin is stabilized to the bony phalanx by fine septi. As an abscess of the pulp space enlarges, the skin reaches its limits of expansion because of these fine septi. As the pressure increases, the blood supply decreases, thereby compromising the nutrient flow to the skin. This also increases the pressure on the nerve endings, which results in severe, throbbing pain.

Progression. If left untreated, a felon may thrombose the digital vessels and necrose the skin and soft tissue. It may spread to the bone of the distal phalanx, leading to osteitis or osteomyelitis. Occasionally, it may cause sequestration of the distal phalanx, pyogenic arthritis of the distal joint, or pyogenic flexor tendon synovitis if the abscess progresses to involve the distal insertion of the profundus tendon. Pyogenic arthritis of a finger joint almost always results in a fusion of the joint. The lysosomal enzymes of the bacteria lead to extensive cartilage destruction, and intra-articular infections need to be treated aggressively—usually with drainage procedures if a stiff finger is to be avoided.

Treatment. The "standard" incision for a felon is controversial. Of utmost importance is division of the septi connecting the skin to the bony phalanx. This is required to adequately drain the abscess and relieve the pressure. Accepted incisions are (1) directly over the "pointing area" if present, (2) lateral midaxial incision, (3) a through-and-through incision, (4) a J-incision, or (5) a fish-mouth incision. The authors prefer the lateral midaxial incision. It avoids incision placement on the most sensitive tactile portion of the fingertip. Incisions on the index, long, and ring fingers are typically on the ulnar side. The thumb and little fingers receive radial incisions. The incision is brought transversely across the pulp space, making sure to divide all septi. A small drain (Penrose) is placed, and soaks are started. Intravenous antibiotics are given during the procedure, and the patient is maintained on oral antibiotic therapy. A loose, bulky dressing is placed in a protective splint fashion. Subsequent care must occur within 48 hours to ensure that the infection is under control. If it is not, further exploration and intravenous antibiotics are indicated.

Sequelae.   Untreated felons often result in osteomyelitis, skin necrosis, and soft tissue breakdown secondary to ischemia. This may even necessitate an amputation at the middle phalanx level to successfully treat the disastrous sequelae.

DEEP SPACE INFECTIONS

Deep space infections account for approximately 8% to 10% of all hand infections. Most occur after penetrating trauma and go unnoticed for 24 to 48 hours because initially there is very minimal, visible skin change. Once a deep space infection develops, surgical drainage and parental antibiotics are necessary to prevent progression.

Web-space collar-button abscess.   After a penetrating injury or infected callous at the base of the finger, the infected material "leaks" across the transverse ligament of the metacarpal bones, creating both palmar and dorsal abscesses. The patient usually shows systemic signs of infection (fever, chills, and increased leukocyte count) and cellulitis within the web space. There also is marked pain, swelling, and tenderness along both the palmar and dorsal aspects of the hand. The abscess between the metacarpal bones separates the fingers, and the patient holds the fingers in a semiflex cascade. Occasionally there are associated tendon signs (see the section on pyelogenic tenosynovitis).

Surgical drainage requires through-and-through drainage to simultaneously drain both cavities (Fig. 4-15). This should be performed through a zigzag incision in the volar between the proximal and digital crease and the midpalmar crease. A straight dorsal incision is used between the metacarpal heads and is extended into the web space as needed.

Midpalmar infection.   An abscess in this location usually is secondary to penetrating trauma. The palmar skin is tense with loss of palmar concavity. Other than palmar swelling, there is a paucity of volar signs. Most of the swelling is dorsal and often painless. Because of the more proximal extension of the ulnar digit

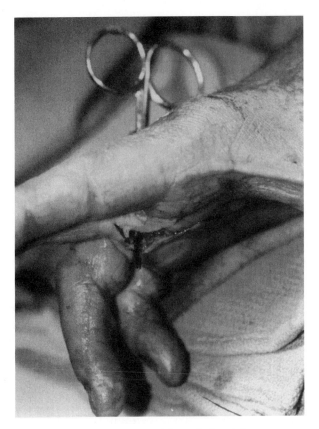

Figure 4-15   A collar-button abscess of the right hand that was not appreciated for approximately 24 to 36 hours needs through-and-through drainage.

bursa along the flexor tendons, infections of this area tend to progress rapidly proximal to the wrist. Drainage is through a transverse incision along the midpalmar crease or parallel to the thenar crease. The latter incision may be helpful if the thenar space also is involved. Drainage, elevation, rest, and perennial antibiotics are required.

Suppurative flexor tenosynovitis.   Pyogenic tenosynovitis accounts for approximately 5% of hand infections. These are severe infections that have a high morbidity rate if not detected and treated aggressively. Most commonly, these show form-penetrating trauma or previous surgery. They also may result from other infections (e.g., felons, septic arthritis, collar-button abscess, or midpalmar space abscess).

Kanaval signs.   Kanavel described the following classic four findings associated with pyogenic flexor tenosynovitis: (1) flexed digit, (2) fusiform swelling of the finger, (3) tendon sheath tenderness, and (4) pain and limitation of passive finger extension. Systemic signs of illness also may be present as well (fever, chills, increased leukocyte count, lymphadenopathy).

Treatment.   A patient with classic findings should be splinted, hospitalized, started on intravenous antibiotics, and have an immediate evaluation by a hand surgeon. Intravenous antibiotics should cover both gram-negative and gram-positive organisms. If this conservative therapy is started aggressively and early, the infection may be controlled. If symptoms improve within 24 hours, drainage is not indicated. The decision to treat an early infection conservatively should be made by an experienced hand surgeon.

If symptoms do not rapidly improve, intraoperative exploration is indicated. General anesthesia usually is employed. Most surgeons favor open drainage and a closed-tendon sheath irrigation employing two incisions. The author's preferred method is to completely open the flexor sheath between the pulleys using a lateral midaxial approach. This incision is carried into the palm across the proximal digital flexion crease with care to avoid the crossing neurovascular bundle (see Fig. 4-10A for release incisions). The incision is then carried in a zigzag fashion to the proximal extent of the infection in the palm. Pressurized, pulsatile antibiotic irrigation is used throughout the length of the tendon. An irrigation catheter may then be placed if the infection is severe. Otherwise, the incisions are closed loosely over a Penrose drain and whirlpools are started. Passive and active therapy are started when symptoms are resolved.

Sequelae.   Undrained purulence and inflammation within a constricting tendon sheath significantly increases the pressure within the sheath. This will decrease nutrient blood flow in an already "compromised" vascular structure, such as the tendon, and can lead to tendon necrosis. The presence of inflammation within the tendon sheath will lead to adhesions that will compromise the delicate gliding mechanism of the flexor tendon with the pulley system and tendon sheath. The functional loss of this tendon system will cause great morbidity and limitations on the hand.

Progressive synergistic gangrene.   Melaney's infection usually is caused by the synergistic action of aerobic beta hemolytic streptococcus and anaerobic nonhemolytic streptococcus. Clostridium species also cause gangrene and mild necrosis. Aggressive surgical debridement, intravenous antibiotics, irrigation with antibiotics, and dressing changes are imperative to save the patient's limb and life.

Pyogenic arthritis. See the section of this chapter that describes the treatment of human bites.

Gouty arthritis. This frequently will simulate the findings of a septic joint (Fig. 4-16). The most important information in making the diagnosis is a previous history of gout. An elevated serum uric acid level also will suggest the diagnosis. Aspiration will confirm the diagnosis using a polarizing scope. X-rays show exten-

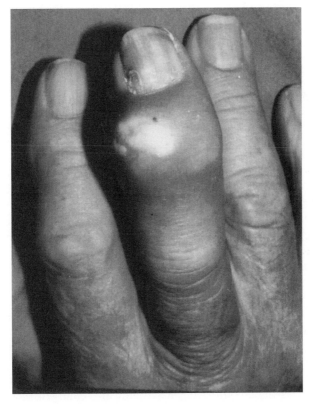

Figure 4-16   Gouty arthritis often is confused with a septic joint. This patient has a large, gouty, arthritic joint requiring drainage and eventual fusion of the finger joint.

sive joint destruction. Occasionally these become infected and require antibiotics, but usually an antiinflammatory medication will resolve the pain and erythema. Debridement and joint fusion may be indicated. The debrided material often is caseous in nature and may be confused with a tuberculous septic joint.

Herpetic Whitlow lesions. This lesion is caused by herpes simplex virus and commonly is seen in medical and dental assistants as well as in immunocompromised patients. The lesion is commonly confused with a perionychia or felon. Unfortunately, incision of the lesion may lead to a secondary infection and a prolonged recovery. The lesion is characteristic. Initial pain is followed by erythema, and tiny vesicles commonly are seen at the periphery of the lesions. These need to be looked for carefully because they are diagnostic. A Tzanck smear confirms the presence of giant cells in the vesicle fluid. Treatment is nonoperative, and the lesion is self-limiting in 3 to 4 weeks. Acyclovir may provide some symptomatic relief and decrease the recovery time.

Chronic Neglected Wounds

Microbiology
    Cultures (including fungal and special stains) should be obtained when the patient first arrives with the injury. These will dictate further therapy for chronic wounds.

Osteomyelitis
    Osteomyelitis usually is secondary to penetrating injuries or open fractures. It occasionally is seen after soft tissue infection (i.e., felons). Treatment includes bone curettage, sequestrectomy, and parental antibiotics. Amputation may be the most appropriate in distal finger bony infections to allow early rehabilitation. Diagnosing osteomyelitis in the environment of a severe soft tissue infection (perionychia or felon) may be difficult. X-rays showing periosteal reaction, an elevated leukocyte count, and an elevated erythrocyte sedimentation rate (ESR) may be helpful. Bone scans usually are not helpful, because they "light up" because of the surrounding soft tissue inflammation. Bone erosion by X-ray and biopsy are definitive.

Microbacterial Wounds

Tuberculosis
    This is becoming more frequent in immunocompromised patients. If a digit is involved, it is uniformly enlarged secondary to periostitis with cortical bone destruction. Bone curettage and antituberculous drugs are indicated. Treatment for tuberculous tenosynovitis includes tenosynovectomy and antituberculous drugs.

Marinum infections
These result from penetrating injuries in a marine environment. They tend to be indolent, requiring multiple surgeries and long-term antituberculous drug therapy.

Fungal Infections
Fungal infections are seen in wounds that are not responsive to the usual therapies.

Candida
This is commonly seen around fingernails and hands that are chronically moist (e.g., from dishwashing, thumbsucking, chronic perionychia). Nail removal and local antifungal agents may be indicated.

Sporotrichosis
This is seen most commonly in gardeners and florists. Treatment is debridement and oral ketoconazole.

Aspergillosis
This is seen in immunocompromised patients. Treatment includes debridement and amphotericin drug therapy.

Other Microorganisms

Anthrax
This is commonly seen after contact with infected livestock (especially cattle). Penicillin is indicated with minimal debridement.

Vibrio
This is seen after lacerations caused by the shells of sea animals (especially crabs and clams). Treatment is with tetracycline and aminoglycosides.

Aeromonas hydrophilia
This microorganism is isolated in stagnant water. It can be very aggressive with fatal septicemia. Treatment includes drainage and aminoglycosides parental antibiotic.

Chemotherapy Extravasation Injuries
Infiltration injuries are best treated acutely by rest, elevation, a splint, and local ice application. Numerous agents, including steroids, have been injected in the surrounding tissue, but may contribute to local tissue damage because of increasing pressure and edema. As with the Brown Recluse spider bites, some physicians recommend early excision of the areas to decrease tissue loss. As a rule, we have been more successful treating the injury with local ice applications for 48 hours, then administering sulfadiazine to prevent secondary infection, and allowing the tissue to demarcate before excision of necrotic tissue and wound closure. The use of dapsone may be as beneficial in these cases as in spider bites, but this needs to be discussed with the treating medi-

cal oncologist. After the wound has stabilized and is debrided, closure can be performed using the most appropriate method (i.e., skin graft, local flaps, or distal flaps).

WOUND COVERAGE OPTIONS
Analysis of Defect

Viability of Tissue

In examining a wound, the viability of the remaining tissue needs to be ascertained. This means examining the edge of the wound, as well as the tissue deep within the wound. Bleeding from the tissue after an abrasion with a sterile gauze is a good sign that the tissue will survive. Muscles that contract when stimulated reveal healthy intact fibers and motor plates. Intact peritenon supplies enough nutrients to keep the tendon from desiccation. If there is any doubt, fluorescein has been shown to reinforce our clinical judgment. If viability is still in doubt, a "second-look" procedure is appropriate within 24 to 48 hours after the tissues have had further time to demarcate.

Tissues Exposed

The exposure of vital structures (i.e., arteries, nerves, tendons, bone) necessitates rapid coverage to avoid desiccation and secondary injury. If tissue viability cannot be assessed early and these vital structures are protected, then temporary wound coverage may "tidy up" a wound and allow later evaluation. Temporary wound coverage includes the use of hydrocolloid gels or temporary allograft coverage.

Degree of Contamination

If heavily contaminated wounds are covered too early, there is a high risk of failure secondary to the bacteria inoculum as well as ongoing tissue necrosis. These wounds require debridement and temporary wound coverage before definitive soft tissue reconstructions.

Size and Location of Wound

Large wounds will not reepithelialize readily, and surgical closure should be considered. Wounds over joints tend to require pliable soft tissue reconstructions to allow motion.

Sensibility

"Like tissue" reconstructions should be considered, especially in the hand. Tissue in the hand has a high density of end-organ receptors. If similar tissue can be employed, the sensibility may be better with reinnervation.

Salvage of Parts

If tissue remnants are available after the injury, they may be used to improve the final result. This can be as simple as replacement of the skin removed by a meat slicer or the use of a retrieved fingertip as a composite graft. More complex uses include employing distal joints of an amputated part to replace injured proximal joints or using finger fragments as a "wrap" to cover a degloved bone of another injured finger.

Treatment Options

An understanding of the real "art" of reconstructive surgery is beneficial in considering the treatment options available (See Box, below).

The choice of "ideal" reconstruction is based on the defect, potential donor sites, and the desires of the patient. The following offers general treatment options. A discussion of specific defects will conclude the discussion.

1. Secondary wound healing may be especially appropriate in fingertip injuries. Wounds will contract to approximately one third of their original size after complete healing.
2. Skin grafting is most appropriate if the vital structures are not exposed and the depth of the wound is minimal. A full-thickness skin graft is more pliable, especially over joints and on the palm. When donor site options are being explored, consider color and the presence or absence of hair follicles, especially with full-thickness grafts. Meshed grafts rarely are used in the hand, except when the bed is draining large amounts of serous fluid; even then, nonexpanded mesh grafts may be the best choice.
3. Local flaps receive their nutrient supply either randomly or in an axial pattern. The flaps constitute an excellent source of similar tissue for reconstruction.
   a. Random flaps receive their blood supply through extensive subdermal plexus. These cannot be extended on the palm of the hand because the blood vessels tend to be oriented more vertically in this area.
   b. Axial flaps take advantage of direct blood supply from perforating vessels (muscular or fascial) that supply specific available

---

The "Art" of Plastic Surgery

1. Analysis of the defect and deformity
2. Consideration of available repair methods
3. Choice of ideal donor area
4. Design, transport, and implantation of the flap
5. The fourth dimension: time

donor area. These flaps leave other tissues available (tendon, nerve, bone) for reconstruction.

4. Distant flaps also are either random based, employing an extensive subdermal plexus, or axial flaps that use a single nutrient vessel.

    a. Random flaps are divided after revascularization by the wound base and edges (10-21 days). Relative ischemia of the flap encourages this neovascularization. Allow the greatest contact between the flap and the defect to ensure a greater surface area for ingrowth. This includes the formation of darts, which will increase the surface area at the edges as well as release cicatricial scarring (Fig. 4-17).

       The distant axial flap is the first choice for a mangled extremity. Coverage is obtained without interfering with the local ves-

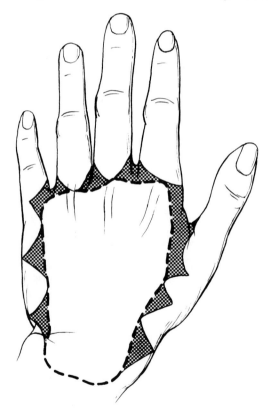

Figure 4-17 The original defect on the dorsum of the hand is outlined by the dashed lines. Extending this in a "dart" fashion to include the dotted shaded area will allow for more rapid ingrowth of new vessels. The flap will also have better drainage for a better cosmetic result.

sels that may be used in later reconstruction (i.e., toe to thumb, toe wrap, functional gracilis transfer). The most common distant axial flap is a free tissue microtransfer commonly known as a "free flap." The blood supply in these flaps is robust. In general, thin fascial free flaps are used (temporalis fascia, lateral arm flap) because of the thin soft tissue requirement in the hand. Other axial distal flaps include flaps from the proximal forearm used to cover hand defects. The venous return in these "reverse" flaps is vena comitantes. The groin flap based on the circumflex iliac artery and the abdominal hypogastric flap based on the perforators of the inferior epigastric artery also are examples of axial pedicle flaps.

Specific Defects and Coverage Options

Fingertips

If the amputated tip is not crushed and is available, a composite graft is possible, especially in children. Random flaps include a cross-finger flap that can be sensate by direct neurorrhaphy (Fig. 4-18) or a VY (Fig. 4-19*A* & *B*) volar pad advancement flap. Distant random

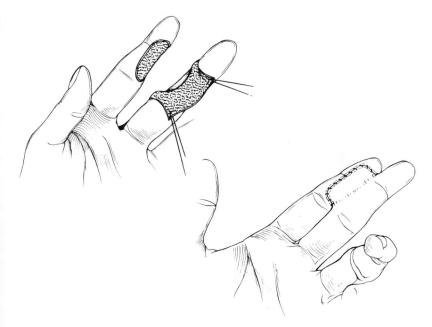

Figure 4-18   Cross-finger flaps are raised, using the adjacent finger dorsal skin to replace skin on the volar surface of the finger. These are divided at approximately 2 to 3 weeks.

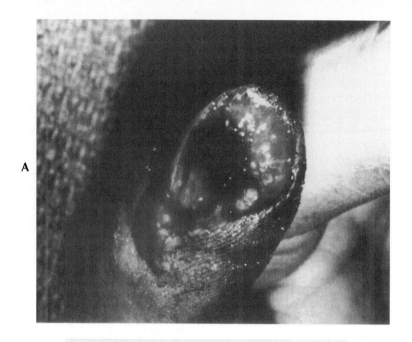

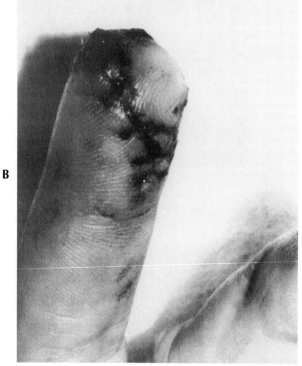

Figure 4-19 **(A)** This patient sustained a sharp injury in a dorsal to volar direction of his index finger. **(B)** The defect was repaired with advancement of the volar skin in a VY fashion.

flaps include the thenar flap (Fig. 4-20) or trunk flaps, including the groin, abdomen, chest, or opposite upper arm. Local axial flaps include the Kutler flap (Fig. 4-21) or a Moberg advancement flap (Fig. 4-22). Distant axial flaps include the neurovascular ulnar ring finger flap (Fig. 4-23), used especially for defects on the thumb or the radial

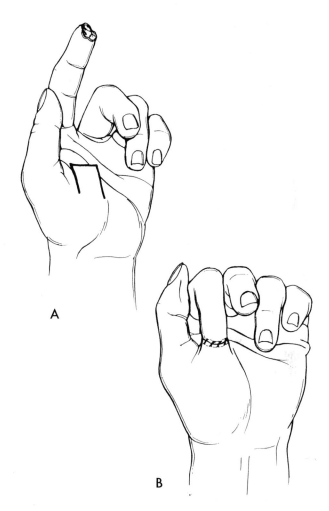

Figure 4-20   The thenar muscle flap is also used in fingertip amputations. The flap is raised along the thenar crease **(A)** and the finger is inserted into this donor flap **(B).**

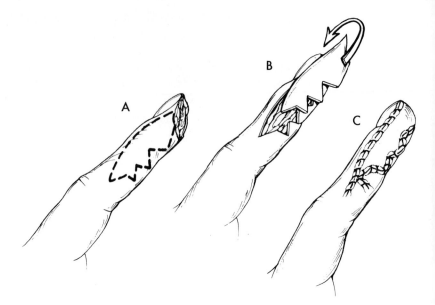

Figure 4-21 A Kutler flap employs the neurovascular bundle along the lateral aspects of each finger **(A).** The flap is maintained on the neurovascular bundle **(B)** and is advanced in suture to cover the fingertip defect **(C).**

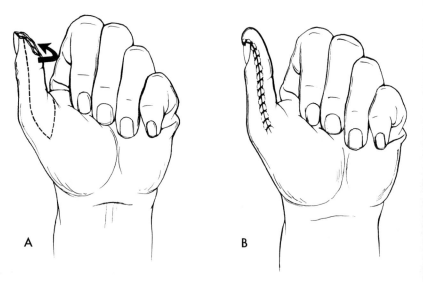

Figure 4-22 A Moberg flap employs both neurovascular bundles on the volar skin surface of the thumb **(A).** The flap is mobilized and advanced over the distal defect **(B)** and sutured into place for immediate soft tissue coverage.

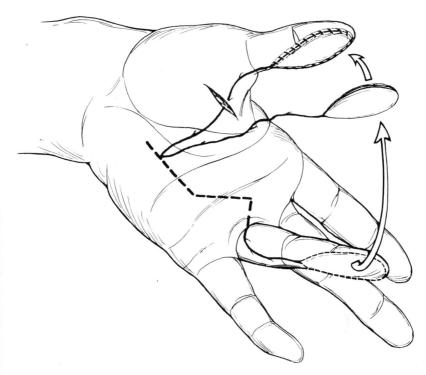

Figure 4-23   An ulnar ring neurovascular flap also may be employed for sensate flap coverage of the volar pad of the thumb. Care must be taken to maintain the neurovascular bundle to continue circulation as well as sensation. The donor site usually is skin grafted.

index where sensation is important, or a toe wrap with or without the toenail.

Finger Defects

Volar finger defects commonly are covered with cross-finger flaps, and dorsal defects are reconstructed with truncal pedicle flaps or dorsal intermetacarpal island flaps (Fig. 4-24*A* & *B*).

Midhand Defects

Palmar midhand defects can be covered with local muscle flaps and full-thickness skin grafts. Local muscle flaps include the pronator quadratus or the abductor digiti minimi (Fig. 4-25*A* & *B*). Larger midhand defects would require a truncal pedicle flap (Fig. 4-26), a free flap (temporalis fascia or sensate dorsalis pedis fasciocutaneous), or a

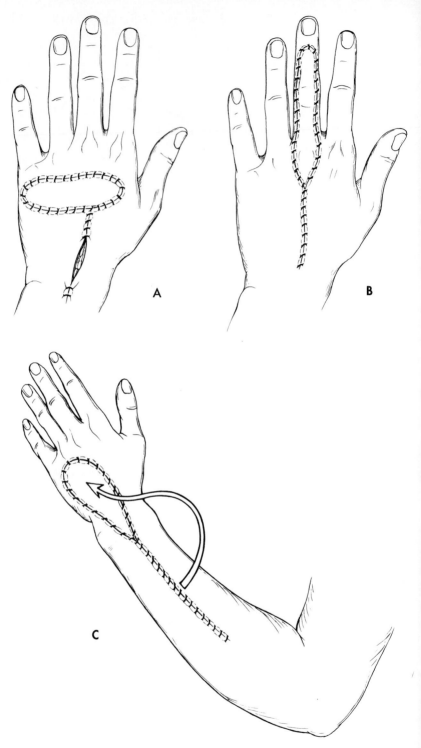

Figure 4-24 The dorsal intermetacarpal island flap is very versatile and can be used in a lateral orientation **(A)** or reversed orientation **(B).** The dorsal interosseous flap may be employed for more proximal dorsal skin defects **(C).**

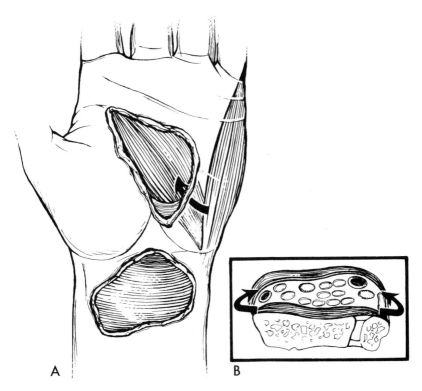

Figure 4-25   Volar palmar defects may be covered by the abductor digiti minimi muscle flap and skin grafting **(A)**. A more proximal defect in the wrist area will require a pronator muscle flap to cover the vital structures in the area **(B)**.

proximal radial (ulnar) reversed forearm flap (Fig. 4-27). There may be some advantages to supplying a fascial layer for tendon gliding, and a reverse interosseous fasciocutaneous forearm flap (Fig. 4-24*C*) has proved beneficial in covering dorsal hand defects, where thin pliable skin also is important.

Forearm Defects

Because these defects usually require more bulk and less sensation, truncal or groin pedicle flaps are very useful. Free flaps may supply motor units (gracilis or latissimus dorsi) or bone (scapula or fibula) for reconstruction.

Elbow Defects

These defects may be filled with local flaps (forearm muscle and split-thickness skin graft, reverse lateral arm fasciocutaneous), distal

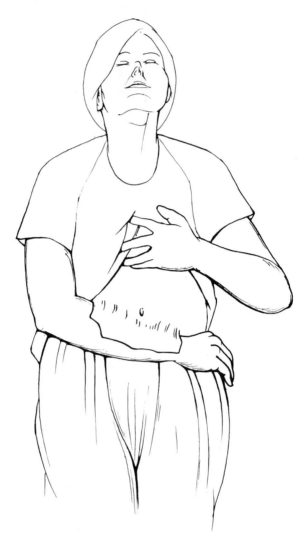

Figure 4-26 Distant pedicle flaps may be employed to resurface forearm and hand defects. In this patient, a superiorly based tailored abdominal flap is employed for a dorsal forearm defect.

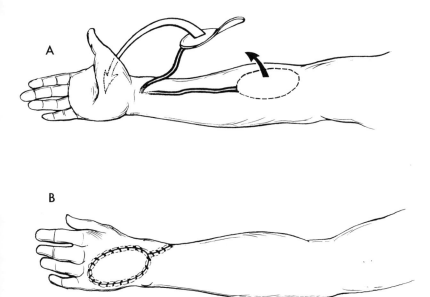

Figure 4-27   A reversed radial forearm flap also may be employed for dorsal hand coverage. The flap is raised and maintained on the radial artery and its venous supply **(A).** It is rotated and inset onto the dorsum of the hand with the donor site usually skin grafted **(B).**

pedicle flaps (truncal), or free flaps (scapular fasciocutaneous, vertical rectus myocutaneous).

SELECTED REFERENCES

Basadre JO, Parry SW: Indications for surgical debridement in 125 human bites to the hand, *Arch Surg* 126:65-67, 1991.

Cohen BE, Cronin ED: An innervated cross-finger flap for fingertip reconstruction, *Plast Reconstr Surg* 72:688-695, 1983.

Dellon AL: The proximal inset thenar flap for fingertip reconstruction, *Plast Reconstr Surg* 72:698-702, 1983.

Dellon AL, Mackinnon SE: The pronator quadratus muscle flap, *J Hand Surg* 9:423-427, 1984.

Early MJ, Barnsly AF: Human bite: a review, *Br J Plast Surg* 37:458-462, 1984.

Green DP: *Operative hand surgery,* ed 3, New York, 1993, Churchill Livingstone.

Hallock GG: Distal-based flaps for hand coverage, *Contemp Orthop* 31:83-89, 1995.

Hoehn J, Elliott R, Edmond J, Spitzer J: Practical management of fingertip injuries, *Surg Rounds* 16-24, August 1983.

Kelleher JC, Sullivan JG, Baibak GJ, et al: Use of a tailored abdominal pedicle flap for surgical reconstruction of the hand, *J Bone Surg* 52A:1552-1562, 1970.

Kelleher JC, Sullivan JG, Baibak GJ, et al: Large combined axial vessel pattern abdominal pedicle flap: indications for its use in surgery of the hand, *Orthop Rev* 11:33-48, 1982.

Kulick MI, Winslow J: Evaluating and treating hand injuries, *Hosp Phys* 26-38, September 1987.

Marty FM, Montandon D, Gumener R, et al: The use of subcutaneous tissue flaps in the repair of soft tissue defects of the forearm and hand: an experimental and clinical study of a new technique, *Br J Plast Surg* 37:95-102, 1984.

Maruyama Y: The reverse dorsal metacarpal flap. *Br J Plast Surg* 43:24-27, 1990.

McGregor IA: Flap reconstruction in hand surgery: the evolution of presently used methods, *J Hand Surg* 4:1-10, 1979.

Newmeyer WL: Management of hand injuries, *Res Staff Phys* 29:72-85, 1983.

Quaba AA, Davison PM: The distally-based dorsal hand flap, *Br J Plast Surg* 43:28-29, 1990.

Rayan GM, Flournoy DJ: Hand infections, *Contemp Orthop* 20:41-54, 1990.

Rees R, Shack RB, Withers E: Management of the brown recluse spider bites, *Plast Reconstr Surg* 68:768-773, 1981.

Roberts RS, Csenscsity TA, Herd CW: Upper extremity compartment syndromes following pit viper envenomations, *Clin Orthop* 193:184-188, 1985.

Schlenker JD, Stasoy E, Lyon JW: The abdominohypogastric flap: an axial pattern flap for forearm coverage, *Hand* 12:248-252, 1980.

Sprenger TR, Bailey WJ: Snake bite treatment in the United States, *J Dermatol* 25:479-484, 1986.

Trott A: *Wounds and lacerations: emergency care and closure,* St. Louis, 1991, Mosqby.

Vogel JE, Dellon AL: Frostbite injuries of the hand, *Clin Plast Surg* 16:565-576, 1989.

Wray RC, Wise DM, Young VL, et al: The groin flap in severe hand injuries, *Ann Plast Surg* 9:459-462, 1982.

Zook EG: Care of nail bed injuries, *Surg Rounds* 44-61, September 1985.

5

Tendon Congruity

David S. Martin, MD
Paul M. Weeks, MD, FACS

STAGED TENDON
RECONSTRUCTION
   Tendon Grafting
   Sources of Tendon Graft
     Material
   Two-Staged Tendon
     Reconstruction
   Pulley System Reconstruction

SUMMARY

SELECTED REFERENCES

Tendon injuries are among the most common and functionally important, specialized tissue injuries encountered in the upper extremity. The extraordinary range of motions accomplished in the hand, from the power grasp of a sledgehammer to the delicate, precise action of threading a needle, require the coordinated, balanced actions of interactive musculotendinous units. Despite the dramatic appearance of large, open, soft tissue wounds, major vascular injuries, and severely comminuted fractures, the ultimate functional outcome following hand injury often is influenced greatly by the degree of musculotendinous dysfunction. Inherent characteristics of the motor system for the hand and fingers contribute both to the controversy and difficulty in successfully managing tendon injuries.

TENDON ANATOMY AND FUNCTION

The muscles that provide motion of the fingers and thumb can be classified as intrinsic and extrinsic. The intrinsic muscles of the hand (Table 5-1) have both their origin and insertion in the hand itself. The lumbricals, dorsal and palmer interossei, intrinsic thenar, and hypothenar muscles constitute this group. The most important intrinsic motor function is that of thumb opposition, which is accomplished by the thenar intrinsic muscles.

Extrinsic muscles generate most of the power for the fingers and the wrist. These large muscles have their fleshy portion proximally in the forearm, have musculotendinous junctions in the mid forearm to distal forearm, and insert through tendons in the fingers themselves where they act synergistically using a complex pulley system.

Volar (Flexor) Muscles

Extrinsic muscles that provide flexion of the wrist, thumb, and fingers are located on the volar (anterior) surface of the forearm (see Fig. 5-1, Fig. 5-2, and Table 5-2).

Name	Origin	Insertion	Action	Nerve
Thenar Muscles				
Adbuctor pollicis brevis	Flexor retinaculum, scaphoid tuberosity, and trapezium	Lateral side of base of first phalanx of thumb	Abducts thumb	Median
Opponens pollicis	Flexor retinaculum and trapezium	Radial side of thumb metacarpal	Abducts, flexes, and rotates thumb metacarpal	Median
Flexor pollicis brevis	Flexor retinaculum and trapezium	Lateral and medial sides of base of thumb proximal phalanx	Flexes and adducts thumb	Median and deep ulnar
Adductor pollicis	Capitate and bases index and long metacarpals	Medial side of base of first phalanx of thumb	Adducts thumb	Deep ulnar
Intermediate Group				
Palmer interossei	Medial side of index metacarpal and lateral side of ring and little metacarpals	Medial side of extensor hood for index finger and lateral side of extensor hood for ring and little fingers	Adduct fingers toward long finger, flexes MCP joints, and extends PIP and DIP joints	Deep ulnar
Dorsal interossei	Metacarpal shafts on adjacent sides of each intermetacarpal space	Lateral sides of index and long finger extensor hoods and medial sides of long, ring, and little finger hoods	Abducts fingers away from long finger, flexes MCP joints, and extends PIP and DIP joints	Deep ulnar

Continued

Table 5-1 Intrinsic Hand Muscles—cont'd

Name	Origin	Insertion	Action	Nerve
Thenar Muscles cont'd				
Lumbricals (index and long fingers)	Radial side of FDP tendons to index and long fingers	Radial side of extensor hood to index and long fingers	Flex MCP joints and extends PIP and DIP joints	Median
Lumbricals (ring and little fingers)	Radial side of FDP tendons to ring and little fingers	Radial side of extensor hood to ring and little fingers	Flexes MCP joints and extends PIP and DIP joints	Ulnar
Hypothenar Group				
Palmaris brevis	Flexor retinaculum and palmar aponeurosis	Skin of medial border of palm	Projects hypothenar eminence	Ulnar
Abductor digiti minimi	Pisiform and tendon of flexor carpi ulnaris	medial side of base of first phalanx of little finger	Abducts little finger and flexes proximal phalanx	Ulnar
Flexor digit minimi brevis	Hook of hamate and flexor retinaculum	Medial side of base of first phalanx of little finger	Flexes proximal phalanx of little finger	Ulnar
Opponens digiti minimi	Hook of hamate and flexor retinaculum	Medial side of base of first phalanx of little finger	Opposes little finger	Ulnar

MCP, metacarpophalangeal; PIP, proximal interphalangeal; DIP, distal interphalangeal; FDP, flexor digitorum profundus.

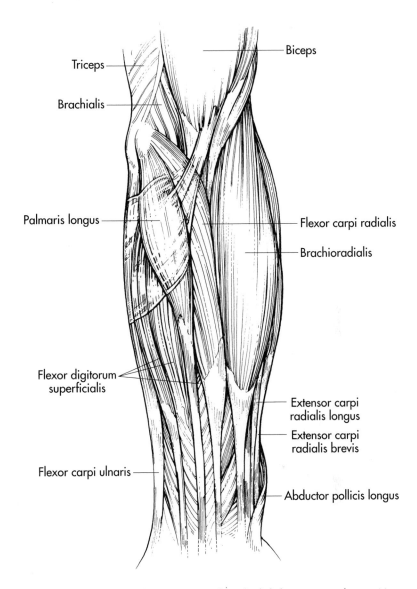

Figure 5-1   The superficial anterior muscles of a left forearm are shown. Note that with the exception of the brachioradialis, the flexor mass arises from the "common flexor origin," consisting of medial epicondyle and proximal ulna.

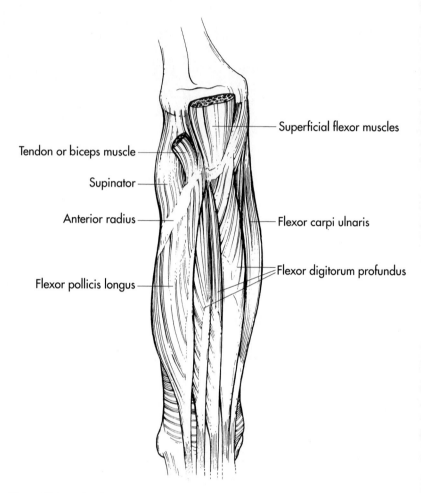

Superficial flexor muscles

Tendon or biceps muscle

Supinator

Anterior radius

Flexor pollicis longus

Flexor carpi ulnaris

Flexor digitorum profundus

Figure 5-2   The deep anterior muscles of a right forearm are shown. The median nerve and ulnar artery travel between the superficialis and profundus muscle bellies.

Wrist Flexors

The flexor carpi radialis (FCR) has as its origin the medial epicondyle of the humerus (common flexor origin) and as its insertion the base of the index metacarpal. It is one of the three most superficial tendons encountered at the wrist and often is visible at rest or during resisted wrist flexion. Its innervation is through the median nerve (C6C7) at the level of the proximal forearm. It travels radial to the carpal tunnel and just ulnar to the radial artery. It acts to flex the wrist

Table 5-2   Anterior Forearm Muscles

Name	Origin	Insertion	Action	Nerve
Superficial Group				
Flexor carpi radialis	Medial epicondyle	BAses of index and long metacarpals	Flexes wrist and abducts hand	Median
Palmaris longus	Medial epicondyle	Transverse carpal ligament and palmer aponeurosis	Flexes wrist	Median
Flexor carpi ulnaris	Medial epicondyle, medial olecranon, and posterior ulna	Pisiform, hamate, and little metacarpal	Flexes wrist and adducts hand	Ulnar
Flexor digitorum superficialis	Medial epicondyle, coronoid process of ulna, and oblique line of radius	Bases of middle phalanges of four fingers	Flexes MCP and PIP joints and wrist	Median
Pronator teres	Medial humerus above epicondyle and medial side of coronoid process of ulna	Lateral side of radius	Pronates forearm	Median

Continued

Table 5-2 Anterior Forearm Muscles—cont'd

Name	Origin	Insertion	Action	Nerve
Deep Group				
Flexor digitorum profundus	Upper anterior and medial ulna, medial coronoid process and proximal ulna, and interosseous membrane	Bases of distal phalanges of all four fingers	Flexes entire finger and wrist	Median and ulnar
Flexor pollicis longus	Anterior shaft of radius and interosseous membrane	Base of distal phalanx of thumb	Flexes thumb and first metacarpal and adducts thumb metacarpal	Median
Pronator quadratus	Distal shaft of ulna	Distal anterolateral border of radius	Pronates forearm	Median

MCP, metacarpophalangeal; PIP, proximal interphalangeal.

and contributes to motions requiring radial deviation, such as hammering.

The flexor carpi ulnaris (FCU) has its origin on the medial epicondyle of the humerus and the posterior ulna and travels across the wrist to insert on the pisiform, little finger metacarpal, and hook of the hamate. It also is one of the most superficial tendons in the forearm and wrist and normally is visible during wrist flexion. Functionally, it is the prime wrist flexor. It is innervated by the ulnar nerve, with branches arising below the elbow (C7C8). Traveling beneath it are the ulnar nerve and the ulnar artery.

The palmaris longus, absent in 15% of the population, is a small muscle originating from the medial epicondyle of the humerus and inserting into the palmer aponeurosis (palmer fascia) just distal to the distal wrist crease. The palmaris tendon is superficial at wrist level and can be seen when resisted flexion of the wrist is attempted. Functionally, it makes a relatively minor contribution to wrist flexion and is considered expendable. It is an excellent choice when a donor tendon is needed for grafting.

Finger Flexors

The index, long, ring, and little fingers each have two primary flexor tendons: the flexor digitorum superficialis (FDS) and the flexor digitorum profundus (FDP).

The flexor digitorum superficialis arises from the common flexor origin at the medial epicondyle of the humerus and anterior radius and traverses the midforearm and the carpal tunnel. The four individual tendons diverge in the palm, and after traveling through the flexor tendon sheath of each finger, split to insert on the radial and ulnar aspects of the bases of the middle phalanges. In the palm, superficialis tendons can be distinguished from profundus tendons by their absence of lumbrical muscles, which originate on the radial aspect of each profundus tendon. In the carpal tunnel, the superficialis tendons from a 2×2 tier, with the FDS to the long and ring fingers typically lying superficial to the FDS tendons to the index and little fingers. In general, the larger, more central fingers have larger caliber flexor tendons. All portions of the FDS (which is one muscle motoring four tendons) are innervated classically by branches of the median nerve in the forearm (C7C8T1); however, variations in innervation are common, and certain FDS slips may be innervated by branches of the ulnar nerve. Each flexor digitorum superficialis tendon splits to encircle its associated profundus tendon at the level of the proximal phalanx, where the profundus becomes the most superficial flexor in the finger. After splitting and encircling the FDP, the FDS reunites to form "campers chiasm" before again diverging to insert on the radial and ulnar aspects of the middle phalangeal base. Both the superficialis and profundus tendons contribute to finger flexion globally, but the best isolated action of the FDS is flexion of the PIP joint while keeping the FDP extended. This motion can be tested by maintaining full extension of the adjacent fingers thereby, restricting excursion of the injured finger's FDP, which cannot flex independently of adjacent FDP tendons (see Fig. 5-11*A*). Isolated PIP flexion cannot be accomplished without the FDS because the FDP inserts across the DIP joint and consequently always moves it at least simultaneously with the other finger joints. The FDS to the little finger may be absent or relatively weak as a normal variant, and comparison to the uninjured hand may be useful.

Flexor digitorum profundus (FDP) tendons arise from a single muscle belly of the FDP in the proximal forearm deep to the FDS and the median nerve. The FDP originates along the medial and anterior proximal ulna and interosseous membrane. These tendons also pass along the midaxial portion of the volar forearm, traverse the carpal tunnel, and then diverge toward each finger, before inserting at the base of the distal phalanx. Each FDP tendon penetrates the center of the FDS to lie superficial to it, beginning at the level of the proximal phalanx. As with the FDS tendons, the caliber of each FDP tendon is larger to the long and ring fingers, smaller to the index, and smallest to the little finger. Although the FDP, like the FDS, contributes to overall finger flexion, its isolated function, which no other flexor tendon can perform, is flexion of the DIP joint. Consequently, testing active DIP flexion after an injury is the most effective method for evaluating FDP integrity (see Fig. 5-11*B*). The innervation of the FDP muscles is classically through the median nerve for the index and long fingers (C7C8) and through the ulnar nerve for the ring and little fingers (C7C8). However, variable patterns of innervation are common.

Thumb Flexion

Flexion of the thumb is accomplished primarily by the flexor pollicis longus (FPL), and to a smaller degree, by the flexor pollicis brevis. The flexor pollicis longus is one of the deepest musculotendinous units in the forearm. It originates from the proximal anterior radius and interosseous membrane and inserts on the proximal portion of the distal phalanx of the thumb. Although it traverses the carpal tunnel, it travels in its own synovial sheath along the deep radial floor of the canal. As with the other digits, the FPL travels through a fibrous digital sheath, but one less complicated than that of the fingers (see Fig. 5-5).

Tendon Orientation at the Wrist Level

A cross-sectional view depicting the orientation of tendons and nerves at the level of the wrist is shown in Fig. 5-3.

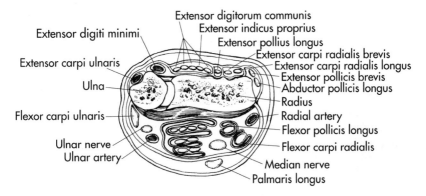

Figure 5-3   Cross-section of the wrist at the level of the distal radius.

Intrinsic Thumb Motion/Opposition

The opposing action of the thumb—the ability to abduct the thumb away from the plane of the remaining digits—is the single most important functional motion in the hand and wrist. A thumb that remains in the plane of the other fingers makes no contribution to the ability to grasp. Although the thumb extensors and abductors, which are detailed in the "extensor" portion of the text, contribute to extending the thumb, it is the action of the intrinsic thenar muscles that allows the thumb metacarpal to become abducted from the palm and rotate into a position facilitating useful opposition.

The intrinsic thenar and hypothenar muscles are listed in Table 5-1. The intrinsic thenar muscles are innervated predominantly by the recurrent motor branch of the median nerve (C8T1), but variable innervation can occur from the deep branch of the ulnar nerve. The slender motor branch of the median nerve diverges from the main portion of the median nerve along its radial aspect, usually just distal to the transverse carpal ligament, before entering and innervating these intrinsic muscles. In a minority of patients, the motor branch of the median nerve actually may penetrate the midportion of the transverse carpal ligament, or may branch from the main portion of the median nerve proximal to the ligament. This nerve typically innervates the abductor pollicis brevis, the opponens pollicis, and the superficial head of the flexor pollicis brevis. Transection of this nerve results in an inability to oppose the thumb and must be recognized.

Also located in the first web space (between thumb and index fingers) are the adductor pollicis and the first dorsal interosseous muscles, both of which are innervated by the deep ulnar nerve. They act to bring the thumb and index into a "key pinch," as if one were grasping a key between the thumb and the radial border of the index finger.

The deep intrinsic muscles in the palm are the lumbricals and the volar and dorsal interossei. Each lumbrical originates on the radial side of the tendon of its flexor digitorum profundus and inserts on the extensor hood for that finger. The lumbricals flex the MCP joints and extend the interphalangeal joints of each finger. The lumbricals also help stabilize the extensor hood throughout its range of motion when acted on by the extrinsic flexor and extensor tendons. The lumbricals to the index and long fingers typically are innervated by the median nerve (C8T1) and those to the ring and little fingers by the deep branch of the ulnar nerve (C8T1).

The three volar and four dorsal interossei originate between adjacent metacarpals and also insert onto the extensor hood. The dorsal interossei abduct the fingers from the axis of the long finger and the volar interossei tend to adduct the fingers in relation to this same axis. They are innervated by the deep (motor) branch of the ulnar nerve (C8T1).

The hypothenar muscles, which are also listed in Table 5-1, include the abductor digiti minimi, flexor digiti minimi brevis, opponens digiti minimi, and palmaris brevis. They aid in rotation and opposition of the little finger from the palm and are innervated by the ulnar nerve (C8T1).

Flexor Tendon Sheath

One of the most important structures ensuring the smooth gliding action of the fingers is the flexor tendon sheath. Its intimate relationship with the flexor tendons allows flexor tendon motion without bowstringing and delicate, supple tendon motion in almost any position. However, its inherent structure also contributes to substantial difficulties in both traumatic injuries and in infection.

The fibrous digital sheath of each finger is comprised of arcuate and cruciate pulleys (designated "A" pulleys and "C" pulleys) through which the flexor tendons glide. These are shown in Fig. 5-4. These pulleys are transverse bands of fibrous tissue of variable thickness (and consequently strength) that allow smooth transmission of flexion forces throughout a variety of finger positions. In general, the A-2 and the A-4 pulleys (at the level of the proximal portion of the proximal phalanx and the middle portion of the middle phalanx, respectively) are the essential pulleys. Their transection, either by trauma or during the process of surgical tendon repair or reconstruction, has serious consequences. Uncoordinated finger motion, bowstringing, and failure of longitudinally transmitted flexor forces to be appropriately directed will result if they are not preserved or restored.

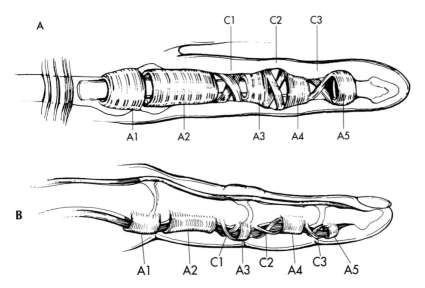

Figure 5-4   The anatomy of the fibrous flexor digital sheath is depicted. The A-2 and A-4 pulleys are considered "essential" to smooth tendon gliding. Intervening areas, including the cruciate pulleys, may be incised to expose the underlying tendons.

The thumb flexor sheath is present, but is much less complicated than that of the other digits. There are two important arcuate pulleys in the thumb, located at the level of the MCP joint and at the interphalangeal joint, that prevent bowstringing (Fig. 5-5). A single cruciate pulley is located between them.

Extensor Muscles

All of the extrinsic musculotendinous units that allow for extension of the wrist, thumb, and fingers are located on the dorsal (posterior) portion of the forearm. Essentially, all extension function in the hand and wrist is extrinsic, with muscles located in the forearm acting through tendons across the wrist on the hand and fingers. All extensor tendons are innervated by branches of the radial nerve (C5C6C7). The extensor surface of the forearm is shown in Fig. 5-6, and the muscles are listed in Table 5-3.

Although the brachioradialis is not an effector of either wrist or finger motion, it is worthwhile to comment on it because of its prominence in the dorsal forearm and its susceptibility to injury from lacera-

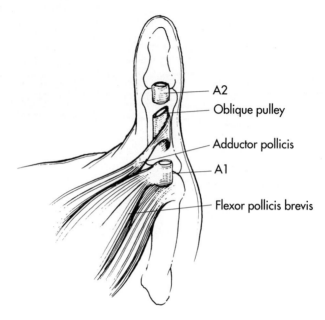

Figure 5-5   The thumb flexor digital sheath is shown. It is composed of two annular pulleys at the level of the MCP and IP joints, respectively, and a single oblique pulley.

tions there. Of the forearm muscles, it has the "highest" origin on the humerus, with its insertion being along the radial (lateral) side of the distal radius. It is innervated by branches from the radial nerve that arise above the elbow. It acts both to assist in elbow flexion and as a supinator of the forearm (thumbs down to thumbs up position). It constitutes a portion of the "mobile wad" of the dorsal forearm and is readily palpable superficially along the dorsal radial aspect of the proximal forearm.

Wrist Extensors

There are three main wrist extensors: the extensor carpi radialis longus (ECRL), extensor carpi radialis brevis (ECRB), and the extensor carpi ulnaris (ECU). The extensor carpi radialis longus (ECRL) earns its designation from its supracondylar humeral origin, whereas the extensor carpi radialis brevis (ECRB) originates along the lateral epicondyle of the humerus (common extensor origin). The ECRL and ECRB insert on the bases of the index and long metacarpals, respectively. The extensor carpi ulnaris (ECU) originates on the lateral epicondyle of the humerus and inserts on the base of the little metacarpal. All wrist extensors are innervated by branches of the radial nerve (C6C7). The most functionally important wrist extensor is thought to be the ECRB.

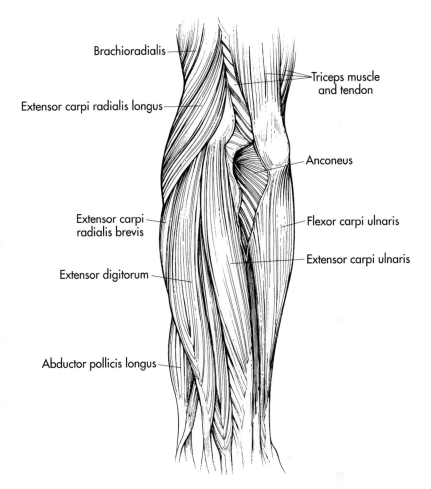

Brachioradialis

Extensor carpi radialis longus

Triceps muscle
and tendon

Anconeus

Extensor carpi
radialis brevis

Flexor carpi ulnaris

Extensor carpi ulnaris

Extensor digitorum

Abductor pollicis longus

Figure 5-6   The muscles of the extensor (posterior) surface of the forearm are shown. The bracioradialis, followed by the extensor carpi radialis longus have the highest origin, arising from the supracondylar humerus, while the extensor carpi radialis brevis and the extensor carpi ulnaris originate predominantly from the lateral epicondyle.

Finger Extensors

The ulnar four fingers share a common extensor muscle–tendon unit, the extensor digitorum communis (EDC). The extensor digitorum communis arises from the common extensor origin (lateral epicondyle of the humerus) and provides four tendons for the four fingers. These tendons are connected on the dorsum of the hand by small transverse bands of tendinous tissue, the juncturae tendinum, which

Table 5-3   Posterior Forearm Muscles

Name	Origin	Insertion	Action	Nerve
Superficial Group				
Extensor carpi radialis longus	Lateral supracondylar ridge of humerus	Posterior base of index metacarpal	Extends and abducts hand	Radial
Extensor carpi radialis brevis	Lateral epicondyle of humerus	Posterior base of long metacarpal	Extends and abducts hand	Radial
Extensor digitorum communis	Lateral epicondyle of humerus	Bases of middle and distal phalanges of the four fingers	Extends fingers and hand	Radial
Extensor digiti minimi	Common extensor tendon	Extensor aponeurosis of little finger	Extends little finger	Radial
Extensor carpi ulnaris	Lateral epicondyle of humerus posterior border of ulna	Base of little metacarpal	Extends and adducts hand	Radial
Deep Group				
Supinator	Lateral epicondyle	Radial tubercle and oblique line of radius	Supinates hand	Deep radial
Abductor pollicis longus	Posterolateral ulna and interosseous membrane	Lateral base of thumb metacarpal	Abducts thumb and hand	Deep radial
Extensor pollicis brevis	Posterior radius and interosseous membrane	Base of proximal phalanx of thumb	Extends thumb proximal phalanx	Deep radial
Extensor pollicis longus	Posterolateral ulna	Base of distal phalanx of thumb	Extends thumb	Deep radial
Extensor indicis proprius	Posterior shaft of ulna and interosseous membrane	Extensor apparatus of index finger	Extends and adducts index finger	Deep radial

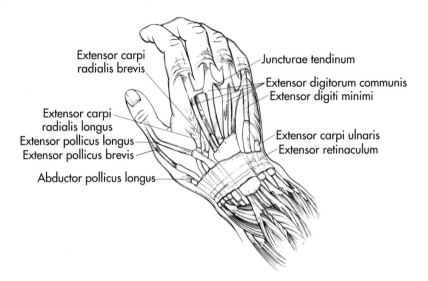

Extensor carpi
radialis brevis

Extensor carpi
radialis longus
Extensor pollicus longus
Extensor pollicus brevis

Abductor pollicus longus

Juncturae tendinum

Extensor digitorum communis
Extensor digiti minimi

Extensor carpi ulnaris
Extensor retinaculum

Figure 5-7   The anatomy of the dorsum of the hand. The extensor tendons travel through the extensor retinaculum in groups as shown. Awareness of their location can assist in tendon retrieval and in surgical approaches to the dorsal wrist.

are shown in Fig. 5-7. Therefore, it is possible for an extensor tendon to one finger to be transected completely but, because of the juncturae distally, motion of an adjacent extensor tendon may exert some—although usually weak—extension of that finger.

Although individual finger extension is less independent than finger flexion, the index and little finger do have independent extensor muscles. The extensor indicus proprius (EIP) and the extensor digiti minimi (or quinti) (EDQ) arise from the lateral epicondyle and have independent insertions on the extensor hoods of the index and little finger, respectively. These tendons are located consistently on the ulnar side of their communis counterparts.

Thumb Extension and Abduction

Extension and abduction of the thumb are accomplished by the following musculotendinous units: The abductor pollicis longus, extensor pollicis brevis, and the extensor pollicis longus. These muscles are listed in Table 5-3. The abductor inserts on the base of the thumb metacarpal, the extensor pollicis brevis onto the base of the proximal phalanx, and the extensor pollicis longus onto the base of the thumb distal phalanx.

Extensor Tendon Orientation at the Wrist

The thumb, finger, and wrist extensor tendons are oriented consistently at the level of the wrist, and an understanding of their relative

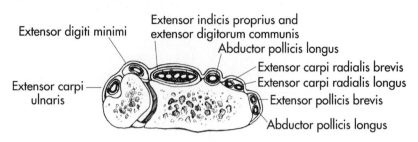

Extensor digiti minimi

Extensor indicis proprius and
extensor digitorum communis

Abductor pollicis longus

Extensor carpi radialis brevis

Extensor carpi
ulnaris

Extensor carpi radialis longus

Extensor pollicis brevis

Abductor pollicis longus

Figure 5-8   Dorsal wrist compartments are shown in cross-section.

Table 5-4   Dorsal Wrist Compartments

First	Abductor pollicis longus
	Extensor pollicis brevis
Second	Extensor carpi radialis longus
	Extensor carpi radialis brevis
Third	Extensor pollicis longus
Fourth	Extensor digitorum communis
	Extensor indicis proprious
Fifth	Extensor digiti minimi
Sixth	Extensor carpi ulnaris

position is important in locating and reconstructing injured tendons. The dorsum of the wrist and its compartments are shown in Fig. 5-8. The extensor tendons have a relatively short retinaculum that is located at the level of the wrist. It is desirable to preserve a portion of the extensor retinaculum during dissection in this area to prevent extensor tendon bowstringing. From radial to ulnar, there are six extensor compartments at this wrist (see Table 5-4).

Finger Extensor Apparatus

The "extensor hood," formed as condensations of the insertions of the extensor tendons, is a more three dimensionally complicated structure than the insertions of the FDS and FDP on the palmer surface. However, there is no true fibrous digital sheath, as is found encompassing the flexor tendons in the digits. Extrinsic extensor forces are kept balanced by the actions of the lumbricals and interossei, which allow a wide range of finger postures. The anatomy of the extensor hood is shown in Fig. 5-9. In general, each extensor hood has strong insertions into the base of the middle phalanx (central slip) and, by consolidation of the lateral bands, into the base of the distal phalanx. Unrecognized injury to portions of the extensor hood and the resultant

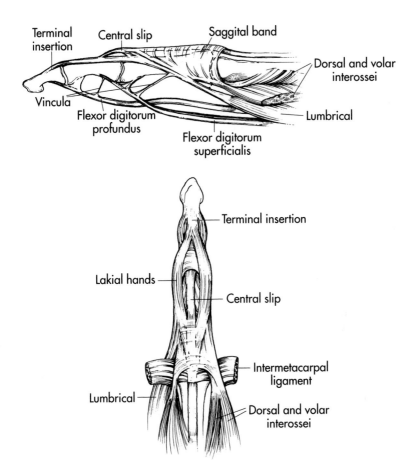

Figure 5-9 The extensor apparatus of a finger. Coordinated interactive motions between lateral forces (from interossei and lumbricals) and between central forces from the extrinsic extensor tendons allow diverse finger motion and position.

imbalance of resting and active forces on the finger ultimately can lead to a variety of abnormal finger postures, such as boutonniere and mallet deformities.

Tendon Nutrition and Healing

Although described more thoroughly in Chapter 1, peculiar tendon anatomy and physiology and their implications for successful healing warrant further brief emphasis. There are several important points.

1. Tendons, particularly flexor tendons, must be capable of gliding to function properly. The typical excursion of flexor tendons often is

several centimeters, whereas that of extensor tendons is less than 1 cm.

2. Tendons are relatively avascular, acellular structures comprised primarily of longitudinally oriented strands of collagen that provide tremendous strength. Longitudinal blood supply in the digit is by a vincular system (dorsal vascular pedicles enter the tendon, perfusing it longitudinally). Optimal repair of injured tendons necessitates a strong and enduring tendon repair that does not compromise tendon vascularity by strangulation.

3. Tendons require long periods of time to regain their tensile strength (typically 6-12 weeks). Excessive premature motion and/or force during healing will lead to tendon repair rupture.

4. Some adhesion formation is necessary at the repair site for tendons to heal, but significant adhesion formation, particularly to the tendon sheath, will impair useful motion.

5. Early controlled (gentle) motion of tendons appears to be fundamentally important, balancing the need for immobilization (to promote healing) and motion (to avoid excessive adhesions and assure gliding).

6. The nature of the initial injury, the adequacy of the surgical repair, and equally importantly, the quality and compliance with a postoperative rehabilitation program determine the amount of useful function regained.

EVALUATION OF TENDON FUNCTION

Diagnosis of tendon injury usually is not difficult. The following concepts, used together, can consistently and accurately diagnose tendon injury in the majority of patients.

History

The patient's description of the injury can give important clues as to the likelihood of tendon injury. Although tendon injuries can occur after blunt (closed) trauma, open injuries with sharp objects of all types are by far a more common etiology for tendon injury and disruption. The mechanism of injury and the position of the hand and/or fingers at the time of injury should be investigated. For example, most flexor tendon lacerations occur with the finger in flexion, with the site of tendon transection lying distal to the site of skin laceration when a resting finger posture is resumed. Similarly, open injuries on the dorsum of the hand, because of the superficial and unprotected position of the extensor tendons, have a high incidence of tendon laceration. As with the aforementioned example, a patient whose hand was clenched in a fist when it struck a glass window may be expected to have sustained an extensor tendon laceration located proximal to the skin laceration.

Any patient with altered sensation and/or evidence of arterial injury should warrant a high index of suspicion for associated tendon injury. Finger lacerations deep enough to lacerate digital nerves usually are deep enough to lacerate a flexor tendon. Similarly, patients attempting suicide who transect the median nerve or the radial or ulnar arteries will have lacerated tendons as well.

It also is worthwhile to query the patient's occupation. Functional requirements for a heavy machine operator are different from those of a retired grandmother. The patient's occupation will influence the amount of time off work before resuming unprotected activity with the injured extremity.

Wound Examination

The patient's wounds should be examined and the length, location, and apparent depth of each wound noted. The amount of contamination present should be assessed, as should the quality and any deficiency of the surrounding soft tissues. The perfusion distal to any wound should be assured and any evidence of threatened tissue viability promptly detected.

Posture

The resting position of the injured hand often can reveal important clues to underlying injuries of the tendons, even without the patient performing any active motion (Fig. 5-10A). This is particularly important in pediatric, intoxicated, demented, or noncompliant patients, who may not be able to perform requested motions. The examiner should note the resting position of the wrist (radial nerve or wrist extensor injuries). The fingers should form a cascade at rest, where the little finger at rest is most flexed, followed by the ring finger, which is slightly less flexed at rest, followed by the long and index fingers. Any finger extended out of its expected position within the cascade is assumed to have a tendon laceration regardless of the nature of the skin laceration. We have observed completely transected FDS and FDP tendons through skin incisions no more than a few millimeters across. Similarly, one may evaluate the tenodesis effect (Fig. 5-10B): altering wrist position will affect the resting position of the fingers. Flexion of the wrist results in relative tightening of the finger extensors and relaxing of the flexors; consequently, the fingers will extend relative to the hand. Similarly, wrist extension should yield comparable smooth

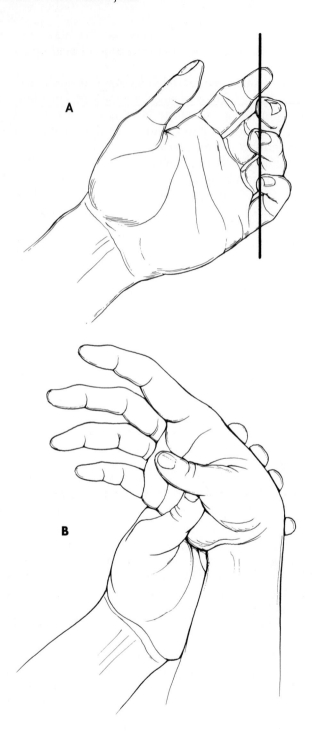

A

B

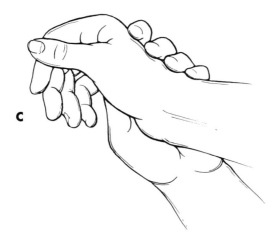

C

Figure 5-10 **(A)** Resting finger cascade. The resting forces exerted by flexors and extensors on the finger normally create the finger postures shown. Deviation from the expected position may indicate underlying tendon injury. **(B)** Tenodesis effect. Flexion of the wrist tightens extensors and loosens flexors; consequently the fingers assume a more extended position, although the normal cascade is preserved. Wrist extension has the opposite effect **(C)**.

flexion of the fingers. It is would be unusual for patients with transected flexor or extensor tendons to exhibit normal finger posture throughout the range of wrist motion. Disproportionate levels of pain during active or resisted motion may signal a partial tendon laceration. The position of the thumb also should be observed. The normal resting position of the uninjured thumb is slightly opposed (out of the plane of the palm), slightly abducted, with 20 to 40° of flexion of the MCP joint. Injuries to the motor branch of the median nerve will allow the thumb to return to the plane of the remainder of the hand; extensor tendon injuries yield excessive resting flexion of the thumb, and flexor injuries yield excessive extension of the thumb, especially if compared with the patients uninjured digit, which often is available for examination.

Active Motion

In patients sustaining open wounds, the hallmark of tendon injury is an inability to actively move a digit or hand in the manner in which a normal hand can move. It is incumbent on the examiner to prompt the patient to move all joints throughout their expected range of motion. This often will be difficult for patients who are in pain, who have moderate swelling or associated fractures, much less in patients with multisystem injuries, underlying medical or psychiatric conditions, or those under the influence of drugs or alcohol.

It is acceptable to provide digital or regional anesthesia to a patient to reduce pain and enhance compliance with testing of motion provided a complete distal neurologic examination has been performed. This usually includes the measurement of two-point discrimination as outlined in Chapter 6. It is not appropriate to anesthetize the hand until this is completed because it will preclude nerve examination until the anesthetic has resolved.

The techniques for testing the FDS and FDP of each finger are shown in Fig. 5-11. These motions isolate the actions of these tendons, and when they cannot be performed, are suggestive of tendon incongruity. The FDS and FDP of each digit should be examined independently. Full flexion of the thumb as well as full opposition to the pulp of the little finger should be elicited. Extensor tendon function should be assessed; however, patients with "weak" extension of a finger may have a lacerated communis tendon and some extension through connections to an adjacent extensor through the juncturae tendinum. Coupled with an abnormal finger posture or uncoordinated motion when testing the tenodesis effect, one can strongly suspect extensor tendon injury.

Flexion and extension of the wrist should be tested with resisted motion. Look for radial or ulnar deviation of the wrist during flexion or extension suggesting injury to radial or ulnar tendons.

Remember that soft tissue injury may help localize but may not adequately predict the extent of underlying tendon injury. It is common for patients to sustain an oblique skin laceration with the location of an underlying tendon laceration lying remote to it. Cursory inspection of the wound itself may reveal an apparently intact tendon, whereas below the surface either proximally or distally lies the site of complete tendon transection. This principle also is important when evaluating those patients who already have undergone closure of the cutaneous portion of their wounds, and a decision must be made whether to explore an already closed wound. It is common for practitioners to report "seeing a cut tendon" in the wound and referring the patient for reevaluation after skin closure. Often the findings on exploration of the wound are inconsistent with those initially reported.

COUNSELING THE PATIENT WITH A TENDON INJURY

From the outset, the examiner should emphasize to the patient that the prognosis after tendon repair is determined mostly by the injury and the patient's postoperative compliance with rehabilitation efforts.

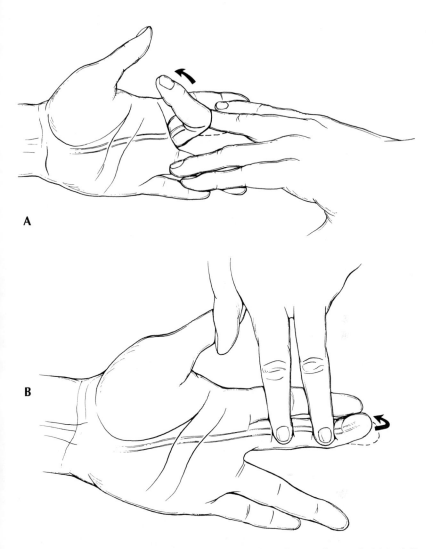

Figure 5-11   (A) Testing FDS function. With the adjacent fingers held in full extension (prohibiting FDP motion), efforts at finger flexion produce isolated FDS motion, as indicated by solitary flexion of the PIP joint. (B) Testing FDP function. Isolated DIP flexion can only be accomplished with an intact FDP musculotendinous unit.

Patients should be aware that although the actual tendon repair often is straightforward, it is their cooperation with splinting and a postoperative rehabilitation protocol that will dramatically influence their chances for a successful recovery. Tendon healing is a lengthy process, and recovery requires patience. Patients should be informed that they will not be able to fully use their fingers for a number of weeks (usually at least 6 weeks for extensor tendons and perhaps 12 weeks for flexor tendons), an upsetting fact considering most people rely on use of their hands for employment and daily activities. We explain the importance of allowing finger motion while avoiding excessive tension on the repair site to avoid tendon rupture. Patients should know that secondary repair of a flexor tendon that has ruptured after primary repair is a lengthy and complicated process that starts over after disruption of the first repair. Even under optimal circumstances, patients sustaining serious tendon injuries will be trying to overcome finger stiffness, poor motion, and the possibility of rupture. Their recovery will be inherently frustrating, but if they are diligent, a satisfactory result can be expected.

PRINCIPLES OF TENDON REPAIR

Standards for the care of tendon injuries are not uniform and are influenced by the timing of injuries, the experience of the practitioners, the presence of other medical or traumatic conditions, and the requirements and desires of the patient. In general, however, certain principles can be provided.

Surgical Exposure

Flexor tendon surgery should be undertaken with proper lighting, instruments, and the use of a tourniquet. The flexor tendons should be exposed using the "zigzag" technique attributed to Bruner, often as extensions of traumatic lacerations, as shown in Fig. 5-12. These incisions cross the axes of joints obliquely, avoiding the scar contracture inherent when volar incisions were made longitudinally along the digit. The tips of the triangular skin flaps often are rounded to minimize flap tip necrosis, while providing excellent exposure of the digital sheath. Other areas of the flexor surface of the hand should be explored widely to allow adequate visualization of injured structures. Other tendon injuries and neurovascular injuries commonly are associated with flexor tendon injuries and should be sought.

Flexor tendon ends that cannot be found proximally are frequently situated either just proximal to the A-1 pulley in the palm, or even as far proximally as the carpal tunnel. Incisions need not connect the site of tendon laceration and the location of the proximal stump; a tendon

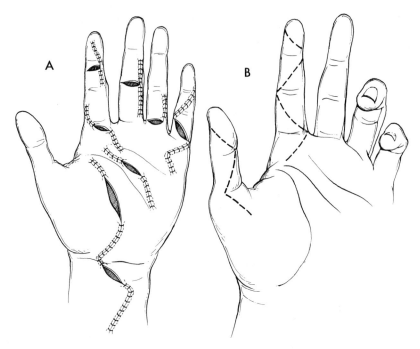

Figure 5-12   Acceptable incisions in hand surgery. Volar "zigzag" incisions (Bruner incisions) permit thorough exposure of underlying structures, while preventing the undesirable scar contracture that can occur using volar longitudingal incisions. Incisions should cross joint creases at a minimum of 45° when possible. Alternatively, lateral axial incisions can also be useful.

retriever or a second counterincision near the A-1 pulley usually will suffice in locating the tendon end. One can look for blood or inflamed synovium, which may suggest the tendon's location. However, care must be taken to avoid reckless, blind, groping for tendon ends in a region containing many vulnerable structures.

Extensor tendons also may retract proximally when lacerated. Tendon ends following more distal lacerations tend not to retract because the juncturae prevent proximal migration. It often is necessary to extend a traumatic dorsal skin laceration to achieve extensor tendon retrieval.

Suture Techniques

As stated previously, tendons are relatively acellular, avascular structures of longitudinally oriented collagen and ground substance. Because simple sutures tend to pull out between the collagen strands, tendon repair using simple interrupted sutures like those routinely used elsewhere in the body is unacceptable, particularly for flexor tendon repairs. A number of suturing techniques have been devised, and some are shown in Fig. 5-13. All are designed to reorient the direction of suture force from a longitudinal axis to a perpendicular axis to avoid

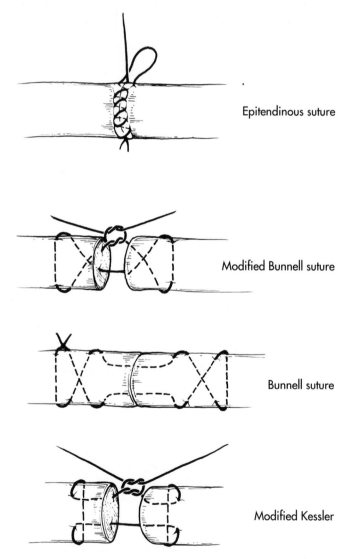

Epitendinous suture

Modified Bunnell suture

Bunnell suture

Modified Kessler

Figure 5-13 Commonly employed tendon repairs. Tendon suturing techniques are employed to convert longitudingal forces that would tend to pull sutures through the tendon to a more transverse orientation.

pulling the sutures through the tendon. The Bunnell technique and similar techniques of lengthy suture weaving have been modified because of their tendency to strangulate the tendon ends (undesirable in an already traumatized region where minimal scarring is sought). We have concluded that carefully placed sutures using the modified Kessler, modified Bunnell (Kleinert), or DOLL technique are equally satisfactory and subject to surgeon preference. One disadvantage of these types of repairs is that they tend to "bunch up" the tendon ends, thereby creating a large "bulb" that may not move smoothly through a tendon sheath. The epitendinous suture may aid in smoothing the edges, but does not reduce the bulk of the tendon repair. Most surgeons overcome this impediment by not excessively tightening the suture, while avoiding any significant gap formation. The epitendinous suture can then smooth the repair edges. For extensor tendon injuries, where repair-site bulk is not as important, forces are reduced and the tendons are broad and flat, simple horizontal mattress sutures often are sufficient, although some surgeons consistently prefer standard tendon sutures for all tendon repairs.

Sutures

Tendons require weeks to heal. The suture material used must therefore be strong enough to not only approximate the tendon ends, but to maintain congruity for several weeks despite early gentle motion. The suture material should be selected to minimize foreign body reaction and scar tissue induction. Experienced hand surgeons debate whether monofilament or other sutures are best; any permanent suture with good strength characteristics probably will suffice. We frequently use 4-0 Ticron, 4-0 Supermid, 4-0 Tevdek, or 4-0 Prolene for flexor tendons in the fingers and similar 4-0 or 3-0 sutures for proximal flexor tendon or extensor tendon repairs depending on the tendon diameter.

Epitendinous Sutures

Epitendinous sutures are small continuous sutures that "tidy up" the edges after a primary tendon repair (Fig. 5-13). They are recommended for flexor tendon repairs in the fingers (where technically possible) to enhance gliding and may even increase the strength of the repair. In other areas, such as the wrist or palm, or on the extensor surface, where there is no fibrous sheath, they are used less consistently, depending on the preferences of the surgeon. We usually use 6-0 nylon.

Partial Tendon Lacerations

Studies have shown that contrary to what would be expected, partially lacerated tendons may have lower rates of rupture when not repaired compared with those that are repaired. In fact, because tendon "bunching" in flexor tendon injuries is undesirable, it often is wise to leave a partially lacerated tendon unrepaired, provided the site of laceration will not "trigger" on the flexor tendon sheath. It has been commonplace, however, when injuries are in less crucial areas, such as the wrist or extensor surface, to repair the lacerated portion of a tendon whose diameter is transected more than 50%. We would not recommend dividing and primarily repairing a partially lacerated tendon.

Where to Repair Injured Tendons

Because the precision with which flexor tendons are repaired determines in part their ability to glide within the flexor sheath and hence, the patients' outcome, it is the standard of care in the United States to repair all flexor tendon lacerations in the operating room with the aid of an adequate anesthetic, a tourniquet, proper instruments, and adequate lighting. Many isolated injuries, including lacerations in the palm, where there is no sheath, may seem ideally suited to closure in the emergency room; however, the proximity of these structures to other important neurovascular structures and the frequent need for proximal and distal dissection provides no protection for the practitioner who elects to perform primary flexor tendon repairs outside a well-supplied and well-staffed operating room.

However, extensor tendon injuries usually are more superficial and often are distant from essential motor and sensory nerve branches and vessels, and their healing is more predictable and tolerant of less precise repairs. For these reasons, repair of simple isolated extensor tendon injuries under favorable conditions is permissible in the emergency department. This assumes that a patient is able to tolerate the procedure under a local anesthetic, and that the surgeon has appropriate instruments, lighting, and sutures to complete the repair. Multiple tendon injuries, heavily contaminated wounds, and other associated injuries mandate care in the operating room. The physician performing the repair must ensure that capable follow-up will be obtained by the patient and that the findings and procedure performed are communicated to the physician responsible for postoperative rehabilitation.

In general, deep forearm or wrist lacerations with tendon involvement should be repaired in the operating room because of the number and depth of tendons lacerated, the importance of thorough exploration before tendon repair, and the concomitant presence of vascular and particularly nerve injuries. Small proximal forearm wounds extending into a muscle belly can be repaired safely in the emergency department with deep and superficial suturing and have a favorable prognosis, provided that there is no evidence of nerve or vascular injury, a minimal degree of wound contamination, and that prompt competent follow-up can be assured.

Timing of Repair of Lacerated Tendons

Optimal timing of flexor tendon repairs is debated by many experienced hand surgeons. There are proponents of immediate operative exploration and repair, citing "one trauma" for the area and the possibility of repairing structures when lacerations are fresh and have less inflammation around them. Others believe that an accelerated inflammatory response is beneficial and prefer to wait several days to repair flexor tendons. Many policies concerning the timing of tendon repairs arise from (1) the surgeon's willingness to perform the repair at the often inconvenient time of consultation (i.e., in the middle of the night or in the middle of other clinical responsibilities) and (2) the availability of operating room facilities and the surgeon's time the following day. At some institutions, all flexor tendon injuries are repaired immediately because no operating room time will be available electively in the next day or two, or the surgeon's operating room schedule and/or clinic commitments are inflexible.

We have concluded that (1) flexor tendons should be repaired "early" (within a few days, optimally within 24 to 48 hours) rather than "later" and that (2) flexor tendons need not be repaired as emergencies under less than optimal conditions for the patient or surgeon in the middle of the night if the first premise still can be fulfilled. We have found that patients who have empty stomachs, are not intoxicated, and have rested, are well satisfied and have a better repair than those done under less favorable conditions. We favor closure of the cutaneous portion of the wound in the emergency room and then arranging for tendon repair the following day. Of course those more severe injuries with devascularized digits, heavily contaminated wounds, or other injuries requiring urgent surgery should be addressed promptly.

Repair of extensor tendon lacerations should be accomplished at the time of emergency room evaluation if the injuries are amenable to repair. Optimally, a qualified person is available to perform a simple primary extensor tendon repair in the emergency room at the time of initial consultation as a single procedure. There is, however, no medically detrimental effect of postponing the primary repair briefly to a more convenient time for the patient or surgeon, if desired.

It should be emphasized that patients must be made aware of the extent of their injuries and the importance of surgery and follow-up. We frequently encounter patients who were advised to see a hand surgeon, but because either they were not counseled emphatically or were not responsible in seeking prompt follow-up, an otherwise simple tendon injury eventually required grafting or tendon transfer because of a delay of several weeks.

Delayed Presentation

It is common for patients to delay in seeing a qualified hand surgeon. This may be the result of patient negligence in seeking any medical care whatsoever, or a delay after being seen by another physician either with or without closure of the overlying skin. Do patients whose tendon repairs have been delayed a week or more fare more poorly if another day or two is allowed before repair? In general, closed wounds that have tendon or nerve involvement should be operated on in the same time frame as one would operate on acute injuries. The patient's fingers already may be stiff, and the patient may be more difficult to initiate into the importance of the rehabilitation effort once the acute injury "scare" is no longer present. Philosophically, we do not believe that breaking the "24 to 48 hour rule" for flexor tendon injuries in these patients will detrimentally affect their result; however, the outcome may be less satisfactory than that of other patients. Any delay outside the standards for acute injuries may subject the surgeon to the scrutiny that perhaps a better outcome could have been achieved with more prompt repair.

In open wounds in which skin closure has been delayed 6 or more hours, we believe that a more aggressive approach is warranted. Open lacerations lead to desiccation of the tendons and tendon sheath, and more importantly, the possibility of wound infection, a devastating occurrence in the vicinity of a tendon injury. Wound infections incite a tremendous inflammatory response that ultimately leads to scarring or worse, to a large open wound with exposed tendon and/or sheath and a large immobile finger. This complication undoubtedly will impair the outcome of what may have otherwise been a straightforward tendon repair. We would advocate prompt operation of these flexor tendon injuries in the operating room, where optimal irrigation and debridement can be performed concomitantly with the tendon repairs. Hospitalization for intravenous antibiotics often is justified.

Neglected Injuries

Patients who, for whatever reason, never seek care for their original injuries, those patients who ignore recommendations for follow-up, and those who rupture a primary tendon repair because of persistent neglect pose a special problem for the hand surgeon. Regardless of the site of the injury, the patient will have some impairment in the range of motion of the digit; where active motion is impaired because of tendon injury, there will be a secondary decrease in passive motion representing joint stiffness. In addition to joint contractures, patients whose flexors or extensors never were repaired often have retracted tendon ends that are heavily scarred and of inadequate length for primary repair. The flexor tendon sheath, if no tendon is present within it, may be contracted and unaccommodating of the original tendon, even if tendon length is sufficient. These patients may only seek care in the emergency room after infection or substantial wound breakdown has occurred. The demonstrated problems with postoperative rehabilitation compliance and follow-up portend a poor prognosis after further reconstruction.

From the outset, it is important to emphasize to the patient and to any family members or friends that are available that simply repairing the tendons is insufficient to obtain a functional hand. Many patients report that "the doctor told me that he/she fixed the cut tendon." Like all patients with tendon injury, these patients must be informed clearly that the repair of the tendons themselves is only one component of their recovery and that it is an inherently prolonged process.

The priorities for care of these patients are:
1. Achieve a noninfected closed wound. This may require admission to the hospital and intravenous antibiotics, local wound care, and/ or incision and drainage in the operating room.
2. Obtain the best possible range of joint motion passively before undertaking any tendon reconstruction. No tendon repair will remain intact—much less achieve motion—across a contracted joint.
3. Create a useful tendon for the motor involved. Primary repair may be possible depending on the operative findings, but frequently the tendon is scarred or frayed and is unsuitable for primary repair. Plans for tendon grafting, Silastic rod placement, or tendon transfer must have been made and discussed at length with the patient. Unfortunately, patients with a pattern of poor compliance often are incapable of conforming to the requirements of sophisticated tendon reconstruction, such as staged tendon grafting.
4. Careful documentation regarding clinical presentation and circumstances should be made in the patient's medical record in anticipation of a less favorable outcome heralded by the poor level of patient cooperation.

FLEXOR TENDON LACERATIONS
Zones of Injury

Verdan described the zones of flexor tendon injury (Fig. 5-14). Observations that injuries where two repaired tendons (FDS, FDP) were expected to glide within a fibrous sheath fared more poorly than any other area led to the term "no man's land," which described the region between the distal palmer crease (beginning of A-1 pulley) and the proximal portion of the middle phalanx (region of A-4 pulley and in-

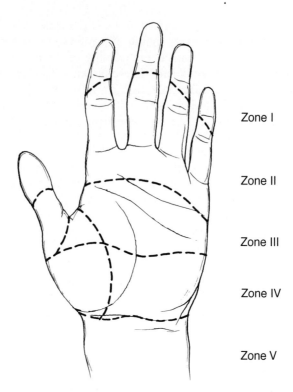

Figure 5-14   Zones of tendon injury. Zone II has been termed "no-mans land" because of the presence of two gliding tendons within the unyielding digital sheath.

sertion of two portions of FDS; Verdan Zone 2). Zone I, located distal to the insertion of the flexor digitorum superficialis, involves the region where the FDP travels singularly through the remaining portion of the flexor digital sheath. Zone III involves those palmer injuries between the distal portion of the transverse carpal ligament and the beginning of the flexor pulley system at A-1 (distal palmer crease). Zone IV injuries occur within the carpal tunnel, and Zone V injuries are proximal to the carpal tunnel in the wrist and distal forearm.

Zone I Injuries

Those tendon lacerations distal to the insertion of the FDS onto the proximal portion of the middle phalanx are considered Zone I. Because tendons move proximally when the fingers are flexed, it is not uncommon for the more distal FDP to be lacerated through a more proximal skin laceration. Typically, the patient will be unable to actively flex the DIP joint of the injured finger. Neurovascular injuries are common because of their proximity to the tendon sheath. The finger is explored using Brunner incisions extended from the patient's original injury. Dissection through the volar soft tissue is performed with care taken to identify and protect the digital nerves and vessels that lie in the soft tissues just lateral and slightly more volar than the sheath itself. The flexor tendon sheath can then be opened with care being taken to protect the A-2 and A-4 pulleys. Some surgeons prefer to open the intervening tendon sheath in a "door" shape that will facilitate closure; others directly incise it. To bring the tendon ends together, flexion of the wrist and finger may be necessary. Typically, the FDP is lacerated near its insertion at the base of the distal phalanx. The proximal tendon may be retrieved using a tendon passer, alligator forceps, or fine hemostat. Counter incisions in the palm just proximal to the A-1 pulley may be necessary to retrieve the proximal tendon end. Once the tendon end is brought into the wound, and passed under the A-2 pulley, a straight (Keith) needle can be placed transversely across the tendon and digital sheath to prevent retraction. Minimize handling of the tendon and particularly avoid crushing it so that no additional adhesion formation will be incited. One may elect to place the tendon suture in the proximal tendon end at this time to avoid any further direct trauma to the tendon. Plans must then be made to repair the FDP either just proximal to or just distal to the A-4 pulley. In instances in which the proximal tendon cannot be advanced through the A-4 pulley and yet the distal portion does not project out proximally from A-4, two choices are available. First, a tiny portion of A-4 may be excised to allow repair, provided that at least 5 mm of A-4 is left in place. Second, the tendon suture may be placed into the distal tendon stump with the tendon withdrawn distally and then tied after the loose tendon ends and the tendon itself have been advanced under A-4.

Occasionally, the FDP will have either insufficient tendon distally to be repaired primarily or will have avulsed a volar chip off the distal phalanx. In either instance, reinsertion of the FDP tendon can be performed by drilling parallel holes from the proximal volar lip out the distal phalanx and through the nailbed, where they can be tied over a button or other suitable bolster. The tendon or the bony fragment must contact a subperiosteal portion of the distal phalanx if the reinsertion is to be successful.

Zone II Injuries

Injuries from the distal palmer crease/beginning of the A-1 pulley and extending to the insertion of the FDS at the proximal portion of the middle phalanx constitute Zone II flexor tendon injuries. These injuries, where gliding of two tendons is to occur within the confines of a relatively unyielding flexor tendon sheath, are both common and difficult injuries. The tendon sheath and skin often are lacerated over the proximal phalanx, with distal tendon stump returning to a more distal position and the proximal stumps retracting proximally. Isolated FDP lacerations or FDS slip lacerations are possible and frequently occur together. Exposure for these injuries is similar to that of Zone I injuries using Brunner zigzag incisions, incorporating the initial laceration when feasible. Care is taken during dissection to evaluate the integrity of each neurovascular bundle in the vicinity of the injury and to avoid iatrogenic injury. Any portion of the flexor sheath may be incised, with the exception of A-2 and A-4 pulleys. Proximal tendon ends, which frequently retract proximal to the A-1 pulley, may necessitate a more proximal incision in the palm or even in the wrist to locate. It is not necessary to connect the finger and palmer incisions. Once located, with the wrist held in flexion, these tendons should be passed back through the flexor sheath using a thin alligator forceps, a small Silastic rod, or even a small red rubber catheter to assist in delivering the tendon end into the digital sheath. The tendon end may then be held in place with a transversely placed straight (Keith) needle. Note that the FDP, which lies deep to the FDS in the palm and proximal finger, becomes superficial after penetrating the FDS tendon, which encircles it completely.

Primary tendon repair is then performed as outlined and should include an epitendinous suture. If the FDS tendons are lacerated at their insertion on the middle phalanx, it may be technically difficult to repair them; however, it usually is possible to reinsert them either onto the periosteum of the middle phalanx or the lateral portion of the distal volar plate. It is not necessary to recreate a connection of the two slips of the FDS before their insertion.

If the tendon ends are not suitable for primary repair (frayed, crushed, etc), minimal trimming of the tendon ends may be accomplished. It has been deemed permissible to shorten the FDS and/or FDP tendons up to 1 cm to facilitate precise repair of uninjured tendon ends. Excessive removal of tendon will substantially alter the fingers biomechanics, leading to premature complete flexion of that digit (with inability to fully flex adjacent digits—the Quadrigia effect) or lead to a finger that cannot be extended fully. Therefore, it is imperative that further tendon trauma be prevented during the exploration, retrieval, and repair of the tendons to avoid the necessity of excessive shortening.

Zone III Injuries

Flexor tendon injuries that occur distal to the transverse carpal ligament and proximal to the A-1 pulley are located in Zone III. They frequently occur after slender penetrating trauma, such as by a knife or glass, or less commonly, after more significant deep transverse lacerations. Tendon repairs in this area have a more favorable prognosis than those in other zones because of the spaciousness of the surrounding soft tissues, but they often are accompanied by injuries to the superficial palmer arch or major branches of the median or ulnar nerves. The superficial palmer arch classically is supplied predominantly from the ulnar artery. The ulnar artery enters the hand through Guyon's canal, between the hook of the hamate and the pisiform, to curve radially across the palm just below the palmer fascia. Similarly, the median nerve—the sensory branches of which leave the carpal tunnel to supply the thumb, index, long, and the radial portion of the ring finger—often are lacerated with injuries in this region.

It can be difficult to identify the individual tendon ends in palmer injuries. The tendons tend to be deep and to retract from the site of injury. The mainstay of successful repair involves adequate incisional exposure under tourniquet, and for distal identification, traction on individual tendon ends with attention to the resultant finger motion. Recall that the presence of a lumbrical arising from a tendon mandates that it be a profundus tendon. Similarly, tendons pass through the carpal tunnel in a predictable topography, with superficialis tendons to the ring and long fingers lying superficial to those to the little and index fingers. The central fingers also have larger tendons than do the peripheral digits. It may be necessary to fully open the carpal tunnel or to make a second incision at the distal wrist to identify and expose the tendon ends. In some patients, the flexor tendons in this region are interconnected loosely by a filmy synovium that may prevent retrieval of a completely transected tendon into the wrist even with traction.

Comparisons of the orientation and caliber of the free tendon ends allow proximal and distal tendons to be paired with confidence. Transected tendon ends may be larger, smaller, cut more or less obliquely, and rounder or flatter than adjacent transected tendons; these observations aid in their correct coaptation. Primary repair is then performed as outlined. Use of an epitendinous repair is optional. Again, careful inspection for adjacent nerve or vascular injuries is mandatory.

Zone IV Injuries

Flexor tendon injuries within the carpal tunnel, from distal wrist crease into the palm, are included in Zone IV. These are unusual injuries because of the depth of the carpal tunnel and the relative protection afforded to these tendons by the overlying ligaments, palmer fascia, and the bony walls of the canal. Lacerations or other injuries in this area often are accompanied by median nerve injury. Careful examination for impaired thumb opposition (intrinsic motor branch of the median nerve (C8T1) or for palmer numbness (palmer sensory branch of the median nerve) should be performed. Repair is similar to that outlined for Zone V.

Zone V Injuries

Injuries proximal to the carpal tunnel constitute Zone V injuries. The lack of adjacent bony protection and the superficial soft tissues covering the tendons, arteries, and nerves in this region often make lacerations severe. Patients seriously attempting suicide and deep glass lacerations account for most cases of "spaghetti wrist," with laceration of all 11 flexor tendons traversing the volar wrist, frequently accompanied by lacerations of the median and ulnar nerves and radial and ulnar arteries. These often are dramatic wounds with profuse bleeding. Hemorrhage usually can be controlled with direct pressure and elevation, and the viability of the hand can be assessed distally. If perfusion to the hand is in jeopardy, the injury becomes a surgical emergency mandating immediate attention in the operating room; this takes priority over all other nerve and tendon injuries. However, injuries may be more superficial, such as simple laceration of the palmaris longus or another wrist extensor. Any patient with wrist laceration should be questioned about and tested for injury to the palmer sensory branch of the median nerve or other nerve injury and should be assessed for possible vascular compromise. It is not uncommon for physicians treating these lacerations to be sufficiently reassured by reduction in bleeding from the wound (due to vessel retraction and vasospasm), while failing to recognize a devitalized hand distally.

Any patient sustaining a laceration to the wrist should be screened for possible suicidal gesture and a psychiatrist consulted if warranted regardless of the severity of the wound itself.

Operative repair of a "spaghetti wrist" necessitates the use of many previously mentioned clues to assure that the repairs are done properly. Briefly, they are as follows:

1. Ensure adequate perfusion to the hand as the first priority in major wrist injuries. An apparently intact artery may be thrombosed and require reconstruction.
2. For devastating injuries, bony stabilization of any radius and/or ulnar fractures should be accomplished before tendon and nerve repairs and may facilitate safe hand revascularization, if time permits.
3. Adequate exposure both proximally and distally is necessary to perform proper tendon repairs.
4. The FCR, palmaris longus (when present), and FCU are the most superficial flexors in the wrist, and will be so on both proximal and distal edges of the laceration.
5. There are nine tendons that traverse the carpal tunnel (Fig. 5-3). These include four finger superficialis flexors, four profundus flex-

ors, and the flexor pollicis longus. The flexor pollicis longus often has its own sheath and usually is the deepest structure along the radial side of the floor of the carpal tunnel and wrist.

6. In addition to the normal orientation of long and ring flexors lying superficial to index and little flexors, the orientation of each tendon's laceration, as well as the caliber of each tendon, give clues to their correct reapproximation.

Despite the number of tendons lacerated, tendon function with injuries at this level often is good, because unrestricted tendon motion can occur without the confines of a flexor sheath. Prognosis after a severe wrist laceration is related more often to return of nerve function for critical sensation and thumb opposition.

Thumb Flexor Tendon Injury

Injury to the flexor pollicis longus tendon is inherently different from that of the extrinsic finger flexors. First, the neurovascular bundles are much closer to the volar axis of the thumb than are those to the fingers, making their concomitant injury common and the possibility of their iatrogenic injury more likely. Second, a less-complicated flexor sheath is present, making primary repair less difficult (Fig. 5-5). As with the fingers, the thumb flexor sheath should be preserved to avoid tendon bowstringing. Third, postoperative rehabilitation is inherently different, as will be discussed.

Thenar and First Web-Space Lacerations

It is common for lacerations of the hand to extend into the thenar musculature. Because these muscles do have broad fascia and ligamentous attachments, the hand surgeon frequently is consulted because of "tendon visible in the wound." It often is possible, under a local anesthetic, to confirm that these lacerations are not extensive and are within the bulk of the thenar muscles themselves, making them amenable to simple primary repair with deep and then superficial sutures. It is permissible to perform these repairs in the emergency room if no other significant injuries are found, particularly injury to the motor branch of the median nerve. As with any injury in the hand, a search for retained foreign bodies should be undertaken when appropriate, because glass, wood, and metal can be concealed easily in the thenar musculature.

SPLINTING AND REHABILITATION FOR FLEXOR TENDON LACERATIONS

Recovery after all types of flexor tendon injuries is determined by the postoperative rehabilitation process. From the preoperative counseling of the patient and family and for weeks after a flexor tendon injury, constant reassurance and encouragement are essential to ensure compliance and, hence, a favorable outcome.

Postoperative Dressing

Immediately after surgery to repair any of the flexor tendons, the patient's tendon repair must be protected. From the time of completion of the repair, it is possible for the patient to rupture the repair. This can be prevented by placing the hand and wrist in a "safe" position (Fig. 5-15). We use a bulky dressing that incorporates a dorsal splint for the fingers and wrist that extends from the proximal dorsal forearm to beyond the fingertips. The hand should be well protected with gauze "fluffs" and overlying padding material. No constricting bandages or splinting materials can be used. The splint material, whether plaster or fiberglass based, must be strong enough to maintain its shape and not crack or bend. Our preferred position is with the wrist in 30 to 40° flexion, with approximately 70° of flexion at the MCP joints, and the PIP joints and DIP joints fully extended. Not only does this position substantially decrease the amount of tension that the patient can generate at the repair site, but it also maintains the MCP joints in a position of maximal collateral ligament tightness (subsequent motion away from this position will be toward collateral ligament laxity rather than toward prohibitive tightness). The PIP and DIP joints are extended to avoid flexion contracture, which can be difficult to correct even with aggressive splinting. The PIP and DIP joints are not strapped to the dorsal splint (any attempted finger flexion would preferably cause PIP or DIP motion and not tension against an unyielding splint). The splint extends beyond the fingertips, thereby reducing the risk of inadvertent forced extension of the fingertips if they are bumped. Hooks or suture loops are applied to the fingernails of affected digits prior to completion of the operation in anticipation of dynamic splinting requirements.

Patients are seen at the next available clinic setting after surgery, preferably within 3 days. A hand therapist should then fabricate a splint, allowing active extension but passive flexion (controlled dynamic splinting). Splints using a "palmer pulley" (Chow modification) promote full PIP and DIP flexion during recovery compared with those whose elastics are attached directly to the splint proximally.

Rehabilitation for Finger Flexor Tendon Repairs

Patients are advanced through the flexor tendon rehabilitation protocol modified from Kleinert (Table 5-5). Many centers have modifications of this protocol that allow gradually increasing wrist and finger extension and gradually increasing active motion over several weeks.

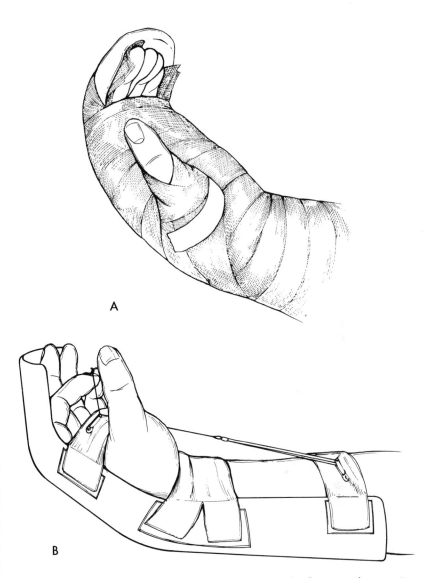

Figure 5-15   **(A)** Immediate postoperative splinting for flexor tendon repairs. Wrist and MCP joint positions are designed to relieve tension along the tendon repair site. **(B)** Dynamic splint for rehabilitation following flexor tendon injury permits full active extension of the PIP qand DIP joints, while allowing full passive flexion of these joints to occur.

Table 5-5   Modified Kleinert Protocol for Rehabilitation Following Flexor Tendon Repair

Time Interval	Management
2–5 days	Constant use of a dorsal wrist splint, maintaining wrist at 20–30° flexion and MP joints at 60–70° flexion, with PIP and DIP joints allowed to extend fully. No strapping fingers to splint.
	Rubberbands to fingertips maintain PIP and DIP joints in full flexion, but allow full active extension. Palmer pulley may be required. Ten repetitions each hour.
	Splint worn constantly except when supervised by therapist. Visits three times per week.
	Passive PIP and DIP flexion under supervision while maintaining MCP joints in full flexion.
1–2 weeks	Continue splinting and observe for any limitation in PIP or DIP extension. Consider increasing MP flexion or using gentle finger extension strap while blocking MP extension.
	Continue active extension/passive flexion exercises.
3 weeks	Modify splint to maintain wrist in 0–30° extension.
	Remove splint under supervision to allow gentle wrist flexion and extension and radial and ulnar deviation.
4 weeks	Begin isolated flexion and extension of PIP and DIP joints while maintaining stabilization of MP joints and wrist.
	Adjust therapy based on any limitations encountered.
6 weeks	Remove splint and evaluate range of motion.
	Adjust exercises and therapy based on limitations present.
7 weeks	Begin flexion against mild resistance, gentle strengthening, and pursue differential tendon gliding.
	Discontinue therapy when active motion reaches plateau, usually 2–3 additional weeks.

MP, metacarpal phalangeal; PIP, proximal interphalangeal; DIP, distal interphalangeal.

All digital flexor tendon injury splints begin with the same joint positions as the initial postoperative splint (Fig. 5-15). It remains imperative to repeatedly counsel patients at each visit about the importance of persistence with their rehabilitation schedules. Those patients who cannot comply with wearing a splint and with exercises should be informed in nonambiguous terms that tendon rupture is a likely sequelae. Many patients who find that the posture of their finger has returned to normal or who have discovered active motion of the fingers are tempted to discard the splint and reject inconvenient visits to the hand therapist. This is to be strongly opposed.

Rehabilitation of Thumb and Wrist Flexor Injuries

The most important factors affecting thumb function are sensibility and stability, which are more important than mobility. Consequently, rehabilitation after flexor pollicis longus lacerations consists of thumb spica splinting for 4 to 6 weeks, after which full active motion is allowed. Similarly, wrist flexor or extensor lacerations are treated with splinting in neutral wrist position for 4 to 6 weeks.

Flexor Tendon Rupture

Rupture of primarily repaired flexor tendons typically occurs 10 to 21 days after repair, coinciding with the period of maximal wound byproduct lysis. When concerns are present that a patient may have ruptured the repair, the examiner should place the wrist in a "protected" position of wrist and MCP flexion and ask the patient to gently flex the involved digit. Any flicker of motion suggests an intact repair. Obviously, any patient who reports "feeling a pop" after attempting full range of motion without a splint and who has no active motion on examination should be assumed to have ruptured the repair.

Tendon repair site rupture is occasionally a normal consequence of an otherwise uncomplicated repair, particularly with current efforts to "walk the line" between achieving motion and avoiding stiffness and tendon adhesions. Usually, patients with recognized rupture should undergo early exploration in hopes of achieving a second primary repair. In patients whose rupture was unrecognized or after secondary rupture, it may be wise to consider placement of a Silastic rod as a "space saver" while full passive finger motion is regained before undertaking definitive tendon grafting.

EXTENSOR TENDON LACERATIONS
General

Extensor tendon injuries tend to be less functionally significant and have a better prognosis than similar flexor injuries, principally because of the relatively shorter excursion required and the absence of a true extensor digital sheath. Extensor tendon injuries are most common on the dorsal hand and wrist. They can be diagnosed in any patient with an open wound who, under adequate local anesthetic, cannot fully extend a finger or thumb, or cannot abduct the thumb.

Extensor tendon injuries frequently are associated with lacerations to either large or tributary branches of the radial sensory nerve and/ or the dorsal sensory branches of the ulnar nerve. Management of injuries to these nerve branches is outlined in Chapter 6, but may necessitate care in the operating room, where extensor tendons can be repaired simultaneously.

Management of open injuries to the extensor apparatus of the fingers is controversial. Coordinated and smooth motion in the finger is determined by the relative contributions in force from the extrinsic and intrinsic muscles inserting, through the extensor hood, onto the middle and distal phalanges, respectively. The biomechanics of the finger extensor system suggest that a delicate balance in intrinsic and extrinsic extensor contributions, with relatively short excursions of each, allows a wide range of finger motions and postures. Consequently, any injury to the extensor apparatus with or without repair, has a propensity to alter the biomechanical interactions of these forces and lead to abnormal finger postures, deformity, and suboptimal motion.

Open Mallet Deformity

Open injuries to the terminal portion of the extensor apparatus near its insertion on the distal phalanx commonly lead to development of a "mallet finger" (Fig. 5-16A). This deformity, which is the result of stretching or detachment of this terminal insertion of the extensor tendon, leaves the DIP joint of the finger in a position of resting flexion from 10 to 40°. The patient is unable to fully extend the finger at the DIP joint and ultimately will be unable to do so passively because of DIP joint contracture. Efforts to directly repair the extensor insertion in isolation often are unsuccessful because of thinning and scar tissue formation at the repair site. Depending on the type of injury, the mainstay of successful treatment of a mallet deformity after open injury, like that following closed injury, is the use of internal or external splinting. Many splints have been used to maintain the DIP joint in extension until healing is complete, the most common being the Stack splint (described in detail later in this chapter). Any external device that prohibits flexion of the DIP without compromising motion of the MCP or PIP joints will be satisfactory. These splints should be used for 6 to 8 weeks after extensor tendon laceration over the DIP joint. Continuous use of a stack splint can lead to maceration of the skin and may complicate wound healing; careful instructions regarding hygiene should be emphasized. Internal splinting, using a "K-wire" across the DIP joint or within the flexor sheath which prevents motion, also is occasionally employed in instances where a Stack splint cannot be used, when there is volar subluxation of the distal phalanx, or when a significant portion of the articular surface is fractured. Any K-wire traversing a joint may permanently damage the joint or cause other complications such as pin tract infections. We prefer to splint the DIP

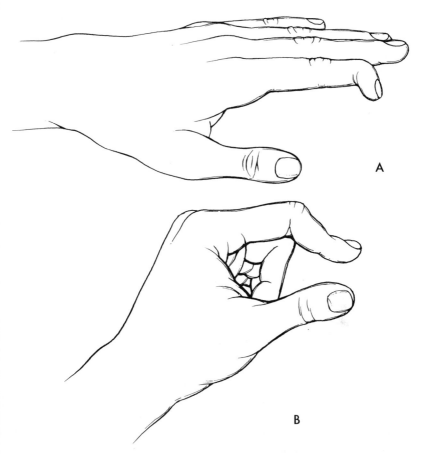

Figure 5-16 (A) Mallet deformity. Loss of integrity of the terminal insertion of the extensor tendon yields the posture shown. (B) Boutonniere deformity. Central slip injury allows subluxation of the lateral bands volarly, anterior to the axis of the PIP joint, where they act to flex rather than extend it.

joint externally in a compliant patient when a significant laceration has occurred. Whether the extensor mechanism is repaired directly or not probably is not the central issue in healing as suggested by operative and nonoperative experience after closed injuries. Motion at the MCP and PIP joints is encouraged and should not be restricted.

Open Boutonniere Deformity

An open boutonniere or buttonhole deformity (Fig. 5-16B) occurs after dorsal lacerations of the finger that transect or badly traumatize the insertion of the central slip of the extensor hood where it inserts onto the proximal portion of the middle phalanx. This injury will then allow the gradual migration of the lateral bands toward the volar surface, anterior to the axis of the PIP joint. This results in an inability to fully extend the PIP joint and ultimately to a fixed flexion contracture of the PIP joint that cannot be extended passively. A compensatory hyperextension of the DIP joint eventually develops as the extensor forces are applied exclusively to the distal phalanx. Central slip injuries often are unrecognized even after open dorsal injuries because the patient may initially exhibit normal finger extension. Until volar (palmer) subluxation of the lateral bands occurs, there will be no boutonniere deformity. The deformity may then develop weeks after blunt injury or after the initial skin laceration has been repaired and is otherwise healing satisfactorily.

Recognition of a possible central slip injury and its propensity for subsequent development of a boutonniere deformity is important. Once the Boutonniere deformity begins to appear, early splinting of the PIP joint in extension until tendon healing is complete (or until sufficient fibrous/scar tissue is present to prevent lateral band subluxation) offers the best prognosis. Any patient with injuries in the vicinity of the central slip who cannot fully extend the PIP joint should be treated for a boutonniere deformity, with a small splint that is fabricated to prevent PIP flexion while allowing full MCP and DIP motion. This should be worn continuously for a minimum of 4 weeks and continued if evidence of recurrent deformity is noticed.

Extensor tendon injuries in the region of the MCP joint often are incomplete lacerations because the extensor "hood" encircles the dorsal portion of the MCP joint, thereby prohibiting circumferential hood laceration. Penetration into the MCP joint should be sought during inspection of any extensor tendon injury overlying the joint, and if encountered, should be treated with vigorous irrigation and antibiotic therapy. A lacerated extensor hood should be repaired primarily, as failure to do so may allow it to sublux radially or ulnarly off the MCP joint and ultimately lead to finger deviation in that direction. Injuries involving the less substantial periphery of the hood can be repaired primarily and gentle active motion resumed using "buddy taping" to an adjacent finger as needed. Those injuries traversing the thick central portion of the tendon, which conveys the greatest strength in tension, should be repaired primarily and the hand treated with splinting as described on the following pages.

Treatment of extensor injuries at the wrist or dorsal hand usually is straightforward. Adequate anesthesia must be provided because extension of the original laceration may be required to retrieve the proximal tendon ends. Full extension of the wrist may facilitate finding the tendon ends, as will finger extension. The varying caliber of extensor tendons between long and little fingers, for example, may justify the use of different suturing techniques and suture sizes (4-0 for the smaller tendons and 3-0 for the larger ones). Lacerated juncturae tendinum need not be repaired. In wounds with portions of extensor tendon absent, the distal tendon ends may be sewn to the tendon of an adjacent finger.

The extensor retinaculum may interfere with gliding after primary repair of the lacerated extensor tendon. It is unwise to fully excise the retinaculum because extensor tendon bowstringing may ensue; however, if the extensor retinaculum will impinge on the tendon repair site, it may be useful to resect either a portion of the distal or a portion of the proximal retinaculum to facilitate unimpeded movement.

Injuries involving the tendons of the first dorsal compartment of the hand and wrist (the abductor pollicis longus and extensor pollicis brevis), the brachioradialis, and/or the wrist extensors or extensor pollicis longus pose special problems in reconstruction. These lacerations commonly have transected the sensory branch of the radial nerve and may have lacerated the radial artery as it extends across the "anatomic snuffbox." We recommend primary repair of these tendons with concomitant sensory nerve repair. Tiny radial nerve branches may be buried proximally to prevent neuroma formation. The thumb should be splinted in extension and abducted from the palm (thumb spica splint) for 4 to 6 weeks, usually allowing motion of the IP joint of the thumb which imparts little excursion/tension of the repaired extensors.

Extensor Tendon Splinting and Rehabilitation

Most extensor tendon injuries do well. Initial splinting should include a well-padded volar splint for all fingers that maintains them with the wrist in neutral and the fingers fully extended (hyperextension of the wrist or fingers is not necessary). The splint should extend beyond the fingertips. A similar removable static splint can be fabricated and worn for a period of 6 weeks, after which active motion is begun.

Dynamic extension splinting, maintaining the fingers in extension with rubberbands while allowing controlled active finger flexion may provide a superior outcome to static splinting. It requires a motivated patient, is higher in cost, and uses more of the patient's and the hand therapist's time. Because static splinting has offered acceptable results, hand surgeons' willingness to routinely adopt dynamic extensor splinting has been inconsistent.

OUTCOME FOLLOWING PRIMARY TENDON REPAIR

Range of motion and strength after primary tendon repair range from near normal to virtually useless depending on the magnitude of injury and the patient's compliance and efforts with rehabilitation. Mutilating injuries with concomitant bone, nerve, and soft tissue injury in patients receiving no rehabilitation fare miserably. Conversely, motivated patients with clean tendon lacerations can regain nearly normal function.

CLOSED TENDON INJURIES
Avulsion Injuries of the Profundus Tendon

Flexor digitorum profundus avulsions occur most commonly when flexion of the DIP is strongly resisted, such as attempting to catch a ledge during a fall. The profundus tendon is avulsed from its insertion into the proximal portion of the volar surface of the distal phalanx. The presence of a bony fragment accompanying the tendon end at the insertion site as seen on X-ray may aid in confirming the diagnosis. The patient will have a painful swollen distal finger and will be unable to actively flex the DIP joint. Treatment involves reinsertion of the profundus tendon, with or without the bony fragment, depending on its size. Occasionally the volar fragment is large enough to accommodate a single screw for fixation. The insertion site is explored via a Brunner incision at the DIP joint level. If screw fixation is not possible, then a form of "pull-out suture" is attached to the terminal tendon and/or bone, and this suture is advanced obliquely across the distal phalanx through two K-wire holes, to exit on the substance of the finger nail. These sutures can then be tied over a button or similar bolster. Attempts to bring the suture ends out the distal pulp at the tip of the finger often are accompanied by pain and skin necrosis despite the use of a bolster or button. The postoperative rehabilitation is similar to that for FDP lacerations, and the pull-out suture is removed at 4 to 6 weeks. Active motion is allowed at 6 weeks with resumption of full power grip at 8 weeks.

Avulsion of the Superficialis

Flexor digitorum superficialis avulsion is an uncommon injury but occasionally occurs through mechanisms similar to those for profundus avulsions, with strongly resisted finger flexion being the culprit. As expected, the patient has a painful swollen finger and cannot independently flex the PIP joint. Exploration under tourniquet control is performed and the tendon reinserted into subperiosteal bone or sutured to the lateral portion of the A-4 pulley.

Pulley Rupture

Rare instances of traumatic closed rupture of the A-2 or A-4 pulleys have been reported after resisted flexion, such as in rock climbers. Patients have experienced swelling and tenderness of the finger in the region of the pulley without loss of FDS or FDP motion. Magnetic resonance imaging scanning has been used to confirm the diagnosis; operative pulley repair or reconstruction using tendon graft are the advocated treatment choices.

Closed Mallet Deformity

Closed mallet finger (Fig. 5-16*A*) implies a flexion deformity of the DIP joint with an inability to fully extend the DIP joint after injury. Most of these injuries occur after axial loading of the digit with forced flexion or occasionally after a direct blow to the dorsal distal phalanx. Patients have resting flexion of the DIP joint greater than that of adjacent or contralateral fingers, and an "extension lag" (inability to fully extend the finger) at the DIP joint. They often are associated with dorsal fractures of the proximal portion of the distal phalanx, indicating that a portion of the bony insertion has been avulsed with the tendon. The examiner should note the relative percentage of the articular surface that has been fractured off the distal phalanx and specifically look for any volar subluxation of the distal phalanx off the axis of the middle phalanx.

Like open mallet injuries, the mainstay of treatment for a closed mallet finger is splinting. The finger must be splinted in full extension continuously for a minimum of 6 weeks, with the splint being removed only to cleanse the finger and with the patient always maintaining the DIP in full extension when the splint is removed. Many modifications of the Stack splints are readily available, prefabricated, and relatively inexpensive. It is a plastic device that comes in different sizes and fits over the end of the finger extending dorsally onto the middle phalanx. It is secured gently around the middle phalanx using a small strap of velcro or similar material. It maintains the DIP joint in full extension but does not restrict PIP or MCP motion, which should be encouraged. The main difficulties with these splints are skin maceration, hygiene, and selecting an appropriate size for the patient's finger depending on the status of swelling. Splinting should be continued after the initial 6-week period if recurrent extensor lag develops after splint removal. The device is extremely effective in minimizing extensor lag although patients may expect 5 to 10° of residual extensor lag. It may be used effectively despite delays treatment of up to 6 months from the time of injury. Surgical intervention has had generally disappointing results when long-term splinting is not used and offers no advantage over conventional closed splinting. The most common reason for treatment failure is patient noncompliance with continuous wearing of the splint. Patients who discard the splint prematurely have a high incidence of recurrent mallet deformity.

In patients whose distal phalanx is subluxed palmerly off the axis of the middle phalanx or in instances where the dorsal bony fragment comprises greater than 30% of the articular surface, operative reduction and fixation of the fragments is justified. Although direct fixation of the palmer fragment to the remaining distal phalanx may be attempted, stable bony reduction often is best accomplished and maintained by placement of a longitudinal K-wire across the DIP joint. If the fragments can be reduced satisfactorily simply with reduction and longitudinal K-wire fixation, we perform no other open intervention at the DIP level. The K-wire is removed at 4 weeks, and the patient is enrolled in a protocol of DIP splinting using a stack splint for an additional 4 weeks. During this time, active MCP and PIP motion are encouraged.

Outcome following treatment of established mallet deformities is generally poor. We have no successful technique for restoring a functioning DIP joint after established contracture has developed, after patients have become hopelessly noncompliant, or when degenerative changes have occurred after distal phalanx fracture. Fusion of the DIP joint in a more useful position of 10 to 20° of flexion is then a useful alternative despite the inherent total loss of motion at the joint that will be required.

Closed Boutonniere Deformity

Acute closed boutonniere deformity (Fig. 5-16*B*) has the lowest rate of emergency room recognition of all tendon injuries. Patients who sustain dorsal or axial load injuries to a finger often will have swelling and tenderness over the central slip insertion onto the middle phalanx without discernable abnormal posture. These patients then subsequently develop progressive PIP flexion, with compensatory DIP hyperextension. On recognition of the deformity, extension splinting of the PIP joint should be undertaken for 4 to 6 weeks or longer if the deformity recurs after discontinuation of the splint. Metacarpophalangeal and DIP motion should be preserved.

TENDON CONSIDERATIONS IN PROBLEMATIC WOUNDS
Tendons Unsuitable for Primary Repair

Considering the serious consequences of tendon healing with substantial adhesion/scar formation, it would be ideal if all transected tendons were lacerated cleanly and precisely with otherwise healthy, uninjured tendon extending in both directions. Unfortunately, it is common for tendons (and their overlying soft tissues) to have been avulsed, deeply abraded, or torn rather then cleanly incised. The tendons themselves may have had dirt, metal, asphalt, or wood fragments impregnated into them, or they may be badly frayed. Management of these injuries is not easy because, unlike many soft tissue injuries, radical debridement of tissue margins and the discarding of a few centimeters of unhealthy tendon will have profound implications for hand biomechanics. As stated previously, excessive shortening of a flexor tendon before repair may result in a flexed finger that reaches full flexion prematurely, thereby preventing full motion or strength in adjacent fingers (quadrigia effect). Full extension after flexor repair or full flexion after extensor repair may not be possible with the limited excursion and stretching ability of the musculotendinous units. Some marginal debridement may be allowed; however, remember that following repair, one should have an appropriately positioned finger (normal cascade) and a nearly full range of passive motion if there is to be any hope of full motion after swelling, stiffness, and eventual healing have taken place. A finger excessively flexed on the operating table will not resume a normal posture with recovery.

Tendons heavily contaminated with particles should be irrigated copiously and extractable particles removed. Although these wounds have a much higher incidence of infection than elective surgical or even clean traumatic wounds, it is not universal, and it is possible to achieve a satisfactory mobile tendon structure despite the presence of residual particles too small to be removed completely.

Heavily Contaminated Traumatic Wounds

Injuries with either a heavily contaminated wound involving the tendon sheath and/or soft tissue loss over the tendon sheath can be some of the most difficult injuries encountered. These wounds can result from industrial crush (burst) accidents, severe degloving injuries, and deep abrasion injuries. In the majority of instances, meticulous debridement of foreign material and copious lavage irrigation can be combined with primary tendon repair, recognizing that a greater chance of wound infection and impaired tendon motion are present. Possible need for tendon replacement with or without Silastic interposition rod would best be deferred until a supple finger with healed overlying soft tissue wounds can be accomplished rather than immediately undertaken in an unfavorable bed.

Gunshot wounds can produce some of the most devastating injuries in the hand. The tendon injuries typically are accompanied by significant bony, nerve, vascular, and soft tissue injury. Isolated low-velocity handgun injuries may create isolated tendon injuries that are amenable to primary repair at the time of irrigation and debridement, although these instances are exceptional. The typical massively traumatized digit, however, is incapable of regaining normal function because of persistent swelling, stiffness, and anesthesia. These fingers fare poorly with complicated tendon reconstruction because of associated joint and soft tissue motion limitations.

Repairs and Wound Infections

The development of a wound infection after tendon repair, particularly flexor tendon repair, is a devastating outcome. Cellulitis and/or a collection of pus leads to pronounced swelling, pain, and inflammation, all of which either increase the likelihood of tendon repair site rupture or prohibit the kind of gentle motion that is so crucial in restoring useful function. As with other finger infections occurring without tendon injury, edema and stiffness can persist long after resolution of the acute stage of the process and despite successful improvement with IV antibiotics.

Deficient Soft Tissue Coverage

Successful motion of the fingers or hand is heavily dependent on a gliding tendon applying force across a mobile joint, with sufficient soft tissue laxity to allow the motion to occur. Any joint or soft tissue impediment to motion of the digit globally or the tendon locally will prohibit effective digital motion. The finest tendon repairs are worthless if this point is neglected; therefore, adequate pliable soft tissue coverage is a prerequisite before acute or delayed tendon repair is undertaken.

Specific options for coverage of soft tissue deficiencies in the upper extremity are covered in Chapters 4 and 10. The principles, however, are as follows:

1. Successful tendon function requires a gliding surface and sufficient soft tissue laxity to allow motion to occur.
2. Tendons themselves, especially when the epitenon (thin fascial covering) is absent, do not heal satisfactorily by secondary intention (granulation). Small dorsal hand wounds involving exposed tendon with intact epitenon can be allowed to granulate and close or be skin grafted, but may occur at the expense of impaired gliding function. This approach is satisfactory dorsally where less gliding is required, but it usually is not satisfactory for palmer wounds. In patients in poor overall health, it is much more common for no granulation to occur whatsoever, leaving a desiccated nonviable tendon in the wound that actually prohibits spontaneous granulation.

Local Care of Exposed Tendons

In instances in which a wound with exposed tendon is to be allowed to heal spontaneously, or in instances in which delayed definitive coverage is planned (such as when a wound is too heavily contaminated to permit coverage or when other injuries preclude safe administration of an anesthetic), care of the exposed tendons is of paramount importance to ensure their survival. Tendons are extremely prone to desiccation and must not be allowed prolonged exposure to the air. The main choices for wound coverage are (1) heavily dampened gauze dressings in the wound that are changed frequently (for large areas of multiple exposed tendons, we routinely ask for "wet-to-wet" normal saline dressing changes every 4 hours with application of more saline every 2 hours in between), or (2) use of one of the hydrocolloid gels, such as Intersite Gel, which maintains a better liquid interface with the tissues and may allow spontaneous granulation to occur in wounds where granulation would not otherwise be expected. It is to be applied to the wound daily or twice daily, and the wound covered with an occlusive dressing, such as Op-Site, through which the wound can be viewed. Hydrocolloid gels are more expensive than saline-gauze dressings but require less frequent nursing care. Although Intersite Gel is used commonly, even in heavily contaminated wounds at other body sites, ensure that no frank infection develops at the wound surface when caring for a contaminated wound bed.

STAGED TENDON RECONSTRUCTION

Although not used commonly for acute injuries, one-stage (tendon graft) and two-stage (Silastic rod insertion followed by delayed tendon grafting) reconstructions deserve consideration when planning the management of complex upper extremity injuries. Conceptually, tendon grafting or Silastic rod placement are used when existing tendon or sheath is either of insufficient quantity or quality to allow smooth unrestricted gliding after primary repair. Unfortunately, instances of traumatic tendon or sheath loss are accompanied by damage or loss of the overlying soft tissue coverage. Complicated tendon reconstruction cannot be undertaken without a healthy overlying soft tissue envelope. For this reason, soft tissue coverage typically is achieved before performing these types of tendon reconstruction.

Tendon Grafting

Tendon grafts can be used when there is insufficient tendon length to allow primary repair, such as after retraction in delayed injuries or repair site disruption. Tendon grafts then allow the sites of tendon repair to be placed intentionally outside the digital sheath (Zone 2), thereby improving gliding. Grafts may be necessary after soft tissue coverage of dorsal hand wounds, where both soft tissue and tendon have been lost, such as in deep abrasion injuries. Because tendon grafts possess no intrinsic blood supply, they require neovascularization from filmy adhesions which develop from surrounding tissues. The dilemma of allowing flimsy adhesion formation to enhance vascularity and yet without restricting motion makes tendon grafting and its postoperative management among the most challenging aspects of hand surgery.

Sources of Tendon Graft Material

Useful lengths of expendable tendon can be obtained from the palmaris longus of either wrist (absent in 15% of individuals). One can detect the presence of the palmaris by asking the patient to flex the wrist against resistance and visually or manually inspecting the middle of the volar forearm. The tendon can be harvested through a small transverse incision at the level of the distal wrist crease. Scissors are used to undermine above and below the tendon. It is not ridiculous to remind the reader to consider the position and appearance of the median nerve at the wrist to avoid careless injury to it. The tendon can then be harvested from the wrist to its musculotendinous junction using a Brand tendon stripper, which is a circular cutting device that dissects and then transects the palmaris via the one wrist incision.

The second most common site of harvest for tendon graft is the plantaris tendon in the lower leg. The tendon can be located just anterior to the Achilles' tendon along the medial aspect of the ankle. As with the palmaris, local dissection is followed by use of the Brand tendon stripper. In patients who have had extensive surgery or tremendous tendon needs, or in instances in which the donor tendon has been transected during harvest, one can harvest a portion of the FCR or other local tendons, leaving at least 50% of their diameter present without detriment. Unfortunately, longitudinal splitting of tendons yields a raw tendon surface not covered with epitenon, which theoretically is more likely to form adhesions along its length than either the palmaris or plantaris tendons. After harvest of the tendon for grafting, it should be placed in a moist gauze sponge and protected until needed.

Two-Staged Tendon Reconstruction

In situations in which the tissues comprising the course of a tendon are unsuitable for primary graft placement, placement of a silastic rod "spacer"—its later replacement with a free tendon graft—may provide useful function. The rod, which is placed into this heavily scarred bed, promotes the formation of a "pseudosheath" through which a tendon graft will ultimately glide. Like tendon grafts, Silastic rods should only be inserted into a clean wound with sufficient soft tissue coverage. Unlike tendon grafts, however, a smooth, unscarred passage is not required, as the presence of the rod will induce sheath formation. Typically, a Silastic rod is inserted from forearm to fingertip within the digital sheath of a previously traumatized finger. Technical details are as follows:

1. The distal end of the rod must not be allowed to freely float in the distal finger tendon sheath, because it might migrate out the distal finger tip. To prevent this, the rod is inserted below the periosteum of the proximal volar distal phalanx or below any remaining FDP tendon and is sutured into place.
2. The proximal end of the rod may be allowed to float in the distal forearm.
3. After rod placement, aggressive passive range of motion is maintained. At approximately 2 months postoperatively, the rod is removed and a tendon graft inserted.

Pulley System Reconstruction

Circumferential tendon or fascial graft material can be used to recreate the essential A-2 and A-4 pulleys either primarily or during insertion of a tendon rod. Pulley reconstruction at the proximal phalanx should encircle the bone under the extensor hood whereas the more distal pulley reconstructions can encircle the bone and extensor apparatus.

SUMMARY

Even with their complicated biomechanics, tendon injuries can be treated successfully with ample rewards for enthusiastic and aggressive attention, surgical technique, and rehabilitation.

SELECTED REFERENCES

Blair WF, Steyers CM: Extensor tendon injuries, *Orthop Clin* 23:141-148, 1992.
Culp RW, Taras JS: *Primary care of flexor tendon injuries.* In Hunter JM, Mackin EJ, Callahan AD, editors: *Rehabilitation of the hand: surgery and therapy,* ed 4, St. Louis, 1995, CV Mosby.
Evans RB: Therapeutic management of extensor tendon injuries, *Hand Clin* 2:157-169, 1986.
Imbriglia JE, Hunter J, Rennie W: Secondary flexor tendon reconstruction, *Hand Clin* 5:395-413, 1989.
Newport ML, Williams CD: Biomechanical characteristics of extensor tendon suture techniques, *J Hand Surg* 17A:1117-1123, 1992.
Nunley JA, Levin LS, Devito D, Goldner RD, Urbaniak JR: Direct end-to-end repair of flexor pollicis longus tendon lacerations, *J Hand Surg* 17A:118-121, 1992.
Steinberg DR: Acute flexor tendon injuries, *Orthop Clin* 23:125-140, 1992.
Stewart KM, vanStrien G: *Postoperative management of flexor tendon injuries.* In Hunter JM, Mackin EJ, Callahan AD, editors: *Rehabilitation of the hand: surgery and therapy,* ed 4, St. Louis, 1995, CV Mosby.
Wehbe MA: Tendon graft donor sites, *J Hand Surg* 17A:1130-1132, 1992.

6

Nerve Injury

Patty K. Young, MD
Susan E. Mackinnon, MD

ANATOMY

Critical assessment and management of peripheral nerve injury involves an appreciation of both the anatomic course of the nerve, as well as its innervation pattern. This chapter describes the most com-

Abbreviations

ADM	Abductor digiti minimi
AIN	Anterior interosseous nerve
APB	Abductor pollicis brevis
APL	Abductor pollicis longus
BR	Brachioradialis
DI	Dorsal interosseous
DIP	Distal interphalangeal
ECRB	Extensor carpi radialis brevis
ECRL	Extensor carpi radialis longus
ECU	Extensor carpi ulnaris
EDC	Extensor digitorum communis
EDM	Extensor digiti minimi
EIP	Extensor indicis proprius
EPB	Extensor pollicis brevis
EPL	Extensor pollicis longus
FCR	Flexor carpi radialis
FCU	Flexor carpi ulnaris
FDM	Flexor digiti minimi
FDP	Flexor digitorum profundus
FDS	Flexor digitorum superficialis
FPB	Flexor pollicis brevis
FPL	Flexor pollicis longus
IP	Interphalangeal
LABC	Lateral antebrachial cutaneous nerve
MABC	Medial antebrachial cutaneous nerve
MCP	Metacarpophalangeal
PIN	Posterior interosseous nerve
PIP	Proximal interphalangeal
PL	Palmaris longus
PT	Pronator teres
II	Index finger
III	Long finger
IV	Ring finger
V	Small finger

mon anatomic relationships. For a list of the abbreviations used throughout this chapter, see the Box above.

Brachial Plexus

Surgical Anatomy

The nerve roots most consistently contributing to the brachial plexus include the fifth to eighth cervical (C5-C8) and the first thoracic (T1). Occasionally, contributions from C4 and/or T2 will be present.

In various combinations that will be described, the roots form trunks. These divide into anterior and posterior divisions, and then recombine to form cords, from which come most of the major nerve branches of the upper extremity. The roots lie between the anterior and middle scalene muscles at the base of the neck. C5, C6, and C7 roots exit the spinal cord above their numbered vertebrae; C8 exits below the seventh cervical vertebra; and T1 exits below the first thoracic vertebra. Consequently, the posterior aspect of the first rib lies sandwiched between the C8 and T1 roots. Just beyond the border of the first rib, the C8 and T1 roots join to form the lower trunk. The middle trunk is the continuation of the C7 root, and the upper trunk is the combination of the C5 and C6 roots.

The trunks lie in the posterior cervical triangle and divide into anterior and posterior divisions at the level of the clavicle. The three posterior divisions join to form the posterior cord (C5, C6, C7, C8, T1) and the anterior divisions of the upper and middle trunks unite to form the lateral cord (C5, C6, C7). The anterior division of the lower trunk continues as the medial cord (C8, T1). The posterior, lateral, and medial cords travel beneath the pectoralis minor muscle, adjacent to the axillary artery. Their position in relation to the axillary artery corresponds to their names (Fig. 6-1).

Nerve Branches of the Brachial Plexus

Roots

There are three nerve branches from the roots; the long thoracic nerve (from C5, C6, C7), the dorsal scapular nerve (from C5, C6), and the nerve to the subclavius muscle (from C5, C6). Occasionally, the latter will arise from the upper trunk. The long thoracic nerve innervates the serratus anterior muscle. The dorsal scapular nerve innervates the levator scapulae and rhomboid muscles.

Trunks

The trunks give rise to one nerve branch. The suprascapular nerve exits the upper trunk proximal to the clavicle, travels deep to the trapezius muscle and through the scapular notch to innervate the supraspinatus and infraspinatus muscles. The scapular notch is located on the superior border of the scapula and is bound by the superior transverse ligament.

Divisions

There are no nerve branches from the anterior or posterior divisions.

Cords

Each cord ends by dividing into two terminal nerve branches. The posterior cord ends as it branches into the axillary and radial nerve. Both the lateral and medial cords contribute terminal branches to the formation of the median nerve, while continuing

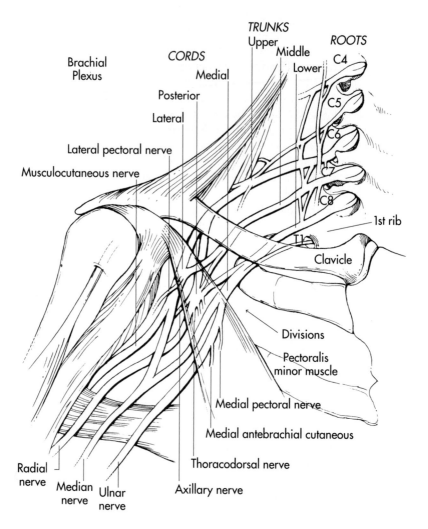

Figure 6-1   Brachial plexus.

distally as the musculocutaneous and ulnar nerve respectively. This configuration results in the classic "M" formation of the musculocutaneous, median, and ulnar nerves.

POSTERIOR CORD

There are two nerve branches from the posterior cord. These include the thoracodorsal nerve to the latissimus dorsi and the subscapular nerve to the subscapularis and the teres major muscles. As the posterior cord terminates, it branches into the axillary nerve and the radial nerve. The axillary nerve travels through the quadrangular space (bounded by the teres minor, the teres major, the humerus, and the long head of the triceps), innervating the teres minor and deltoid muscles.

LATERAL CORD

The lateral pectoral nerve is the single nerve branch from the lateral cord. It supplies innervation to both the clavicular and sternocostal heads of the pectoralis major muscle. The two terminal branches of the lateral cord include its contribution to the median nerve and the musculocutaneous nerve. The latter nerve travels along the undersurface of the biceps muscle, innervating the coracobrachialis, brachialis, and biceps muscles, terminating in the forearm as the LABC. The LABC supplies sensory innervation to the lateral forearm.

MEDIAL CORD

Two nerve branches arise from the medial cord. The medial pectoral nerve supplies innervation to the pectoralis minor and the sternocostal head of the pectoralis major muscles. It does not innervate the clavicular head of the pectoralis major. The MABC also arises from the medial cord, supplying sensory innervation to the posterior elbow and the volar, medial forearm. The two terminal branches of the medial cord include its contribution to the median nerve and the ulnar nerve.

Radial Nerve

Surgical Anatomy

The radial nerve is the terminal branch of the posterior cord (C5, C6, C7, C8). It lies posterior to the axillary artery at its origin. In the proximal axilla, at the distal edge of the pectoralis major muscle, the radial nerve turns at a right angle to course toward the spiral groove. It then travels in the spiral groove along the posterior aspect of the humerus. From this point, it courses through the triceps muscle bellies, then crosses the musculospiral groove, and enters the anterior aspect of the arm by piercing the lateral intermuscular septum approximately 10 cm proximal to the lateral humeral epicondyle. Two to 3 cm proximal to this epicondyle, the nerve lies lateral to the brachialis and the biceps tendon and medial to the origin of the BR muscle, coursing distally at the level of the elbow to lie in the groove between the biceps and the BR. Over the next 5 cm, the nerve divides into the sensory radial nerve and its deep motor branch, the posterior interosseous nerve (PIN). The PIN enters the supinator muscle beneath its leading edge, known as the arcade of Frohse. At the distal portion of the supinator, it gives off multiple branches to the extensor muscles of the forearm. It continues along the interosseous membrane, then travels on the radial side of the fourth extensor compartment adjacent to Lister's tubercle and the terminal branches of the anterior interosseous artery, terminating in the dorsal wrist capsule and intercarpal ligaments (Fig. 6-2).

Functional Anatomy

The radial nerve innervates the long, lateral, and medial heads of the triceps muscle, BR, ECRL, and ECRB. The PIN innervates the supinator, EDC, EDM, ECU, anconeus, APL, EPL, EPB, and EIP. It terminates with innervation to the dorsal wrist capsule and intercarpal ligaments.

Median Nerve

Surgical Anatomy

The median nerve originates from terminal branches of the lateral and medial cord (C5, C6, C7, C8, T1). The sensory component of the median nerve originates from the lateral cord, whereas the motor component for the median innervated intrinsic muscles originates from the medial cord. The median nerve, once formed, generally lies anterior to the axillary artery, crosses the medial intermuscular septum, and enters the forearm superficial to the brachialis muscle, lying medial to the biceps tendon and brachial artery in the antecubital fossa, deep to the lacertus fibrosis. The nerve then travels between the muscular origins of the deep and superficial heads of the pronator teres and the FDS, giving off the anterior interosseous nerve (AIN) branch. The median nerve continues distally between the FDS and FDP muscles. Near the wrist, it becomes more superficial, lying between the tendons of the FDS and FCR muscles. It then passes deep and medial to the PL tendon, entering the hand beneath the transverse carpal ligament, giving off a motor branch to the thenar muscles and continuing distally to give off branches to the first and second lumbricales and provide sensory innervation to the radial three and one-half digits (Fig. 6-3).

Functional Anatomy

In the forearm, the median nerve innervates all the flexors (except for the FCU and the FDP to the ring and small fingers); these include the PT, FCR, PL, and FDS. The AIN branch of the median nerve innervates four muscles: FDP to the index and middle fingers, FPL, and pronator quadratus. Intrinsic muscles of the hand innervated by the median nerve are the first and second lumbricales and the thenar muscles, APB, superficial head of FPB, and opponens pollicis. (Twenty percent of the time the opponens pollicis will be innervated by the ulnar nerve and 5% of the time the APB is innervated by the ulnar nerve.)

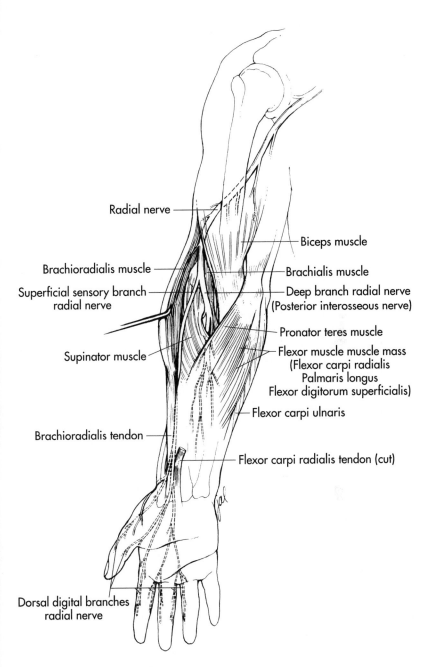

Radial nerve

Brachioradialis muscle

Superficial sensory branch
radial nerve

Supinator muscle

Brachioradialis tendon

Dorsal digital branches
radial nerve

Biceps muscle

Brachialis muscle

Deep branch radial nerve
(Posterior interosseous nerve)

Pronator teres muscle

Flexor muscle muscle mass
(Flexor carpi radialis
Palmaris longus
Flexor digitorum superficialis)

Flexor carpi ulnaris

Flexor carpi radialis tendon (cut)

Figure 6-2   Radial nerve.

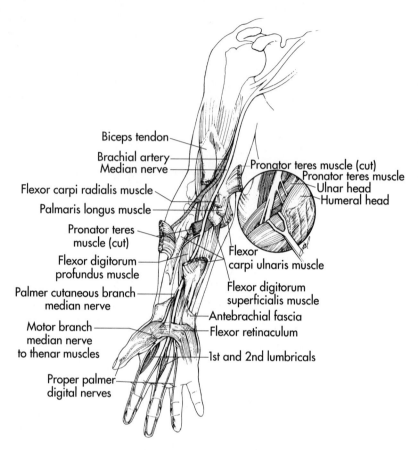

Biceps tendon

Brachial artery
Median nerve

Flexor carpi radialis muscle

Palmaris longus muscle

Pronator teres
muscle (cut)

Flexor digitorum
profundus muscle

Palmer cutaneous branch
median nerve

Motor branch
median nerve
to thenar muscles

Proper palmer
digital nerves

Pronator teres muscle (cut)
Pronator teres muscle
Ulnar head
Humeral head

Flexor
carpi ulnaris muscle

Flexor digitorum
superficialis muscle

Antebrachial fascia
Flexor retinaculum

1st and 2nd lumbricals

Figure 6-3   Median nerve.

Ulnar Nerve

Surgical Anatomy

The ulnar nerve is the terminal branch of the medial cord (C8, T1). It lies medial to the axillary artery, travels between the medial head of the triceps and the humerus, and then passes inferiorly and medially to the medial humeral epicondyle to lie in the postcondylar groove in the olecranon. It proceeds distally between the two heads of the FCU, traveling down the forearm deep and lateral to this muscle and between the muscle bellies of the FDP and FDS. Approximately 9 cm proximal to the wrist, the ulnar nerve gives off the dorsal cutaneous branch, leaving the terminal motor and sensory branches. These branches pass deep to the antebrachial fascia and the transverse carpal ligament. The motor fascicles are ulnar to the sensory fascicles in the forearm and just proximal to the wrist. They then move deep to the sensory fascicles on crossing the pisohamate ligament. The deep motor branch then travels radial to the sensory fascicles as it enters the tunnel between the pisohamate ligament and the FDM muscle. It travels beneath the fibrous edge of the FDM, lying superficial to the opponens digiti minimi and radial to the ADM. The sensory branch continues distally and lies superficial to the FDM.

Functional Anatomy

The ulnar nerve innervates nothing in the arm. Its innervation pattern in the forearm and hand includes the FCU, FDP to the ring and small fingers, palmaris brevis, ADM, FDM, opponens digiti minimi, third and fourth lumbricales, deep head of the FPB, adductor pollicis, and palmar and dorsal interossei (Fig. 6-4).

Medial Antebrachial Cutaneous Nerve (MABC)

Surgical Anatomy

The MABC is a terminal branch of the medial cord. It travels medial to the biceps muscle and divides into anterior and posterior branches in the proximal to midarm region. Each branch then travels anterior/posterior to the basilic vein, coursing anterior and lateral to the medial humeral epicondyle. The posterior branch crosses the region of the medial humeral epicondyle and courses over the posteromedial aspect of the olecranon. The anterior branch continues down the medial forearm.

Functional Anatomy

The posterior branch provides sensation to the posterior aspect of the elbow and forearm. The anterior branch provides sensation to the medial volar third of the forearm.

Lateral Antebrachial Cutaneous Nerve (LABC)

Surgical Anatomy

The LABC is the cutaneous continuation of the musculocutaneous nerve. It lies adjacent to the cephalic vein at the junction between the lateral and middle third of the forearm.

Functional Anatomy

The LABC provides sensation to the distal radial forearm. Approximately 75% of the time, there is extensive overlap in sensory territory with the radial sensory nerve.

Radial Sensory Nerve

Surgical Anatomy

The radial sensory nerve is the superficial branch of the radial nerve. Initially, it lies beneath the BR muscle, superficial to the radial artery.

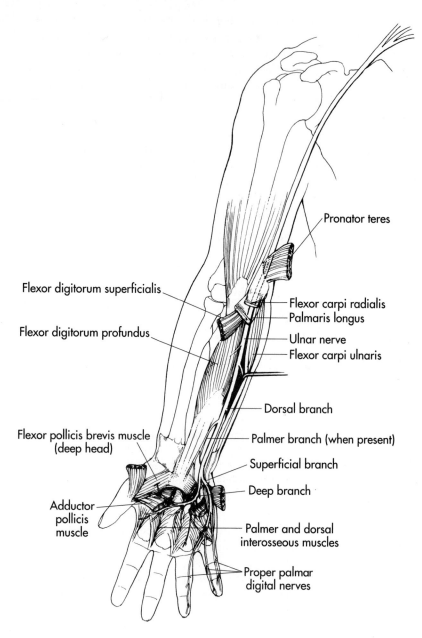

Figure 6-4   Ulnar nerve.

It becomes subcutaneous as it emerges between the tendons of the ECRL and the BR, most commonly at the junction of the distal and middle thirds of the forearm. Terminal branches are sent along the distal dorsoradial aspect of the forearm and wrist and to the dorsal aspects of the thumb, index, middle, and ring fingers through the dorsal digital branches.

Functional Anatomy

The radial sensory nerve provides sensation to the dorsoradial wrist and hand, and the dorsal aspects of the thumb, the proximal index and middle fingers, and the proximal, radial half of the ring finger. There is extensive overlap in sensory territory with the LABC and slight overlap in sensory territory with the dorsal cutaneous branch of the ulnar nerve.

Dorsal Cutaneous Branch of the Ulnar Nerve (DCU)

Surgical Anatomy

The DCU is a branch of the ulnar nerve, arising approximately 9 cm proximal to the wrist, exiting from beneath the flexor carpi ulnaris, coursing along the dorsoulnar aspect of the wrist and hand, sending terminal dorsal digital branches to the small and ring fingers.

Functional Anatomy

The DCU provides sensation to the dorsoulnar wrist and hand, and the dorsal, proximal aspects of the small finger and ulnar half of the ring finger.

Palmar Cutaneous Branch of the Ulnar Nerve (PCU)

Surgical Anatomy

The PCU arises from the ulnar nerve at a variable site in the mid to distal forearm, travels distally with the ulnar nerve, and passes through the volar carpal ligament to enter the ulnar aspect of the palm. The incidence of this nerve is very low.

Functional Anatomy

The proximal ulnar aspect of the palm receives its sensory innervation from the PCU.

Palmar Cutaneous Branch of the Median Nerve (PCM)

Surgical Anatomy

The PCM arises from the median nerve in the distal third of the forearm and courses distally parallel to the median nerve, and superficial and ulnar to the FCR tendon. It then pierces the radial border of the antebrachial fascia, the volar carpal ligament, or the transverse carpal ligament at the level of the wrist and divides into lateral and medial branches in the radial aspect of the palm.

Functional Anatomy

The PCM supplies sensation to the proximal two fifths of the radial palm and the thenar eminence.

CLASSIFICATION OF NERVE INJURIES

There are several patterns of nerve injury that may vary from fascicle to fascicle and along the longitudinal axis of the nerve. An understanding of the type of nerve injury is important in planning patient management. Six types of nerve injury have been described.

Neurapraxia (First Degree Injury)

This involves a localized conduction block along a discrete area of the nerve. Segmental demyelination may or may not be seen histologically. Because there is no axonal damage or subsequent regeneration, a Tinel's sign will not be present. The patient should completely recover within 3 months. Examples of a first degree injury include tourniquet palsy, localized pressure palsy, and early nerve entrapment syndromes.

Axonotmesis (Second Degree Injury)

This involves axonal damage with Wallerian degeneration distal to the site of the injury. The endoneurium and perineurium are intact. Proximal nerve regeneration results in a Tinel's sign, which will advance distally as the nerve regenerates at the classic rate of 1 inch/month or 1 to 1.5 mm/day. Because the endoneurium is not injured and the axonal sprouts do not have to regenerate through scar tissue, recovery will be complete. Examples of second degree injuries include stretch and injection injuries.

Third Degree Injury

With this injury, scarring in the endoneurium has occurred. Because of this, regeneration will occur through some degree of scar tissue with the potential for an incomplete recovery. In addition, if the injury involves fascicles with mixed sensory and motor fibers in the same fascicle, mismatching of nerve fibers to inappropriate distal receptors is likely. Thus, recovery may vary from nearly complete to poor, depending on the degree of endoneural scarring and how pure or mixed the fascicle is. Recovery will occur at 1 inch/month and with an advancing Tinel's sign. Examples of third degree injuries are stretch and injection injuries.

Fourth Degree Injury

In this injury, the nerve is in continuity. At the level of the injury, however, complete scarring has occurred. As a result, nerve regeneration is not possible. Wallerian degeneration will occur distal to the site of injury, while proximal to the site of injury regenerating nerve fibers will be trapped in scar. A Tinel's sign will be present at the level of injury and will not advance distally. No recovery occurs without surgical repair. Examples of fourth degree injuries include stretch injury, failed primary nerve repair, and injection injury.

Neurotmesis (Fifth Degree Injury)

In this injury complete transection of the nerve exists. No recovery occurs without surgical repair.

Sixth Degree Injury

This involves a mixed pattern of injury within the nerve. Some fascicles may have normal function, whereas others show varying degrees of injury (I, II, III, IV, V). The pattern of recovery will be mixed, with complete recovery in the fascicles having first or second degree injuries, partial recovery in the fascicles with third degree injury, and no recovery in the fascicles containing a fourth or fifth degree injury. The surgical challenge is in protecting normal or recovering fascicles, while repairing/grafting nonrecovering fascicles. This type of injury is seen with neuroma in continuity.

EVALUATION OF SENSORY AND MOTOR FUNCTION

A detailed physical examination is vital for the accurate diagnosis of a peripheral nerve injury. Both the motor and sensory examination will vary with the type and severity of the nerve injury. With nerve compression, for example, the functions may remain intact, but are diminished both qualitatively and quantitatively. In contrast, with either partial or complete nerve transection, absence of some or all of its function occurs. Table 6-1 lists the critical points of the examination for the assessment of the major motor and sensory nerves of the upper extremity. See also the section on brachial plexus.

Motor Evaluation

Injury of motor nerves manifests itself as either muscle weakness or paralysis. This can be assessed manually by a physical examination and quantitated by measurement of pinch and grip strength.

Sensory Evaluation

The evaluation of sensory function depends on an accurate history of the injury and a physical examination. With an open wound and a patient report of altered sensation, a high degree of suspicion for nerve injury exists and dictates surgical exploration (except for missile injury). Physical examination of sensory testing includes the assessment

Table 6-1   Critical Physical Examination Points for Unambiguous Diagnosis of Peripheral Nerve Injury

Motor Evaluation	Sensory Evaluation
1. Radial nerve a. Elbow extension b. Wrist extension c. Extension of fingers at MCP joints d. Thumb extension at the IP joint 2. Median nerve: intrinsic a. Thumb palmer abduction 3. Median nerve: extrinsic a. Flexion DIP all fingers b. Flexion PIP of index finger (isolated) c. Flexion IP of thumb d. Flexor carpi radialis 4. Ulnar nerve: intrinsic a. First dorsal interossei b. Hypothenar muscles 5. Ulnar nerve: extrinsic a. Flexion PIP of small finger (isolated) b. Flexor carpi ulnaris	1. Radial nerve: Dorsal radial aspect of hand—near first web space 2. Median nerve: Pulp of index finger and thumb 3. Ulnar nerve: Pulp of small finger 4. Palmer cutaneous branch of median nerve: Proximal palm near thenar eminence/crease 5. Dorsal cutaneous branch of ulnar nerve: Dorsal ulnar region of hand 6. Digital nerve: Adjacent to DIP flexion crease—distal third of middle phalanx and proximal third of distal phalanx, not tip of finger

MCP, metacarpophalangeal; DIP, distal interphalangeal; PIP, proximal interphalangeal; IP, interphalangeal.

of innervation density and threshold measurements of vibration and pressure. Two-point discrimination (2PD) measures innervation density and reflects the number of intact innervated receptors. Threshold measurements indicate how normally these innervated receptors are functioning. When testing sensation, the digit being tested must be immobilized to prevent proprioceptive feedback.

Two-point discrimination is evaluated both for slowly adapting receptors (static 2PD) and quickly adapting receptors (moving 2PD). Static two-point discrimination is measured by holding two points against the skin for several seconds; moving two-point discrimination is assessed by moving two prongs longitudinally along the finger pulp. The patient then indicates whether she or he feels one or two prongs. The smallest distance in which the patient responds correctly on two of three trials is recorded.

Threshold measurements are performed for both vibration (quickly adapting receptors) and pressure (slowly adapting receptors). Vibration threshold can be evaluated with a tuning fork or quantitated with a vibrometer. The smallest vibration stimulus perceived by the patient is noted as the baseline vibration threshold and is recorded in microns of motion. Semmes–Weinstein monofilaments quantitatively assess pressure thresholds. The nylon monofilaments are applied perpendicularly to the skin with increasing pressure until bending occurs. The force required to bend the monofilament is recorded numerically on each probe. The smallest numbered monofilament that can elicit perception is recorded.

When there has been actual nerve fiber loss, two-point discrimination will be abnormal. When nerve fiber loss has not occurred, but nerve damage is present from ischemia or mechanical injury, two-point discrimination may be normal, but threshold testing will be abnormal.

ELECTRODIAGNOSIS

There are specific indications for electrical testing in the evaluation of peripheral nerve injury. However, the limitations of these studies must be appreciated.

Indications

1. To compliment the clinical evaluation when establishing the diagnosis.
2. To rule out systemic conditions and associated neuropathies.
3. To assess for the presence of cervical radiculopathy.
4. To evaluate nerve recovery after an injury.
5. To stage the degree of peripheral nerve compression.
6. To obtain objective, serial measurements to evaluate results of treatment.

Limitations

1. The recording electrode detects electrical activity in the fastest conducting fibers and may not reveal conduction problems in one or two severely impaired fascicles.
2. The EMG needle samples 6 to 30 muscle fibers in its proximity and may not detect muscle fibers undergoing denervation in other areas of the muscle belly.
3. Peripheral vasoconstriction related to temperature changes or apprehension of the patient can cause variation in conduction velocity measurements.
4. Anatomic variation with overlap of sensory nerve territory may result in false results of sensory nerve evaluation.
5. Anatomic anomalies also may confound EMG evaluation.

6. Unless performed segmentally, latency testing over prolonged distances is inaccurate (i.e., from the elbow to wrist).
7. Coexisting peripheral neuropathy makes interpretation of results difficult.
8. The results are examiner dependent.

Specific Electrical Tests

Nerve Conduction Studies

Routine studies characterize conduction in large-diameter, myelinated nerve fibers. Because of this, normal values may be present in the face of partial nerve injury when a few undamaged large fibers remain intact. When correlated with the physical examination, nerve conduction studies are helpful in determining the degree of peripheral nerve dysfunction, the presence of segmental demyelination or axonal degeneration, the site of injury, and whether the injury is unifocal, multifocal, or diffuse. The information obtained narrows the differential diagnosis, aides in formation of a treatment plan, and assesses functional recovery.

Terminology

Electrical stimulation of a motor or sensory nerve elicits an evoked depolarization potential that propagates both proximally and distally along the nerve. Recordings of the nerve response can be orthodromic (direction of physiologic conduction) or antidromic (direction opposite to physiologic conduction). Conduction recordings typically are orthodromic for motor nerve, and either orthodromic or antidromic for sensory nerves, depending on the specific nerve studied.

COMPOUND MUSCLE ACTION POTENTIAL (CMAP)

A typical, normal recording of an electrically stimulated motor nerve is a biphasic action potential with a large upward (negative) deflection followed by a smaller downward (positive) deflection. The motor response, which is designated as the M-wave or CMAP, represents the sum of the individual muscle fiber action potentials.

SENSORY COMPOUND NERVE ACTION POTENTIAL (SNAP)

The action potential recording for a sensory response typically is either triphasic (orthodromic) or biphasic (antidromic). The sensory response, which is referred to as SNAP, represents the sum of the action potentials of the individual nerve fibers.

LATENCY

The interval of time between the onset of the stimulus and the evoked motor/sensory response is termed latency. With motor nerve conduction, there is a lag time for stimulus transmission across the motor end plate. To account for this nerve-receptor lag time, distal motor latency can be obtained by stimulating the most distal site along the motor nerve near the muscle belly. This reflects the conduction time in the most distal segment of the motor nerve. Nerve-receptor latency measurements for sensory nerves are not required.

CONDUCTION VELOCITY (CV)

Motor nerve CV reflects the CV of the fastest nerve fibers. In a injured motor nerve, a few intact fibers may yield an entirely normal nerve CV. In sensory nerves, the CV also represents the CV of the fastest sensory fibers. However, the CV of slower-conducting fibers can be estimated by differing the way in which the latency is measured.

Nerve conduction velocity is calculated indirectly by dividing the measured distance between the proximal and distal stimulating sites by the latency. For calculation of motor nerve CV, the distal motor latency is subtracted from the motor latency, thereby excluding the nerve-motor end plate lag time.

$$CV \text{ (m/sec)} = \frac{\textit{distance (mm) between proximal and distal stimulation sites (motor)}}{\text{proximal latency (m/sec)} - \text{distal latency (m/sec)}}$$

AMPLITUDE

Amplitude measurements are made from baseline to peak or from negative to positive peak (peak to peak) for motor action potentials, and peak to peak for sensory action potentials. The amplitude of the M-wave is an estimation of the number of muscle fibers activated by stimulation of the motor nerve, while the amplitude of the SNAP reflects the number of nerve fibers activated. However, the latter is influenced strongly by the distance between the nerve and the recording electrode—greater distance results in a decrease in amplitude.

Electromyography (EMG)

Evaluation of muscle activity by measuring and recording muscle fiber action potentials in response to electrical stimulation allows for the assessment of both the condition of the muscle and the peripheral motor nerve. The EMG electrode needle samples only muscle fibers in its immediate proximity, and thereby detects only very localized activity. On insertion of the needle electrode into the muscle, the fibers are stimulated mechanically. The result is a burst of action potentials. This burst of activity normally lasts from 300 to 500 m/sec. Prolonged insertional activity may be seen with early denervation, inflammatory myopathies, and myotonic disorders. Decreased insertional activity is seen with fibrosis and fatty replacement of muscle. After cessation of insertional activity, any subsequent spontaneous electrical activity generally is abnormal, because normal muscle is electrically silent at rest. With voluntary muscle contraction, motor unit action potentials are generated and recorded.

Terminology

An evaluation of the motor unit action potentials that are generated by voluntary muscle contraction and any recorded spontaneous activity of the muscle fibers facilitates the diagnosis and management of the patient, particularly when correlated with the findings of the physical examination. This section discussed only the terminology relevant to peripheral nerve injury.

MOTOR UNIT POTENTIAL (MUP)

The action potential generated by the muscle fibers from one motor unit is referred to as the motor unit potential (MUP). The MUP is characterized by its duration, configuration, amplitude, and variability in shape at consecutive discharges (firing pattern). Individual MUPs can be assessed with weak voluntary contraction, which results in visibly separated action potentials on the tracing. With moderate voluntary contraction, more motor units are activated and the MUPs will overlap. Strong voluntary contraction results in an interference pattern in which action potentials obliterate the baseline. The duration of the MUP is an indicator of the size of the motor unit territory within a radius of approximately 2.5 mm from the electrode. The MUP amplitude is determined by both the muscle fiber density and the distance between the recording electrode and the active muscle fibers. The configuration or shape of the MUP reflects the synchrony of the action potentials from the muscle fibers nearest the recording electrode. Polyphasic and serrated MUPs demonstrate reduced muscle fiber synchrony, as seen with reinnervation patterns or myopathies. The shape of the MUP also is influenced by age, activity level, temperature, muscle-to-muscle variation, and position of the electrode.

FIBRILLATIONS AND POSITIVE SHARP WAVES

Both of these represent abnormal spontaneous activity that occurs because of denervated muscle fibers. Fibrillations and positive sharp waves have different wave characteristics, but both are the result of spontaneously firing action potentials from denervated muscle fibers and have the same clinical significance. They generally appear 2 to 5 weeks after a second degree or higher-order peripheral nerve injury and also can be seen in primary muscle disease.

Interpretation of Test Results

The type and degree of peripheral nerve injury, the time since the onset of injury, and the coexistence of neuromuscular disease affect the interpretation of nerve conduction studies.

Neurapraxia

During the time of localized conduction block, before recovery, conduction velocity will slow across the area of injury. When motor fibers are involved, EMG will demonstrate decreased recruitment of motor units, with decreased duration and amplitude of MUPs. There will, however, be no signs of denervation.

Axonotmesis

With axonotmesis, conduction failure will exist across the site of injury. For approximately 7 days after the injury, conduction velocity in the distal nerve segment will be maintained, but CMAPs and SNAPs will progressively decrease in amplitude with distal stimulation, until ultimately conduction ceases. Electromyographic studies will demonstrate denervation with fibrillations and positive sharp waves 2 to 5 weeks after the injury of a motor nerve. Reinnervation changes take at least 6 to 8 weeks or longer to develop, depending on the level of motor nerve injury in relation to the muscle. With reinnervation, MUPs will be present, and will show increased amplitude and firing instability (desynchronization) with a polyphasic or serrated appearance. Because recovery is complete, conduction velocity will return to preinjury levels, fibrillations and positive sharp waves will disappear, and the MUP firing pattern will again become synchronous.

Third degree nerve injury

Nerve conduction studies and EMG findings will be similar to axonotmesis, except that recovery is incomplete. Nerve conduction velocity will not return to preinjury levels across the site of injury, because of the presence of persistent scarring. With a mixed nerve injury, recovery may be poor and fibrillations and positive sharp waves may persist.

Fourth and fifth degree nerve injuries

In these injuries, conduction failure will exist across the site of injury. Conduction velocity in the distal nerve segment will be maintained for up to 7 days, but ultimately will progress to complete failure of transmission. During this time, CMAPs and SNAPs will show progressively decrease in amplitude with distal stimulation. Electromyographic studies will demonstrate denervation with fibrillations and positive sharp waves within 2 to 5 weeks after the injury. No MUPs will be on the EMG and no evidence of reinnervation will occur.

Sixth degree nerve injury

Electrophysiologically, the findings will vary with the degree of injury in each fascicle. Recovery is partial, and findings will show evidence of denervation and reinnervation patterns.

NERVE REPAIR

The goal of nerve repair is to direct the proximal regenerating fibers into the distal nerve with a minimal loss of regenerating units at the suture line.

Basic Principles (Overview)

1. Quantitative preoperative and postoperative assessment of both sensory and motor systems is essential. The sensory system is evaluated by measuring vibration or pressure stimulation, static and moving two-point discrimination, and pain and temperature perception. The motor system is assessed by appraisal of muscle wasting and quantification of muscle strength by pinch or grip measurements.
2. Microsurgical technique requires appropriate magnification, instrumentation, and suture materials.
3. The nerve repair must be tension free.
4. An interposition nerve graft must be used if a tension-free repair is not possible.
5. The extremity should be in a neutral position for nerve repair or grafting. Postural positioning of the extremity to facilitate an end-to-end repair is inappropriate.
6. When conditions permit, a primary end-to-end repair should be performed.
7. Critical assessment of the proximal and distal nerve stumps for evidence of damage should be performed. The damaged nerve must be resected.
8. If the proximal extent of nerve damage cannot be ascertained at the time of injury, the nerve ends should be approximated, and a formal nerve repair or graft performed at a later date. This may be as early as 3 weeks, or when the wound permits. The delay allows for demarcation of the injury, while approximation of the nerve ends prevents shortening.
9. An epineural repair should be performed unless the internal topography of the peripheral nerve dictates a group fascicular repair.
10. The potential surgical result will be maximized with postoperative motor and sensory reeducation.

Timing of Nerve Repair

The timing of the nerve repair is dictated by the nature of the nerve injury. The reader is referred to discussions of specific types of nerve injuries later in this chapter.

Primary Versus Secondary Nerve Repair

The majority of acute nerve lacerations can be repaired primarily. Primary nerve repair should not be undertaken when the extent of longitudinal damage to the nerve endings cannot be determined, when there is actual nerve loss, or in the presence of an avulsion injury, a closed injury, an injection injury, or a gunshot/shotgun wound injury. These situations call for delayed repair and expectant observation. If a clean transection injury of the nerve has occurred, then primary end-to-end repair may be performed. Both fascicular and epineural repair techniques can be used, depending on the fascicular arrangement of the nerve and the location and nature of the injury.

Group Fascicular Versus Epineural Repair

A group fascicular repair may be performed when the internal topography of the nerve is known, as is the case with the recurrent motor branch of the median nerve, the deep motor branch of the ulnar nerve in Guyon's canal, and the dorsal cutaneous branch of the ulnar nerve in the forearm. Injuries in the distal aspect of the extremity are more amenable to group fascicular repair, because the nerve fascicles are polyfascicular and often are aligned in a group fascicular pattern. When the nerve injury is acute, the fascicular orientation of the proximal and distal segments are usually easily matched. However, when there is any concern about the motor/sensory orientation, there are techniques that can be used for identification, including anatomic clues (surgical identification of fascicles going to specific muscles or cutaneous territories), topography maps, awake stimulation, and enzyme staining. The last two techniques are helpful only in proximal nerve stumps. Chemical enzyme staining techniques are helpful in identifying proximal motor (acetylcholinesterase, choline acetyl-transferase, and choline acetylcholinesterase) and sensory (carbonic anhydrase) fascicles. However, this technique is pathologist or technician dependent and is not yet universally available.

Awake stimulation is very useful in determining motor and sensory fascicular grouping in the proximal stump. Either a local or IV regional anesthetic is used. The area of nerve injury is explored, and the damaged nerve identified. The nerve end is sharply transected until a normal fascicular pattern is identified. The tourniquet is then deflated, and the proximal portion of the nerve is stimulated. Stimulation of sensory fascicles is interpreted by the patient as an electrical or burning pain in a specific cutaneous distribution. In contrast, the patient perceives stimulation of the motor fascicles as a dull, nonspecific stimulus, generally localized to the midportion of the muscle belly of the corresponding motor nerve. Stimulation should be initiated with very low amplification settings and first performed on the fascicles thought to be motor. Once the patient reports a sensory response, the same stimulus is then transferred to the supposed sensory portion of the nerve. If this is indeed the sensory component, the patients perception/response will be much greater, sharper, and superficial, confirming the supposition that there are sensory fascicles. With the identification of the fascicles, a prioritization of function can be determined for major nerves and reconstruction directed at maximizing important function.

When well-defined groups of fascicles are not present and their function is primarily mixed sensory and motor, or when the topography cannot be determined, an epineural repair should be performed. Injuries in the proximal aspect of the extremity are managed by epineural repair because the fascicular pattern is often monofascicular or oligofascicular.

NERVE GRAFTING
Role of Nerve Grafting

When an end-to-end nerve repair cannot be performed without tension at the repair site, a nerve graft is indicated. There is disagreement over the critical length of the gap between the nerve ends that would necessitate a nerve graft. No tension should be allowed at the site of repair because this will lead to scarring and incomplete recovery. Only minimal length may be gained by mobilization of the nerve proximally and distally. For injuries in the ulnar nerve close to the region of the cubital tunnel, additional length (approximately 3 cm) may be obtained by anterior transposition of the nerve. Extreme postural positioning of the extremity to facilitate an end-to-end repair will jeopardize the recovery.

Technique of Nerve Grafting

The injured nerve site is prepared by resection of the neuroma in continuity or the proximal neuroma and distal glioma. The proximal nerve end is transected sharply until a normal fascicular pattern is identified. The polarity of the donor nerve graft is reversed. This minimizes loss of regenerating axons through small branches within the donor nerve. In addition, the graft is not necessarily placed in the normal anatomical route, but rather, at the site of shortest distance between the proximal and distal nerve stumps. The length of the graft should be designed to ensure that the repair is tension free. The extremity is moved through a range of motion to ensure a tension-free repair with movement. Thus, immobilization for more than 2 weeks is not needed. This prevents unnecessary scarring and tethering of the nerve graft in the tissue bed.

Prioritization of Function

The sensory and motor fascicles between the graft and the proximal and distal repair sites should be matched as accurately as possible. Awake stimulation, enzyme staining, or known anatomic topography can be useful in identifying proximal motor and sensory groups, so that direct matching of the motor and sensory fascicle through the graft can be attained. This allows for preservation of both motor and sensory function in a situation in which each is deemed equally important. For the distal nerve stump, the fascicular motor and sensory alignment can be determined quite easily by anatomic dissection. This allows the graft to be placed with precision so that all innervation is directed into the restoration of critical motor or sensory function by excluding either the (less important) distal motor or sensory fascicles from the repair. Examples of prioritizing critical nerve function at the expense of less important nerve function are listed below. (Also see the section on brachial plexus injuries for prioritizing functions.)

Radial Nerve Grafting

In the radial nerve, the proximal fibers are mixed motor and sensory. Distally, the radial sensory nerve can be identified and followed proximally to the distal nerve stump. By excluding the superficial radial nerve from the graft, all regenerating fibers are directed into the distal motor fascicles. This maximizes functional recovery at the expense of the less important radial sensory innervation.

Median Nerve Grafting

Injuries of the median nerve at the distal forearm and wrist level that require a graft for repair usually are operated on at a time after injury that precludes recovery of muscle function. In this situation, the dissection is carried into the hand to determine anatomically the fascicles destined for specific digits and to exclude the motor fascicles to the thenar muscles. The nerve graft then connects the proximal median nerve to the distal median nerve segment, allowing all regenerating fibers to travel to the digits for sensory reinnervation. This results in good sensibility recovery and localization. A tendon transfer for recovery of thumb opposition will be required.

Ulnar Nerve Grafting

The ulnar nerve at the wrist is composed of approximately 40% motor fibers and 60% sensory fibers. The topography of the ulnar nerve in the forearm is well known, and the sensory and motor fascicles are located in distinct positions. This allows for excellent functional recovery if the motor/sensory alignment is correct. Proximally, the motor group of fascicles is located between the two sensory groups of fascicles. After the dorsal cutaneous branch has separated from the main nerve in the midforearm, the motor group is aligned medial and slightly dorsal to the remaining sensory group. On reaching Guyon's canal, the motor group passes dorsal and radial to the sensory group. Correct orientation of the distal groups of fascicles is determined by exploration of Guyon's canal. Correct orientation of the proximal motor/sensory fascicles can be determined anatomically, with reassurance obtained by use of chemical staining or awake stimulation. Therefore, both motor and sensory recovery can be anticipated with nerve grafting.

DONOR NERVE GRAFTS

Donor nerves are those that, when sacrificed, result in minimal functional loss. The nerves typically available for use as donor grafts are the sural nerve, the LABC nerve, and the anterior division of the MABC nerve. In rare instances, the terminal sensory branch of the PIN, the posterior cutaneous nerve of the forearm, the posterior cutaneous nerve of the thigh, and the lateral femoral cutaneous nerve of the thigh also may be used for nerve graft material. Additionally, donor nerve may be obtained from an expendable portion of a nerve in an established nerve injury to reconstruct its more critical components (examples are given below).

Common Donor Nerves

Sural Nerve

This nerve provides 30 to 40 cm in length of nerve graft material. Anatomically, the sural nerve travels from the lateral aspect of the ankle, posterior to the lateral malleolus, toward the popliteal fossa. Harvesting of this nerve results in numbness along the lateral aspect of the foot that diminishes in time to an area approximately 2 to 3 cm in diameter. Either a longitudinal incision or a stepladder technique of multiple small transverse incisions overlying the course of the nerve may be used for harvesting. The longitudinal incision ensures that all communicating branches are identified, maximum donor nerve is obtained, and that no damage is done to the sural nerve during the dissec-

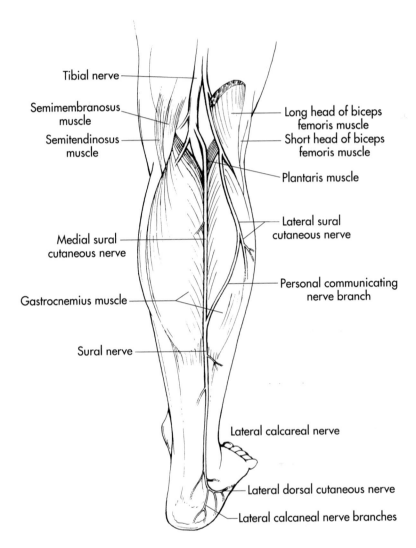

Figure 6-5   Surnal nerve.

tion. However, the stepladder incisions result in a superior cosmetic result (Fig. 6-5).

Lateral Antebrachial Cutaneous Nerve (LABC)

This nerve provides 4 to 8 cm of nerve graft material. The LABC is found in the volar forearm, lying adjacent to the cephalic vein. At this level, it often has two branches, both of which may be harvested. Identification of the site of dissection is determined easily by marking out the forearm longitudinally into thirds. The LABC will be found at the junction of the lateral and middle thirds of the forearm, adjacent to the cephalic vein and on the volar border of the brachioradialis muscle. Either a transverse or longitudinal incision may be used, although the former has a superior cosmetic result. The resulting sensory deficit will be an area of numbness along the lateral aspect of the forearm that will diminish in size with time (Fig. 6-6).

Medial Antebrachial Cutaneous Nerve (MABC)

A total of 18 to 20 cm of nerve graft material may be obtained from this nerve. Both anterior and posterior branches will be found adjacent to the basilic vein, medial to the biceps muscle in the arm. Usually just the anterior branch is harvested because the sensory loss along the volar forearm results in a minimal deficit. The posterior branch, however, supplies important sensibility along the posterior aspect of the elbow and forearm, and in most instances should be preserved. On rare occasions, it also may be harvested if necessary. The resulting extensive sensory loss will decrease over 2 to 3 years (Fig. 6-6).

Examples of Donor Nerve From Nerves With Established Injury

Radial Sensory Nerve

For proximal radial nerve injuries that require grafting, the radial sensory nerve may be used as donor nerve material. It is appropriate to exclude the radial sensory nerve branch from the regenerating proximal nerve so as not to loose advancing motor fascicles to cutaneous reinnervation. By excluding the radial sensory nerve branch, all of the regenerating fascicles will advance through the motor branches. In this situation, the radial sensory nerve may be neurolysed proximally, excised, and used for donor material.

Cutaneous Nerve Branch from Median Nerve to Third Web Space

When an established median nerve injury is present and no sensation in the median nerve distribution exists, the cutaneous nerve branch destined for the third web space can provide ample nerve graft material. This cutaneous branch can be neurolysed proximally for approximately 24 cm before reaching any major plexus formation in the proximal forearm. This graft material can then be used to reconstruct the five digital nerves to the thumb, index, and radial long digits, while sacrificing the sensory reinnervation to the digital nerves to the third web space.

Dorsal Cutaneous Branch of the Ulnar Nerve

In established ulnar nerve injuries requiring grafting for reinnervation, the dorsal cutaneous branch can be used as donor nerve material.

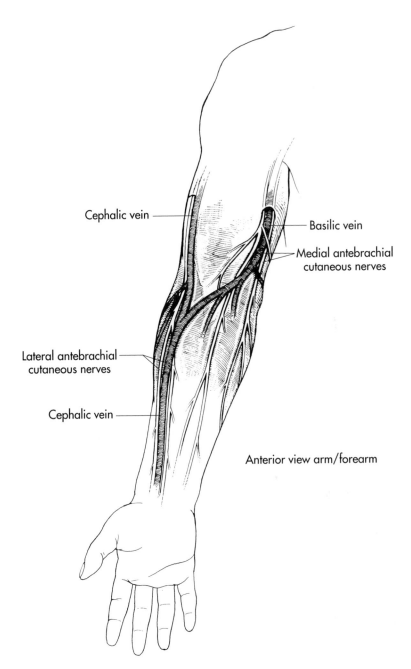

Cephalic vein

Basilic vein

Medial antebrachial
cutaneous nerves

Lateral antebrachial
cutaneous nerves

Cephalic vein

Anterior view arm/forearm

Figure 6-6   Lateral antebrachial and medial antebrachial cutaneous nerves.

This cutaneous branch can be neurolysed proximally from the main ulnar nerve for a long distance. By excising and excluding the sensory nerve component from the repair, the motor fascicles will not be lost to the cutaneous branches, and the dorsal cutaneous branch itself can be used as the donor nerve for the repair.

ACUTE NERVE INJURIES
Open Nerve Injuries

Clinical suspicion of nerve injury necessitates surgical exploration of the open wound. If a clean division of the nerve is identified, a microsurgical repair is performed. If the nerve ends are damaged and the extent of injury can be determined, the damaged portion is sharply transected. Otherwise, scar tissue will form at the site of the repair and prevent the distal migration of the regenerating axons. If a clean partial transection of the nerve is found, those fascicles remaining intact are left alone, whereas the transected ones are repaired.

When the injury to the nerve appears to involve a long segment, as with actual loss of nerve tissue or an avulsion injury, it generally is best to delay the repair for 3 to 4 weeks, thereby allowing for full demarcation of the extent of damage. If at the time of initial exploration the proximal and distal nerve ends can be approximated, retraction of the nerve ends will be prevented. This will decrease the length of nerve graft needed at the second operation.

Primary nerve grafting rarely is indicated because the longitudinal extent of nerve injury is not known in the proximal and distal nerve segments. If the extent of nerve damage is underestimated at the time of the nerve graft, the final result will be compromised because of the time spent waiting to assess the results of the graft. In addition, valuable donor nerve will have been used.

When the wound has healed, a secondary nerve graft may be carried out in as few as 3 weeks. However, if the injury involves extensive damage to the soft tissue, reconstruction should be delayed until the soft tissue permits. This time frame allows for definition of the zone of injury in the nerve before the development of extensive scar formation (Fig. 6-7).

Closed Nerve Injuries

These include injuries result from direct blows, bony fractures, avulsion trauma, and so on. Generally, primary surgery is not indicated in closed nerve injuries. Because the nerve is in continuity, functional recovery may occur. However, if the patient is undergoing operative exploration for an associated injury in the extremity, such as a humerus fracture reduction-fixation, then the injured nerve should be explored. Otherwise, the patient is observed over a 3-month period. If clinical or

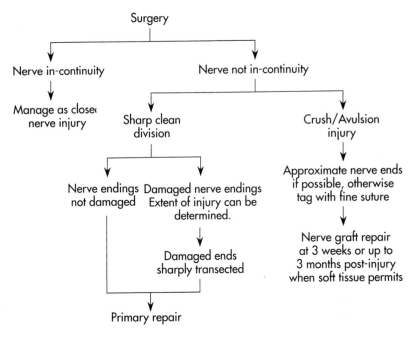

Figure 6-7   Open nerve injury algorithm.

electrical evidence of recovery is seen by 3 months, the patient is followed expectantly on a monthly basis until recovery occurs. If the patient fails to show continued improvement in an anatomically sequential pattern progressing from proximal to distal, surgical repair is undertaken. Caution must be undertaken with a very proximal nerve injury (i.e., brachial plexus). If a patient with such an injury demonstrates a nonanatomic return of function with good distal nerve recovery in the presence of an isolated lack of proximal recovery, this would imply a less severe injury to the nerves innervating the distal muscles and a more severe injury to the nerves innervating the proximal muscles. In this case, surgical intervention for reconstruction of the damaged elements would be indicated. Similarly, if the patient fails to demonstrate any clinical or electrical evidence of recovery by 3 months, surgical exploration is performed. At the time of surgery, the nerve is evaluated with intraoperative electrodiagnostic studies across the site of the injury. If a nerve action potential is recorded, then neurolysis alone is performed. If no electrical activity is recorded, then the area of injury is excised and grafted.

An exception to expectant management of closed nerve injuries is considered when the nerve is located at an anatomic site known to be susceptible to nerve entrapment. When this occurs, the nerve may be decompressed so that nerve recovery may progress without the superimposed effects of nerve compression. An example would be a traumatic injury to the hand or forearm with acute carpal tunnel syndrome (Fig. 6-8).

Civilian Gunshot and Shotgun Wounds

The nerve injuries in these types of wounds usually are associated with a significant component of first, second, and third degree injury from the blast effect. A significant percentage will recover spontaneously. Thus early exploration is only indicated if an associated vascular or skeletal injury is present. These injuries are managed as closed injuries, with expectant observation for the first 3 months, as noted above.

NERVE INJECTION INJURIES

The spectrum of nerve injury is broad, and may involve first, second, third, fourth, and sixth degree injury patterns. To exert damage, the substance must be injected intrafascicularly. Extrafascicular injections will not result in injury. The degree of injury is drug-dose related. This can be seen with drugs that are not otherwise neurotoxic because of the associated carrier agents that are combined with the drug. The clinical picture directly following nerve injection is classic, with complaints of immediate, severe pain at the injection site and radiating pain throughout the nerve distribution. Motor weakness or loss also may be seen, depending on which nerve is damaged. Early exploration is indicated only for those areas of known potential for nerve compression, such as the cubital tunnel, proximal forearm, or the carpal tunnel. For other areas of injury, a 3-month observation period is indicated for assessment of potential electrical or clinical recovery. Should this not occur, surgical exploration is warranted. Management of the injury would be similar to that used for neuroma in continuity. Amitriptyline (Elavil) and carbamazepine (Tegretol) are useful for the treatment of associated pain.

CLINICAL PRESENTATION OF ACUTE PERIPHERAL NERVE INJURY

The clinical signs and symptoms are those of complete nerve injury. Assuming normal anatomy, this results in loss of function extending from the level of injury distally. Recovery will be complete for all first degree nerve injuries. For second degree or higher-level nerve injuries, the level of injury is critical in determining the prognosis for recovery. The management of the lesion depends on the nature of the injury, as described for open, closed, missile, or acute compression injuries. Discussion of tendon transfers for persistent palsies follows.

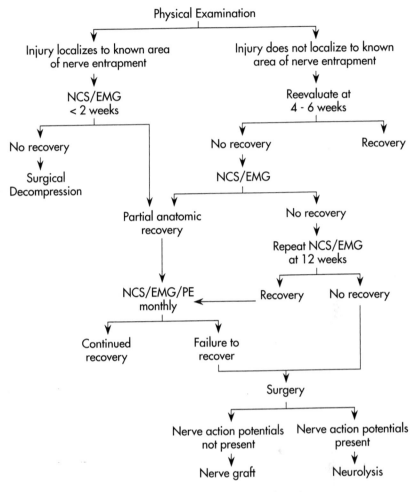

Figure 6-8 Closed nerve injury algorithm.

Radial Nerve Injury

Level of Injury

Upper arm level

A very proximal radial nerve injury must be distinguished from an injury to the posterior cord. Both will result in paralysis of the triceps muscles. However, the deltoid muscle (axillary nerve) and the latissimus dorsi muscle (thoracodorsal nerve) will remain intact in an isolated radial nerve injury that does not involve the posterior cord. Injuries to the radial nerve at this level are very rare.

Most commonly, the radial nerve is injured at the midhumeral level in the upper arm, sparing the innervation to the triceps muscles. This injury is proximal to the take off of nerve branches to the BR and ECRL muscles. The resulting clinical picture of radial nerve palsy (excluding the triceps muscles) is lack of wrist extension, MCP joint extension of the fingers and thumb, and thumb abduction. Supination of the hand is weak, but not lost, because of persistent function of the short head of the biceps. With full elbow extension, the function of the biceps muscle will be blocked, and the patient will be unable to supinate the hand. Sensory innervation in the distribution of the radial sensory nerve is also absent.

Elbow and proximal forearm level

Injury to the radial nerve at this level occurs distal to the nerve branches supplying innervation to the BR and the ECRL muscles, and proximal to the division of the radial nerve into its superficial and deep branches. The resulting paralysis primarily affects the muscles innervated by the PIN. When the ECRL muscle is intact, it is difficult to assess the presence of an intact ECRB muscle. The function of the ECRB muscle usually is absent at this level of radial nerve injury, although it may be intact. In either case, the resulting clinical picture of PIN paralysis is the same. The patient is able to radially deviate and radially dorsiflex the wrist because of the intact ECRL muscle. However, the patient cannot dorsiflex the wrist in a neutral plane, extend the MCP joints of the fingers and thumb, or abduct the thumb. Supination of the hand is weak, and loss of sensation in the radial distribution of the hand is present.

Midforearm level

An injury to the radial nerve in the midforearm level occurs distal to the division of the radial nerve into its deep and superficial branches, and may result in sparing of the sensory innervation of the radial sensory branch. The function of the ECRB muscle is likely to be intact. The resulting motor paralysis is one of PIN palsy, as described previously.

Wrist level

At the level of the wrist, only the sensory innervation of the radial nerve would be lost. This is not a significant functional deficit.

Prognosis for Recovery (In Second Degree or Higher-Level Nerve Injury)

Because radial innervated muscles receive their neural input relatively proximal in the upper extremity, the prognosis for muscle recovery after nerve repair is good. The distance between the nerve injury and the motor end plates is relatively short. Axons, regenerating at a rate of 1 inch/month, have adequate time to reinnervate the muscles before permanent loss of motor end plates and muscle fibrosis. In addition, most of the extensors innervated by the radial nerve function synergistically, so that mismatching of motor fascicles is of little consequence. Full recovery will occur with second degree nerve injuries and good recovery should occur with surgical repair of third degree or higher-level nerve injuries when repaired in a timely fashion.

Intraoperative Management

If operative exploration is required and the injured nerve is found to be in continuity, intraoperative nerve conduction studies should be performed. Neurolysis alone is carried out if action potentials are recorded across the site of injury. If no action potentials are generated with intraoperative nerve conduction studies, or if the injured nerve is transected, the nerve is repaired surgically (see sections on Nerve Repair and Nerve Grafting.) Because the fascicles are mixed motor and sensory in the proximal radial nerve, an epineural repair is performed at this level. All regenerating fibers should be directed into motor fascicles by excluding the radial sensory nerve (see Nerve Grafting-Prioritization of Function-Radial Nerve Grafting.). This maximizes functional motor recovery. For distal radial nerve injuries, a grouped fascicular repair is performed, allowing preservation of both sensation and motor function.

Median Nerve Injury

Level of Injury

Upper arm level

Injury to the median nerve at this level causing a complete median nerve palsy results in loss of thumb opposition, palmar thumb abduction, thumb IP joint flexion, FDS function, and FDP function to the index and middle fingers. Distal interphalangeal and PIP middle finger flexion may be weak or absent, depending on the degree of ulnar innervation of the FDP muscle to this digit. Forearm pronation is weak. The resulting functional deficit from denervation of the median forearm flexors is loss of power grip. Lumbrical function to the index and middle fingers will be weak or absent, so that full extension of these digits, with MCP joint flexion, may be poor. Ulnar-deviated wrist flexion will be present because of intact ulnar innervation to the FCU muscle and FDP muscle to the ring and small digits. Critical sensation in the distribution of the median nerve will be lost.

Elbow level

Branches of the median nerve to the PT muscle usually originate above the elbow, so that injury to the median nerve at this level generally spares forearm pronation. Otherwise, the resulting paralysis of the median innervated forearm and intrinsic muscles is identical to that for a higher-level injury, as described previously. Critical sensation of the median nerve also is lost.

Wrist level

Injury to the median nerve at the level of the wrist spares the forearm flexors, so that the resultant clinical picture is lack of thumb opposition and palmar thumb abduction and weakness of the lumbricales to the index and middle fingers. Absence of sensation in the median nerve distribution is present.

Prognosis for Recovery (In Second Degree or Higher-Level Nerve Injury)

The level at which the median nerve is injured is critical to the prognosis for recovery. Proximal median nerve injuries in the arm and at the level of the elbow will result in full recovery of forearm muscles in a second degree nerve injury, and generally will result in adequate recovery of forearm muscles after nerve repair of third degree or higher-level nerve injury, but will have poor to no recovery of the median innervated intrinsic muscles of the hand. This, in part, is the result of the long distance that regenerating axons must travel to reinnervate the intrinsic muscles of the hand. This time period allows for loss of motor end plates and development of muscle fibrosis, so that reinnervation cannot occur. In addition, the intrinsic muscles of the hand do not act in a synergistic fashion, as do the FDS and FDP, and require greater innervational input to function efficiently. Tendon transfers usually will be required to restore the lost median intrinsic function of the hand.

When the level of median nerve injury is at the wrist, full recovery can be expected for second degree nerve injuries. For third degree or higher-level nerve injuries, the prognosis for recovery of median innervated muscles of the hand after nerve repair is good. This is because of the short distance from the level of injury to the intrinsic muscles and because all the regenerating motor fascicles will be directed into the intrinsic muscles at the time of repair.

Intraoperative Management

At the time of operative exploration, if the injured nerve is in continuity and intraoperative nerve conduction recordings reveal action potentials, neurolysis alone is performed. If no action potentials are generated with intraoperative nerve conduction studies or if the injured nerve is not in continuity, a group fascicular repair should be done when the level of the injury is distal forearm or wrist and the potential for intrinsic muscle function exists. However, if the prognosis for intrinsic muscle recovery of the hand is poor, as in proximal median nerve injuries or late presentation of the patient, then the nerve repair should direct all the regenerating fascicles into the distal median nerve segment destined for sensory innervation (see section on Nerve Grafting-Prioritization of Function-Median Nerve Grafting.). This allows for preservation of critical sensory function. Thumb opposition can be obtained with tendon transfers.

Ulnar Nerve Injury

Level of Injury

Upper arm level

Injuries to the ulnar nerve at this level generally occur after the take off of the MABC, so that posterior elbow and medial volar forearm sensation is preserved. A complete, proximal ulnar nerve palsy results in lack of neutral wrist flexion, DIP small finger flexion, abduction and opposition of the small finger, and adduction of the thumb. Weakness of DIP joint flexion of the ring finger usually is present. Paralysis of the palmar and dorsal interossei muscles prevent crossing of the fingers. Weakness or paralysis of the lumbricales to the small and ring fingers also will be present, resulting in an inability to flex the MCP joints and extend the PIP and DIP joints of these digits. Instead, the MCP joint does not flex until IP joint flexion has been completed, causing the fingers to curl into the palm when attempting to grasp an object. There may be variable involvement of the ring and middle finger lumbricales depending on the contribution of ulnar or median nerve innervation to these muscles. The resulting deficit to the patient with paralysis of the ulnar intrinsics of the hand is loss of precision grip and loss of distal stability and rotation for tip pinch between the thumb and index finger. In addition, patient attempts to flex the wrist will result in radially deviated flexion because of paralysis of the FCU muscle. Loss of critical ulnar sensory innervation also will be present.

Elbow and proximal forearm level

Injuries to the ulnar nerve at this level generally spare the innervation of the FCU muscle because the major motor branches to this muscle usually originate above the elbow. With an ulnar nerve paralysis at this level, neutral wrist flexion will be possible. Otherwise, the resulting paralysis of the ulnar innervated FDP to the ring and small fingers and the ulnar intrinsic muscles of the hand is identical to that for a higher-level injury, as described previously. Ulnar sensation to the hand is absent.

Wrist level

At this level of injury, ulnar innervation to the FCU and the FDP to the ring and small fingers remains intact. Paralysis of the ulnar intrinsics of the hand, with intact FDP function to the ring and small fingers, leads to formation of the "claw hand." With paralysis of the lumbricales to the ring and small fingers, the stability of the MCP joint is lost. This allows the unopposed radial innervated extensor muscles to pull the MCP joint into hyperextension, while the intact FDP and FDS flex the PIP and DIP joints. Variations in innervation of the lumbricales may result in clawing of the middle, ring, and small fingers, or the small finger alone. As with more proximal ulnar lesions, abduction and opposition of the small finger, adduction of the thumb, and paralysis of the interossei will be present. Sensation along the dorsal aspect of the hand in the distribution of the dorsal cutaneous branch of the ulnar nerve will be intact, whereas ulnar sensation to the ulnar one-and-a-half digits will be lost. (Again, this assumes normal anatomy.)

Potential for Recovery (In Second Degree or Higher-Level Nerve Injury)

The level of injury to the ulnar nerve is critical to the prognosis for recovery. In a proximal ulnar nerve injury at the level of the upper arm, some return of function of the FCU and FDP muscles is likely to occur. However, recovery of ulnar intrinsic muscle function of the hand will not occur with this level of injury, because of the long distance through which the regenerating axons must travel and the need for precise innervation of the ulnar intrinsic muscles of the hand. Loss of motor end plates and muscle fibrosis will have begun to occur by the time the regenerating axons reach the intrinsic muscles of the hand. For second degree ulnar nerve injuries at the level of the elbow and proximal forearm, recovery of FDP function and sensation will occur, and partial to near complete recovery of the ulnar intrinsic muscles may occur. Likewise, for third degree injuries at this level, the prognosis for recovery is good after nerve repair. Full recovery should be expected with second degree ulnar nerve lesions at the level of the wrist. For third degree or higher-level nerve injuries, the prognosis for recovery after nerve repair is good.

Intraoperative Management

Neurolysis is performed when the injured nerve segment is in continuity and demonstrates action potentials with intraoperative nerve conduction studies. The lack of action potential generation with intraoperative nerve conduction or a transection of the ulnar nerve necessitates surgical repair. For proximal ulnar nerve lesions in the arm, group fascicular repair is performed. This will allow for return of function to the FCU and FDP muscles and critical ulnar nerve sensation. Tendon transfers will be required for the ulnar intrinsic muscle loss. For ulnar nerve lesions at the level of the elbow, forearm, or wrist, group fascicular repair also is performed. Partial to near complete recovery of ulnar intrinsic muscle function is likely, depending on the time of presentation of the patient. Excellent return of critical ulnar sensory innervation should occur. (See Section on Nerve Grafting-Prioritization of Function-Ulnar Nerve Grafting.)

NERVE COMPRESSION INJURIES
Acute Nerve Compression

The pathologic process involves local demyelination of large myelinated fibers in the periphery of the nerve, sparing the small diameter fibers and those fibers located in the center of the nerve. Neurapraxia is a form of acute nerve compression noted clinically by a motor deficit and mild to moderate sensory changes. The earliest test to indicated decreased nerve function with this type of nerve injury is an increase in the vibratory threshold stimulus. Recovery of function usually is complete.

Acute Compartment Syndrome Nerve Injury

The type of nerve injury initially seen is similar to that seen with acute compression, but ischemia is the primary etiology. Both the degree and duration of the pressure determines whether the injury is irreversible. After 8 to 10 hours, irreversible Wallerian degeneration occurs within the nerve, after 6 hours, irreversible muscle damage occurs. Clinically, the initial findings from physical examination include pain with passive muscle stretching and diminished perception to vibratory stimulation. Decreased sensation then occurs, followed by weakness and/or diminished muscle function. Distal pulses rarely are absent.

Chronic Nerve Compression

The type of nerve injury, the clinical presentation, and the degree of recovery after treatment depend on the severity and duration of the compression. Nerve injury may vary from demyelination to Wallerian degeneration without regeneration. In the early stages of compression, symptoms of pain and burning are transient and are brought on by positioning or repetitive movements. Provocative tests of the extremity (i.e., wrist flexion, elbow flexion, etc.) or direct pressure over the nerve may be used to elicit symptoms. In moderate nerve compression, symptoms may progress to weakness and episodic, abnormal sensibility. At this stage, intraneural fibrosis has occurred, but Wallerian degeneration has not. With severe nerve compression, persistent paresthesia is present. Muscle wasting and abnormal two-point discrimination occur with the presence of Wallerian degeneration.

After surgical decompression of the nerve, improvement may be rapid or may take many weeks to months as the nerve regenerates through areas of structural damage. With severe compression, recovery may be incomplete. However, a total absence of recovery is very unlikely, because the continuity of the sensory and motor fascicles with the neuronal cell body is maintained.

NERVE ENTRAPMENT INJURIES (CHRONIC COMPRESSION SYNDROMES)

Trauma to the upper extremity leading to direct injury, avulsion, or compression of the peripheral nerve is most likely to occur at potential anatomic sites of entrapment. Knowledge of the location of these potential sites of entrapment/injury and the associated clinical findings is of paramount importance in diagnosing and treating these nerve injuries. An acute open nerve injury or a closed nerve injury that fails to recover should be approached in a surgical fashion similar to that described for nerve entrapment injuries—all potential sites of compression within the area of injury should be released.

Median Nerve Entrapment at the Wrist (Carpal Tunnel Syndrome)

Carpal tunnel syndrome (CTS) refers to the entrapment and compression of the median nerve within the carpal tunnel at the level of the wrist. It results in a broad range of symptoms involving the distribution of the motor and sensory median nerve innervation within the hand. The most common symptoms include hypesthesia or paresthesias in the distribution of the median nerve, which at times may awaken the patient from sleep and cause weakness and/or clumsiness when attempting to use the hand. The above symptoms are aggravated with repeated use of the hand. The patient may have a history of a distal radius fracture or work involving repetitive wrist motion.

Surgical Anatomy

The carpal tunnel is formed by the carpal bones on its deep surface; the hook of the hamate and the pisiform on its ulnar side; the tubercle of the trapezium and the distal pole of the scaphoid on its radial side; and the transverse carpal ligament on its superficial surface. The proximal extent of the tunnel is not well defined because the antebrachial fascia blends distally with the transverse carpal ligament. The carpal tunnel ends distally when the fat surrounding the superficial palmar arch is reached. This tunnel is a potential site of compression of the median nerve, as it travels within its unyielding boundaries.

The motor branch usually comes from the radial side of the median nerve, although variations in its take off have been well described. Division of the transverse carpal ligament should be carried out along its ulnar-most border. In patients with thenar muscle atrophy, the presence of a separate fibrous tunnel where the motor branch enters the thenar muscles may be present. If found, it should be released.

Care should be taken to avoid injury to the palmar cutaneous branch of the median nerve during the surgical incision. This nerve runs deep to and parallel with the tendons of the PL and the FCR. An incision in the radial axis of the ring finger, well ulnar to the PL tendon and the thenar crease, is least likely to injure the palmar cutaneous branch of the median nerve.

Diagnosis

Examination of the patient will show positive findings with provocative tests. This includes the production of a Tinel's sign (lancing paresthesias in the distal distribution of the median nerve) with percussion of the median nerve at the wrist and Phalen's sign (reproduction of the symptoms) when the wrist is flexed and held in position. Weakness of the thenar muscles also may be present. Advanced signs include abnormal static two-point discrimination (greater than 6 mm), abnormal moving two-point discrimination (greater than 4 mm), and thenar muscle wasting. A minimal degree of nerve compression is present when the patient reports intermittent symptoms and a positive Phalen's or Tinel's sign is present. The degree of compression is moderate when thenar muscle weakness also is present. An advanced degree of compression occurs when symptoms are persistent in nature, static and moving two-point discrimination are abnormal, and thenar muscle wasting is present or EMG demonstrates denervation potentials in the thenar muscles.

Treatment

For a minimal or moderate degree of carpal tunnel syndrome, conservative treatment with night splinting is indicated. After a 3-month period, if the patient is improving, the same regimen is continued. If the patient fails to respond to conservative therapy, surgical release of the carpal tunnel is indicated. If surgery is contraindicated, cortisone injections into the carpal tunnel may provide relief of symptoms for up to 3 months. For patients with an advanced degree of compression, surgery may be undertaken without a trial of conservative therapy.

Postoperative Management

For 3 weeks, a volar splint is worn at night and, as needed for comfort, during the day. During this time, the patient is encouraged to move his/her fingers and wrist. This allows for excursion of the median nerve, preventing adherence of the nerve to surrounding structures.

Median Nerve Entrapment in the Distal Arm/Proximal Forearm (Pronator Teres Syndrome)

This syndrome involves compression of the median nerve at one or more of multiple potential sites of compression in the distal arm and proximal forearm. These sites of compression include the lacertus fibrosis; high origin of the PT muscle; a fibrous arch between the deep and superficial head of the PT muscle; the arch of the FDS muscle; crossing branches of the ulnar collateral vessels; anomalous muscles; and rarely a supracondylar process and the ligament of Struthers.

Patients usually report an aching pain in the volar distal arm and/ or proximal forearm. They also may report numbness and tingling in the distribution of the median nerve in the hand. These symptoms frequently are aggravated by activity or work. A history of trauma involving crush injury to the forearm, supracondylar fracture, or posterior dislocation of the elbow, or a work history in which the arm is used in a repetitive or forceful pronation–supination motion may be given. Persistent symptoms of carpal tunnel syndrome after carpal tunnel release often are associated with pronator teres syndrome.

Surgical Anatomy

Five of the potential sites of compression will be discussed. One or more fibrous arches may be present in a single patient, allowing for multiple sites of potential compression of the median nerve. Discussion of the anatomy of the potential sites of compression follows, from proximal to distal.

Supracondylar process and Struthers ligament

Struthers described a variation of the normal anatomy found in 3% of cadaver dissections. A supracondylar bony process may exist on the medial aspect of the distal humerus. Struthers ligament travels from this supracondylar process to the medial humeral epicondyle, creating a tunnel through which the median nerve passes. Entrapment and compression of the median nerve at this level rarely occurs in the absence of trauma.

Lacertus fibrosus

The median nerve crosses the elbow superficial to the brachialis muscle and deep to the bicipital aponeurosis and lacertus fibrosis. The lacertus fibrosis is continuous with the fascia of the superficial head of the PT muscle, forming a fibrous sheath beneath which the median nerve travels distally. A potential site of compression of the median nerve is formed by the fibrous arch of the lacertus fibrosus.

High origin of the pronator teres muscle

A high origin of the superficial head of the PT muscle has been found in 20% of cadaver dissections, arising 2 cm proximal to the medial humeral epicondyle. As the median nerve passes deep to the superficial head of the pronator, it may potentially be compressed against the underlying trochlear process of the humerus. This compression would be potentiated by PT muscle hypertrophy and brought on by elbow extension and forearm pronation.

Fibrous arch between the deep and superficial heads of the pronator teres

Potential sources of compression exist as the median nerve travels distally between the superficial and deep heads of the PT muscle. The superficial head of the PT arises from the medial humeral epicondyle. Its overlying aponeurotic fascia is continuous with the lacertus fibrosis, forming a fibrous sheath beneath which the median nerve passes. The deep head of the PT arises from either the coronoid process of the ulna or from the interosseous membrane, or both. A fibrous arch may be formed at the point where the deep head and the superficial head of the PT joint, with its fibrous component lying beneath the superficial head of the pronator and/or on the ulnar side of the deep head of the pronator. This arch, when present, is a potential source of compression of the overlying median nerve.

The arch of the flexor digitorum superficialis muscle

As the median nerve continues to travel distally in the proximal forearm, it passes deep to the FDS muscle and superficial to the FDP muscle. The fascia of the FDS muscle may form a distinct fibrous arch, under which the median nerve may be compressed.

Diagnosis

Symptoms include aching pain in the forearm, generally exacerbated by activity involving forceful pronation of the forearm. In addition, numbness and tingling in the distribution of the median nerve may be present. Reproduction of symptoms with forced supination and gentle pressure over the median nerve just proximal to the leading edge of the PT muscle is diagnostic in the majority of patients. On physical examination, functional evaluation of the muscles of the forearm may suggest the site of compression of the median nerve. Intensification of symptoms when the elbow is flexed against resistance (between 120 and 135° of flexion) suggests entrapment at Struthers ligament. Aggravation of symptoms with forceful pronation of the forearm while the elbow is extended implies compression beneath a high origin of the superficial head of the PT muscle. Entrapment beneath the lacertus fibrosis is suggested by resistance to active elbow flexion and forearm supination when the forearm is in the pronated position. Resistance to forceful pronation of the forearm with the wrist in a flexed position suggests compression beneath the PT muscle in the proximal forearm. Entrapment at the FDS arch is suggested by resisted flexion of the middle finger sublimis. Resistance to the aforementioned movement is secondary to the onset or exacerbation of pain in the proximal forearm.

Nerve conduction velocity studies may localize the level of the median nerve compression and confirm the clinical diagnosis. Electromyography also may assist in the diagnosis. However, negative electrodiagnostic test results are the most frequent finding. This should not exclude the diagnosis if the clinical findings are consistent with this syndrome.

Treatment

Exercises to stretch tight pronator teres muscles usually will relieve the symptoms. For patients who work in a pronated position, frequent short breaks during the day to supinate the forearm are encouraged. This is particularly important with keyboard operators. Surgical decompression of the median nerve in this syndrome rarely is necessary, but would involve a thorough exploration for all potential sites of entrapment. Each site of potential compression should be divided, and the tendon of the PT muscle should be released and step lengthened to ensure complete release of the median nerve. Failure to do so may result in inadequate treatment and persistence of symptoms postoperatively.

Postoperative Management

Early postoperative movement is key to a successful result and is begun 48 hours after surgery.

Anterior Interosseous Nerve Entrapment (Anterior Interosseous Nerve Syndrome)

Compression of the anterior interosseous nerve (AIN) in the proximal forearm leads to a decrease or loss of function in the muscles innervated by this nerve, as manifested by an inability to flex the IP joint of the thumb and the DIP joint of the index and middle fingers. The latter finding of middle finger involvement is variable. Typically, the patient reports weakness and/or loss of coordination in the use of the fingers. Very rarely does the patient report pain in the proximal forearm. A history of trauma involving a crush or avulsion injury to the forearm, a supracondylar fracture, or posterior dislocation of the elbow may be given.

Surgical Anatomy

The AIN arises from the median nerve as it passes between the superficial and deep heads of the PT muscle. If it lies in relation to one of the fibrous arches of the PT or the FDS arch, it may be compressed or injured at one or more of these sites. In addition, variations of anatomy and/or vessels in the region may contribute to compression of the AIN in the proximal forearm.

Diagnosis

On examination, the patient will demonstrate an inability to pinch the thumb and index fingers into a round "O." When attempting to perform this maneuver, the DIP joint of the index finger and the IP joint of the thumb will hyperextend secondary to loss of function of the FDP to the index finger and the FPL. The pronator quadratus is difficult to test. Electromyography may demonstrate denervation in the pronator quadratus, FDP to the index finger, and the FPL.

Treatment

Surgical decompression of the AIN requires exposure of the median nerve from proximal to the elbow distally to the level of the FDS. As with pronator teres syndrome, all potential sites of compression of the median nerve proximal to the take off of the AIN should be released, including the FDS arch when necessary.

Postoperative Management

This is identical to the postoperative management already described for pronator teres syndrome.

Ulnar Nerve Entrapment at the Wrist

Compression of the ulnar nerve at the wrist rarely occurs within Guyon's canal. The etiology of the compression may be repeated blunt trauma, fractures of the hook of hamate or distal radius, carpal dislocations, burns to the palm, tumors, anomalous vessels or muscles, or a fibrous edge to the palmaris brevis. Patients typically report numbness and tingling in the small and ring fingers and weakness or clumsiness of the hand. The symptoms may vary, depending on whether the compression involves the ulnar motor branch, the sensory branch, or both. Ulnar intrinsic muscle atrophy may or may not be present. In long-standing cases, clawing (MCP joint hyperextension, PIP and DIP joint flexion) of the ring and small fingers may be present. Variations in innervation of the lumbricales may result in clawing of the middle, ring, and small finger, or the small finger alone.

Surgical Anatomy

In the distal third of the forearm, distal to the take off of the dorsal ulnar sensory branch, two main fascicular nerve groups are present within the ulnar nerve. The ulnar fascicular group contains motor fibers to the ulnar intrinsic muscles of the hand, and the radial fascicular group contains sensory fibers to the little and ring fingers. When the ulnar nerve enters Guyon's canal and passes distal to the pisiform, the motor fascicles move deep to the sensory fascicles, forming the deep and superficial branches of the nerve. Distally, the motor branch becomes radial to the sensory branch as it passes between the origins of the FDM and the ADM. Ultimately, it travels beneath the FDM to supply the interosseous and lumbrical muscles of the hand. The sensory branch continues distally to overly the superficial aspect of the hypothenar muscles.

Guyon's canal is triangular in shape. The roof is formed by the palmar carpal ligament, the tendinous insertion of the flexor carpi ulnaris into the pisiform bone, and the pisohamate ligament; the radial wall is formed by the hook of the hamate and the insertion of the transverse carpal ligament; and the ulnar wall is formed by the pisiform bone and the fibrous connections to the pisohamate ligament.

Diagnosis

A detailed sensory and motor examination is performed. Sensibility testing should not only include the ring and small fingers, but the dorsum of the hand. The latter aids in localizing the site of the nerve lesion. If the sensation on the dorsum of the hand is diminished, an ulnar nerve lesion proximal to the takeoff of the dorsal sensory branch of the motor nerve is suggested. Motor evaluation should include the ulnar intrinsics of the hand and the FDP. The latter muscle should be functioning normally with ulnar nerve entrapment at the wrist. Pinch and grip strength should be measured. In addition, a positive Tinel's sign usually will be present over the ulnar nerve at the level of the pisiform.

The primary diagnostic difficulty is the exclusion of a more proximal nerve lesion. A thorough examination of the upper extremity will aid in identifying muscles that have weakness or wasting, in addition to those traditionally innervated by the ulnar nerve. Variations in the motor and sensory innervation of the ulnar nerve must be known.

Treatment

When the site of the lesion has been localized to the wrist, surgical exploration and release of Guyon's canal is performed. The incision used is the same as for carpal tunnel release. Potential sites of entrapment include the palmar carpal ligament, interdigitating fibers inserting along the pisiform, and a fibrous origin of the FDM. All of these potential sites of compression must be explored and excised if present. If the etiology of the ulnar nerve compression is a ganglion or anomalous muscle, these are excised. Similarly, a nonunion of a fractured hook of hamate may be excised subperiosteally.

Postoperative Management

This is identical to that described for carpal tunnel release.

Ulnar Nerve Entrapment at the Elbow (Cubital Tunnel Syndrome)

This syndrome refers to entrapment of the ulnar nerve within the cubital tunnel. Many types of trauma may result in the compression of the ulnar nerve in this region, including direct soft tissue injury, elbow dislocation, supracondylar fractures, and fractures of the lateral or medial humeral epicondyle. Additional etiologies include rupture of the biceps tendon, arthritis, congenital anatomic variations, external compression, tumors, and occupations in which repetitive flexion–

extension, pronation–supination movements are performed or in which the elbow is maintained in a flexed position while resting on a desk.

Patients typically report numbness and tingling in the little and ring fingers. They also may complain of pain along the medial aspect of the elbow or forearm, which may radiate proximally into the arm or distally into the forearm and ulnar digits. Weakness or clumsiness of the hand also may be reported. Activities requiring elbow flexion typically exacerbate these symptoms. In some cases, wasting of the ulnar innervated intrinsic muscles of the hand may be present.

Surgical Anatomy

The cubital tunnel begins at the level of the elbow in the region bounded by the medial humeral epicondyle, the postcondylar groove in the olecranon, and the overlying fascia connecting these two bony prominences. This fascia continues distally as it extends over the two heads of the FCU, forming the distal extent of the cubital tunnel. A thickening in the leading edge of the two heads of the FCU, known as Osborne's band, may be present and may contribute to nerve compression in this region. An additional potential site of compression is the "arcade of Struther's," located approximately 8 cm proximal to the medial epicondyle when present. This is a thick fascial shelf that runs from the medial head of the triceps to the medial intermuscular septum. The ulnar nerve travels adjacent to the medial head of the triceps and the medial intermuscular septum, and may become tethered/compressed by this overlying fascia if it is not released completely at the time of surgical decompression.

Diagnosis

An examination may reveal a Tinel's sign over the ulnar nerve at the elbow or a positive elbow flexion test. The latter is a provocative test, in which elbow flexion elicits or aggravates symptoms of numbness and tingling in the little and ring fingers. Direct manual compression over the ulnar nerve at the elbow is an additional provocative test that also may intensify symptoms. Weakness of the ulnar intrinsics of the hand may be present, as indicated by the patient's inability to completely cross the index and long fingers. Electrodiagnostic test results may reveal prolonged motor latency in ulnar nerve conduction or fibrillations within the ulnar intrinsic muscles of the hand. Sensibility testing of the little and ring fingers also should be performed.

Treatment

The choice of treatment is initially based on the degree of severity of the nerve compression. For patients with mild compression (i.e., intermittent paresthesias and subjective weakness), nonoperative treatment is chosen. This includes removable elbow pads, alterations in sleeping position by keeping the elbow extended and the arm by the patient's side, and adjustments in the work environment to facilitate an upper extremity posture of 30° elbow flexion and a wrist neutral position (e.g., use of a telephone head set). If after 3 months the symptoms and signs have not worsened, the same regimen is carried out for an additional 3 months. For patients with a moderate degree of ulnar nerve compression (e.g., measurable weakness in pinch or grip strength), a trial of nonoperative treatment may be undertaken. If this should fail, or if the patient is unable to appropriately restrict activities, surgical decompression should be considered. When a severe degree of nerve compression is present (e.g., abnormal two-point discrimination muscle atrophy), surgical decompression is necessary.

Multiple surgical techniques have been described for decompression of the ulnar nerve. We recommend anterior submuscular transposition. Full release of all potential sites of compression should be performed, including release of the fascia spanning the medial head of the triceps to the medial intermuscular septum for 8 cm proximally, division of the roof of the cubital tunnel, division of the fascia overlying the two heads of the FCU, excision of the intermuscular septum, and release of the periosteal origin of the FCU. The latter two steps prevent proximal and distal kinking of the transposed ulnar nerve.

Postoperative Management

The patient is splinted at 70 to 90° elbow flexion, with the wrist pronated for 48 hours. During the first 3 postoperative weeks, the upper extremity is kept in a sling at night. Early movement during the day allows for excursion of the ulnar nerve and prevents scarring/adhering of the nerve to surrounding structures. At 3 weeks postoperatively, the elbow is fully extended, and by 4 weeks, strengthening exercises are instituted.

Radial Sensory Nerve Entrapment in the Forearm (Wartenberg Syndrome)

Compression of the radial sensory nerve as it emerges between the tendons of the ECRL and the BR in the forearm is referred to as Wartenberg syndrome. Characteristically, patients complain of pain over the dorsoradial aspect of the hand. The pain may be aggravated by writing, pinching, gripping, or movements of the wrist. Less commonly, complaints of numbness and tingling or burning along the dorsoradial aspect of the hand may be reported. A history of trauma to the forearm, or an occupational history of repetitive pronation–supination of the forearm or radial deviation–ulnar deviation of the wrist is common.

Surgical Anatomy

Most commonly, the superficial radial nerve emerges from beneath the BR at the junction of the middle and distal thirds of the forearm.

As it passes superficially between the tendons of the BR and the ECRL, it pierces a bridging fascial band. At this site, the sensory nerve is subjected to compression when the forearm is pronated. Distally as the nerve crosses the dorsoradial aspect of the wrist, it may be subjected to stretch injury with ulnar wrist flexion. Combined compression and stretch forces occur when the forearm is in hyperpronation, and the wrist is deviated ulnarly.

Diagnosis

Examination of the wrist will reveal a positive Tinel's sign along the course of the radial sensory nerve. Provocative testing with forceful ulnar deviation of the wrist while the forearm in hyperpronation generally elicits numbness and tingling in the distribution of the radial sensory nerve. A positive "pseudo" Finkelstein's sign also will be present. This is assessed by asking the patient to grasp the thumb between the fingers, and then to ulnarly deviate the wrist. A positive sign occurs when this maneuver elicits pain in the distribution of the radial sensory nerve. This finding also may be present in first dorsal extensor tenosynovitis, but other findings consistent with this diagnosis will not be present in Wartenburg syndrome, such as tenderness to palpation of the first dorsal compartment over the radial styloid and pain with resisted thumb extension. Examination of the sensation in the radial sensory nerve distribution may reveal asymmetry between the hands, and, in advanced cases, moving two-point discrimination will be abnormal. Special electrodiagnostics may be of benefit in evaluating the function status of the radial sensory nerve. A radial sensory nerve anesthetic block in the forearm that alleviates the symptoms would corroborate the diagnosis.

Treatment

Conservative treatment that consists of removal of constricting wristwatches and jewelry, as well as wrist immobilization with splinting in a neutral position, may resolve the patients symptoms. Splinting the forearm in supination is useful but is not tolerated well by patients. If this fails or if symptoms return after resumption of active wrist motion, surgical decompression is performed.

At the time of surgical exploration, care should be taken to avoid injury to branches of the LABC. The fascia spanning the tendons of the BR and the ECRL is incised proximally for 6 to 8 cm. The fascia of the BR tendon also is incised down to its insertion, allowing the tendon to pull away from the nerve. Alternatively, a portion of the tendon may be excised to decompress the nerve. An intraneural neurolysis may be done if needed.

Postoperative Management

A resting wrist splint is given to the patient. A light surgical dressing is worn for 1 week, and early movement is encouraged. During the first postoperative week, gentle ranging of the wrist and digits is begun so that the nerve will not adhere to surrounding tissues. During the third postoperative week, the patient begins scar massage in an effort to prevent cicatrix formation between the skin and the underlying nerve.

Radial Nerve Entrapment in the Proximal Forearm (Radial Tunnel Syndrome and Posterior Interosseous Nerve Syndrome)

There are multiple sites of potential compression of the radial nerve in the forearm, one of which (the arcade of Frohse), may be involved in both radial tunnel syndrome (RTS) and posterior interosseous nerve syndrome (PINS). The distinguishing feature between these two syndromes is the lack of motor paralysis in RTS, as originally described by Roles and Maudsley. The RTS is characterized by an aching pain in the extensor–supinator muscle mass in the proximal forearm. Radiation of the pain to the distal arm and distal forearm may occur. There are no sensory changes distally in the distribution of the radial nerve. In PINS, patients also report pain in the region of the extensor–supinator muscle mass. In addition, weakness and/or atrophy of some or all the muscles innervated by the PIN may be present. As with the RTS, there are no sensory complaints. The distinction between these two entities is more historical than real.

Surgical Anatomy

Two to 3 cm proximal to the lateral humeral epicondyle, the radial nerve gives off branches to innervate the BR and the ECRL. At this point, the radial nerve enters the proximal extent of the radial tunnel, lying lateral to the brachialis muscle and the biceps tendon, medial to the origin of the BR muscle, and anterior to the lateral humeral epicondyle. As the radial nerve travels distally, it runs deep to the ECRB. In this region, the radial nerve sends a motor branch to the ECRB, then divides into the superficial radial nerve and the PIN. The PIN then passes between the two heads of the supinator muscle. A fibrous arch, the arcade of Frohse, spanning the two heads of the supinator muscle, may be present. This is the distal extent of the radial tunnel. The radial nerve may be compressed by fibrous bands lying anterior to the radial head near the proximal portion of the tunnel; the radial recurrent vessels; the overlying ECRB muscle belly; a fibrous arch from the ECRB compressing the radial nerve against the arcade of Frohse; and the arcade of Frohse itself. The later is the potential site of entrapment of the PIN.

Diagnosis

The diagnostic features of RTS and PINS will be discussed separately.

RTS

Tenderness may be elicited with palpation of the radial nerve in the region of the extensor–supinator muscle mass. In addition, resisted supination producing pain in the extensor–supinator muscle mass may be present. A provocative test to elicit reproduction of the patient's symptomatology and to distinguish RTS from lateral humeral epicondylitis (tennis elbow) is performed by having the patient extend the middle finger against resistance. If this generates pain in the extensor–supinator muscle mass at the level of the radial head, the results are positive. In contrast, the pain in tennis elbow is generated over the lateral humeral epicondyle. Electrodiagnostic testing should be normal in pure RTS.

PINS

In PINS, point tenderness in the extensor–supinator muscle is present. Depending on the site of compression of the PIN, some or all of the muscles innervated by the PIN may be weak or paralyzed. The extensor carpi radialis longus and brachioradialis are not affected when normal anatomy is present. Sensation in the distribution of the radial sensory nerve is unaffected.

A patient with a complete lesion of the PIN presents with a classic hand position, in which the digits are held in flexion at the MCP joints. The patient is unable to extend the MCP joints but has the ability to extend the PIP and DIP joints because of the intrinsic muscles of the hand. The thumb lies volar to the plane of the metacarpals because of paralysis of the APL and the EPB. The IP joint of the thumb may be held in neutral position by the action of thumb intrinsic muscles, but the ability to hyperextend is lost because of paralysis of the EPL. The wrist is unable to extend in a neutral position, but will extend to the radial side because of paralysis of the ECU and persistence of intact innervation to the ECRL.

A partial lesion of the PIN may result in a "pseudoclaw hand." This results from an inability to extend the MCP joints of the small and ring fingers. The absence of hyperextension of the MCP joints will readily reveal that an ulnar claw hand is not present. Multiple clinical pictures may be seen in a partial lesion of the PIN because of the variable muscles affected. Electromyography can be very beneficial in this situation.

Treatment

For RTS, a trial of conservative treatment is indicated, including immobilization with splinting. Failure of conservative treatment warrants surgical decompression. Operative intervention is indicated in cases of PINS. For both syndromes, all potential sites of entrapment are identified surgically and divided and/or excised. Additional dissection distally is indicated in PINS. The PIN is dissected distally completely through the supinator muscle until it exits from the distal portion. Fibrous bands within the body of the supinator or along its edge may be present and require resection. For pure RTS, in which weakness and paralysis of the muscles innervated by the PIN is not part of the clinical picture, this additional dissection is not necessary.

Postoperative Management

For 2 days postoperatively, the patient wears a posterior splint, holding the elbow in 60 to 90° of flexion with the wrist in the neutral position. At 2 days, wrist and elbow movement is begun to allow gliding of the nerve and prevent adhesion formation to surrounding tissues. Gentle resistance exercises of the thumb, fingers, wrist, and forearm are started during the third postoperative week.

Radial Nerve Entrapment in the Brachium

There is no syndromic name associated with radial nerve entrapment in the arm. The majority of injuries to the radial nerve at this site result from associated skeletal injury, missile wounds, injection trauma, and crush trauma, and are not related to nerve entrapment. However, compression palsies of the radial nerve do occur and may be secondary to entrapment by the lateral intermuscular septum. In general, the radial nerve palsies associated with compression at this proximal site resolve spontaneously and do not require surgical intervention. Should the palsy fail to resolve, surgical exploration with release of the intermuscular septum should be performed.

MULTIPLE CRUSH SYNDROME

Multiple crush syndrome refers to compression of a peripheral nerve at two or more sites of entrapment, resulting in a variable symptom complex. Each compression site itself may be insufficient to cause electrical changes of nerve compression, but the sum of multiple compression sites leads to symptomatic neural dysfunction. Because the entrapment will not cause sufficient compression to result in Wallerian degeneration, muscle wasting and abnormal two-point discrimination may not be present. The diagnosis requires a detailed physical examination, with use of provocative tests and assessments of sensory threshold changes and muscle strength. Treatment is directed at the conservative management of each entrapment site. If conservative management fails, judicial surgical treatment with release of the more severely compressed sites may be considered. Multiple crush syndrome may occur in the following situations.

Multiple Anatomic Regions

In the upper extremity, the most common series of anatomic regions causing compression across a peripheral nerve are (1) C5, C6, C7 roots, the brachial plexus upper trunk, the median nerve in the fore-arm, and the median nerve in the carpel tunnel and (2) C8, T1 roots, the brachial plexus lower trunk, the ulnar nerve in the cubital tunnel, and the ulnar nerve in Guyon's canal.

Multiple Anatomic Structures

There are multiple potential sites of compression along a peripheral nerve in a given anatomic region. These potential sites of compression have been discussed for median, ulnar, and radial nerve entrapment syndromes.

BRACHIAL PLEXUS INJURY

Plexus injuries may include any of the six injury patterns described in the section on Electrodiagnosis. However, in plexus injuries, man-agement approaches may be based on three broad categories of nerve injury: root avulsion, nerve interruption, and nerve in continuity le-sions. Treatment depends on type of injury, level of the injury, degree of recovery, and functional priorities of the upper extremity.

Localizing the Level of Injury

Although a confusing array of motor and sensory deficits may be present with a plexus injury, a thorough, systematic physical examina-tion of the patient, proceeding from proximal to distal, will aid in lo-calizing the level of injury. Knowledge of the plexus anatomy and its innervation patterns is required. Electrodiagnostic studies are used to support the diagnosis and to evaluate progressive recovery or lack of recovery over time.

Root Avulsion

Loss of function of the muscles innervated by nerve branches di-rectly off the roots of the plexus is suggestive of a proximal root avul-sion injury. The integrity of both the long thoracic nerve (C5, C6, C7) and the dorsal scapular nerve (C5, C6) can be assessed clinically. Palsy of the serratus anterior muscle results in winging of the scapula, and atrophy of the rhomboid muscles may be visualized and palpated. If these muscles are not functioning, it indicates the presence of nerve root avulsion with no proximal nerve at that level for reconstruction. If these muscles are functioning when diffuse palsy is present elsewhere, it suggests that a proximal nerve stump is viable and reconstruction possible.

The presence of Horner's syndrome in conjunction with brachial plexus injury suggests root avulsion or traction injury at the C8, T1 level. Horner's syndrome results from the associated injury to the cervical sympathetic fibers. Physical findings of Horner's syndrome include enophthalmus, ptosis, myosis, and anhydrosis.

The location of the root avulsion with respect to the dorsal root ganglion may be classified as preganglionic or supraganglionic lesions (those with the roots avulsed proximal to the ganglion), or postganglionic or infraganglionic lesions (those with the roots avulsed distal to the ganglion). Because the nerve roots in supraganglionic lesions have been avulsed proximal to the dorsal root ganglion, no proximal nerve tissue remains, and surgical repair is not possible. With infraganglionic lesions, surgical repair is possible because nerve fibers remain proximal to the site of the avulsion.

Both supraganglionic and infraganglionic lesions will lead to complete loss of motor and sensory function. However, in supraganglionic lesions, the sensory fibers remain attached to their neurons in the dorsal root ganglion. Because of this, no Wallerian degeneration will occur in the sensory fibers and sensory nerve conduction studies will be normal, even though the patient will have no sensation. Thus, the level of the avulsion can be determined based on the clinical examination and the presence or absence of normal sensory nerve conduction studies.

Trunk Injury

When a plexus injury has occurred, loss of function or wasting of the supraspinatus and infraspinatus muscles (suprascapular nerve; C5, C6) suggests injury to the upper trunk. In a patient with a diffuse plexus injury who demonstrates recovery of all the muscles except for the supraspinatus and infraspinatus, a superimposed traction injury to the suprascapular nerve at the level of the scapular notch may be present.

Division Injury

There are no nerve branches from the divisions. Localization of injury to this site is not possible.

Posterior Cord Injury

Loss of function or wasting of the latissimus dorsi muscle (thoracodorsal nerve), the deltoid muscle (axillary nerve), and the triceps (radial nerve) suggests injury to the posterior cord. If the triceps demonstrate recovery of function, but the deltoid muscle does not recover, entrapment or damage to the axillary nerve within the quadrangular space may be present.

Lateral Cord Injury

Injury to the lateral cord results in loss of musculocutaneous nerve function and sensation in the thumb and index fingers. In addition, an injury proximal to the lateral pectoral nerve branch will result in paralysis of the clavicular head of the pectoralis major muscle. The sternocostal head of the pectoralis major muscle may continue to function because of intact innervation by the medial pectoral nerve from the medial cord. An injury to both the lateral and medial cord would result in paralysis of both heads of the pectoralis major muscle.

Medial Cord Injury

Isolated injury to the medial cord results in loss of ulnar nerve function and intrinsic median nerve function in the hand. The medial pectoral nerve from the medial cord innervates the sternocostal head of the pectoralis major muscle, but paralysis would not occur because of overlapping innervation to the sternocostal head by the lateral pectoral nerve.

Treatment of Plexus Injuries

The principles of management for isolated peripheral nerve injuries also apply to the management of plexus injuries. See the section on Acute Nerve Injuries for management of open, closed, and missile injuries. An algorithm for the treatment of closed brachial plexus injuries is shown in Fig. 6-9.

During the first 3 months after a closed brachial plexus injury, the patient is managed expectantly. Physical therapy is instituted to maintain a full range of passive motion of all joints. Electrodiagnostic studies are obtained 6 weeks after the injury to establish baseline function and to ascertain the presence of fibrillation potentials and positive sharp waves. These signs of denervation require a minimum of 3 weeks to develop.

Three months after the injury, the patient is evaluated for evidence of clinical and electrical recovery. If recovery is present and progressing in a defined, anatomic, sequential pattern, the patient is followed expectantly on a monthly basis until recovery is complete. If there is no clinical or electrical evidence of recovery or if the patient demonstrates nonanatomic return of function with good distal recovery in the presence of isolated lack of proximal recovery, surgical intervention is indicated. If an avulsion injury is suspected, a myelogram should be obtained. The accuracy of predicting a root avulsion with a myelogram is improved with the use of a postmyelogram computed tomography (CT).

Surgical intervention should be undertaken by the sixth month. Any further delay will compromise the chances for functional recovery, and by 12 to 18 months after denervation, muscles will have undergone irreversible fibrosis. This explains the poor prognosis for functional recovery of the intrinsic muscles of the hand when a high, proximal median or ulnar nerve or plexus injury is present. Regenerating axons

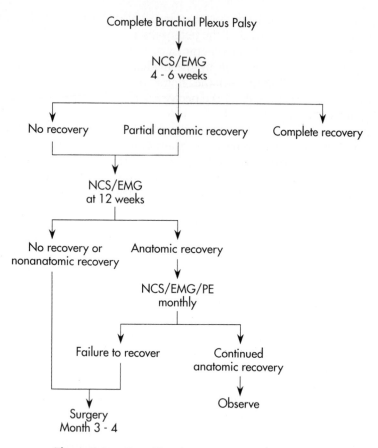

Figure 6-9 Closed brachial plexus injury algorithm.

travel distally at a rate of approximately 1 inch/month. Several months is required for the regenerating axons to travel the length of the upper extremity. Thus, even though nerve repair is successful, the excessively long period of dennervation may lead to failure because of muscle fibrosis and the inability of the muscle to respond to reinnervation.

Reconstruction Priorities

In patients with a complete brachial plexus palsy, restoration of critical motor function is the main priority. The most significant motor function is elbow flexion (musculocutaneous nerve), followed closely by shoulder abduction (axillary and suprascapular nerves). Elbow flexion has priority over shoulder abduction because the upper extremity can maintain some degree of function with elbow flexion alone. The reverse is not true.

The area of critical sensory function depends on the absence of motor function within the hand. In patients with a complete brachial plexus palsy, the restoration of protective sensation to the medial border of the forearm and hand takes priority. Reinnervation of sensory fibers to the medial cord would be performed. However, if the patient has the potential for recovery of motor function to the thumb and index finger, then the area of priority of critical sensory restoration changes. Attempts to restore sensation to the thumb and index finger by sensory reinnervation of the lateral cord would be indicated.

Surgical Management

Primary Nerve Repair

Primary neurorrhaphy rarely is possible in plexus injuries. With an open injury to the plexus, if a sharp transection is identified, primary nerve repair may be performed. Because of the proximal level of the injury, an epineural repair is appropriate.

Neurolysis

Neurolysis frequently is used in plexus surgery. Many injuries involve in continuity lesions. If an element of the plexus demonstrates an injury and remains in continuity, intraoperative nerve stimulation and recording is necessary to assess the degree of injury. If a nerve action potential is recorded, neurolysis is performed. The neurolysis separates the nerve fascicles from the surrounding scar and may facilitate recovery of the nerve fibers.

Nerve Grafting

Nerve grafting frequently is performed in plexus surgery both for segmental loss of nerve tissue and for severe in continuity lesions. Should an in-continuity lesion fail to demonstrate an action potential with intraoperative nerve stimulation, then excision and grafting of that element of the plexus is indicated. Neurolysis is used frequently in this setting to define good proximal and distal nerve tissue. Ideally, the proximal and distal nerve segments will have the appropriate match of nerve fibers, such as grafting from the C5 or C6 root to the musculocutaneous nerve. Mismatching of motor fibers can occur when an appropriate match between the proximal and distal nerve segments cannot be obtained. For example, mismatching of motor fibers occurs when grafting a portion of the posterior cord (C5, C6, C7, C8) to the axillary nerve to reinnervated the deltoid. If the injury to the axillary nerve is isolated at the quadrangular space, a nerve graft between the proximal and distal axillary nerve segments will restore the continuity of the appropriate motor fibers. Because of the high priority of function of the axillary and musculocutaneous nerves, if the appropriate proximal nerve tissue is not viable, then grafting to other available proximal motor nerve tissue is indicated.

Neurotization

Neurotization is the transfer of a normal proximal nerve to the distal segment of an injured nerve to restore critical motor or sensory function. The donor nerves are considered to be of less significant functional value than the injured nerve. When no proximal nerve tissue is available for reconstruction in a plexus injury, such as an avulsion injury, neurotization provides a means of reinnervating critical areas of function. Critical motor function for the upper extremity includes shoulder abduction (axillary and suprascapular nerves) and elbow flexion (musculocutaneous nerve). The most commonly used donor motor nerves are the medial pectoral nerves and the intercostal and rectus nerves. Critical protective sensibility along the ulnar border of the forearm and hand can be restored with neurotization of the cervical sensory plexus or the greater auricular nerve to the medial cord. These same sensory donor nerves can be neurotized to the lateral cord to provide sensation to the thumb and index finger, if restoration of motor function of these digits is anticipated.

Postoperative Management

During the first postoperative week, a shoulder immobilizer is worn. This is later changed to an external prosthesis that provides shoulder stability and static elbow flexion. The shoulder is kept adducted for 1 month to allow the pectoralis major tendon to heal. Physical therapy to maintain full range of motion of the joints is continued. Depending on the extent and level of injury, it will take 18 to 24 months to assess the final degree of nerve regeneration.

Additional Reconstruction Options

Muscle transfers, tendon transfers, or free muscle grafts should be considered when there is a lack of significant functional recovery after brachial plexus surgery. Lack of motor reinnervation may be the result of loss of motor end plates and muscle fibrosis, rather than the failure of nerve regeneration. In this situation, the nerve graft could be used to innervate a free muscle transfer.

Shoulder Reconstruction

With proper patient selection, shoulder mobility may be maintained by multiple muscle transfers, if partial recovery of brachial plexus lesions has occurred. When these muscle transfers are not possible or if total paralysis of the shoulder muscles is present with no chance for recovery, glenohumeral arthrodesis is indicated.

Tendon Transfers for Elbow Flexion

Tendon transfers for the restoration of elbow flexion are warranted when nerve repair or neurotization has not been successful. The prerequisites for tendon transfers are discussed in the section on Tendon Transfers for Peripheral Nerve Palsies. Options for transfer include the latissimus dorsi, pectoralis major, triceps, and flexor forearm muscles (Steindler Flexorplasty).

TENDON TRANSFERS FOR PERIPHERAL NERVE PALSIES
General Principles

Maximum passive range of motion must be achieved and maintained in all joints of the wrist and hand before any tendon transfer. The donor tendon chosen for transfer must be expendable. Each joint must have one remaining adequate extensor and flexor for acceptable function. Adequate, comparable force of muscle strength must be present for the tendon to function in its new location. The range of excursion of the transferred tendon must be adequate to perform its intended new function. This effective range may be amplified by freeing the muscle from its investing fascial attachments or by changing the muscle from a monoarticular to a multiarticular muscle that moves multiple joints in parallel. Finally, if possible, a tendon of synergistic function is preferable.

Early Tendon Transfers

Tendon transfers carried out at the time of nerve repair may be indicated in certain situations. With a proximal median nerve palsy, in which recovery of intrinsic function of the thumb will not occur, an early tendon transfer is appropriate. Restoration of thumb opposition with an EIP tendon transfer to the APB should be performed. There is nothing to be gained by delaying tendon transfer in this situation. An argument also may be made for an early tendon transfer in radial nerve palsy. Transfer of the PT tendon to the ECRB tendon will function as an internal splint and allow for wrist extension while awaiting reinnervation of the radial extensors. This tendon transfer is ideal because minimal motor reeducation is required, the surgical dissection is limited, and the PT retains its original function after transfer. Potential drawbacks may include decreased wrist extension during pronation and decreased wrist flexion during supination.

Radial Nerve Palsy

Timing of Tendon Transfers

Because radial nerve repairs have a good prognosis for recovery, most tendon transfers should be delayed until adequate time has been allowed for nerve regeneration. If a poor prognosis is expected because of the extent of an injury or pronounced delay in presentation by the patient, then early definitive tendon transfers may be indicated.

Deficits

The patient may show lack of wrist extension, finger extension at the MCP joints, thumb extension at the MCP joint, and thumb abduction.

Tendon Transfers

Multiple transfers have been proposed; the following include the most often used transfers. Where multiple options are enumerated, our preference is listed first. We do not use the FCU for restoration of finger extension because it is the prime ulnar stabilizer of the wrist and its transfer may result in radial deviation of the wrist.

Wrist Extension
    PT to ECRB

Finger Extension
    FDS III and IV to EDC
    FCR to EDC
    FCU to EDC

Thumb Extension
    PL to EPL

Posterior Interosseous Nerve Palsy

Timing of Tendon Transfers

This is identical to that for radial nerve palsy.

Deficits

The patient may show radial dorsiflexion of the wrist and lack of finger extension at the MCP joints, thumb extension at the MCP joint, and thumb abduction.

Types of Tendon Transfers

Multiple transfers have been purposed. The following include the most often used transfers. Where multiple options are enumerated, our preference is listed first.

Wrist Extension
    PT to distal ECRB

Finger Extension
    FDS III and IV to EDC
    FCR to EDC

Thumb Extension
    PL to EPL
    BR to EPL

High Median Nerve Palsy

Timing of Tendon Transfers

Because recovery of median intrinsic function of the hand is unlikely to occur after nerve repair of a proximal median nerve injury, opponensplasty can be undertaken at the time of nerve repair. However, tendon transfer to restore power grip because of paralysis of the FDS, FDP to the index and middle fingers, and the FPL should be delayed after nerve repair. Adequate time should be allowed for reinnervation of these muscles because the prognosis for recovery of the forearm flexors is good. Again, if long after the injury, the patient will have poor prospects for recovery because of the time delay, all necessary tendon transfers should be undertaken. In this situation, repair of the median nerve should focus solely on reestablishment of critical median sensory innervation. If sensation cannot be restored in the distribution of the median nerve, tendon transfer for opponensplasty is not indicated, because the patient will not use these digits for precision pinch.

Deficits

The patient may show loss of palmar thumb abduction, thumb opposition, thumb IP joint flexion, FDS function, and FDP to the index and long fingers. Generally, flexion of the long finger is possible because of ulnar nerve contributions to the FDP to this digit. However, considerable weakness of this digit usually is present. In addition, forearm pronation is weak. The primary deficit resulting from dennervation of the forearm median innervated flexors is loss of power grip.

Types of Tendon Transfers

Numerous types of opponensplasty techniques have been described. Our choices for tendon transfer for high median nerve palsy are listed in preferential order.

Thumb Opposition
  EIP to APB
  FDS IV to APB
  PL to APB
  ADM to APB
Thumb IP Flexion
  BR to FPL
  ECRL to FPL
Index and Long Finger Flexion
  Side-to-side tenodesis of ring/small FDP to index/long FDP
  ECRL to FDP of index and long fingers (This transfer is reserved
    for those individuals who have no chance of recovery of the

index and long FDP and who need radial side power, e.g., manual laborers.)

Low Median Nerve Palsy

Timing of Tendon Transfers

The prognosis is good for recovery of the median intrinsics of the hand after nerve repair. Generally, opponensplasty is delayed until adequate time has passed for reinnervation. However, if the patient does not seek treatment until such a time that recovery of muscle function is precluded opponensplasty should be performed in conjunction with median nerve exploration and reestablishment of median nerve sensation. An early tendon transfer may be performed using the PL to the APB at the time of carpal tunnel release if atrophy of the thenar muscles is present. This may augment the functional recovery while reinnervation of remaining musculature is taking place.

Deficits

The patient may show loss of palmar thumb abduction and thumb opposition and weakness of the index and possibly the long finger lumbricales. The latter functional loss usually is compensated for by the ulnar innervated intrinsics.

Types of Tendon Transfers

Our choices for tendon transfer for low median nerve palsy are listed in preferential order.

Thumb Opposition
  EIP to APB
  FDS IV to ABP
  PL to APB
  ADM to APB

High Ulnar Nerve Palsy

Timing of Tendon Transfers

Because a proximal ulnar nerve palsy has a good prognosis for recovery of function of the FCU and the FDP to the small and ring fingers, but a poor prognosis for recovery of the ulnar intrinsics to the hand, an early tendon transfer for restoration of thumb adduction and index finger abduction is appropriate. This will allow for thumb adduction for key pinch and thumb to index finger tip pinch. If recovery of the FCU and the FDP to the small and ring fingers does not occur after an adequate time period after nerve repair, tendon transfers should be performed to reestablish function.

Deficits

The patient may have paralysis of the FCU, resulting in radial deviation of the wrist with flexion, as well as loss of small and ring finger

DIP joint flexion; loss of thumb adduction with the inability to perform key pinch; loss of index finger abduction, which combined with lack of thumb adduction results in an inability to precisely pinch the tips of the index and thumb; lack of integrated action of MCP joint and IP joint flexion of the small and ring fingers because of paralysis of the lumbricales to these digits, resulting in uncoordinated grasping; and paralysis of the interossei and hypothenar muscles, with an inability to abduct and adduct the fingers. All of these deficits cause loss of power grip and precision grip. There is no claw deformity of the hand with high ulnar nerve paralysis.

Types of Tendon Transfers

There are numerous types of tendon transfers described for improvement of these deficits. The patient's needs will dictate which transfer is appropriate (i.e., power versus precision restoration). A representative sample is listed.

Small and Ring Finger DIP Flexion
Side-to-side tenodesis of long finger FDP to small and ring finger FDP
Wrist Flexion
None
PL to FCU insertion
Index Finger Abduction
EIP to APL
Accessory slip of APL with free PL tendon graft to 1st DI (with arthrodesis of thumb MCP)
Thumb Adduction
FDS of long finger to bony abductor tubercle of thumb proximal phalanx
ECRB with free PL tendon graft to AP
EDC of the index finger with free PL tendon graft to bony adductor tubercle of thumb proximal phalanx

Low Ulnar Nerve Palsy

Timing of Tendon Transfers

The prognosis is good for recovery of ulnar intrinsic muscles after nerve repair for a low ulnar nerve palsy. If recovery fails to occur after nerve repair or if nerve repair is unlikely to result in recovery in a chronic, established deficit, then tendon transfers for restoration of function are performed.

Deficits

The deficits are identical to those listed for a high ulnar nerve injury, except that innervation to the FCU and the FDP to the small and ring fingers is intact. Because of the intact FDP function, a claw hand deformity will develop. This is the result of paralysis of the lumbricales to the small and ring fingers, which permits the unopposed action of the radial innervated EDC to hyperextend the MCP joints, while the intact FDP and FDS flex the PIP and DIP of the small and ring fingers.

Types of Tendon Transfers

Methods used to prevent the development of the claw hand and tendon transfers used to correct existing claw hand are listed here. For tendon transfers restoring lost ulnar intrinsic function, see the previous section.

Static Control of Clawing (prevention of MCP joint hyperextension)
   Lumbrical bar splint
   Zancolli capsulodesis of the MCP joint
   Bunnell A1/A2 pulley release
   Parkes static volar tenodesis: free tendon graft from central slip insertion to deep transverse ligament
Dynamic Control of Clawing (Tendon transfers are performed for restoration of lumbrical function, thereby coordinating MCP and PIP flexion. Both FDS and ECRL are used frequently, but only ECRL will increase grip power).
   FDS of long finger split into four slips to radial lateral band of each finger
   FDS of long and ring finger split into two slips each to A1 or A2 pulley
   ECRL or ECRB with free tendon grafts to radial lateral bands of long, ring, and small fingers, and ulnar lateral band of index finger
   ECRL with free tendon grafts to A2 pulley of all four fingers

PAINFUL SEQUELAE OF PERIPHERAL NERVE INJURY
Neuroma

After nerve injury, the proximal nerve will regenerate in an attempt to restore neural continuity. If the sprouting axons make the appropriate sensory or motor connections distally, then functional recovery will occur. If these regenerating axons do not connect with the appropriate distal connections, they will branch irregularly and become contained in a disorganized mass at the proximal nerve stump. This mass of entangled axons and scar tissue is a neuroma.

Diagnosis

Neuromatous pain is characterized by a discrete area of tenderness corresponding to the localized nerve injury. Percussion at the site of the neuroma will produce paresthesia in the distribution of the injured nerve. Alleviation of the pain with a diagnostic nerve block is helpful in the evaluation of the etiology of the pain and in the localization of the specific sensory nerve involved. This should be repeated to exclude potential placebo effect. Patients who do not tolerate nerve blocks are not likely to be good candidates for surgery.

Treatment

After a neuroma has been diagnosed, nonoperative treatment options may be considered. Desensitization techniques, such as light touch, massage, vibration, transcutaneous electrical nerve stimulation, and additional desensitization modalities, may benefit some patients. In general, if conservative management is going to be effective, the therapist will note improvement within a few weeks. If conservative management is unsuccessful in a carefully selected patient, operative intervention is indicated. The ultimate goal of surgical treatment is to relieve the pain and restore critical sensory nerve function.

Surgical Management Algorithm

Within the hand, if the appropriate distal nerve stump is accessible, the neuroma should be excised and the nerve repaired or grafted. If the distal nerve segment is not available and the sensory function of the injured nerve is critical, grafting with innervated free tissue transfers should be considered. If the sensory function of the injured nerve is not critical or prior neuroma treatment with nerve grafting has failed, then the proximal nerve stump should be transposed to an area not subjected to mechanical stimulation, such as bone or muscle. Proximal nerve stumps in the hand should be transposed into bone or forearm muscle, because the muscle within the hand lacks sufficient bulk to pad the nerve stump. With radial sensory and lateral antebrachial cutaneous nerves, where sensation is not critical, the proximal nerve stump should be transposed and buried within the BR muscle (Fig. 6-10). The results of surgical treatment are better in patients treated for the first time (primary neuroma) than in patients with recurrent neuromas.

Neuroma In Continuity

Neuromas may develop within a nerve that anatomically remains in continuity to some degree. This type of injury is a sixth degree nerve injury. There are essentially three general situations in which this occurs: (1) a partially lacerated nerve, in which the regenerating axons of the lacerated fascicles do not connect with the appropriate distal fibers, but instead escape into the surrounding tissue, forming a neuroma along the lateral aspect of the nerve, (2) a transected nerve previously repaired, in which some of the regenerating axons escape through the sutured area, forming a neuroma at the site of the repair, (3) a nerve subjected to repeated trauma, such as crush, pressure, or friction, caus-

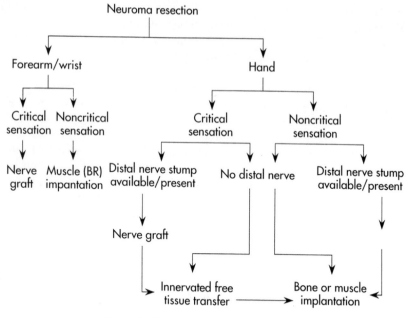

Figure 6-10   Painful neuroma algorithm.

ing injury within the nerve and the development of scar tissue, which prevents the regenerating axons from traveling distally. These axons may then become entrapped within the scar tissue and form a "neuroma" within the body of the nerve. The latter example is not, by definition, a true neuroma.

Diagnosis

The clinical presentation and diagnostic evaluation of a painful neuroma in continuity is similar to that described for neuromas, except that sensation usually will be altered rather than absent. With an incontinuity injury, hyperalgesia in the distribution of the partially injured fascicles may be present.

When evaluating the patient, a detailed examination should assess the function in each group of fascicles within the injured nerve. Those components of the nerve that are functioning appropriately must be distinguished from those that are not. The type of sensibility remaining or the lack of sensibility, and/or the degree of motor loss must be assessed. Electrodiagnostic studies will aid in this evaluation.

Treatment

Nonoperative treatment modalities are not likely to be successful for resolution of painful neuromas in continuity.

Surgical management algorithm

The preoperative assessment of the type of sensibility present in the remainder of the nerve will influence surgical management. If the patient's response to a light touch is diminished and nonpainful, neurolysis of the involved fascicles is all that is required surgically. However, if a light touch is exquisitely painful with the presence of hyperalgesia, excision and nerve grafting should be considered at the time of surgical intervention. If exploration of the nerve demonstrates only marked scarring around the nerve, and the fascicles appear normal after neurolysis, then neurolysis may be all that is required to relieve the patients symptoms. When no sensation (or motor function) is present, a fourth or fifth degree injury exists. This requires resection of the injured segment and repair or grafting. Therefore, the preoperative clinical examination and electrodiagnostic studies will distinguish those parts of the nerve that have no function and require nerve grafting from those parts of the nerve that remain in continuity but have altered sensibility that will influence surgical management. For smaller cutaneous nerves that mediate noncritical sensation (e.g., radial sensory nerve, palmar cutaneous branch of the median nerve), nerve grafting is not performed. In these situations, either neurolysis or resection of the nerve and transposition in a proximal location is recommended.

Reflex Sympathetic Dystrophy (Sympathetic Maintained Pain Syndrome)

Reflex sympathetic dystrophy (RSD) commonly refers to a pain syndrome that is maintained by an abnormality in the response of the sympathetic nervous system to any number of precipitating factors. Common precipitating factors include nerve compression, complete or partial nerve division with hyperalgesia, fracture, soft tissue trauma, and surgery. The pain syndrome may be maintained by several factors at once, such as chronic inflammation, arthritis, disuse stiffness, neuroma, nerve compression, psychogenic or nonorganic functional factors, and secondary gain, or any combination of these factors. The three diagnostic criteria for RSD are (1) diffuse pain, usually out of proportion to the precipitating injury and often nonanatomic in distribution, (2) diminished function, and (3) objective evidence of autonomic dysfunction, with skin and/or soft tissue trophic changes with or without vasomotor instability. The three stages of RSD are early, intermediate, and late. In the early stage, sympathetic overactivity with vasomotor instability is present. Skin and soft tissue changes vary between redness, warmth, cyanosis, and sweating. Edema also is present classically. This stage can last from weeks to months. The intermediate stage develops when edema and vasomotor activity has lessened. Pain is less marked and usually is elicited by attempts at activity or movement of the joints. Stiffness and atrophy of the skin and soft tissue is present, typically with a cool, pale extremity. This stage may last for several months. In the late stage, diffuse atrophy, fibrosis, and stiffness are present, with a variable degree of pain. The chronic pain may result in the manifestation of functional or psychogenic problems.

Diagnosis

An examination reveals a relevant history and the presence of the three aforementioned diagnostic criteria. Radionuclide scintigraphy with three-phase bone scanning provides an objective marker of RSD in the hand. Diffuse increased uptake of technetium-99 tracer in the delayed image is considered diagnostic for RSD. Ultimately, however, RSD is considered a clinical diagnosis.

Treatment

Although no treatment has proven completely satisfactory, the best chance for success is early diagnosis and aggressive treatment. The first priority is to diagnose all the components of the pain syndrome. Treatment of any underlying surgical problem or associated systemic illness is then carried out. Psychosocial issues may need to be addressed as well. Desensitization therapy, nerve blocks, and physiotherapy may be helpful. Permanent surgical sympathectomy is considered only after underlying precipitating factors have been treated, when the pain persists despite full conservative therapy with repeated blocks, and when the patient has demonstrated consistent, positive responses to sympathetic nerve blocks. In the late stages of RSD, no treatment may be useful.

Prognosis

The prognosis relates to the stage of RSD. The earlier that treatment is instituted, the better the prognosis. Comparison of therapeutic modalities and treatment results is difficult because of inaccurate and overdiagnosis of RSD.

RESULTS OF NERVE REPAIR AND GRAFTING

Reported results of nerve repair and grafting are difficult to compare because of the variabilities in techniques used to quantitate motor and sensory recovery. The four broad categories that affect the end results of surgical repair/grafting are patient factors, injury pattern, surgical technique, and postoperative rehabilitation.

Patient Factors

Age and patient compliance are very important in determining functional recovery. Several studies have shown that after peripheral nerve division and repair, reorganization of the central cortex of the brain occurs. Older patients may have a decreased potential for this central reorganization, whereas young children with nerve repair have excellent functional recovery because of the ability of the central cortex to adapt more easily. These cortical changes return closer to normal with reeducation and rehabilitation; thus, the importance of patient compliance cannot be overemphasized. In addition, related illnesses, such as diabetes and alcoholism, may have an adverse effect on the end results of nerve regeneration.

Injury Pattern

Patients with proximal nerve injuries are less likely to achieve good functional recovery because these injuries tend to be more severe (avulsion traction versus sharp laceration), involve a greater longitudinal extension of injury, and by their very location, result in increased distance and time to reinnervation of motor end plates and sensory receptors. All of these factors are associated with greater loss of neurons centrally. In addition, reinnervation of motor end plates may be fruitless, because successful reinnervation of motor fibers is time dependent. Further, because the nerve fascicles in the proximal extremity tend to have mixed motor and sensory fibers, there is a greater opportunity for mismatching of these fibers within a given fascicle. This results in misdirection of critical sensory or motor reinnervation.

In the distal extremity, functional recovery is more likely to be good because injuries tend to have less longitudinal damage and are more likely to be sharp, the motor and sensory fascicles are organized more discretely, and the distance between the level of the injury and the motor end plates and sensory receptors is less.

Surgical Technique

The following key factors influence ultimate recovery:
1. Microsurgical expertise.
2. Tension at the repair site.
3. Underestimation of the longitudinal extent of nerve injury.
4. Inappropriate sensory and motor fascicular alignment.
5. Prolonged immobilization leading to scar formation and prevention of gliding of the nerve at the repair site.

Postoperative Sensory and Motor Reeducation

Motor and sensory reeducation is critical in achieving maximal functional recovery.

SENSORY REEDUCATION

With sensory reeducation, the patient is taught to interpret abnormal sensory impulses generated after peripheral nerve repair. The central transmission of these sensory impulses is different after repair of the nerve injury because (1) axons may be misdirected to a different cutaneous region (e.g., axons that previously transmitted sensation from the middle finger may now transmit sensation from the thumb after a median nerve repair); (2) fewer axons will have regenerated distally; (3) regenerating axons may reinnervate a different peripheral receptor than that innervated before the injury (e.g., a quickly adapting fiber that formerly innervated a Meissner corpuscle, coding for moving touch and vibration, may reinnervate a slowly adapting Merkel cell-neurite complex, coding for constant touch and pressure). The sensory perception of the patient may, therefore, be altered with respect to location, quantity, and mechanical transduction capacity. Sensory reeducation teaches the patient to interpret the altered profile of sensory impulses. A better level of functional sensation is achieved and is accomplish sooner than without sensory reeducation.

Pattern of Sensory Recovery

A consistent pattern of sensory recovery after peripheral nerve repair was found by Dellon. The first sensation to recover is that of pain and temperature. This is followed by touch perception in the following order: vibratory touch, moving touch, and then constant touch. In the course of sensory reeducation, specific sensory exercises are performed at the appropriate time, coinciding with the pattern of sensory recovery.

Early Phase Reeducation

In this phase, the patient is able to ascertain moving and constant touch, but has not yet developed two-point discrimination. Reeducation is directed at teaching the patient to discriminate between a constant and a moving touch, and to correctly localize the area touched.

Late Phase Reeducation

This phase of reeducation improves the sensory discriminatory abilities of the patient.

Reeducation of Unpleasant Sensations (Desensitization)

Desensitization is effective for the treatment of dysesthesia, the unpleasant sensation felt as the nerves regenerate in a previously anesthetized area. Patients with hyperalgesia or long-standing neuromatous pain do not respond well to desensitization. Through desensitization techniques, the brain learns to filter out the unpleasant sensations while allowing perception of meaningful sensory messages. Transcutaneous nerve stimulators may be helpful in some patients, but vibration stimulation is helpful in most. Pharmaceutical intervention with antineuropathic medication may be of added benefit in these patients.

MOTOR REEDUCATION

The three phases of motor rehabilitation are facilitating active motion, increasing strength, and improving coordination and dexterity. The timing of the various phases differs, depending on the surgical procedure (e.g., nerve repair, neurotization, tendon transfer, or free muscle transfer). The following phases correspond to tendon and free muscle transfers.

Phase I: Immobilization

This phase generally lasts 4 weeks. Appropriate immobilization allows for healing of the tendon and muscle before any stress is placed on the repair site. Active mobilization of uninvolved joints and control of pain and edema are therapies instituted during this phase.

Phase II: Active Movement and Reeducation

Active motion begins at 4 weeks to minimized scar formation and facilitate a gliding tendon system without placing unnecessary stress on the repair site. Massage and compression therapy assist in minimizing scar formation. Reeducation is directed at teaching the patient to perform the desired motor movement in an unconscious fashion. Biofeedback may facilitate this goal.

Phase III: Strengthening and Coordination

At the sixth week, resistance exercises and passive stretching exercises are begun. Exercises isolating the involved muscle are used to prevent stronger muscles from compensating for the injury by performing the desired function. To improve dexterity, gross prehensile activities are first performed. The patient should strive for accuracy in performing an activity before advancing to exercises that increase the speed with which the activity is completed.

SELECTED REFERENCES

Brand PW: Tendon grafting. Illustrated by a new operation for intrinsic paralysis of the fingers, *J Bone Joint Surg* 43B:444-453, 1961.

Brooks AL, Jones DS: A new intrinsic tendon transfer for the paralytic hand, *J Bone Joint Surg* 57A: 730, 1975.

Bunnell S: Opposition of the thumb, *J Bone Joint Surg* 20:269-284, 1938.

Bunnell S: Surgery of the intrinsic muscles of the hand other than those producing opposition of the thumb, *J Bone Joint Surg* 24:1-31, 1942.

Burkhalter WE, Christensen RC, Brown PW: Extensor indicis proprius opponensplasty, *J Bone Joint Surg* 55A:725-732, 1973.

Camitz H: Über die Behandlung der Opposition slahmung, *Acta Chir Scand* 65:77, 1929.

Chuinard RG, Boyes JH, Stark HH, Ashworth CR: Tendon transfers for radial nerve palsy: use of superficialis tendons for digital extension, *J Hand Surg* 3:560-570, 1978.

Dellon AL: Musculotendinous variations about the medial humeral epicondyle, *J Hand Surg (Br)* 11:175-181, 1986.

Dellon AL: Operative technique for submuscular transposition of the ulnar nerve, *Contemp Orthop,* 16:17-24, 1988.

Dellon AL, Curtis RM, Edgerton MT: Evaluating recovery of sensation in the hand following nerve injury, *Johns Hopkins Med J* 130:235-243, 1972.

Huber E: Hilfsoperation bei median Uslahmung, *Dtsch Arch Klin Med* 136:271, 1921.

Jones R: On suture of nerves, and alternative methods of treatment by transplantation of tendon, *Br Med J* 1:679-682, 1916.

Mackinnon SE, Dellon AL: Results of treatment of recurrent dorsal radial wrist neuromas, *Ann Plast Surg* 19:54-61, 1987.

Mackinnon SE, Dellon AL, editors: *Surgery of the peripheral nerve.* Thieme, New York, 1988.

Mackinnon SE, Holder LE: The use of three-phase radionuclide bone scanning in the diagnosis of reflex sympathetic dystrophy, *J Hand Surg (Am)* 9:556-563, 1984.

Merzenich MM, Nelson RJ, Stryker MP, et al.: Somatosensory cortical map changes following digital amputation in adult monkey, *J Comp Neurol* 224:591-605, 1984.

Milford LW: *Radial nerve palsy.* In Edmonson AS, Crenshaw AH, editors: *Campbell's operative orthopaedics.* ed. 6, CV Mosby, St. Louis, 1980, pp. 297-300.

Omer GE Jr: *The palsied hand.* In Evartx CM, editor: *Surgery of the musculoskeletal system.* ed 2, Churchill Livingstone, New York, 1990.

Parkes A: Paralytic claw fingers—a graft tenodesis operation, *Hand* 5:192-199, 1973.

Riordan, DC: Tendon transfers for nerve paralysis of the hand and wrist, *Curr Pract Orthop Surg* 2:17-40, 1964.

Roles NC, Maudsley RH: Radial tunnel syndrome: resistant tennis elbow as a nerve entrapment, *J Bone Joint Surg* 54B:499-508, 1972.

Rudge P, Ochoa J, Gilliatt RW: Acute peripheral nerve compression in the baboon. Anatomical and physiological findings, *J Neurol Sci* 23: 403, 1974.

Saha AK: Surgery of the paralyzed and flail shoulder, *Acta Orthop Scan* Suppl 97, 1967.

Starr CL: Army experiences with tendon transference, *J Bone Joint Surg* 4:3-21, 1922.

Struthers J: On a peculiarity of the humerus and humeral artery, *Monthly J Med Sci* 28: 264-267, 1848.

Szabo RN, Gilberman RH, Williamson RV, Dellon AL, Yaru NC, Dimick MP: Vibratory sensory testing in acute peripheral nerve compression, *J Hand Surg (Am)* 9:104, 1984.

Zancolli EA: Claw-hand caused by paralysis of the intrinsic muscles. A simple surgical procedure for its correction, *J Bone Joint Surg* 39A:1076-1080, 1957.

7

Hand Fractures and Dislocations

Philip E. Higgs, MD, FACS

The treatment of fractures of the hand and fingers is integral to most plastic surgery practices and to all hand surgery practices. Although they are among the most common fractures, unfortunately they frequently are dismissed as minor injuries with little potential consequence. The contrary is certainly more correct. Improperly treated or neglected hand fractures may lead to significant disability. This chapter presents a rational approach to the management of hand and finger fractures.

When treating any injury of the hand, the first consideration is long-term restoration or normal hand function. An excellent result is normal hand function, not a perfect X-ray. With this in mind, our management sequence is as follows:

1. **History** is taken to determine the nature of the injury and the causal mechanism. This provides an initial impression of what is injured, the force transmitted to the injured part, and what treatment was provided.

2. **Symptom** complaints are noted. Not all abnormalities noted on an X-ray will be related to the current problem. Although it is important to note all abnormalities, it is essential that symptoms correlate with the X-ray abnormalities identified.

3. **Physical Examination** is recorded. A thorough examination notes any deformity, swelling, or tenderness. Joint stability is tested except in special cases, such as suspected collateral ligament ruptures at the metacarpal phalangeal (MP) joint of the thumb. Neurovascular status and tendon function is tested and noted.

4. **X-rays** are obtained and should include adequate numbers of views to provide complete characterization of the fracture. This usually includes at least a posterior–anterior, lateral, and oblique views, but may include other views if necessary.

Once a diagnosis is established, treatment is directed to obtain the best long-term function. Although this long-term function at outcome takes priority, other considerations include the shortest treatment course, the best short-term results, and which treatment is most compatible with the patient's lifestyle and occupation. Keep in mind that there usually is more than one treatment option, and the expected outcome from any treatment choice may not be entirely predictable or clear. The patient deserves to be informed and should participate in the treatment decision-making process. Conservative options may include splinting, casting, or buddy taping, with or without closed reduction. Surgical options may include closed procedures with percutaneous fixation or open procedures with wire, plate, screw, or external fixation. If a surgical solution is selected, additional scarring is an unavoidable consequence. Therefore the benefits of open intervention must be sufficient to overcome this.

In treating hand fractures, the following guidelines should be kept in mind.

1. **Frequent early follow-up.** Early follow-up is vital to the outcome of fracture management. With conservative treatment methods, it allows for an early repeat X-ray evaluation to detect any change in fracture alignment. This facilitates changes in treatment before fracture healing progresses to the point at which cor-

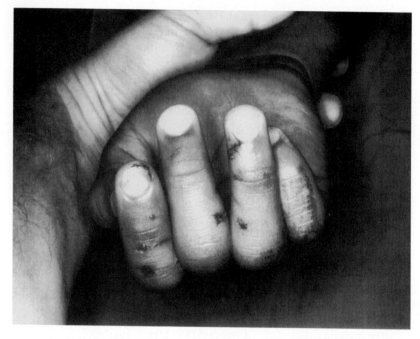

Figure 7-1 Proximal rotational deformity causes distal scissoring.

rection of problems becomes difficult. In all cases, early evaluation will detect unsatisfactory rehabilitation efforts and provides an opportunity to change the rehabilitation protocol or to reinforce the importance of compliance to the patient.

2. **Early motion produces early return of function.** One of the most important steps in rehabilitating a hand fracture is reestablishing motion at the earliest opportunity. Involved joint motion should begin within days of the injury or surgery. Rigid fixation of unstable fractures facilitates early motion. For stable fractures, motion should also begin within days of the injury.

3. **Consequences of hand fractures may take 6 to 12 months to resolve.** Individuals unaccustomed to treating or managing hand fractures often expect pain, swelling and stiffness to dispel within weeks of the injury. Although this may be the time frame for some patients, more often it will be 6 to 12 months before the injury heals. It is useful to inform patients that some scarring created by the injury often will persist and produce a permanent enlargement, especially around joints. This is not to say that the involved hand cannot be of use for this period of time. In most cases, patients are using their hands for regular activity within 8 to 12 weeks of the injury.

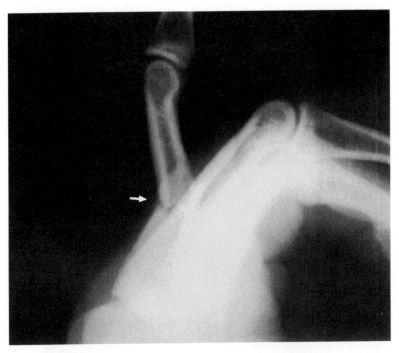

Figure 7-2 Proximal phalangeal fractures often occur with volar angulation. The magnitude of the angulation will result in an equal magnitude of lost flexion.

4. **The more proximal the fracture, the more significant rotational deformities become.** Residual rotational deformities in the distal phalanx will have almost no consequence. However, the same cannot be said for metacarpal fractures. Because of amplification to the length of the finger, a 5° rotation of a metacarpal fracture will translate into more than 1 cm of scissoring at the end of the finger (Fig. 7-1), whereas the same 5° rotation in the distal phalanx will produce no scissoring at all.

5. **Dorsal angulation of the proximal phalanx means loss of flexion.** Dorsal angulation of proximal phalangeal fractures results in loss of flexion at least as great as the angulation. Full flexion of the MP joint is the maximal mechanical flexion allowed by the joint. Fully flexing the joint in the presence of a dorsally angulated fracture, as shown in Fig. 7-2, results in a loss of flexion equivalent to the angle of fracture.

6. **Examination of MP joint of the thumb should not stress the collateral ligaments until a ligamentous injury has been ruled out.** If the ulnar collateral ligament of the MP joint of the thumb is torn or involved with an avulsion fracture, stress testing may cause the

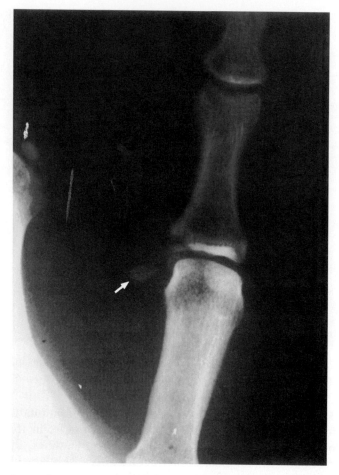

Figure 7-3 The proximally displaced bone fragment is attached to the ulnar collateral ligament, indicating the need for surgical repair.

ligament and fracture fragment to reflect superficial to the adductor aponeurosis. This will convert the injury into one that requires open repair and reapproximation of the ligament and fragment to the proximal phalanx of the thumb (Fig. 7-3).

FRACTURES OF THE DISTAL PHALANX

Closed fractures of the distal phalanx rarely need specific intervention. The discomfort often can be treated by the use of protective splints and finger caps. Transverse fractures with minimal contact between major bony fragments should be reduced. Significant nailbed injuries also should be repaired. In the case of open fractures, debridement, irrigation, and repair of lacerations are essential to the treatment of the fracture. This should be done under sterile conditions, which may require treatment in the operating room. However, if such conditions can be achieved in the emergency department, satisfactory results may be obtained, usually in a more timely fashion.

Tuft Fractures

The most common fracture of the distal phalanx is the tuft fracture. The usual history reveals a crushing-type injury. Patients often report that the fingertip was caught in a door or piece of machinery.

The patient may report significant pain in the fingertip, which can persist for several weeks after the injury. These injuries frequently involve lacerations that may or may not penetrate the nailbed. For closed injuries, the most frequent finding would be a subungual hematoma. A general assessment of the extent of the subungual hematoma should be made, and careful inspection of the base of the nail should be performed to ascertain whether the nail plate has been avulsed from its proximal bed. Avulsion of the nail plate implies significant lacerations of the nail matrix itself. Although X-rays are not particularly helpful in treating tuft fractures, an X-ray is warranted to rule out midshaft distal phalanx fractures with significant bony displacement and to rule out proximal avulsions.

Treatment of tuft fractures falls into two categories. For those fractures without significant nailbed injuries, treatment may be entirely conservative, with the use of protective splints or finger caps to treat the discomfort of the injury. Surgical intervention in simple closed tuft fractures without nailbed injuries is rarely, if ever, indicated. In those fractures that do involve significant nailbed lacerations, removal of the nail plate is indicated, with careful repair of the germinal and sterile matrix using fine suture and loupe magnification. Once the nail plate has been removed, it is advisable to save the nail plate for use after repair of the nailbed to stent the repair. This also will hold open the eponychial fold, preventing synechia. Little, if any, follow-up therapy is necessary. The patient should be examined within 7 to 10 days for wound inspection and to evaluate the progress of range of motion of the distal interphalangeal joint. Motion is encouraged immediately after injury and repair. If a satisfactory range of motion is not achieved, then referral to a hand rehabilitation therapist is in order.

The patients usually are able to return to limited light use of the involved digit within 2 to 3 weeks, and to full use within 6 weeks without serious discomfort. Full recovery and resolution of all discomfort in the finger usually takes several months. The patient must be advised that growth of the nail plate may be arrested for some time after the injury. When growth resumes, there often will be a ridge in the nail

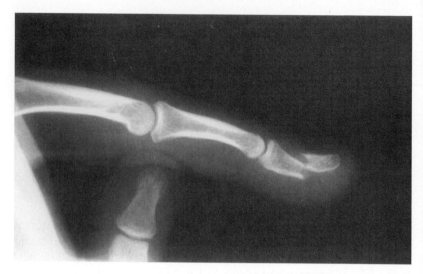

Figure 7-4   Distal phalangeal fractures with little or no bony contact will benefit from closed reduction.

that is followed by a smoothing over time. The patient also should be informed that some permanent nail deformity may follow.

Shaft Fractures

Shaft fractures of the distal phalanx usually do not require any intervention. The history and symptoms frequently are similar to those of tuft fractures, and examination also is generally unremarkable except for swelling and tenderness. Nailbed disruptions and subungual hematomas tend to be less frequent. X-rays are useful in shaft fractures, primarily to determine the extent of bony displacement. Initial treatment consists of a closed reduction under a digital block anesthetic when bony contact has been lost between the two segments of the shaft fracture (Fig. 7-4). When significant bony contact remains, conservative treatment with protective splints or finger caps will suffice to treat the patient symptomatically. If the proximal nail has been avulsed from the nail fold, it is useful to reduce the nail plate and hold it with one or two sutures. This helps maintain reduction of the distal phalanx fracture as well.

Occasionally, in very proximal shaft fractures in which it is difficult to maintain reduction, a longitudinal K-wire may be placed for fracture fixation. Follow-up in the case of conservatively treated fractures should be within 7 to 10 days to determine the range of motion of the IP joint involved. When adequate range of motion is not being initiated

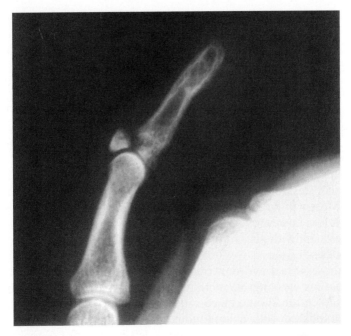

Figure 7-5   This avulsion has resulted in a mallet deformity.

by the patient, referral to a hand therapist is indicated. Attempts at range of motion exercises usually are begun within a few days of injury. Return of limited use of the digit may be accomplished within 2 to 3 weeks, and full use within 6 to 8 weeks. Full recovery may take several months.

Proximal Avulsion Fractures of the Distal Phalanx

Special considerations are appropriate for both volar and dorsal avulsions from the distal phalanx, because these areas involve the insertion of the extensor and flexor tendons, respectively.

The history may vary in the case of avulsion fractures, but most patients report a strike on the end of the finger by a ball in athletic endeavors. In the case of volar avulsions, the history is often of a vigorous grasping activity followed by pain. Signs and symptoms include pain and swelling at the area of the distal interphalangeal joints. In most cases, no significant deformity may be found on examination, except for the loss of extension or flexion.

The most common avulsion of the distal phalanx is from the dorsal surface at the attachment of the extensor tendon. This may produce a mallet deformity (Fig. 7-5). The initial X-ray should be examined carefully to determine whether the major phalangeal fragment maintains joint congruity. Loss of joint parallelism implies subluxation of the phalanx. In cases in which parallelism of the joint does remain, the fracture may be treated conservatively with extension splinting for 6 weeks. After the 6 weeks of extension splinting, the splint is gradually weaned off the finger, with replacement of the splint on a full-time basis if extension lag recurs at the distal interphalangeal joint. When necessary, the splint is replaced for 2 weeks before weaning is tried again. This process could continue for up to 12 weeks, at which time further efforts at splinting would be abandoned.

After prolonged splinting approximately 20 to 30% of patients will have some residual extension lag at the distal interphalangeal (DIP) joint. Most will be 15° or less and will not have any functional problems. A few, however, will have severe extension lag or persistent pain. In these individuals, improvement may be obtained with DIP arthrodesis.

In those dorsal avulsion fractures in which the major distal fragment has lost its congruity with the distal interphalangeal joint, operative intervention should be considered for reduction of the joint. This is accomplished with a longitudinal Kirschner wire (K-wire) which holds the fragment in place. The pin is left in place for 6 weeks, after which it is removed and the joint is treated as it would be for a mallet deformity after 6 weeks of splinting. The patient will be unable to use the involved digit for heavy labor for at least 6 to 8 weeks from the time of initial treatment, and full recovery takes several months.

Volar avulsions may imply a volar plate injury or flexor tendon avulsion. The more proximal volar avulsions are usually from the attachment of the volar plate. In most cases, these are relatively minor injuries that can be treated conservatively with early range of motion exercises. Avoidance of hyperextension of the volar joint should be emphasized during the initial treatment period.

More distal avulsions would be representative of avulsion injury of the flexor digitorum profundus. These injuries usually occur with a grasping-type activity, followed by pain at the distal interphalangeal joint or along the flexor tendon sheath of the involved digit. On examination, the patient is unable to actively flex the distal phalanx. X-rays may be unremarkable, but sometimes reveal an avulsion fragment within the flexor tendon sheath itself (Fig. 7-6).

Treatment of avulsed flexor digitorum profundus tendons with or without a fragment involves reinsertion of the tendon. The follow-up will be as in a flexor tendon advancement or insertion protocol (see Chapter 5). The patient can be expected to return to limited use of the digit in 6 to 8 weeks and full use in 8 to 12 weeks. Full recovery will take 3 to 4 months.

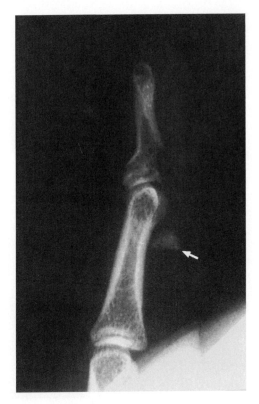

Figure 7-6   Avulsion of the flexor digitorum profundus may include a bony fragment that will usually be seen in the flexor tendon sheath.

Dislocations of the Distal Interphalangeal Joint

Dislocations of the distal interphalangeal joint are uncommon. In our practice, the most common mechanism of injury is motor vehicle accidents or significant falls. The patient usually is seen in the emergency department with pain in the affected fingers. Physical examination reveals obvious distortion at the distal interphalangeal joint. X-rays confirm subluxation or dislocation (Fig. 7-7). Treatment consists of a digital block followed by manual distraction of the distal phalanx and reduction of the joint. After reduction, active motion in the joint is verified. Dislocations may be associated with disruption of either the extensor tendon or the flexor tendon. If active motion verifies that the tendons remain intact, postreduction care consists of early active motion. The patient may have limited use of the involved fingers for 3 to

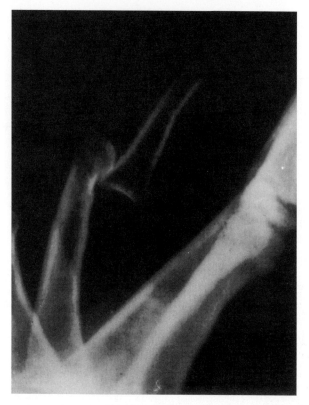

Figure 7-7   Dislocation of the distal interphalangeal joint.

4 weeks; it will take months for the result of the injury to become evident. Early motion is vital in these patients because there is a tendency to develop significant stiffness at the distal interphalangeal joint if motion is not initiated early.

Crush Injuries of the DIP Joints

Severe crush injuries of the distal interphalangeal joints are usually the result of mechanical injuries at a job site. The patient may have a closed wound, but often this is an open injury. Examination usually reveals a painful, swollen joint that may be markedly distorted. X-rays typically demonstrate severely comminuted fractures of the distal interphalangeal joint (Fig. 7-8). It is useful to inform patients from the outset that permanently restricted motion is likely following these injuries.

Treatment will vary depending on the degree of comminution of the

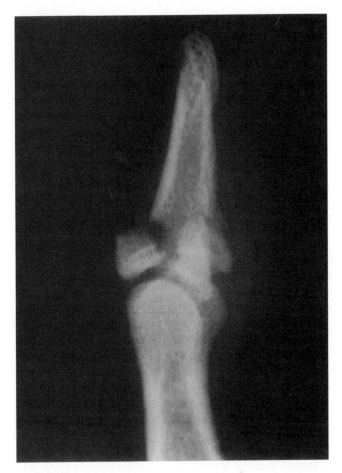

Figure 7-8   Severely comminuted DIP fractures are best treated with splints.

joint. In those joints with minimal comminution, screw or pin fixation may reconstitute a joint and facilitate efforts to regain motion in the distal interphalangeal joint. In severely comminuted joints, the problem often is best addressed with simple splinting, allowing the joint to autofuse or develop a pseudarthrosis. In the case of a pseudarthrosis, however, the joint may go on to be painful in the future and eventually require a formal fusion.

MIDDLE PHALANGEAL FRACTURES

In addressing middle phalangeal fractures, attention must be paid to angulation, rotation, and displacement of the fractures. Although rotation is of only minimal concern, displacement and angulation can affect both the cosmetic appearance of the finger and ultimate function. The flexor and extensor tendon involvement becomes an issue in middle phalanx fractures. Their close proximity to the underlying phalanx makes them subject to tendon adhesions that ultimately influence the outcome of any fracture involving the middle phalanx. In addition, two joints—the proximal interphalangeal joint and the distal interphalangeal joint—are subject to capsular fibrosis that creates joint stiffness after injuries to the middle phalanx. Swelling and subsequent collagen deposition in and about joint structures produce stiffness in joints even when not directly involved with the initial trauma or fracture.

Distal Middle Phalanx Fractures

The most common fracture of the middle phalanx is a transverse distal fracture. This fracture tends to be severely angulated and very difficult to reduce. It frequently heals with significant stiffness, especially at the distal interphalangeal joint, because of joint capsular fibrosis and tendon adhesions. Examination reveals a contused, painful phalanx that may show visible signs of deformity. X-rays often will demonstrate a dorsally tilted distal fragment within 1 cm of the distal interphalangeal joint. Closed reduction may be attempted in the emergency room under a digital block anesthetic. However, these efforts usually are not successful. The finger should be splinted for comfort until definitive treatment can be obtained. This usually requires open reduction and internal fixation in the operating room. If the fracture can be reduced under closed manipulation in the emergency room and remains stable, then early gentle motion may be initiated at the distal interphalangeal joint and proximal interphalangeal joint, along with very close follow-up and repeat X-rays to ascertain whether reduction has been maintained. Fractures that are unstable or cannot be reduced are managed with open reduction and internal fixation. This may be accomplished under digital block or regional anesthesia. Fixation methods include crossed K-wires, tension band wiring, screws, or small plates. Postoperative and rehabilitation periods should include immediate active motion followed by passive motion exercise typically beginning at 3 weeks. Percutaneous K-wires generally are removed between 4 and 6 weeks. This is followed by intensive hand therapy for 3 to 4 weeks to maximize range of motion. The patient can return to light use of the hand in 3 to 4 weeks if adequate fixation is obtained and in 4 to 6 weeks for less rigid forms of fixation, such as K-wires, or when no fixation was used. Return to full use will be at 8 to 12 weeks, and full recovery cannot be expected for several months.

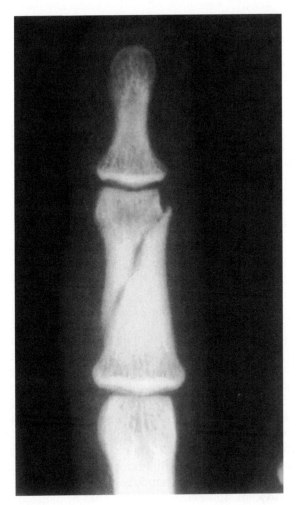

Figure 7-9   Common oblique fracture of the middle phalanx.

Shaft Fractures

Shaft fractures of the middle phalanx generally are transverse or oblique. The oblique, or spiral, fractures are seen somewhat more commonly than the transverse fracture (Fig. 7-9). Physical examination may reveal only tenderness at the fracture site, but X-rays will demonstrate the spiral nature. These, as opposed to the more distal fractures, tend to be somewhat more stable and often are minimally displaced.

Those fractures that are minimally displaced or that can be reduced under digital block and maintain reduction can be treated conserva-

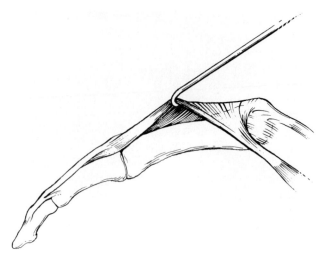

Figure 7-10 Elevation of lateral bands facilitates exposure of fractures in the distal half of the proximal phalanx.

tively with early motion and buddy taping. Follow-up should be within 7 to 10 days, with repeat X-rays to confirm that fracture reduction remains adequate. It should be pointed out that the fracture reduction does not have to be perfectly anatomic and that motion in the digits without evidence of scissoring is more important than perfect fragment alignment on an X-ray. Angulation of more than 10° is reason for consideration of reduction and, if unstable, rigid fixation. Otherwise uncomplicated spiral or oblique fractures that shorten less than 4 to 5 mm typically do not impair ultimate function. The posttreatment course should include intensive hand therapy to minimize both tendon adhesions and joint stiffness. Attention should be directed to both extension and flexion.

In those fractures that remain unstable or that cannot be reduced by closed measures, open reduction is indicated. The approach to the fracture is through a dorsal incision using either a digital or regional anesthetic. Tourniquet control is essential to facilitate dissection and visualization. The extensor tendon may be elevated by incising just volar to the lateral bands, elevating the extensor tendon off the middle phalanx, exposing the fracture (Fig. 7-10). The preferred fixation method for oblique fractures is placement of lag screws. The technique for placement and lagging of screws is described in detail in the section on screws and plates. Plates generally are difficult to apply to the middle phalangeal fractures because of the close adherence of the overlying extensor tendon to the fracture itself. If plates are selected for fixation, use of very small microplates will minimize interference with the extensor tendons. In those fractures that cannot be treated adequately with screws or plates because of comminution or the direction and nature of the fracture, adequate fixation may be achieved using crossed K-wires. These should be avoided if possible because the pins tend to interfere to a greater extent with the collateral ligament system, especially at the distal interphalangeal joint. This increases the likelihood of permanent stiffness. Fixation with K-wires also tends to be less rigid, limiting immediate postoperative motion. Furthermore, pin tract infections, although easily managed in most cases, are not a rare complication.

There are a few occasions where cerclage or tension band wiring may be applied usefully to fractures of the middle phalanx, especially those that are nearly transverse (see the section on fixation methods). The postoperative follow-up for all open reduction, internal fixation fractures of the middle phalanx includes intensive hand therapy within a few days of surgery. Intensive therapy should continue throughout the recovery period. When used, K-wires should be removed at 4 to 6 weeks. Return to light use may be allowed in 4 to 6 weeks, full use in 8 to 12 weeks. The patient should be informed that it will be 9 months to a year before full recovery can be anticipated. Occasionally, secondary procedures, such as tenolysis or capsulotomies, may be required to achieve maximal return of function.

Proximal Middle Phalangeal Fractures

Fractures in the proximal portion of the middle phalanx present unique problems. Like the proximal fractures of the distal phalanx, the volar fractures and the dorsal fractures must be addressed separately. The dorsal fractures generally are an avulsion-type fracture at the insertion of the central slip of the extensor mechanism. These are unusual fractures and usually are picked up by X-ray. Visualization of dorsal avulsion fragments implies a central slip injury and should be treated as a closed boutonniere injury. The finger should be splinted in extension at the PIP joint. Extension splinting will be maintained for 6 weeks, at which time intensive hand therapy is necessary to achieve return of flexion at the proximal interphalangeal joint. In some instances, the return of flexion is unsatisfactory, and it may become necessary to perform capsulotomies. Full use of the digit can be obtained in 8 to 12 weeks, and complete recovery may take 9 months to 1 year.

The volar fractures appear as either a large volar fragment or a

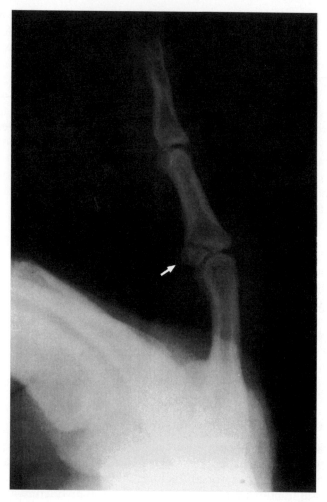

Figure 7-11 Fracture at the insertion of the volar plate with minimal displacement.

crush injury to the volar lip of the middle phalanx. Examination may show some deformity and difficulty in flexion. X-rays confirm the fracture; in particular, they may show dorsal subluxation of the middle phalanx. Fracture dislocation injuries are the most serious injuries. Full motion of the PIP joint is difficult, if not impossible, to restore.

Volar lip fractures (Fig. 7-11) without subluxation of the middle phalanx may be treated initially with extension block splinting (See

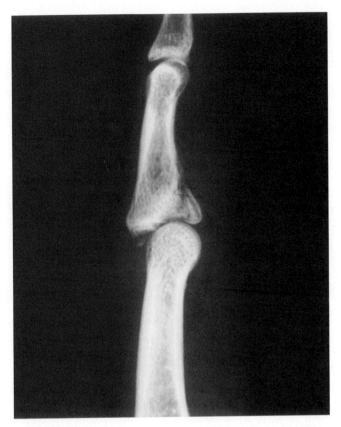

Figure 7-12   Subluxation of the middle phalanx will require ORIF on this fracture.

Chapter 12). Active flexion and limited extension exercises should begin immediately. The splint is modified to gradually allow full extension over a 3-week period. Repeat X-rays are essential to rule out developing subluxation of the phalanx. Return to light use can be achieved in 4 to 6 weeks, full use in 8 to 12 weeks. Complete recovery will take 9 months to 1 year, especially reduction of the swelling at the joint itself. Some degree of thickening of the PIP may be permanent, and the patient should be informed of this possibility at the outset.

Volar fractures that involve subluxation of the phalanx are a much more serious problem (Fig. 7-12). These must be reduced and, if closed reduction fails, open reduction and internal fixation is indicated. These fractures are best approached from a volar aspect of the joint. The

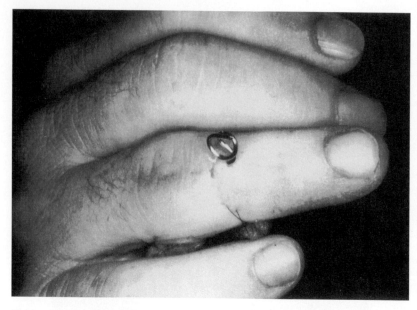

Figure 7-13   Buttons can be used as a tie holder or as shown here, the K-wire can be used to immobilize the PIP joint.

flexor tendon sheath is elevated off the volar plate of the proximal inter-phalangeal joint, exposing the volar plate and fracture. The fracture is approached distally, with care being taken to avoid separation of the fracture from the volar plate attachment. Suture or wire is woven into the volar plate and brought through a drill hole in the fragment. The drill hole is continued through the dorsum of the phalanx. Suture is tied over a button at that location, reducing the fracture fragment vo-larly. The dorsal subluxation is reduced and then held in place with a transarticular K-wire with the joint in 30° of flexion. The K-wire should be driven through the dorsal aspect of the middle phalanx into the proximal phalanx. This K-wire may be used in place of a button for the tie-over of the wire or suture placed in the volar fragment (Fig. 7-13).

Fractures that involve severe crush injuries of the volar lip of the middle phalanx can be approached volarly as described earlier. However, with severe comminution or crush-type injuries, debridement of the volar fragments may be necessary. A bony groove or trough is cre-ated in the volar aspect of the middle phalanx, and the volar plate is advanced into the groove using a technique described by Eaton and Malerich. The technique is similar to that already described for a frac-

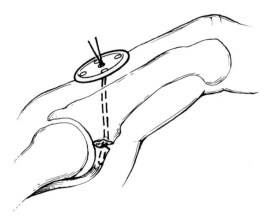

Figure 7-14   The volar plate is advanced into the groove produced in the volar lip of the middle phalanx.

ture fragment (Fig. 7-14). A suture is woven through the volar plate and brought out through a drill hole in the phalanx. It is tied over a button or the transarticular K-wire which holds the joint in 30° of flexion. Postoperatively, motion is begun at the MP and DIP joints. Motion at the proximal interphalangeal joint is impossible and should be protected during exercise periods to prevent fracture of the transarticular K-wire. The K-wire is removed in 3 to 4 weeks, and flexion is begun immediately after removing the transarticular K-wire. During a 2- to 3-week period, gradual extension is achieved with hand therapy. Return to limited use of the digit occurs at 6 to 8 weeks, full use at 10 to 12 weeks. Full recovery will take 9 months to 1 year.

Satisfactory reduction will not be achieved either by open or closed methods in the severely crushed proximal interphalangeal joint (Fig. 7-15). In our experience, these fractures are best treated by intraoperative placement of a transverse K-wire in the distal portion of the middle phalanx. The K-wire is brought out of either side of the digit, and a 90° bend placed in the wire on both sides. A loop is then placed in the wire itself. This loop provides for attachment of a traction apparatus that is fabricated by the hand rehabilitation therapist. This apparatus (Fig. 7-16) allows for flexion at the proximal interphalangeal joint while maintaining a slight amount of traction across the joint. Intensive hand therapy continues for 6 weeks, at which point the traction is discontinued and hand therapy without the traction apparatus is continued. A return to light activity can occur in 8 to 12 weeks; return to full activity will take 12 to 16 weeks. Final recovery will require approximately 1 year. This traction method has produced good results,

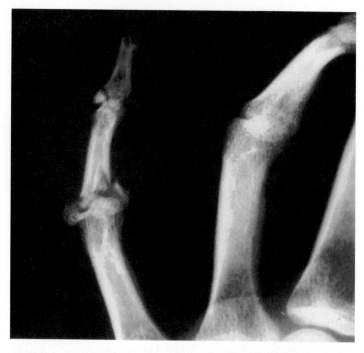

Figure 7-15 Crushed PIP joints are difficult to treat with methods other than traction.

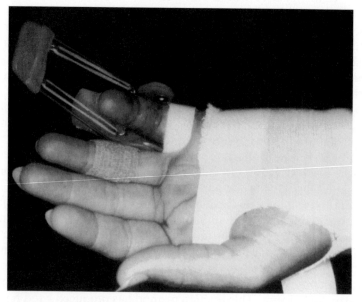

Figure 7-16 This low profile splint supplies traction for the crushed PIP joint and allows motion at the PIP joint by use of a hinge.

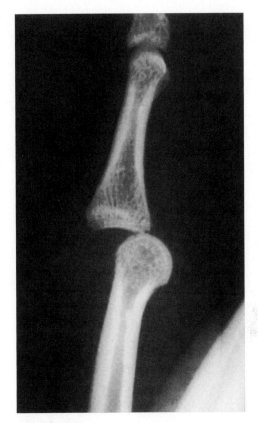

Figure 7-17   Dorsal PIP joint dislocations usually can be reduced readily by manipulation.

especially compared with what might be expected with these severely crushed joints.

Proximal Interphalangeal Dislocations

Proximal interphalangeal (PIP) dislocations happen relatively frequently. Most are athletic injuries that occur while the patient is playing basketball or softball. The majority of these are reduced in the field and are reported or considered as a "jammed finger." A few do make it to a physician, and X-rays reveal the dislocation. The dislocations may be dorsal (Fig. 7-17) or volar (Fig. 7-18).

Reduction of the joint is facilitated by a digital block anesthetic. After the patient is anesthetized, reduction can be achieved by digital pressure. For volar dislocations, however, closed reduction may be difficult or impossible. Although this is rare, the extensor mechanism

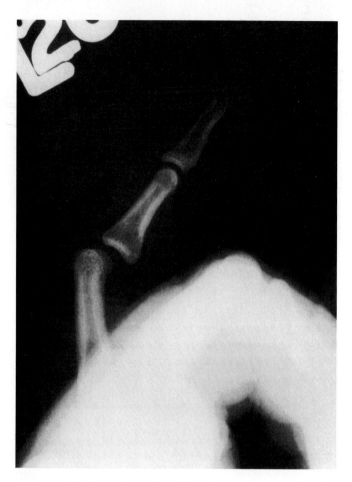

Figure 7-18   In this figure, the volar dislocation is maintained by the trapped condylar head on the proximal phalanx, which is caught protruding through a tear in the extensor mechanism.

may tear dorsally during volar dislocation. This allows the head of the proximal phalanx to project through the tendon mechanism. The condyl of the proximal phalanx then prevents easy reduction because it is trapped by the extensor tendon (Fig. 7-18). Reduction can be achieved easily by making a dorsal incision, lifting the lateral band trapping the head of the proximal phalanx over the condyle, and then repairing the tear in the extensor mechanism.

Volar dislocations also may result in disruption of the central slip insertion. If open reduction is necessary, the central slip insertion should be inspected closely. For closed injuries not requiring open reduction, injury to the central slip is suspected if extension of the PIP joint cannot be achieved with the MP joint fully flexed. This is not always a reliable test, and patients suspected of having sustained a volar dislocation of the PIP joint should be observed closely for any sign of developing boutonniere deformity.

Postreduction care consists of early hand therapy. Motion must be maintained to full flexion and full extension. This is achieved by initiating motion therapy within days of the injury. The exception to this rule is the individual with an injury to the central slip, which requires splinting in extension for 6 weeks.

Proximal Phalangeal Fractures

Proximal phalangeal fractures are in an area where rotation begins to play an important role in potential postinjury disability or loss of function. Angulation of the more proximal fractures of the proximal phalanx can result in a loss of range of motion at the MP joint equal to or greater than the degree of angulation that the fracture subtends. As in areas over the middle phalanx, tendon adhesions remain a significant consideration and problem postinjury. The extensor and flexor tendons remain in close contact with the underlying phalanx; adhesions are frequent and must be addressed early. In addition, capsular fibrosis leading to stiffness of the PIP and MP joints also is a major concern and must also be addressed early with hand therapy. The primary goals of treatment of proximal phalangeal fractures are the reduction to a functional position and early motion to prevent both strongly adherent tendon adhesions and joint capsular fibrosis limiting motion at the PIP and MP joints. Adjacent fingers also may be involved with some capsular fibrosis. Range of motion in these digits should not be neglected.

Distal Fractures

Distal fractures of the proximal phalanx often are intraarticular and involve condylar head fractures in which one or the other condyle fractures off (Fig. 7-19). This creates a displacement through the joint that ultimately may lead to traumatic arthritis at the proximal interphalangeal joint. The patient is seen in the acute phase, with ecchymoses, swelling, and tenderness about the distal end of the proximal phalanx. Typically, there is some inhibition of motion secondary to pain and swelling. X-ray confirms the nature of the fracture, which often is a single oblique fracture splitting off one condylar head, but may include severe comminutions or both condyles.

Intraarticular fractures that are not displaced may be treated conservatively. However, early motion is essential to help minimize joint

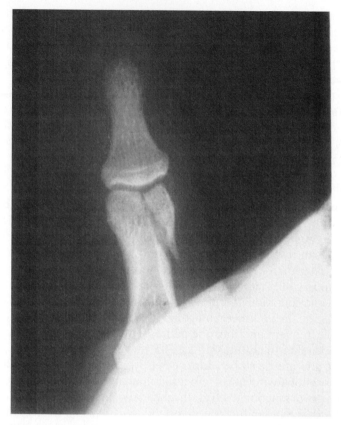

Figure 7-19   Fractures of the condylar head can be fixed with a single lag screw.

stiffness and reconstitute the cartilaginous surface. In these cases, the fractured finger may be buddy taped to an adjacent finger and early protected motion begun. The patient should be instructed to avoid heavy lifting or significant use of the hand for any work or recreational activities. Active range of motion is strongly encouraged. Early follow-up should include repeat X-rays to confirm that no further displacement of the involved fragment has occurred.

Fractures with more than 1 mm of displacement at the intraarticular surface, especially those that are displaced in a longitudinal direction, creating a step off, should be considered for open reduction and internal fixation. Initially, these fractures are treated by simple splinting. This is adequate until arrangements can be made for elective open reduction and internal fixation. The fracture is approached from a dorsal incision. The retinacular ligament is incised just volar to the lateral bands that are elevated to expose both the proximal interphalangeal joint and the fracture itself. The dorsal capsule can be incised, but care should be taken to avoid injury to the central slip insertion on the middle phalanx. The fracture is then reduced under direct vision and the articular surface checked for congruity. The fracture may be fixed in this position with a bone clamp and lag screws placed to hold the fragment in its anatomic position. Reduction and fixation are verified under fluoroscopy or with intraoperative X-rays. In the immediate follow-up period, the patient begins active range of motion exercises administered by a hand therapist. The patient can expect to return to light activity with the hand in 4 to 6 weeks and may return to full use of the hand in 8 to 12 weeks. The patient is advised that final recovery, as in most hand injuries, will take 9 months to 1 year and that some permanent loss in range of motion may occur.

Severely comminuted distal fractures of the proximal phalanx with destruction of the phalangeal head are unusual. These may be treated in the manner already described for severe crush injuries of the PIP joint with traction on the middle phalanx. Basically, a transverse K-wire is placed in the middle phalanx to which a splint, fabricated for early motion at the proximal interphalangeal joint, may be attached.

Midshaft Fractures

Shaft fractures of the middle phalanx usually are oblique or spiraling. In comminuted fractures, multiple longitudinal and oblique fragments occur. The spiral fractures, oblique fractures, and butterfly or three-part fractures of the shaft of the middle phalanx may remain relatively stable. Shortening can be accepted, if it is less than 3 to 4 mm. In patients who require fine use of their digits, such as professional musicians, this degree of shortening may be unacceptable. X-rays characterize the fracture well and should be examined carefully to determine whether there is significant angulation at the fracture site itself. Stable fractures can be managed with 6 weeks of buddy taping.

When angulation greater than approximately 10° exists, we recommend open reduction and internal fixation. These fractures are approached through a dorsal incision. Fractures that need to be visualized in the proximal third of the shaft require approach through a tendon-splitting incision. This is accomplished by making a longitudinal incision in the extensor tendon down its center. The tendon is repaired after fracture fixation using nonabsorbable horizontal mattress sutures. The more distal fractures, however, still may be approached by elevating the extensor tendon, first incising just volar to the lateral bands. The oblique, spiral, and butterfly fragments generally are treated best with lag screws (Fig. 7-20). Please refer to the section on

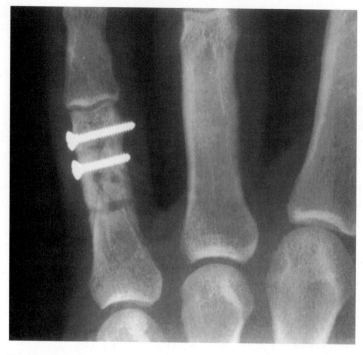

Figure 7-20 Lag screws easily reduce oblique or butterfly fragments.

screws and plates for a description of the operative methods of placing lag screws. In the more transverse fractures, lag screws become difficult or impossible to place to achieve satisfactory fixation. Under these circumstances, attempts are made to place small plates on the dorsum of the phalanx (Fig. 7-21). Other considerations for fixation when plates or screws are not feasible are the placement of tension band wiring or crossed K-wires. The use of tension band wiring presupposes that the comminuted fracture is not severe. Before fixation, verify the absence of any rotational deformity by flexing the PIP joints and observing for any evidence of "scissoring" or overlap of the fingers distally.

Fractures that are severely comminuted can often be treated with the placement of crossed K-wires, which help prevent dorsal angulation and maintain alignment of the finger. In the immediate postoperative period, the patient is referred to the hand rehabilitation center for active range of motion exercises. These are started within a few days of surgery. Patients with fractures that have been treated conservatively should also begin early range of motion exercises. Three follow-up X-rays are taken 1 week apart to determine that there has been no change in fracture configuration or reduction. K-wires are removed in 4 to 6

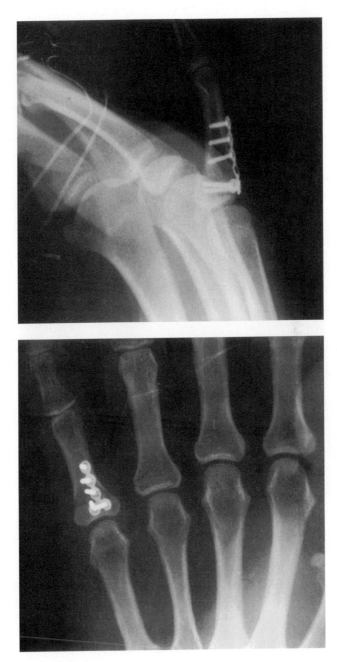

Figure 7-21   Small plates currently available with low profile screws will adequately fix proximal phalanx transverse fractures.

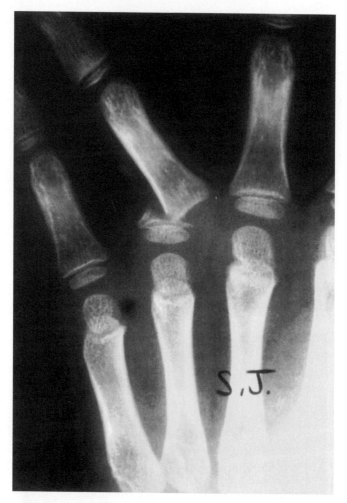

Figure 7-22   This is a common fracture in children and, once reduced, is usually stable. Reduction is accomplished easily by placing a pencil in the long/ring web space and squeezing the distal portion of the digits together.

weeks. Light activity is begun between 4 and 6 weeks, when rigid fixation methods, such as lag screws or plates, have been used, and 6 to 8 weeks when K-wires or tension band wiring has been used. The patient can expect to return to full work activity, depending on the nature of the job, in 8 to 12 weeks. Full recovery requires 9 months to 1 year.

PROXIMAL FRACTURES OF THE PROXIMAL PHALANX

Proximal fractures of the proximal phalanx are frequently transverse in nature and significantly angulated (Fig. 7-22). These are well characterized on X-rays, but be sure to obtain multiple views, because one or two views may not adequately demonstrate the fracture. Transverse fractures in children tend to be stable once reduced, but are often unstable in adults. Attempts at conservative treatment of transverse fractures, and in particular, attempts at closed reduction, are often unsuccessful because of the difficulty in obtaining control of the more proximal fragment that is essentially floating loose on the MP joint. Fractures with more than 10° of angulation are considered for open reduction and internal fixation. These fractures are approached dorsally and a tendon-splitting incision is used, exposing both the MP joint and the fracture. The fracture may then be reduced under direct vision and fixed, preferably with small plates if enough bone stock is present proximally to allow for screw placement. Please refer to the section on screws and plates for the technical details of plate fixation on the phalanges. If the proximal fragment is too comminuted or small for plate fixation, adequate fixation may be obtained by using crossed K-wires. Attempts are made to place the K-wires well away from the collateral ligaments of either the PIP or the MP joints. The K-wires do not provide rigid fixation, but do prevent the angulation from recurring if adequately placed. The K-wires are driven from proximal to distal catching the shoulder of the proximal fragment. They are then preferably driven out the distal fragment and withdrawn distally to minimize interference with the extensor tendon mechanism. The tendon-splitting incision is repaired with nonabsorbable horizontal mattress sutures. The patient is begun on active range of motion exercises in the early postoperative period. For patients who have had K-wire fixation, the wires are removed in 4 to 6 weeks and hand therapy efforts are intensified after removal of the pins. The patient can expect to return to light activity in 4 to 6 weeks and full activity in 8 to 12 weeks. Final recovery, however, will take 9 months to 1 year.

INTRAARTICULAR FRACTURES OF THE MP JOINT

Intraarticular fractures of the proximal phalanx are considered for open reduction and internal fixation when displacement of the fracture, especially in longitudinal directions, exceeds approximately 1 mm. These intraarticular fractures should be evaluated closely on the X-ray to determine the location of the fractured fragment. The fracture may extend through a sagittal plane, which allows one to approach the fracture through a dorsal incision. However, many intraarticular fractures of the proximal portion of the proximal phalanx are volarly located. These are difficult to visualize from a dorsal incision, and a volar approach, as later described, should be considered. For fractures that are approached dorsally, a longitudinal, tendon-splitting incision is used. Lag screw fixation generally will hold the fracture after its has been reduced under direct vision. This requires careful inspection of the intraarticular portion of the fracture to be sure that joint congruity has been reestablished. The tendon-splitting incision is repaired with nonabsorbable sutures, and the patient begins early active motion exercises in the immediate postoperative period. Passive motion exercises can begin within 3 to 4 weeks to supplement the active motion exercises begun in the early postoperative period.

Volar fragments, especially the large avulsion fractures, can be approached from a volar incision. A zigzag incision is made over the area of the A-1 pulley. The A-1 pulley is then split, allowing retraction of the flexor tendons to one side or the other. This exposes the volar plate, which is incised longitudinally along its edges to expose the fracture and the joint. The fracture is reduced under direct vision and, generally, screw or K-wire fixation is possible from this location (Fig. 7-23). As in all cases, early active motion exercises are begun in the immediate postoperative period, and intensive hand therapy continues for 4 to 6 weeks. The patient may return to light activity in 4 to 6 weeks and heavy use in 8 to 12 weeks. Full recovery may be expected in 9 months to 1 year.

Small avulsion fractures of the proximal phalanx (Fig. 7-24) are treated conservatively with simple buddy taping to an adjacent finger. This provides support for the collateral ligaments and allows early motion.

Fracture dislocations of the proximal phalanx at the MP joint are unusual in absence of severely comminuted fractures with major intraarticular fragments. These fractures should be approached as already described for intraarticular fractures of the joint, achieving joint congruity and adequate fixation to allow for early motion. Severely crushed joints may be treated with a traction apparatus as already described for the proximal interphalangeal joint by placement of a transverse K-wire in the distal portion of the proximal phalanx. A hinged splint is fabricated by the hand rehabilitation therapist for immediate motion. Adequate follow-up of these proximal phalanx fractures is of vital importance to the ultimate outcome and function. Early active motion is encouraged very strongly, and intensive hand therapy is promoted throughout the first 2 months.

MP Joint Dislocation

Dislocations of the MP joint are rarely seen in the office or emergency department. Most are reduced in the field or spontaneously reduce. If they do not reduce, these dislocations present special problems similar to those of volar dislocation at the PIP joint. At the MP joint, the dorsal dislocation is most likely to result in reduction problems

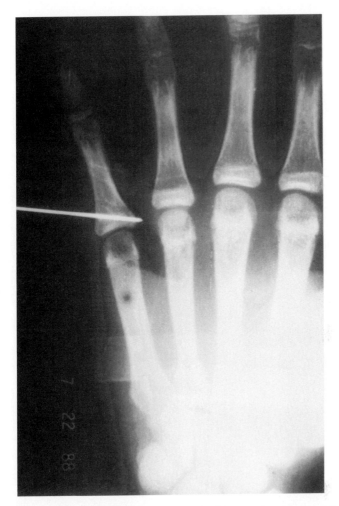

Figure 7-23 Volar fragments can be approached by incising the A-1 pulley and reflecting the volar plate distally. A K-wire may then be driven retrograde for fixation of volar fragments.

(Fig. 7-25). In these cases, the metacarpal head first disrupts the loose proximal attachments of the volar plate that protrude volar to the flexor tendons. The tendons then produce a loop extending dorsal to the head of the metacarpal. Attempts at closed reduction generally result in just tightening this loop, thereby making closed reduction impossible.

Reduction is accomplished through a volar incision at the distal

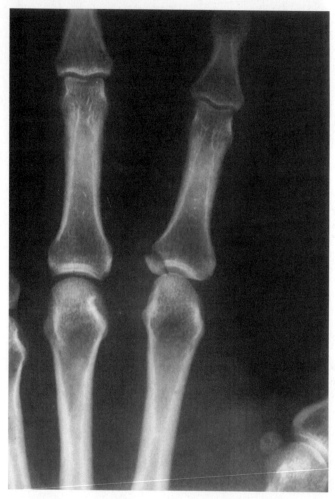

Figure 7-24   Small avulsions at the base of the proximal phalanx are best treated with buddy taping and early motion.

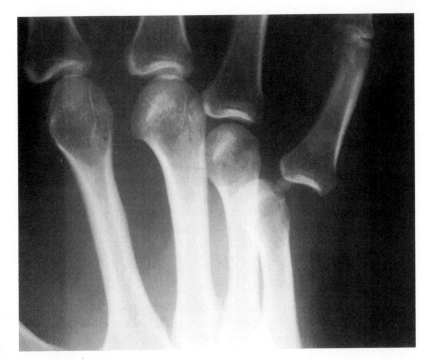

Figure 7-25   With dorsal dislocation of the MP joint, the metacarpal head may be trapped by the flexor tendons.

palmer crease. Generally, a Brunner incision is used. The cartilagenous surface of the metacarpal head will be seen immediately or on incising the A-1 pulley of the flexor tendon sheath. Once the A-1 pulley is incised, the flexor tendons can be lifted over the head of the metacarpal, allowing easy reduction of the joint. Postoperative care consists of early motion exercises. Recovery is complete in 6 weeks.

METACARPAL FRACTURES

Fractures of the metacarpal, particularly the little finger metacarpal, are very common in a hand surgery practice. The mechanism of injury frequently is punching a person, wall, window, or door. Hence, the injury is commonly called "boxer's" fracture. Typically, this injury results in a fracture of the head of the little finger metacarpal, but fractures throughout the length of the metacarpal, including its base, may be induced by this mechanism. In addition, any crushing mechanism or direct blow to the hand may be responsible for fractures of the metacarpal.

Angulation of these fractures tends to be less of a concern than angulations in the phalanges. The more serious problem that results from inadequate reduction of metacarpal fractures is malrotation. Displacement and shortening can be of concern in some individuals, but to a much lesser degree than the problems created by rotation. As already noted, small-angle rotational deformities of the metacarpal are amplified by the entire length of the finger, translating into significant displacements at the fingertip. The result is scissoring and functional limitations. Fractures near the metacarpal head frequently produce significant stiffness in the MP joints at this location, particularly in extension. In addition, fractures of the distal end of the metacarpals that are left unreduced may create cosmetic deformities by reducing the profile of the MP joint on the dorsum of the hand. For those fractures that are more proximal, angulation becomes more of a concern than does it does near the MP joints. Angulation in a more proximal fracture may produce lumps in the palm of the hand, which may interfere with gripping or holding on to objects with force.

DISTAL METACARPAL FRACTURES

The boxer's fracture or the fracture of the head of the little finger metacarpal is one of the most frequent fractures to the metacarpal (Fig. 7-26). Many surgeons believe that dorsal angulation of boxer's fractures up to 60° is acceptable and does not interfere significantly with function. At our institution, fractures with less than 30° of angulation are managed with splinting. We begin to be concerned for fractures with between 30 and 45° of angulation. Greater than 45°, we recommend reduction by closed or open methods. The more proximal the fracture, the more that angulation may interfere with hand function. For interior digits, angulated fractures may produce significant deformities across the dorsum of the hand. Therefore, angles of 20° or more are of concern in the ring, long, and index fingers.

Attempts at conservative treatment with closed reduction can be made, but these fractures tend to be unstable and the initial angulation often recurs. Reduction can be accomplished with a hematoma block at the fracture, followed by flexion of the MP joint to 90°, distal traction, and dorsal displacement of the fracture apex. Patients often are placed in an ulnar gutter splint initially, and may be treated with the splint for 3 to 4 weeks. However, this can result in significant stiffness and is not a practice we recommend. For fractures proximal to the head of the metacarpal of the index, long, ring, or little fingers, a Galveston splint (Fig. 7-27) can be used to maintain reduction once a closed reduction has been accomplished. The Galveston splint needs to be adjusted carefully to avoid pressure necrosis beneath the pressure pads, in particular on the dorsum of the hand. In addition, the splint

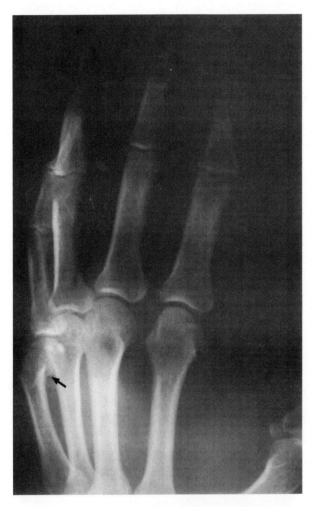

Figure 7-26   The most common fracture of the metacarpals is the distal meta-carpal of the little finger, commonly called a "boxer's fracture."

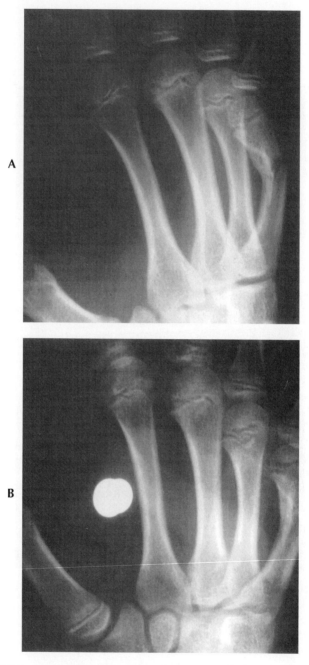

Figure 7-27 More proximal fractures of a metacarpal often can be treated with a Galveston splint. **(A)** Proximal angulated fracture. **(B)** X-ray with Galveston splint in place.

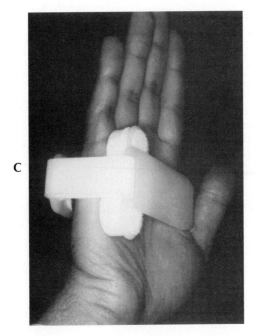

Figure 7-27—Cont'd   **(C)** Galveston splint.

will have a tendency to slide off to one side or the other of the metacarpal on the dorsum of the hand and should be adjusted carefully, with
marks placed on the skin so the patient can adjust the splint if necessary. Although motion at the MP joint is inhibited by the splint, it is
sufficient for satisfactory recovery of motion once the splint is discontinued at 4 to 5 weeks postinjury. We begin active range of motion
exercises immediately, and once the splint has been discontinued, vigorous therapy is begun to achieve better motion at the MP joint. For
more distal metacarpal head fractures, control of the distal fragment is
nearly impossible with the bulky Galveston splint. For these patients,
simple buddy taping and early motion may be satisfactory.

Fractures that are unstable or have more than 30 to 45° of angulation are considered for open reduction and internal fixation. In some
cases, closed reduction may be accomplished under fluoroscopic control, with a single or crossed K-wires placed percutaneously across the
fracture to maintain fixation. If this is not possible, then open reduction is performed. The fracture is approached through a dorsal incision
that retracts the extensor tendon and hood mechanism to one side to
expose the fracture. The fracture is fixed with lag screws, plates, or K-
wires (Fig. 7-28). Careful attention to reduction is imperative during
the fixation phase of an open reduction and internal fixation. The MP

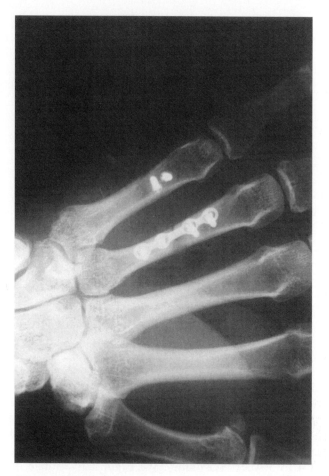

Figure 7-28 Metacarpal fractures may be fixed with lag screws, as seen in the little finger metacarpal, or plates as demonstrated here on the ring finger metacarpal. Crossed K-wires can be used when plates or screws are not usable.

joint should be flexed and rotational deformity at the fracture site corrected before fixation. Once the fracture has been fixed rigidly, periosteum and surrounding soft tissue is closed over any fixation device to prevent tendon adhesions. The patient is referred to a rehabilitation center for immediate range of motion therapy. Light use of the hand can be initiated in 3 to 4 weeks with rigid fixation and 4 to 6 weeks with K-wire fixation. The patient can return to full work activity in 8 to 12 weeks, but final recovery from the fracture will take 6 months to 1 year. If K-wires are used, these are left in place for 4 to 5 weeks.

Fractures of the metacarpal shaft tend to be transverse or oblique.

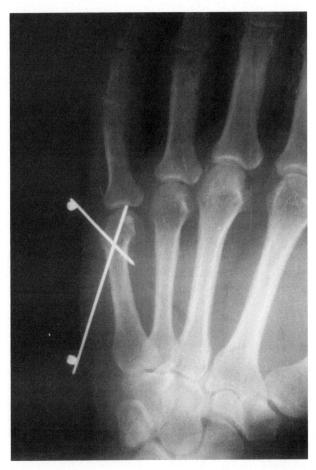

Figure 7-28—Cont'd   For legend see opposite page.

The transverse fractures tend to be unstable, and both types are subject to rotational deformities at this level. Care should be taken to assess the fracture for any rotational deformity. When these fractures are minimally displaced and rotational deformities are not present, conservative treatment with a wrist cock-up splint that extends to, but does not include, the MP joints can be used. Shortening of 4 to 5 mm generally will not produce any significant functional problems. This may not be true, however, for certain patients, such as professional musicians. In these patients, any degree of shortening should be corrected.

Early motion of the MP joints is begun to prevent joint stiffness. A

Galveston splint also may be used successfully at this level. Close follow-up is necessary to confirm that a rotational deformity does not develop and that the fracture remains reduced. Fractures that are unstable or rotated require open reduction, internal fixation. Fixation methods, in order of preference, are lag screws, plates, and K-wires. For metacarpal fractures in the midshaft portion, especially for interior digits of the long and ring fingers, fixation may be accomplished by transversely placed K-wires that pass through the adjacent metacarpals on either side of the fracture. To fully control the fragments, two K-wires should be placed distal to the fracture and, in some cases, proximal to the fracture as well. In any case, at least one pin will be necessary proximal to the fracture to adequately control the reduction. Early motion exercises are begun after surgery. Joint stiffness usually is not a problem, but extensor tendon adhesions at the fracture site may prevent full recovery of range of motion in the fingers. Early motion and hand rehabilitation therapy should be an essential part of treatment of these fractures. The patient may return to light activity in 4 to 6 weeks and heavy activity in 8 to 12 weeks. Final recovery will take 6 months to 1 year.

PROXIMAL METACARPAL FRACTURES

Fractures of the proximal metacarpals of the fingers are less common injuries. Those that do occur are most frequently at the little and ring fingers. These fractures may or may not be intraarticular, but the intraarticular extension of the fracture must be assessed carefully. Fractures of the little finger base (Fig. 7-29*A*) that involve significant offset of the articular surface should be considered for open reduction and internal fixation to preclude the development of painful arthritis at this joint in the future. This may necessitate evaluation by computed tomography (CT) scan.

Fractures of the little finger base are approached through an incision directly over or ulnar to the CM joint of the metacarpal. For intraarticular fractures, the joint should be opened to determine adequate reduction of the joint surfaces. The fractures may then be fixed by any convenient method. Although lagged screws are the preferred method, plates or K-wires may be adequate. If the fracture is comminuted severely, transverse K-wires between the little and ring finger metacarpals will provide adequate fixation and prevent collapse of the metacarpal (Fig. 7-29*B*). Range of motion in the fingers is begun immediately after the surgery. We generally keep the patient in a wrist cock-up splint for the first 3 weeks to allow additional immobilization of the fractured area.

The hand surgeon treating fractures at the base of the little finger

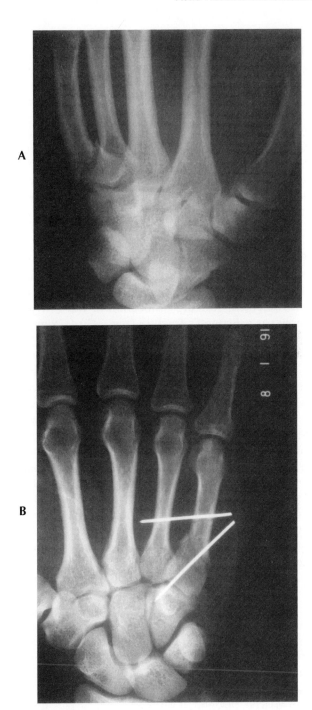

Figure 7-29   Proximal metacarpal fractures. **(A)** Fracture at the base of the little finger metacarpal. **(B)** Fixation is achieved with K-wires.

metacarpal should be aware that fracture of the hamate may be associated with these injuries. Any fracture of the hamate should be reduced with care to reestablish the joint surface at the same time surgery is performed on the metacarpal. If the joint is crushed sufficiently to preclude adequate reduction, consideration should be given to a primary arthrodesis.

Fractures of the ring and long finger metacarpal bases are encountered less frequently. When they do occur, reduction and fixation may be accomplished through dorsal exposure directly over the involved metacarpal. Fractures of this nature that we have treated have been fixed easily with K-wires or screws and generally heal without any long-term problems because of the minimal motion normally at these joints.

THUMB METACARPAL FRACTURES

Fractures of the thumb metacarpal often present a special problem. The majority of the fractures seen in the thumb metacarpal are at its base. The two-fragment fracture dislocation of the CM joint of the thumb is known as a Bennett's fracture (Fig. 7-30A). Significant concerns with this fracture are its intraarticular nature and displacement. Stabilizing ligaments remain with the ulnar fragment, allowing the major portion of the metacarpal to sublux radially. Any significant displacement or evidence of subluxation of the major fragment is an indication for open reduction and internal fixation. Bennett's fractures are approached through a radial incision along the metacarpal base. The thenar musculature is then reflected off the metacarpal, exposing the fracture fragments. The fracture is reduced under direct vision. The reduction is verified by intraarticular inspection of the joint surfaces. After achieving joint congruity, the fracture is fixed with screws or K-wires (Fig. 7-30B). The thumb is held in a spica splint for 3 to 4 weeks. When the splint is removed, motion at the CM joint is allowed unless restricted by K-wires. K-wires are removed at 4 to 6 weeks. Light activity may begin at 4 to 6 weeks and heavier activity at 8 to 12 weeks. Final recovery can be expected in 6 months to 1 year.

A very similar fracture is Rolando's fracture, which involves a comminuted intraarticular fracture of the base of the thumb. Fractures that involve three or four fragments may be candidates for open reduction and internal fixation using several screws or K-wires (Fig. 7-29). For more severely comminuted fractures at the base of the thumb metacarpal, the reduction of the fracture and the joint may be best obtained through ligamentotaxis. This is accomplished by placing traction on the thumb and then holding the metacarpal out at length with transverse K-wires placed through the thumb metacarpal into the index metacarpal. It is held in this position for 4 weeks. The pins are then

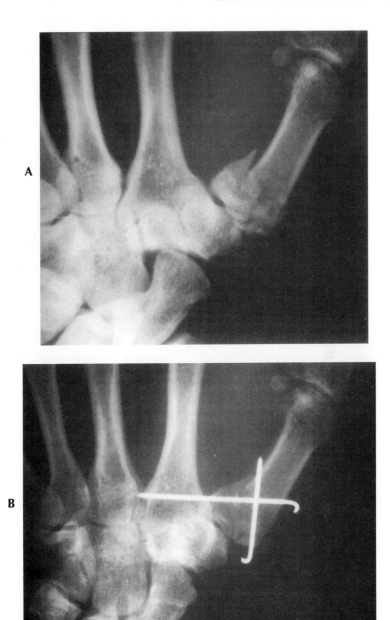

Figure 7-30   Bennett's fractures **(A)** are fracture/dislocations of the thumb metacarpal base. As near anatomic reduction as possible is indicated to prevent traumatic arthritis. **(B)** Fixation is achieved with K-wires.

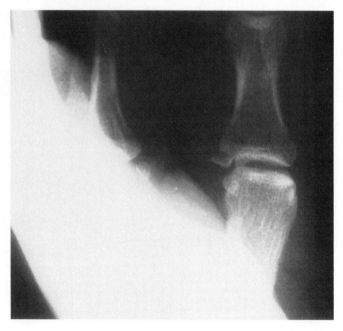

Figure 7-31   Thumb MP ulnar collateral ligament avulsions such as this should not be stressed. Instead the thumb should be immobilized for 6 weeks.

removed and motion is allowed. Fractures that are severely comminuted may ultimately develop painful arthritis of this joint, requiring either arthrodesis or arthroplasty.

THUMB METACARPAL JOINT INJURIES

Because of the prehensile use of the thumb, the MP joint is subjected to forces not commonly applied to the other digits. Injuries to the ulnar collateral ligament of the MP joint, known as "Gamekeeper's thumb," commonly occur in skiers. Pain at the MP joint of the thumb after trauma should be evaluated cautiously. An X-ray should be obtained before an examination that stresses the collateral ligaments of the joint. This will prevent turning an injury that may be treated nonoperatively (see Fig. 7-31) into one that requires operative repair (see Fig. 7-3). If a minimally displaced fragment is seen on X-ray, the thumb may be placed in a spica splint for 6 weeks. If no fragment is seen, the joint is tested for stability of the MP joint. Stener has described a lesion in which the ulnar collateral ligament is trapped proximal and superficial to the adductor aponeurosis. This may be palpated in some cases or, if an avulsion fragment is present, may be seen on X-

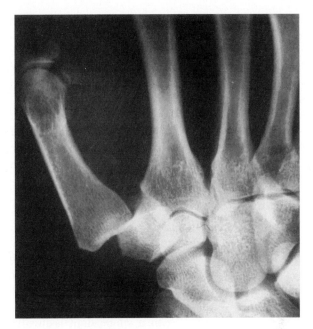

Figure 7-32   Thumb CM joint dislocations should be reduced and held for 6 weeks. If the reduction cannot be maintained, a ligamentous repair will be necessary.

ray with the fragment displaced markedly proximally. If a Stenner's lesion is present, or if the joint "opens up" more than 30°, operative repair is indicated. The collateral ligament is approached through an incision over the ligament. A nonabsorbable suture is woven into the ligament and then passed through the base of the metacarpal at the insertion site of the ligament. The suture is passed to the radial side and then out through the skin, where it is tied to a button. The MP joint is fixed in place with a transarticular K-wire. The wire and button are removed in 6 weeks.

Dislocation of the carpal metacarpal joint of the thumb also may produce long-term problems if not treated adequately. Pain at the CM joint after trauma should raise the suspicion of fracture or dislocation. Dislocation can be seen readily on X-ray, but may be easily missed without careful scrutiny (Fig. 7-32). Reduction is attempted with injection of a local anesthetic into the periarticular structures. If the joint can be reduced and remains stable, placing the thumb in a spica splint for 6 weeks will be adequate treatment. However, if the stabilizing ligaments of the CM joint have been injured sufficiently, long-term stability of the joint will be compromised. In this situation, reconstruction of the anterior oblique ligament, as described by Littler and Eaton, should be considered. The joint is approached through an incision along the radial border of the thumb metacarpal. The thenar musculature is elevated. One half of the flexor carpi radialis is harvested, leaving its insertion on the index metacarpal base intact. The slip of FCR is then passed through a hole that is drilled in the base of the thumb metacarpal. The joint is reduced and held in reduction using a transarticular K-wire. The FCR slip is then tightened and sutured to itself, the insertion of the abductor pollicis longus, and the intact portion of the FCR. The K-wire is removed after 6 weeks and rehabilitation efforts begun.

LOSS OF BONE

Loss of bony substance sometimes accompanies such injuries as gunshot wounds or severe motor vehicle accidents. This problem also may accompany severe industrial injuries from such machinery as a punch press (Fig. 7-33). When only small bone segments are lost, the ends may be trimmed appropriately, reduced, and fixed, as if it were a simpler fracture, with K-wires or plates. However, for large defects, shortening is not an option. When a single digit is involved and in addition to bone loss, the MP and/or PIP joints have been destroyed, amputation is considered. This option, however, rarely is considered for the thumb. When amputation is not considered, or is rejected, replacement for lost bone will need to be obtained. The most acceptable replacement will be autogenous bone graft.

Small quantities of bone may be obtained from the distal radius. An incision, approximately 3 cm long, is made just proximal to Lister's tubercle. The abductor pollicis longus muscle is retracted, and the underlying distal radius is exposed through the periosteum for an area large enough to obtain the desired graft. Using a 4-mm chisel, a 4 × 10 mm cortical window is made in the radius. Using a curette, cancellous bone is removed from the radius for use as a graft. The cortical window is not replaced. The wound is closed in a simple manner.

Larger quantities of bone or substantial cortical struts may be obtained from the iliac crest. An oblique incision is made over the iliac crest lateral to the anterior iliac spine. Dissection is taken to the crest, where the periosteum is incised along the anterior border of the crest for a distance of approximately 6 cm. Care should be use to avoid the lateral femoral cutaneous nerve, which usually is located medial to the anterior iliac spine. After incising the periosteum, a subperiosteal dissection is performed for a distance that is just sufficient to allow the placement of a curve osteotome no more than 1 cm down the crest. Perpendicular cuts with an osteotome are made in the iliac crest. If

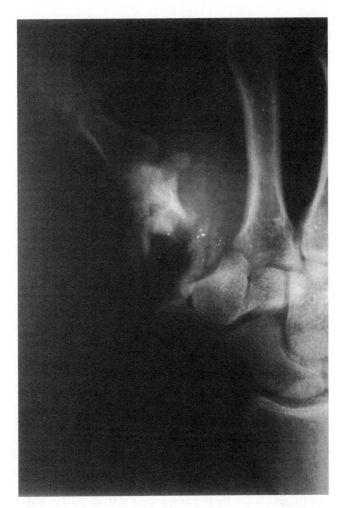

Figure 7-33   With complete or near complete bone loss, bone grafts from the iliac crest or other source will be necessary for repair and to prevent collapse. Initial treatment may be external fixation until a bone graft can be accomplished.

only cancellous bone is to be obtained, the two perpendicular cuts are approximately 2.5 cm apart. If cortical bone is needed, the cuts are made to accommodate the desired size of bone. A transverse cut may be made with a curved osteotome on the anterior surface of the iliac bone. When only cancellous bone is to be obtained, the crest between the perpendicular cut is reflected to allow access to cancellous bone which is removed with a curette. Otherwise the crest is removed for use as a cortical strut. Substantial pieces of bone may be obtained and shaped for grafting. To close, the reflected crest is sutured in place with absorbable suture. A closed suction drain is left, if necessary, and removed the following day.

LATE PRESENTATION

Ideally, fractures are fixed within the first 10 days of injury. Beyond this, fibrous healing makes movement of the fracture increasingly difficult. However, fractures may be treated primarily as late as 3 weeks after the injury without any substantial adverse effects. At 3 weeks, it is more difficult to move the fracture fragments and obtain good reduction. However, these goals can usually be achieved. After 3 weeks, correction of malignments increasingly requires an osteotomy. At this point, the benefits of surgery should be weighed carefully against any apparent functional loss that may result from malunion. As in the case of many fractures of the little finger metacarpal, substantial angulation or radiographic malalignment may not result in any noticeable loss of function.

FIXATION METHODS

For unstable fractures, a method of fixation to maintain alignment, after either closed or open fracture reduction, is necessary. A variety of traditional and modern methods of fixation are available. The most traditional fixation method is a splint or plaster cast. Currently, most hand fractures are splinted or casted judiciously because these methods can result in postinjury stiffness. Exceptions will be discussed in greater detail, but include mallet deformities, closed boutonniere deformities of the fingers, and ligamentous injuries of the thumb. Some physicians have achieved acceptable results using ulnar gutter splints to repair metacarpal fractures. Our choice of splinting for metacarpal fractures is currently the Galveston splint (Fig. 7-27).

More rigid fixation methods allow for earlier active range of motion exercises, which help minimize stiffness in both the affected and adjacent joints in any hand, finger, or wrist fractures. Rigid fixation methods include K-wire fixation, screw fixation, plates, wire fixation, and external fixators. In addition, some fractures are best treated with traction devices that will be discussed at the end of this section.

K-Wire Fixation

One of the simplest methods of fixation is K-wires. K-wires come in a variety of sizes ranging from small (0.028-inch diameter) to pins that may be ⅛″ or larger in diameter. To repair hand fractures, the four diameters used most often are 0.028 through 0.065 inch. K-wires should be inserted using a powered driver, a variety of which are avail-

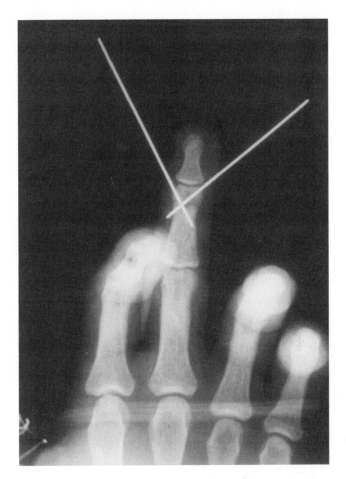

Figure 7-34 Crossed K-wires will effectively fix the fracture, but may cause increased stiffness in an adjacent joint.

able. The most common method of K-wire fixation uses crossed K-wires. Although the fixation is not entirely solid, it does prevent recurrent angulation, rotation, or displacement, and will maintain alignment while the fracture heals. Using the power driver, the K-wires are placed in a crossed manner in such a way that they do not interfere with or penetrate the joint capsule, collateral ligaments of the adjacent joints, or extensor mechanism (Fig. 7-34). Unfortunately, this is not always possible. When impingement on adjacent structures is unavoidable, postinjury stiffness is more likely. The K-wires may be buried beneath the surface or left penetrating the skin. Exposed wires are cov-

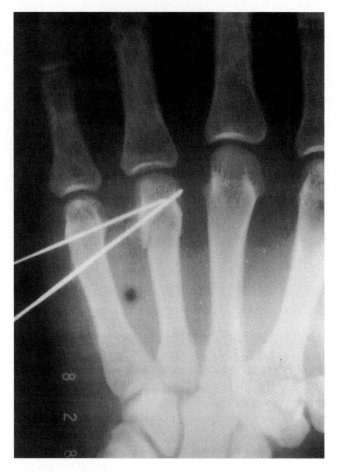

Figure 7-35 Transverse K-wires may be used for fixation, as shown here, and may be placed percutaneously.

ered with a small plastic ball or plastic caps that fit over the K-wire itself. This helps prevent inadvertent abrasions and scratches from the end of the K-wire. Exposed K-wires also are treated with a daily wound care regimen that includes cleaning around the pin with peroxide and then applying an antibiotic ointment or antiseptic solution.

The K-wire also can be placed longitudinally, typically traversing one or more joints. In this case, we splint the affected joints until the K-wire is removed so that the wire does not fracture. Transarticular K-wires that are not splinted run the risk of metal fatigue or fracture from small motions at the involved joint. When longitudinal K-wires are used, further stabilization may be necessary. For example, a single

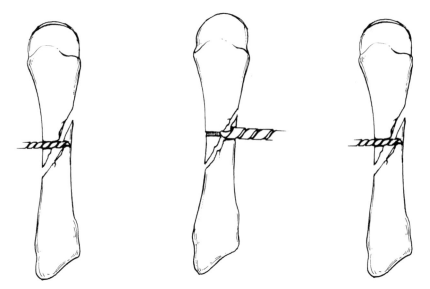

Figure 7-36   Screws provide solid fixation and when lagged provide fracture compression.

crossed K-wire may be used with transverse fractures of the middle phalanx.

Transverse K-wires are used infrequently to repair finger injuries. However, for metacarpal fixation, they may be used effectively by traversing a fragment of the fracture and passing it into an adjacent metacarpal (Fig. 7-35). K-wires generally are removed between 4 and 6 weeks. Exposed pins are removed easily in the office without an anesthetic. Those that are buried just beneath the skin and are palpable in the office may be removed under local anesthetic without difficulty. Potential complications from K-wire fixation include erosion of buried pins, which may be followed by wound infections, and pin tract infections.

Screw Fixation

Screws are very effective in fixing fractures, especially those with an oblique orientation. If lag screws are available, these may be used. If a lag screw is not specifically available (as is often the case), a lag effect can be achieved by overdrilling the outer cortex (Fig. 7-36). Proper placement of the screws requires near-perfect reduction of the fracture that is maintained with bone clamps. Fracture reduction should be assessed under fluoroscopy, and any intraarticular component of the fracture also should be inspected carefully to ascertain that joint congruity has been restored. Remember that after the screw holes have been placed and the screws threaded, further adjustment of the reduction will be impossible. After the fracture has been reduced and stabilized with a bone clamp, a drill of an appropriate size for the anticipated screw is selected. A drill hole is placed perpendicular to the oblique fracture. A depth gauge is then used to determine the length of the screw that will be necessary to effect the repair. The screw hole is then tapped, unless self-tapping screws are used. Next, the outer cortical hole, where the head of the screw will lie, is enlarged to equal the diameter of the screw threads. The appropriate size screw is placed through this hole and then snugged up. This allows for compression of the fracture once the screw has been placed. A second screw is placed in a similar fashion to adequately fix the fracture. After the fracture has been fixed with the screws, reduction is again verified. Attempts are made to close periosteum over the screw head and the fracture site.

It generally is not necessary to remove these screws. On occasion, a patient may feel some discomfort or the screws may loosen over time to the point where removal is indicated. This usually can be accomplished as a minor surgical procedure.

Two other screws are worth mentioning, although they are more commonly used for fractures of the wrist, especially fractures of the scaphoid, than for fractures of the hand or fingers. These are the Herbert screw and the Accutract screw. The Herbert screw has two sets of threads, one on the leading edge of the screw and one on the trailing edge, which have different pitches (Fig. 7-37). This allows for compres-

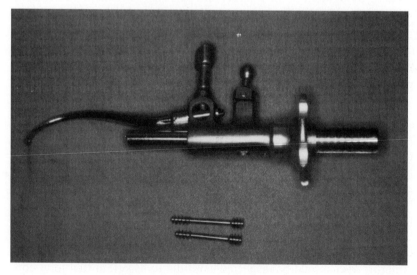

Figure 7-37   Herbert screws and jig.

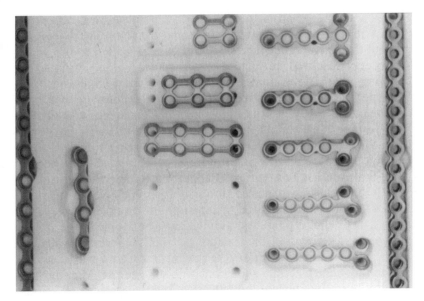

Figure 7-38   Plates may be obtained in a variety of shapes and sizes.

sion of the fracture when the screw is tightened. The Accutract screw, which is tapered, has a variable pitch running through the length of the screw. Both screws come with and without cannulation. The variable pitch and alternating pitch of these screws was designed to compress the fracture without a lagging procedure. Research into the performance of the Herbert screw indicates that while compression is obtained, the compression is not as high as that obtained using lag screws. Both screws may be difficult to remove if it should become necessary to do so after a fracture has healed.

Plate Fixation

A variety of small metal plates are available for fixation of fractures, some of which are shown in (Fig. 7-38). Plates offer a form of very rigid fixation that allows for early active and passive range of motion to help minimize joint stiffness. The plates come in a variety of shapes and sizes and are fixed to underlying bone using screws. Plate application is similar to that of screw placement in that the first step is accurate reduction of the fracture. Of all fixation methods, placement of the plate is perhaps most dependent on accurate reduction of the fracture. After the fracture has been reduced, it is held together with bone clamps while the plate is applied to achieve fixation. A plate of the appropriate size matches the bone that is being reduced and is able to incorporate any fragments to achieve permanent reduction. Some attention should be given to the fact that the plate must be held in place with screws. In comminuted fractures, the plate may be ideal for holding the fracture, but there may not be any stable bone to which screws may be affixed. In such cases, alternative methods will need to be chosen to achieve fixation. For fractures that can be held using plate fixation, the plate is bent carefully to follow the normal contours of the bone. Again, we stress the importance of adequate reduction before plate fixation. One should not attempt to bend the plate into place using a screw. The plate should lie flat on the bone in the proposed position before the drilling of screw holes or the placement of screws. After the plate has been adjusted appropriately and the fracture reduced, the first screw is placed through one of the holes in the plate. A pilot hole is drilled, followed by tapping and placement of the screw. Screws that penetrate the fracture line must be avoided. Not only is the bone stock absent at the fracture site, but the screw actually can cause further displacement of the fragment by acting as a wedge. Screws should be placed in good bone with solid cortex. After the fracture has been fully plated, the reduction and plate placement should be carefully assessed under fluoroscopy. The joint distal to the fixation should be taken through the normal range of motion to verify that no residual rotational deformity or impingement on the plate exists. If problems are discovered at this point in the operation, the plate must be replaced or alternative methods selected. Plates are covered with soft tissue when possible and rarely have to be removed. Occasionally loosening of the plate or patient complaints that seem to refer to the plate, require removal of the hardware in a minor surgical procedure.

Wire Fixation

A 24- or 25-gauge wire is sometimes used to fix fractures. The wire may be placed in a cerclage fashion or in a tension band fashion (Fig. 7-39). These methods may provide adequate fixation of less comminuted fractures. In certain cases, a cerclage wire may be useful in a fracture that shows significant comminution. The cerclage wire should be placed carefully to prevent the flexor and extensor tendons from being trapped in the circumferential wire. Although the wires generally do not require removal, they may be removed in a minor surgical procedure after the fracture has healed, if necessary. Wires may be used to supplement fixation with K-wires by providing some compressive force while the K-wire stabilizes in rotation.

External Fixation

External fixation is a common fixation method in long bones, especially those of the lower leg, wrist, and forearm. It is used less fre-

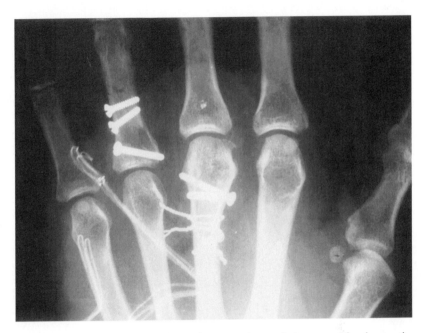

Figure 7-39   Cerclage wires shown here may be used alone or with other methods of treatment.

quently as a fixation method for fingers. In fractures that need rigid fixation that cannot be accomplished by any other method, an external fixator for the fingers may be used. One method of external fixation is with transverse K-wires that are first left exposed and then incorporated into a small chest tube that is subsequently filled with methyl methacrylate (Fig. 7-40). Two K-wires should be placed proximal and two distal to the fracture to prevent rotation. This may provide adequate fixation, especially on a temporary basis. When applying this method, the fracture ends must remain aligned. Some external fixation devices available on the commercial market may be applied to K-wires that have been placed transversely using clamping devices. These fixation methods are used to maintain bony length in fractures with significant bone loss and when early placement of plates is contraindicated because of soft tissue injury. This is commonly seen after gunshot wounds or saw injuries that result in loss of both soft tissue and bone.

Traction

Although traction of fractures is not specifically a rigid fixation method, it is very useful, particularly for significantly comminuted fractures of joints. Our most frequent use of this technique follows

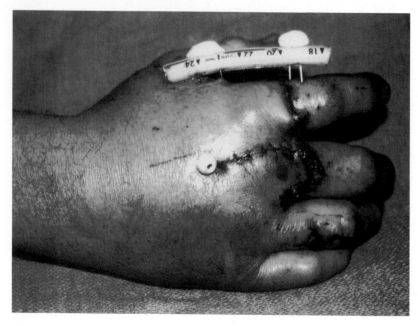

Figure 7-40 External fixation can be obtained with K-wire, chest tube, and methyl methacrylate.

crushing injuries to the PIP joint. In cases of severe joint crushes, traction allows for early motion and subsequent molding of the comminuted joint fragments into a shape that allows some motion in the postinjury phase. The traction device is created by inserting a transverse K-wire distally. This is left exposed on either side of the digit and has loops bent into both sides (Fig. 7-11). Rubberbands are applied through the loops and passed to a hinged splint that is fabricated by the hand therapist to allow motion at the injured joint (Fig. 7-16). The traction unloads the joint and allows for early remodeling. It is left in place for 4 to 6 weeks. The pin is then removed in the office after first cutting off the loop on one side.

SUMMARY

The most successful postinjury results are achieved by minimizing joint fibrosis and adhesions of extensor or flexor tendons to the fracture site, as well as by maintaining anatomic reduction. Fracture reduction ideally is achieved within 3 weeks of the injury and preferably within approximately 10 days. With adequate fixation, motion at involved joints is begun within days of the fixation application. The use of screws and plates provides the most rigid fixation and allows early active, as well as gentle, dynamic motion in the early postoperative period.

SELECTED REFERENCES

Brennwald J: *Principles and techniques of AO/ASIF fracture fixation.* In Grenn DP editor: *Operative hand surgery.* New York, 1993, Churchill Livingstone, pp. 759-765.

Dray GJ, Eaton RG: *Dislocations and ligament injuries in the digits.* In Green DP editor: *Operative hand surgery.* New York, 1993, Churchill Livingstone, pp. 767-798.

Schenck RR editor: Intra-articular fractures of the phalanges, *Hand Clinics* 10(2): 169-339, 1994.

Stern PJ: *Fractures of the metacarpals and phalanges.* In Green DP editor: *Operative hand surgery.* New York, 1993, Churchill Livingstone, pp. 695-758.

Weeks PM: *Acute bone and joint injuries of the hand and wrist.* St. Louis, 1981, CV Mosby.

Weeks PM, Wray RC: *Management of acute hand injuries.* St. Louis, 1978, CV Mosby.

8

The Injured Wrist

V. Leroy Young, MD
Philip E. Higgs, MD, FACS

GENERAL MANAGEMENT PRINCIPLES

Most carpal injuries involve bone and/or ligamentous damage sustained as a result of loading the wrist in extension, which most frequently happens when a person falls on an outstretched hand. Achieving a good final outcome after a carpal injury depends largely on quick and accurate diagnosis of the problem, followed by appropriate treatment and early restoration of the active range of motion. In most instances, treatment is guided by the need for reduction of fractures or joint dissociations (as well as maintaining the reduction), reinsertion or reconstruction of ligaments, and preservation of the blood supply to bones and soft tissues. Proper management of soft tissues also is important, and septic arthritis, which is a devastating complication, must be prevented at all costs by vigorously cleaning open injuries or surgical wounds. The overriding objective of managing carpal injuries is to restore a wrist that is free of pain, anatomically aligned, and able to tolerate the stresses of movement. Unfortunately, the chances of a good outcome generally are poor when treatment of wrist fractures, dislocations, or instabilities is delayed or performed improperly.

The physician should inform and educate patients about their problems, the treatment options, the expected outcomes, and the potential complications. The physician is primarily an educator, and the patient has the right to choose the treatment that seems best suited to his or her overall situation. This decision may involve input from a spouse or other family members. The patient's life style must be considered in determining the most appropriate treatment. Considerations include work activities, recreational interests, and the status of the noninjured hand and wrist. Be compassionate, but also be objective, sincere, and as accurate as possible when assessing a wrist injury and selecting a treatment course that will yield the best outcome for each individual patient.

WRIST ANATOMY
Carpal Bones

The eight carpal bones lie between the long bones of the forearm and the metacarpals. They allow the motions of flexion, extension, and ulnar and radial deviation. Because of the configuration of the carpal bones, the carpus is more stable in flexion than extension. For this reason, most carpal injuries are caused by the transmission of force across the wrist when the wrist is in a hyperextended position.

The wrist has two rows of four bones each (Fig. 8-1). The proximal carpal row consists of the scaphoid, lunate, triquetrum, and pisiform. The three major proximal row bones (scaphoid, lunate, and triquetrum) are relatively mobile. The scaphoid and lunate articulate with

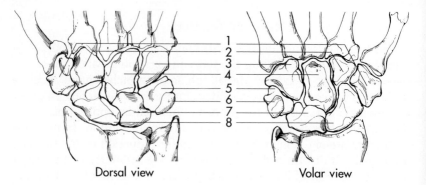

Dorsal view   Volar view

Figure 8-1   The carpal bones. Distal carpal row: 1 = trapezium; 2 = trapezoid; 3 = hamate; 4 = capitate. Proximal carpal row: 5 = triquetrum; 6 = pisiform; 7 = lunate; 8 = scaphoid.

the radius; the triquetrum does not directly articulate with the ulna because the triangular fibrocartilage articular disk covers the major portion of the distal surface of the ulna.

The distal carpal row, which articulates with the proximal carpal row and the metacarpals, consists of the trapezium, trapezoid, capitate, and hamate. These four bones form a relatively rigid row.

The blood supply of the carpal bones is of great importance when planning treatment of fractures because these bones do not exist in a well-vascularized soft tissue milieu, but rather as discrete elements within the joint fluid environment of the wrist capsule. The vascular supply enters individual carpal bones at discrete points, and interruption of bony continuity may devascularize bone fragments.

Carpal Joints

The wrist is composed of several joints, some of which are extrinsic (articulating with structures outside the carpal rows) and some of which are intrinsic (within the carpal row). The extrinsic joints are the distal radioulnar joint, radiocarpal joint, and carpometacarpal joints (first, second, and third). The intrinsic joints are the midcarpal joint and the pisotriquetral joint.

As a pivot joint, the distal radioulnar joint (DRUJ) is formed by the ulnar head and the sigmoid notch of the distal radius. An interosseous membrane and the triangular fibrocartilage complex (TFCC) loosely hold the radius and ulna together. An important functional movement of the wrist is rotation, and it occurs at the DRUJ. The loose capsule surrounding the joint allows rotation of the radius about the ulna. (This joint is described in more detail later in this chapter.)

The radiocarpal joint is formed distally by the scaphoid, lunate, and triquetrum bones and proximally by the expanded end of the radius and the most radial portion of the TFCC. This joint permits free movement in flexion and extension, in radial and ulnar deviation, and in pronation and supination. The joint capsule is supported by the dorsal and volar radiocarpal and ulnocarpal ligaments. This joint is sealed into a single unit that normally does not communicate with other joints.

The first, second, and third carpometacarpal (CMC) joints are complex. In many individuals, the second and third CMC joints communicate with the midcarpal joint. Details of the anatomy of these joints can be found in other chapters in this book.

The midcarpal joint is formed by the triquetrum, lunate, and scaphoid in the proximal carpal row and the hamate, capitate, trapezoid, and trapezium in the distal carpal row. Between these bones of the midcarpal joint lies a very irregular and extensive cavity, which contains proximal interconnections between the scaphoid and lunate and between the lunate and triquetrum. Three distal interconnections of the cavity lie between the four bones of the distal carpal row. In many people, the joint space between the trapezium and trapezoid, or between the trapezoid and capitate, communicates with the cavities of the carpometacarpal joints. In some individuals, the cavity of the midcarpal joint communicates with the joint cavity formed between the hamate and the fourth and fifth metacarpals. The midcarpal joint always is separated from the cavity formed between the first metacarpal and carpus.

The articulation between the pisiform and the volar surface of the triquetrum forms the flat, planar pisotriquetral joint. In approximately one third of people, this joint communicates with the radiocarpal joint.

Carpal Ligaments and Wrist Stability

There are two types of carpal ligaments: (1) extrinsic ligaments, which connect the radius or ulna to one or more carpal bones and (2) intrinsic ligaments, which connect one carpal bone to another.

Extrinsic Ligaments

The carpal bones are held in position by volar and dorsal radiocarpal and ulnocarpal ligaments. They maintain the stability of the wrist while allowing forces to be transferred between the hand and forearm. These extrinsic ligaments, which are external to the synovial lining of the carpal bone compartments, have the function of guiding the excursion of the proximal carpal row on the distal carpal row. In general, these ligaments connecting the radius or ulna to the carpal bones run in oblique directions.

The volar radiocarpal ligaments are the most important for maintaining the functional alignment of the radiocarpal joint and wrist stability. The major volar radiocarpal ligaments, shown in Fig. 8-2, are the radiolunotriquetral (sometimes called the long radiolunate), the short radiolunate, the radioscapholunate, and the radioscaphocapitate. The radiolunotriquetral is the largest wrist ligament. It arises from the radial styloid and attaches to the volar surfaces of the lunate and triquetrum bones. The short radiolunate ligament also originates from the radius and inserts broadly on the volar surface of the lunate. It is believed to play an important role in lunate stability. The radioscapholunate ligament originates on the distal articular surface of the radius and inserts into the scapholunate articulation. This ligament transmits blood vessels to the scaphoid and lunate. The fibers of the radiosca-

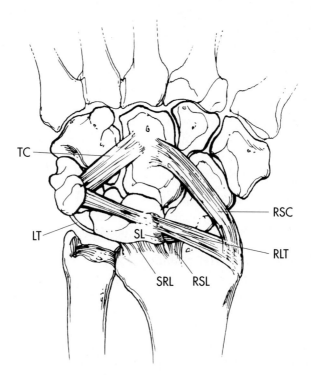

Figure 8-2 The volar extrinsic ligaments that play major roles in maintaining wrist stability: RSC = radioscaphocapitate ligament; TC = triquetrocapitate; RLT = radiolunotriquetral ligament; RSL = radioscapholunate ligament; SRL = short radiolunate ligament. Together the radioscaphocapitate and triquetrocapitate form the arcuate ligament complex. The most important intrinsic ligaments are also shown: SL = scapholunate ligament and LT = lunotriquetral ligament.

phoid portion are longer than those of the radiolunate portion, which allows for differences in the range of motion of the two bones.

The radioscaphocapitate ligament, which is the only ligament connecting the distal carpal row to the forearm, is the most radial extrinsic ligament and perhaps the strongest. Arising from the volar surface of the radial styloid, it crosses the proximal carpal row and inserts on the radial volar surface of the capitate. Its function is to loosely bind the distal carpal row to the radius. It also acts as a "sling" to stabilize the waist of the scaphoid.

The most important dorsal extrinsic ligament with respect to wrist stability is the dorsal radiocarpal ligament, which can be divided into three major parts: the radioscaphoid, the radiolunate, and the radiotriquetral (Fig. 8-3). Taken together, these form a thin, wide structure that connects the dorsal aspect of the distal radius with the dorsal proximal carpal row.

The arcuate ligament (also referred to as the deltoid ligament) actually is a ligament complex, with an ulnar and a radial limb that both insert on the capitate. Together, these two ligaments are shaped like a "V." The ulnar limb, or triquetrocapitate ligament, runs from the volar

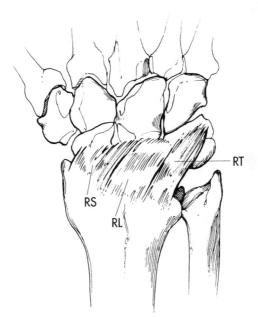

Figure 8-3   The dorsal radiocarpal ligament, which is the most important dorsal ligament for maintaining wrist stability. The dorsal radiocarpal ligament has three portions: RT = radiotriquetral; RL = radiolunate; and RS = radioscaphoid.

aspect of the triquetrum to the capitate. The radial limb is the radio-scaphocapitate ligament, which has been described previously. The arcuate is a major stabilizer of the distal carpal row and helps link the distal and proximal carpal rows. As such, the arcuate plays the primary role in maintaining midcarpal stability.

The wrist also is supported by the triangular fibrocartilage complex (TFCC), which serves as the primary uniting structure of the distal radioulnar joint and is the most important stabilizer of the ulnar carpus. The most prominent structure within the TFCC is its articular disk (also called the TFC proper) that lies between the ulna and the ulnar side of the carpus. The lunotriquetral intrinsic ligament attaches to an extension of the TFC complex, as do the dorsal and volar radioulnar ligaments, which are thickenings of the TFCC. These radioulnar ligaments connect to the base of the ulnar styloid and the radius. More detailed anatomy of all these TFCC structures is described later in this chapter.

Small radial and ulnar collateral ligaments also connect the bones of the forearm to the carpal bones. However, these collateral ligaments do not play important roles in wrist stability.

Intrinsic Ligaments

Intrinsic ligaments connect the carpal bones to one another and are contained within the synovial lining of the carpus. Their function is to limit the relative motion between the carpal bones within the proximal or distal carpal rows. Complete disruption of any of these intrinsic ligaments can cause instability by allowing the carpal bones to move out of their normal anatomic alignments.

The intrinsic ligaments of the proximal carpal row are the most often injured, even though they are quite strong. These short ligaments, which are only about 1 to 2 mm thick, connect the volar and dorsal surfaces of the carpal bones and insert around the proximal aspects of the bones. Their function is to transmit forces from one bone to the next in the carpal rows. The scapholunate and lunotriquetral ligaments provide maximal rotational constraints, unite the proximal carpal row as a stable rotational unit, and are the most important ligaments for maintaining carpal stability. Hyperextension injuries of the wrist often involve the scapholunate and lunotriquetral ligaments.

Stability of the distal carpal row is provided by intrinsic ligaments that join the trapezium and trapezoid, the trapezoid and capitate, and the capitate and hamate. These intrinsic ligaments tightly bind the bones of the distal carpal row; consequently, the distal carpal row functions as a unit. The hamatocapitate, which is the strongest ligament in the distal row, binds the capitate and hamate surfaces, serves as a "shock absorber," and allows only a few degrees of rotation in a normal wrist. Because these distal row intrinsic ligaments typically do not extend from dorsal to volar surfaces, continuations of the midcarpal joint space can connect with the carpometacarpal joint spaces through the distal carpal row.

General Wrist Mechanics

The wrist (carpal unit) has two primary mechanical functions. It transmits generated or applied forces from the hand to the forearm, and it controls or adjusts movements of the hand. With respect to the transmission of forces, the radius normally carries the major portion of a transmitted load.

A complex interaction of motions occurs when the wrist is deviated from radial to ulnar. The proximal carpal row rotates dorsally, while simultaneously translocating in a radial direction. This combination of motions is called the rotational shift of the carpus. The center of this wrist motion is in the head of the capitate bone.

The wrist can be viewed as a four-link system. The radius and ulna form the most proximal link, and the metacarpals form the most distal link. In between are the proximal and distal carpal rows. The distal carpal row usually moves as a unit with the metacarpals, but the relationship of this unit can be disrupted by trauma. The proximal carpal row plays the central role in stabilizing the wrist. The scaphoid and lunate are considered an intercalated segment. This intercalated segment would collapse under axial loading forces if not for the scaphoid bone, which acts as a bridge between the proximal and distal carpal rows.

This linked system of the wrist has four central elements: the radius, the lunate, the capitate, and the third metacarpal. In a normal wrist, they are in near colinear alignment. These structures primarily are responsible for controlling wrist flexion and extension through the lunocapitate articulation. The lunate is especially important in maintaining the alignment of the four central elements of the carpus, and instability typically results if the anatomic position of the lunate is disrupted by injury. A deviation of more than 5 to 10° either way between these links should be viewed as a joint system that is either diseased, lax, or damaged.

PATIENT HISTORY

Each patient being evaluated for a possible wrist injury should be approached in a systematic and comprehensive manner to ensure reproducibility and minimize the risk of overlooking some important component of the history or physical examination. Have an approach in mind, and then proceed in an orderly, sequential fashion to exclude possibilities as you work to establish a correct diagnosis. Treat the patient only after you have sufficient information to feel comfortable with the diagnosis.

When evaluating a patient with an injured wrist, take care not to focus entirely on one anatomic problem. This might lead to overlooking a more pressing injury. First exclude the existence of any other significant problems that could be a threat to life, vision, or loss of an extremity.

The patient's evaluation begins with a thorough and systematic history that should include the who, what, when, where, and why details of the patient and the injury. Possible issues to explore are listed in Table 8-1.

Table 8-1   Issues to Explore in the Patient History

WHO	Patient's age
	Right or left handed
	Place of employment
	Type of job performed
	Previous employment
	Recreational interests
	Previous injuries and their treatment
	Any medications taken
	History of any medical problems unrelated to the wrist
WHAT	Exactly what happened when the injury was sustained?
	What was the specific position of the wrist when the injuring process began? Hyperextension, flexion, radial or ulnar deviation?
	What was the direction and degree of stress to which the wrist was subjected?
	What were the intensity, duration, and location of the pain that occurred when the injuring event happened?
	What are the duration and frequency of pain since the injury?
	What, if any, movements or activities relieve or exacerbate the pain?
WHERE	Did the injury occur at home, at work, as a result of sports activity?
WHEN	When did the injury occur?
	Was any treatment rendered immediately afterward?
	What treatments have been used since the injury occurred?
WHY	Was a fall involved in the injury?
	Was the patient tired when the injury occurred?
	Was the patient inexperienced at performing a task or having problems with equipment?

When asking these types of questions, be aware that different personality types will provide vastly different descriptions of the same injury. For example, if a patient states that the wrist was crushed, try to determine what the individual really means. On further questioning, some may say that a book fell on their wrist, whereas others may say that a large machine fell on their wrist.

When inquiring about the precise movements and/or position of the wrist when the injury occurred, it is extremely important to have the patient be as specific as possible. Different types of movements may produce a different injury pattern or fracture. For example, forces applied when the wrist is in supination or extension typically produce perilunate injuries, whereas pronation and flexion forces usually injure the ulnar side of the wrist.

Along with eliciting details of the wrist injury, obtain a more generalized medical history and ask specifically about prior wrist pain or injuries, orthopedic and rheumatologic disorders, the presence of any acute or chronic medical diseases, and family history of orthopedic problems.

PHYSICAL EXAMINATION

Once the history is completed, a thorough physical examination is performed. A primary objective of the physical examination is to pinpoint the anatomic source of pain and/or tenderness as closely as possible to localize the site of a bone or soft tissue injury.

The most common symptoms of injuries to the wrist are pain, localized tenderness, swelling, loss of motion, and instability. In many instances, a physical examination and radiographs will lead to diagnosis of a fracture, dislocation, or complete ligament disruption and joint dissociation. Localized tenderness usually identifies the involved bone or joint; the ligaments surrounding that joint must then be assessed by ligament stress. To allow full stress testing of a joint, analgesia may be required if the pain is too severe to adequately evaluate ligament continuity. This also is true when positioning the injured area for certain diagnostic maneuvers such as those required for stress view radiographs.

The physical examination should begin in a very general manner. If the injury is confined to the wrist, the upper extremity should be exposed at least to the elbow; if there is any question of a more proximal injury, the shoulder also should be exposed.

Both wrists must be examined because anatomic variants may produce false-positive results. When evaluating the wrist for injury, the patient's forearm, wrist, and hand must be completely relaxed. The best way to relax an injured wrist is to lay the forearm on a soft examination table. Then gently hold the patient's distal forearm and hand to support the wrist while you position it as desired.

Initial Inspection

Begin the examination away from any tender or painful area as you look for swelling, discoloration, the presence of calluses or trophic changes, and any apparent abnormalities, such as a carpal boss, nodule, or mass. Note and record any erythema, abrasions, lacerations, or scars.

Functional Testing

Perform a full active and passive range of motion (ROM) examination on both wrists that includes wrist extension and flexion, radial and ulnar deviation, and forearm pronation and supination. Normal ranges of motion are as follows:

Wrist Extension ~ 60°
Wrist Flexion ~ 70°
Wrist Radial Deviation ~ 20°
Wrist Ulnar Deviation ~ 30°
Forearm Supination ~ 80°
Forearm Pronation ~ 80°

Compare the range of motion of the injured wrist with the contralateral wrist. Motion testing of the elbow, shoulder, and neck also may be necessary if more proximal areas of the extremity might have been injured.

Other functional tests to perform are grip and pinch strength measurements to assess gross motor strength.

Palpation of Significant Wrist Structures and Provocative Tests

Systematically palpate the bony and soft tissue structures of the wrist to localize areas of tenderness and pain as well as to identify any crepitus. Whenever possible, the movements and palpations described below should be repeated more than once to confirm any abnormalities.

Several provocative tests often are used to reproduce pain and the sound of clicks or clunks that indicate wrist instabilities. A finding of clicking or clunking sounds is most significant when they correlate with the reported symptoms and are produced when the patient actively moves his or her wrist. Production of such sounds through passive movement by the examiner is less important unless the passive motion also reproduces the clinical symptoms. Many individuals have "loose" joints that can make painless sounds. This finding is sometimes misinterpreted by inexperienced physicians.

A division of the wrist into five zones of examination can ensure that palpation of all important structures is conducted in a systematic manner. These zones are: (1) radial dorsal, (2) central dorsal, (3) ulnar dorsal, (4) radial volar, and (5) ulnar volar. The following can be done in any order. Remember that dozens of important structures in the wrist must be assessed, and physicians should develop a consistent examination routine so that nothing is overlooked.

Radial Dorsal Examination

Palpable features in the radial dorsal zone are the radial styloid, the scaphoid, the trapezium, the base of the first metacarpal, and the first carpometacarpal (CMC) joint. Soft tissue structures within this zone include the extensor pollicis longus and extensor pollicis brevis and abductor pollicis longus (the tendons of the first dorsal compartment).

The scaphoid lies just distal to the radial styloid, and its tuberosity is more prominent in extension and radial deviation. The waist of the scaphoid is palpable deep in the anatomic snuffbox, which lies at the base of the thumb between the tendons of the first dorsal compartment and the extensor pollicis longus. When the thumb is extended, the snuffbox appears as a depression bounded by these tendons. Tenderness in the snuffbox may indicate a fracture of the scaphoid, trapezium, or radial styloid, as well as scaphoid nonunion or de Quervain syndrome. A finding of pain in the snuffbox must be compared with the uninjured wrist because minor snuffbox tenderness is commonly present in normal wrists.

The trapezium and scaphotrapezial joint are found just distal to the scaphoid along the axis of the thumb. The trapezium can be distinguished from the first metacarpal by gently rotating the thumb.

Perform a grind test of the first CMC joint (Fig. 8-4). The first carpometacarpal joint can be identified by slowly moving your finger proximally along the dorsomedial aspect of the first metacarpal. The small depression you will feel is the first CMC joint. A positive grind test is indicated by the production of pain and crepitus felt by both the patient and physician. Results of a grind test usually will be positive in cases of scaphoid injuries, as well as carpometacarpal arthritis. Carpometacarpal arthritis is distinguished from scaphoid injuries by the presence of tenderness over the volar aspect of the CMC joint. Pain caused by a grind test must also be differentiated from pain that originates at the scaphotrapezial joint, which is one joint more proximal. X-rays will assist in the differential diagnosis.

Palpate the extensor pollicis brevis, abductor pollicis longus, and extensor pollicis longus tendons for tenderness, crepitus, or nodules. De Quervain tenosynovitis is a common cause of pain in this area. Other symptoms of de Quervain syndrome are tenderness on the radial

1. Stabilize the patient's hand with your left hand and place your middle finger on the first CMC joint.
2. Grasp the patient's thumb with your right hand, as if making a fist around it.
3. Push the thumb toward the trapezium and rotate it several times while also palpating the CMC joint. Move the thumb through a full range of motion.
4. A gritting or grinding sensation of bone on bone felt by both the patient and physician indicates a positive grind test. The patient also will feel pain.

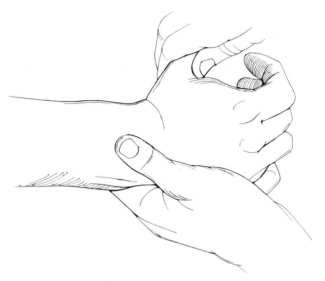

Figure 8-4   Grind Test.

side of the wrist and in the anatomic snuffbox, as well as pain that is exacerbated by active extension and abduction of the thumb. Swelling over the first dorsal compartment also may be evident. Another sign of de Quervain syndrome is a positive Finklestein's test result (Fig. 8-5). The results of Finklestein's test for both wrists should be compared.

Central Dorsal Examination

This zone includes the lunate, the scapholunate joint, the capitate, and the base of the second and third metacarpals and their CMC joints. Important soft tissue structures include the extensor digitorum communis tendons, the extensor pollicis longus, and the distal aspect of the extensor carpi radialis brevis and longus.

The lunate, which is most prominent when the wrist is flexed, is

1. Have the patient flex the thumb into the palm.
2. Have the patient close the fingers over the thumb, as if making a fist.
3. Have the patient deviate the wrist ulnarly.
4. This maneuver will produce excruciating pain in the first dorsal compartment in cases of de Quervain's syndrome.

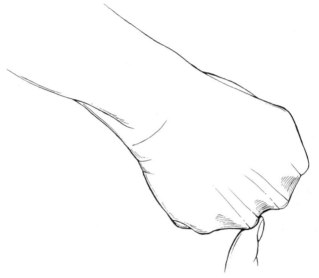

Figure 8-5   Finklestein's Test.

palpated on the dorsum of the wrist by applying pressure just ulnar to Lister's tubercle (located on the dorsal aspect of the distal radius). Pain on palpation in the area of the lunate may indicate injury to the scapholunate or lunotriquetral ligaments or a lunate fracture or dislocation. Lunate tenderness, along with localized swelling or synovitis, are common in Kienböck's disease.

The capitate lies just distal to the lunate beneath a mild depression found between the lunate and the base of the third metacarpal. When the wrist is in full flexion, the capitate is the most prominent bony landmark on the dorsum of the wrist.

The extensor carpi radialis longus and brevis are found just radial to Lister's tubercle. On the ulnar side of Lister's tubercle is the extensor pollicis longus, which is prominent when the interphalangeal joint of the thumb is hyperextended. The extensor digitorum communis is ul-

1. Place the fingers of one of your hands on the dorsal aspect of the radial border of the patient's distal forearm. With the thumb of the same hand, apply pressure to the volar aspect of the scaphoid at the base of the thenar eminence (the distal pole of the scaphoid). *(Use your right thumb when examining the right scaphoid bone and your left thumb when examining the left scaphoid bone.)*
2. Use your opposite hand to range the patient's hand from an ulnar extended position to a radial flexed position while maintaining pressure on the scaphoid with your thumb.
3. When positive, this test produces a painful and palpable "clunk" and may also cause displacement of the proximal pole of the scaphoid out of the scaphoid fossa of the radius. If pain is produced over the dorsum of the wrist during the scaphoid shift test, rotary subluxation of the scaphoid is the probable diagnosis.

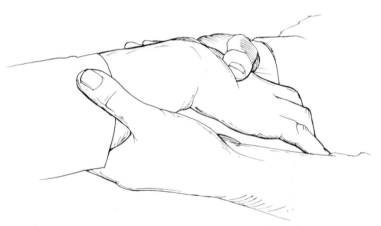

Figure 8-6   Scaphoid Shift Test (Watson's Test).

nar to the extensor pollicis longus. If any of these tendons are tender, localized inflammation or impingement should be suspected.

To evaluate scapholunate joint integrity, perform a scaphoid shift test, which is also called scaphoid ballottement (Fig. 8-6). The dorsal pressure applied during this provocative test prevents normal flexion at the scaphoid bone and thereby stresses the periscaphoid ligaments. This test is positive and, if it produces a palpable clunk, pain, and an increased size of the scapholunate depression, indicative of joint dissociation. The clicking associated with scapholunate instability represents the scaphoid jumping back into its normal relationship with the lunate.

If palpation of the scapholunate joint produces tenderness in the dorsal aspect of the joint, the cause may be occult ganglia, which frequently cause chronic wrist pain. They should be palpable as pea-sized tender nodules in the distal aspect of the scapholunate joint that usually become more prominent with wrist flexion.

Ulnar Dorsal Examination

The ulnar dorsal zone contains the hamate, the triquetrum, the lunotriquetral joint, the distal radioulnar joint, the ulnar head and styloid, and the base of the fourth and fifth metacarpals. The major soft tissue structures are the triangular fibrocartilage complex (TFCC) and the extensor carpi ulnaris tendon.

The hamate can be felt proximal to the base of the fifth metacarpal. The triquetrum is best located with the wrist in radial deviation; it lies in a sulcus between the hamate and ulnar styloid.

The lunotriquetral joint should be located and palpated. Dissociations or sprains of this joint are indicated by tenderness and possibly a wrist click. Instability of this joint is diagnosed with a lunotriquetral ballottement test, which is positive when this maneuver produces pain, crepitus, and increased motion in the lunotriquetral joint (Fig. 8-7).

The distal radioulnar joint (DRUJ) is found just radial to the ulnar head. Disorders of the DRUJ produce pain when the forearm is rotated. Note any changes in the relationship between the distal radius and ulna, which may indicate subluxation or dislocation of the ulna. Also pay attention to signs of crepitus or clicking, which suggest arthritis. Palpate the DRUJ as follows:

1. Hold the wrist in a neutral position and stabilize the patient's radius with one hand.
2. Grasp the ulnar head between your thumb and index finger with the other hand and move it first in a dorsal direction and then volarly several times.

Pain in the area of the ulnar head may indicate a triangular fibrocartilage complex injury, distal radioulnar joint arthritis, tenosynovitis of the extensor carpi ulnaris tendon, dislocation of the ulnar head, or a fracture involving the distal ulna.

The TFCC lies just distal to the radioulnar joint. Extreme tenderness in this area usually indicates either a tear of the TFCC or lunate chondromalacia caused by ulnocarpal abutment.

The extensor carpi ulnaris tendon lies ulnar to the ulnar styloid. Subluxation of this tendon is identified by a sudden palpable snap that occurs when the patient actively moves the wrist to a position of ulnar deviation and supination. If palpation reveals tenderness of this ten-

1. Grasp and stabilize the patient's lunate between the thumb and index finger of one of your hands.
2. Grasp the triquetrum and pisiform bones between the thumb and index finger of your other hand.
3. While holding the lunate stable, move the triquetrum first in a dorsal direction and then volarly several times in an attempt to displace the triquetrum and pisiform.
4. If this test produces pain, crepitus, and increased motion (laxity), a lunotriquetral ligament injury should be suspected.

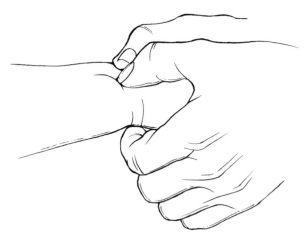

Figure 8-7   Lunotriquetral Ballottement Test.

don but there is no palpable snap or obvious deformity, the cause may be tenosynovitis.

Radial Volar Examination

The structures palpated in the radial volar zone are the scaphoid tuberosity, the tubercle of the trapezium, the flexor carpi radialis, the palmaris longus (which is not present in all individuals), and the long flexors of the fingers (which are difficult to identify individually).

The scaphoid tuberosity is located just distal to the radial styloid and is most prominent when the wrist is deviated radially. The tubercle of the trapezium lies distal to the scaphoid along the same axis as the index finger. A fracture of the trapezial ridge will produce tenderness on palpation, but diagnosis cannot be confirmed without special radiographic views.

The flexor carpi radialis tendon lies ulnar to the scaphoid tuberosity. This tendon disappears into a synovial tunnel when it reaches the trapezium. The area over this synovial tunnel will be tender in cases of tenosynovitis.

More than 85% of people have a palmaris longus tendon, which is identified by having the patient flex his or her wrist while opposing the thumb and little finger.

Ulnar Volar Examination

The ulnar volar zone contains the pisiform, the hook of the hamate, and the flexor carpi ulnaris tendon.

The pisiform is the bony prominence found at the base of the hypothenar eminence. The pisiform should be mobile and easily ballotted against the triquetrum when the wrist is relaxed. When pisotriquetral arthritis is present, this ballottement will produce pain and possibly crepitus.

Just radial and distal to the pisiform is the hook of the hamate. A fracture should be suspected when there is isolated tenderness over the hook of the hamate, but special radiographic views are necessary to confirm the diagnosis.

The flexor carpi ulnaris tendon inserts into the pisiform. This tendon can be located by having the patient make a clenched fist and then actively flex the fist while ulnarly deviating the wrist.

Neurovascular Evaluation

Several neurovascular examinations assess arterial patency and sensation. Ulnar and radial artery patency are evaluated with Allen's test (Fig. 8-8). The ulnar nerve and artery can be identified by using a gentle rolling motion to palpate Guyon's canal, which lies between the pisiform and the hook of the hamate. Allen's test is positive when capillary refill in the fingers is delayed after the arteries are occluded and released.

A neurological examination should include percussing for a Tinel's sign over the median and ulnar nerves at the wrist, the median nerve in the forearm, and the ulnar nerve at the elbow (Fig. 8-9). A Tinel's sign is positive if the tapping over the nerve elicits paresthesia along the nerve's distribution.

Compression of the median nerve because of increased pressure in the carpal tunnel is identified by a positive Phalen's test. Phalen's test should be done at the same time as the elbow flexion test, which elicits evidence of ulnar nerve compression. The two tests are performed by having the patient hold the wrists together in full volar flexion for at least 60 seconds, as illustrated in Fig. 8-10. A positive response to Phalen's test is the production of numbness or tingling along the median

1. Hold the patient's hand in supination and have the patient clench the fist.
2. Squeeze the blood out of the patient's hand and wrist by using both of your index fingers to occlude the radial and ulnar arteries **(A).**
3. Have the patient open the hand and extend the fingers (but not hyperextend them).
4. Release the occlusive pressure on the radial artery and look for a quick return of normal color (indicating blood flow) to the fingers **(B).**
5. Repeat Steps 2 and 3, release the occlusive pressure on the ulnar artery, and look for a quick return of blood flow to the fingers.
6. An Allen's test is positive when there is delayed capillary refill in the fingers after the arteries are occluded and released.

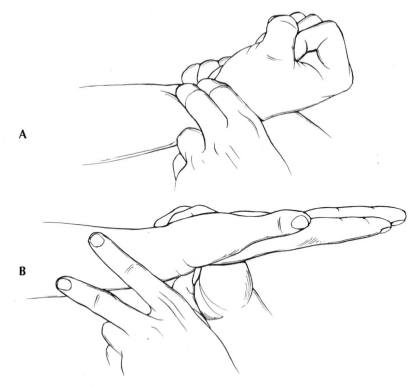

A

B

Figure 8-8   Allen's Test.

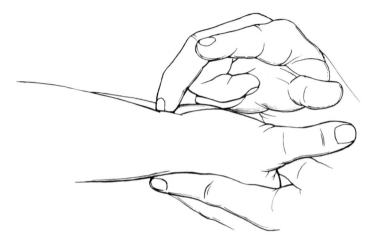

Figure 8-9   Percussing for Tinel's sign at the ulnar nerve in the wrist.

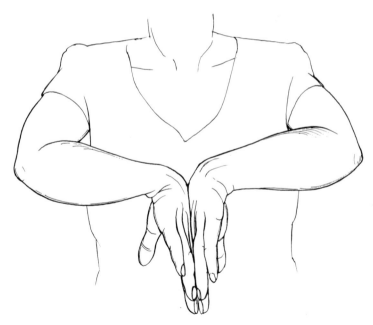

Figure 8-10   Phalen's test and the elbow flexion test can be performed at the same time.

nerve distribution when the wrist is in flexion. The elbow flexion test result is positive when the raised and flexed elbows produce numbness or tingling in the distribution of the ulnar nerve.

The straight arm-raising test also should be performed to determine whether there are signs of nerve compression in the neck or shoulder. This is done by having the patient simultaneously raise both arms straight above his or her head and hold them there for 1 minute. A positive response to this test is indicated by numbness, tingling in the fingers, and/or a tired feeling in the upper extremity.

Sensation should be evaluated with some objective method, such as a static or moving two-point discrimination test, vibratory testing, or the Semmes–Weinstein method.

If an injury involving the carpal tunnel or Guyon's canal is suspected, specific tests of intrinsic muscle function should be done to check for median or ulnar nerve entrapment.

Four-View Wrist Series and Stress View Radiographs

When the physical examination has been completed, a tentative diagnosis usually can be entertained. Some of the imaging techniques described in Chapter 3 often are required to confirm the diagnosis, typically beginning with a standard four-view wrist series, which consists of radiographs taken in posteroanterior (PA), lateral, and two oblique views; all views are obtained with the wrist in a neutral position. An anteroposterior (AP) view with the elbow extended and the wrist in neutral often is the best way to visualize the intercarpal joints. The heads of the metacarpals should be included on all projections.

For many wrist injuries, obtaining a true neutral position radiograph of the carpus and distal radioulnar joint (DRUJ) is critical for evaluating the positions of the carpal bones and the relative lengths of the radius and ulna. To obtain a true neutral X-ray, the patient sits with the forearm on the X-ray table and places the palm on the X-ray cassette. The shoulder is abducted 90°, the elbow is flexed 90°, and the forearm is in a neutral position with the radius and the third metacarpal in the same axis. In some instances, radiographs of the contralateral, asymptomatic wrist may be necessary for comparison purposes.

To obtain a true lateral radiograph, the axis of the third metacarpal and the axis of the distal radius should be in alignment. Lateral view X-rays are necessary for measuring the scapholunate and capitolunate angles. They also help diagnose instability involving the perilunate ligaments.

Figure 8-11*A* is a neutral PA view that illustrates the carpal arcs evident on a normal X-ray. Figure 8-11*B* shows a disrupted alignment of the carpal bones. The four-view wrist series should reveal fractures,

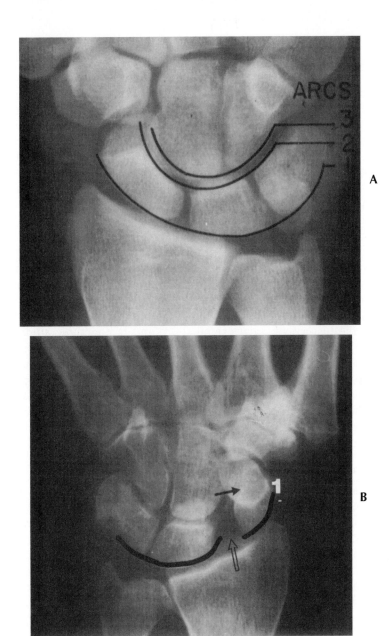

Figure 8-11 Neutral posteroanterior views of the wrist illustrate normal **(A)** and disrupted **(B)** carpal arcs. **(A)** Three normal carpal arcs are evident. Arc 1 joins the outer proximal convexities of the scaphoid, lunate, and triquetrum; arc 2 joins the distal concavities of the same three carpal bones; and arc 3 joins the proximal convexities of the capitate and hamate. **(B)** Arc 1 is disrupted because of rupture of the scapholunate ligament. A gap between the scaphoid and lunate is evident (*open arrow*). The scaphoid appears somewhat foreshortened (rotated) and has the configuration of a signet ring (*arrow*). This latter finding is called a "ring sign." (Reprinted with permission from Gilula LA: Carpal injuries: analytic approach and case exercises, *AJR Am J Roentgenol* 133:503-517, 1979).

fracture fragments, frank dislocations, subluxations, various arthritides, Kienböck's disease, static instability patterns, and carpal bossing.

More detailed information regarding the stability of a joint can be obtained with stress view radiographs, which are indicated when the patient's history and physical examination are suggestive of dynamic instability patterns or ligamentous injuries but the plain films are normal. Many views are possible in an instability series; the most important are:

- Posteroanterior (PA) and lateral views in radial and ulnar deviation
- PA and lateral views in flexion and extension
- Clenched-fist anteroposterior (AP) views with the wrist in neutral, radial deviation, and ulnar deviation positions.

These various wrist positions can demonstrate abnormal carpal alignments that result from injured ligaments or nonunited and malunited fractures that produce instability but are not revealed on standard X-rays. Carpal instability also can be diagnosed with fluoroscopy and/or cineradiography.

If the history, physical examination, and radiographic studies do not establish a diagnosis, additional imaging methods should be used, including bone scans, computed tomography, magnetic resonance imaging, arthrography, and arthroscopy. Remember that the diagnostic use and therapeutic interpretation of each of these imaging modalities requires clinical correlation. A diagnosis rarely should be based on imaging test results alone.

FRACTURES OF THE CARPAL BONES
Diagnostic Principles

Fractures of the carpal bones usually result from an acute, severe injury. The primary symptom is pain of either acute or gradual onset. Symptom onset related to a specific event probably represents an acute injury rather than a chronic process, such as osteoarthritis, although preexisting chronic damage may first be diagnosed during injury evaluation. The patient's description of a wrist injury provides important information and should help to suggest which bone has been injured. For example, scaphoid fractures commonly result from a fall on the thenar eminence of an outstretched hand. The location and duration of the pain also are important in making a diagnosis, as are activities that exacerbate symptoms. Ulnar-sided wrist pain aggravated by gripping a golf club, for instance, is a common complaint after hamate fractures.

Carpal fractures are characterized by pain, tenderness, swelling, and guarded motion of the wrist. Associated soft tissue injuries also may be present. When a bony injury is suspected, an attempt should be made to palpate the individual carpal bones, the CMC joints, and the distal surfaces of the radius and ulna. Palpation always should begin away from the area of maximal tenderness.

Imaging Studies

Using the appropriate tests, bony injuries can be diagnosed with a high degree of reliability. A standard four-view wrist series should be obtained first, because these views reveal the gross bony outline and demonstrate most injuries to wrist bones. Some soft tissue detail also is provided. For example, the radial wrist soft tissue fat stripe often is displaced after a scaphoid fracture. Nondisplaced carpal fractures may not appear as lucencies on plain X-rays until bone resorption occurs at the fracture site, which may take up to 2 weeks.

Computed tomography (CT) provides a detailed image of fracture sites and the three-dimensional relation of fracture fragments. Magnetic resonance imaging (MRI) offers specific information on both bones and soft tissue structures (Fig. 8-12). In addition, MRI can demonstrate the presence of cystic lesions within the wrist capsule or carpal bones, as well as information about marrow edema or the vascular status of bone fragments. A bone scan done immediately after an acute injury is justified sometimes by a particular need to determine whether a serious injury has been sustained.

Carpal bone fractures must be distinguished from bony contusions or bruises, with which patients also experience pain or swelling after a specific event. The diagnosis is one of exclusion. Most imaging results usually are negative in the case of contusions or bruises, with the possible exception of a bone scan or MRI. This diagnosis can be made only after sufficient time has elapsed to demonstrate that there has been no fracture.

General Fracture Treatment Guidelines

In most instances, the return to function after a carpal bone fracture has a much greater chance of success if treatment addresses the need for early and accurate reduction of the fracture to reestablish normal anatomy. Accurate anatomic reduction of a carpal fracture is the best way to avoid the development of traumatic arthritis later. Once reduced, the alignment of bones or articular surfaces must be maintained to give bony and ligamentous structures sufficient time to heal.

Remember that carpal bones heal primarily through the contributions of medullary callous formation. This process is slower than periosteal healing and is motion intolerant, which means that immobilization is always required after reduction. For many types of fractures, active motion can be started after 6 to 8 weeks, and fracture-site tenderness will diminish as bony healing progresses. However, there should always be X-ray evidence of bony union before movement is

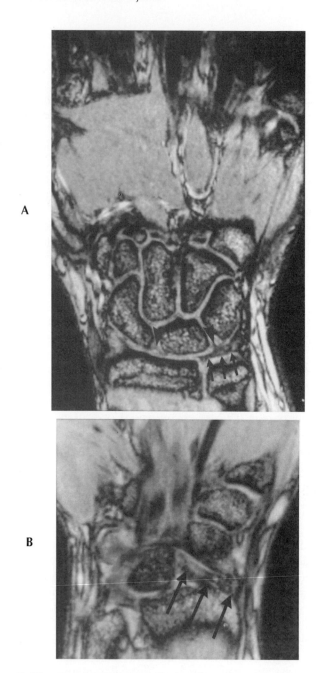

Figure 8-12 Coronal GRE MRI of a healthy wrist. MRI allows direct visualization of both bony and soft tissue structures. **(A)** The scapholunate and lunotriquetral intrinsic ligaments of the proximal carpal row (*arrowheads*) and the TFC articular disk (*arrows*). **(B)** Extrinsic carpal ligaments such as the radioscaphocapitate.

begun. This can be seen on plain film X-rays but will be apparent earlier on CT. A bone scan remains positive long after bony union is achieved. Because immobilization typically causes stiffness, dynamic splinting may be necessary once therapy is begun to restore motion.

If stability can be achieved with closed reduction of fractures or dislocations, the fracture fragments or reduced dislocation and the surrounding joints must be completely immobilized with a cast. Even when casted, displaced fractures are likely to remain unstable after closed reduction. In these cases, immobilization in a cast plus internal fixation, usually with percutaneous Kirschner wires (K-wires) placed under fluoroscopy, will be required for proper healing to occur.

To completely stabilize many fractures, open reduction and internal fixation may be necessary, especially when multiple bones are fractured or when the fracture pattern is complex, remains displaced, or is associated with ligamentous damage. Depending on the location of the fracture, internal fixation may necessitate the use of K-wires, screws, or plates (either neutralization, compression, buttress, or strut plates).

Accurate fracture reduction sometimes must be accompanied by management of ligamentous disruptions. If a ligament has been a-vulsed from its origin or insertion, it can be reattached with bone anchors and/or sutures. If a ligament has been avulsed while attached to a large bony fragment, reattachment of the fragment will require the use of pins, wires, or screws. Reconstruction with tendon grafts may be necessary if a portion of the ligament is lost.

If a fracture is severely communited, repair may be impossible and proximal carpal row carpectomy or primary or delayed arthroplasty may be required. In some cases, motion must be sacrificed and arthrodesis performed to obtain an otherwise functional wrist that is pain free, strong, properly aligned, and stable.

If articular cartilage is lost, an immediate or delayed arthroplasty (with autogenous tendon or fascia) or arthrodesis of the joint is required.

Scaphoid Fractures

Among the carpal bones, the scaphoid is fractured most often because it has a long lever arm and its radial aspect is unprotected. In addition, the scaphoid occupies the unique position of serving as the bridge between the proximal and distal carpal rows. These factors make the scaphoid more susceptible to injury.

Diagnosis

The most typical cause of a scaphoid fracture is a fall on an outstretched hand. Patients have pain at the radial aspect of the carpus that may become more severe in resisted pronation. Extreme tenderness in the anatomic snuffbox is a frequent clinical finding, and in some patients, swelling may obliterate the normal concavity of the snuffbox. Results of the first carpometacarpal (CMC) joint grind test usually are positive.

Imaging studies

Most scaphoid fractures can be seen on the standard four-view wrist series, although the entire bone is difficult to see and a nondisplaced fracture may not be apparent until there is bony resorption at the fracture site. For these reasons, a PA radiographic view with the wrist in ulnar deviation should be obtained to improve visualization of the scaphoid and demonstrate nondisplaced fractures. The "navicular fat stripe" (a collection of fat between the radial collateral ligament and the abductor pollicis longus and extensor pollicis brevis tendons) often is displaced immediately after a scaphoid fracture.

When a scaphoid fracture is accompanied by a ligament injury that leads to scapholunate dissociation and/or rotary subluxation of the scaphoid, the more distal fracture fragment may be displaced radially, whereas the proximal fragment and the lunate slide toward the ulna. Avulsion fractures of the radial styloid process and the triquetrum also may be present when scaphoid fractures are associated with severe scapholunate dissociation.

A bone scan almost always is abnormal in cases of scaphoid fracture. A negative bone scan obtained 72 hours after the injury therefore excludes an occult scaphoid fracture. Computed tomography can be helpful in identifying hard-to-see fractures, assessing the position of the fracture and the reduction of fragments, and evaluating the progress of healing. An MRI can show the vascular status of the fragments, avascular necrosis, or marrow edema (Fig. 8-13).

It is not always possible or advisable to obtain these types of expensive imaging studies. If a patient's history and physical examination are consistent with a scaphoid fracture but routine X-rays fail to show a fracture, the patient should be placed in a short-arm thumb spica cast and additional radiographs should be obtained after 2 weeks. By this time, bony resorption at the fracture site will be evident.

Scaphoid fractures in children are less common than in adults and also differ in the site of fracture. Children do not seem to fracture the proximal pole of the scaphoid; instead, fractures typically involve the distal pole or dorsoradial aspect of the bone.

Treatment

The location, configuration, and degree of fragment displacement of scaphoid fractures are important considerations when selecting the most appropriate treatment.

The location of the fracture is important because it affects the vascular supply to the fragments. Fractures may occur in the distal third, waist (middle third), or proximal third of the scaphoid bone (Fig. 8-14). On the volar aspect of the distal scaphoid is the scaphoid tubercle. Approximately 70% of scaphoid fractures are through the waist, 20% are in the proximal third, and 10% are in the distal third. Among scaphoid waist fractures, approximately 30% are unstable.

A scaphoid fracture is considered unstable if the fragment displacement is more than 1 mm. Malunion or nonunion is common, as is an increased rate of pseudoarthrosis, when displaced fractures (> 1 mm) are not reduced accurately with either closed techniques and percutaneous K-wire fixation (guided under fluoroscopy) or open reduction and internal fixation. Other causes of nonunion are fractures of the proximal pole and cases in which treatment has been delayed more than 4 weeks.

The distal third of the scaphoid receives a reliable vascular supply because the tubercle of the scaphoid is attached to the transverse carpal ligament. Fractures of the distal third therefore are unlikely to be

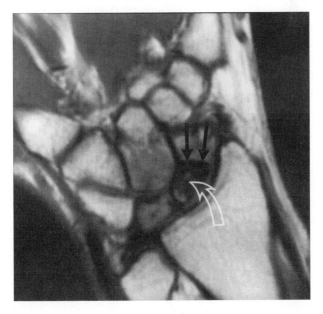

Figure 8-13   Coronal T1 weighted MRI of the wrist demonstrates fracture of the scaphoid waist (*arrows*). The proximal fracture fragment has a very low signal intensity, which indicates abnormality in the marrow space (*open arrow*). Additional MRI sequences would be needed to differentiate this marrow space abnormality from a healing reaction, avascular necrosis, or marrow edema.

devascularized. The risk of interruption of the vascular supply increases as the fracture site progresses proximally. The proximal pole of the scaphoid seems to receive no direct blood supply. Because of this, there is a high incidence of delayed healing in fractures of the proximal third, and avascular necrosis of the scaphoid can develop. Patients with avascular necrosis complain of radial-sided wrist pain and swelling and may note decreased sensation along the median nerve distribution. A truly avascular scaphoid bone would not be detected by a bone scan, but an MRI should be able to identify this serious fracture complication.

Scaphoid fracture configuration may be horizontal oblique, vertical oblique, or transverse (Fig. 8-15). The vertical oblique fracture pattern is inherently unstable and requires internal fixation. Horizontal oblique fracture patterns are usually stable, as are some transverse patterns, and may be treated by cast immobilization only. However, some transverse fractures of the scaphoid represent partially reduced transscaphoid perilunate fracture dislocations, and serious ligament injuries should be suspected in these cases. Transscaphoid fracture dislocations are much more extensive injuries than a scaphoid fracture alone and require more aggressive management. If there is any question about the configuration or alignment of a fracture, obtain a CT scan to define the fracture anatomy.

Table 8-2 outlines the average duration of immobilization for different patterns and locations of scaphoid fractures. Standard casting for nondisplaced distal fractures of the scaphoid is a short-arm

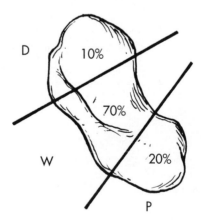

Figure 8-14   Division of the scaphoid bone into thirds: D = distal third; W = waist (middle third); and P = proximal third. The percentage number shown on each division indicates the percentage of scaphoid fractures associated with the three areas.

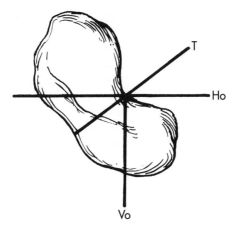

Figure 8-15 The various scaphoid fracture configurations: Vo = vertical oblique; Ho = horizontal oblique; and T = transverse.

Table 8-2 Treatment Plans for Different Patterns of Scaphoid Fractures

Site or Type of Fracture	Likelihood of Stability after Reduction without Fixation*	Duration of Immobilization
Distal third	Depends on fracture configuration	6–8 weeks
Middle third		
Transverse	Shear forces destabilize	6–12 weeks
Horizontal oblique	Stable	6–8 weeks
Vertical oblique	Longitudinal shear destabilizes	10–12 weeks; X-ray surveillance for healing
Proximal third	Depends on fracture configuration	10–12 weeks; monitor for avascular necrosis

*Fractures in which there is a displacement of fragments greater than 1 mm or dorsal tilting of the proximal fracture fragment always should be considered unstable.

thumb spica cast that maintains the wrist in a neutral position. Because the distal pole of the scaphoid receives a robust blood supply, stable fractures of the distal pole should heal in 6 to 8 weeks.

Closed reduction

Displaced fractures can sometimes be reduced through manipulation by using traction on the thumb while molding the snuffbox. Another closed reduction technique is to hold the wrist in flexion and apply longitudinal traction while putting manual pressure on the proximal carpal row. This latter method is especially useful if the lunate is rotated out of its anatomic position.

A more seriously displaced scaphoid fracture that is not accompanied by instability of the lunate sometimes can be reduced successfully with K-wires that are placed under fluoroscopy. In this procedure, one or two wires are passed through the distal fragment, from distal to proximal, and brought out at the fracture line before reduction. The wires should be positioned through a volar approach made radial to the flexor carpi radialis tendon.

A long-arm thumb spica cast that holds the wrist in a neutral position is appropriate for immobilizing scaphoid fractures of the waist or proximal third, or those in which a displaced or angulated fracture has been reduced by manipulation. The metacarpal of the third finger is aligned with the radial shaft, and the thumb is held in full volar abduction (with the distal joint left free). This position should close any fracture gap. In addition to being snug, the cast must be well molded between the thenar and hypothenar eminences. The long-arm cast can be replaced with a short-arm thumb cast after 4 weeks; this short cast should be changed every 4 to 6 weeks. The average healing time is 8 to 12 weeks for a scaphoid fracture of the proximal pole or waist.

Open reduction

Successful reduction of some scaphoid fractures can be difficult to achieve with closed techniques. This is particularly true if a scaphoid fracture is severely displaced, if the fracture pattern is vertical oblique, or if the fracture is associated with instability of the lunate caused by a hyperextension injury. Unstable fractures must be reduced openly and fixated to restore the normal scaphoid length. Otherwise, carpal collapse may result.

Open reduction techniques typically incorporate the use of internal K-wires or a lag or Herbert screw, which provides both fixation and compression. The use of compression screws can prevent the need for prolonged plaster cast immobilization. When instability of the lunate also is present, the lunocapitate joint also should be reduced and fixed along with the scaphoid fracture. Open reduction and internal fixation are followed with a bulky dressing until the swelling subsides (usually 7-10 days after surgery). The surgical dressing is then replaced with a short-arm thumb spica cast that holds the wrist in a neutral position until evidence of bony union is apparent on X-rays.

If bony union of a scaphoid fracture has not occurred within an expected interval, electrical stimulation may be applied. The duration of electrical stimulation necessary to achieve healing in approximately 75% of scaphoid nonunions is 4 to 6 months.

Late treatment of scaphoid fractures

Patients sometimes present months or even years after an injury with an untreated scaphoid fracture that has begun causing acute pain. Such cases indicate malunion or nonunion of a previously unrecognized scaphoid fracture. This serious situation requires debridement, possibly osteotomy, and bone grafting. Grafting of the distal two thirds is easiest through a volar approach, whereas a dorsal approach is preferred for fractures of the proximal third.

Capitate Fractures

Fractures of the capitate are uncommon, but the body or neck of the capitate can be fractured. Although the capitate, like the scaphoid, acts as a lever arm, it is isolated to a single carpal row and is protected by bones on either side. Capitate fractures almost always occur in combination with other injuries, such as major ligamentous (perilunate dislocation), bony (scaphocapitate syndrome), or bony and ligamentous (transscaphoid perilunate dislocation) injuries.

In scaphocapitate syndrome, a fracture at the waist of the scaphoid is associated with a fracture at the neck of the capitate and rotation of the proximal capitate fragment. The mechanism of injury is either transmission of force through the scaphoid into the capitate or direct injury to the capitate after carpal destabilization secondary to the scaphoid fracture. This pattern of injury may accompany a perilunate dislocation (see the discussion later in this chapter). After a perilunate dislocation is reduced, only the scaphoid fracture may be seen on X-rays. Because a nonreduced capitate fracture is poorly visualized on plain radiographs, the possibility that a capitate fracture exists alongside a scaphoid fracture in cases of perilunate dislocation must be considered. If the entire capitate bone cannot be visualized clearly on plain films, a CT scan should be obtained to eliminate the possibility of overlooking a capitate fracture.

Diagnosis

Patients with capitate fractures report a history of trauma to the hand and present with pain localized to the capitate bone, loss of motion, and swelling. Capitate fractures can result from direct blows to the dorsal aspect of the wrist or hyperextension injuries of the wrist when it was in a neutral position or radial or ulnar deviation.

Imaging studies

Most capitate fractures are apparent on close examination of standard four-view plain radiographs. Computed tomography is useful for evaluating equivocal plain films and for determining the alignment of capitate fragments and the extent of injury. An MRI is the best way to demonstrate avascularity or edema of the capitate proximal pole.

Radiographic evaluation of capitate fractures is very important. If collapse or gross disruption of the articular surface of the proximal pole is present, closed fracture reduction is not an option.

Treatment

Treatment of capitate fractures consists of closed reduction of the fracture and any associated injuries, followed by immobilization with a long-arm thumb spica cast in a neutral position for 4 weeks. This is followed by a short-arm thumb cast for several more weeks until bony union is apparent on X-rays. Percutaneous K-wire fixation (placed under fluoroscopy) also should be used if there is a suspicion that proper alignment may not be maintained after reduction.

If acceptable reduction is not attained by a closed technique, or if a capitate fracture is displaced, open reduction and internal fixation with K-wires are required. A dorsal or combined volar–dorsal approach is used. The quality of the bone and the condition of the articular surface are important. If bone quality is poor or if the cartilage is destroyed, a procedure is performed in which some of the soft-tissue attachments to the fragments are preserved in an attempt to maintain the vascular supply to the capitate. Cancellous bone grafting is occasionally necessary.

Much like the scaphoid bone, the vascular supply of the capitate enters through its waist. Because of this, avascular necrosis and nonunion can occur with proximal fractures.

Late treatment of capitate fractures

Patients sometimes present with chronic complaints because of an earlier capitate fracture that was unrecognized. If the wrist is stable and generally pain free, the patient may be allowed to resume normal activities with the knowledge that arthritis is likely to result and will probably eventually require a fusion procedure. If the wrist is unstable and/or painful, a four-corner arthrodesis (fusion of the triquetrum, lunate, capitate, and hamate) or total wrist fusion should be performed.

If a patient sustained a previously unrecognized injury leading to scaphocapitate syndrome, and the proximal fragment of the capitate fracture is rotated in a volar direction, the capitate may act as a mechanical block to wrist flexion. Excision of this bony fragment and replacement with an anchovy tendon graft may improve wrist motion. It must be noted that altered wrist-force transmission patterns after proximal-pole excision coupled with the ligamentous injuries commonly associated with scaphocapitate syndrome are likely to result in arthritis or considerable instability.

Hamate Fractures

Hook of the hamate fractures are not uncommon, but they often are overlooked by inexperienced physicians. Fractures most frequently occur at or near the base of the hook and typically are caused by a fall, by sudden extension when the wrist is loaded, or by direct trauma and the transmission of forces to the hypothenar eminence from equipment such as bats, golf clubs, or rackets. Fractures of the hamate body are less common than those of the hook, but body fractures can occur medial or lateral to the hook. The dorsal surface of the body also may fracture, especially in injuries involving dorsal dislocation of the fourth or fifth metacarpal bones.

Diagnosis

The typical clinical picture is one of pain in the hypothenar eminence, as well as tenderness when the volar area over the hook of the hamate is palpated. Decreased grip strength or weakness in the intrinsic muscles is often present, especially if the injury also involved the ulnar nerve, which is in close proximity to the hook of the hamate. Most patients with ulnar nerve injury have numbness or tingling in the ring and/or little fingers. Patients with old, untreated fractures of the hook of the hamate may present with chronic pain and tenderness in this area.

Imaging studies

Fractures of the hook of the hamate are difficult to see on plain-film X-rays, but they sometimes can be visualized with a carpal tunnel view. Obtaining this radiographic view can be difficult in the patient with an acute injury because it produces severe pain. Fractures of the hook of the hamate, as well as dorsal fracture dislocations of the hamatometacarpal joint, almost always will be detected on a CT scan, and all fractures older than 72 hours will be evident on a bone scan.

Treatment

For acute undisplaced fractures of the hook of the hamate, immobilization with a short-arm spica cast (with the thumb free) in a neutral wrist position should be tried for 6 weeks or until bony union is evident on X-rays. However, there is a good chance that immobilization will not be effective for hook fractures.

The use of open reduction and K-wire fixation often is unsuccessful in healing acute hook fractures that are displaced. Consequently, this procedure should not be attempted. For displaced hook fractures or undisplaced fractures that do not heal and remain painful after immobilization, the fracture fragment should be excised.

Fractures of the body of the hamate require either closed reduction plus K-wire fixation or open reduction and internal fixation with either K-wires, a T-plate, or cancellous screws.

For patients with long-standing untreated hook fractures, excision of the nonunited fragment usually produces a good outcome. However, the chronic injury may cause rupture of the flexor tendons to the fourth and fifth fingers, as well as neuropathy of the deep branch of the ulnar nerve. These patients do less well. In cases of an old, untreated dorsal fracture dislocation of the hamatometacarpal joint, arthrodesis of the joint is required.

Lunate Fractures

The lunate is the keystone of the carpus and is supported by both radial and ulnar structures. Isolated fractures of the lunate are rare.

Diagnosis

Patients with lunate fractures experience dorsal pain over the central aspect of the wrist and tenderness when the lunate is palpated. They typically have a positive response to lunotriquetral ballottement (see Fig. 8-7).

Imaging studies

A four-view standard wrist series will detect most lunate fractures. If X-rays are not conclusive, diagnosis can be assisted by a bone scan or CT scan, which is the best way to illustrate the extent of bony disruption.

Treatment

Open reduction and internal fixation of lunate fractures are recommended, followed by a bulky surgical dressing for 7 to 10 days. Once the swelling subsides, this dressing is replaced with a short-arm spica cast until evidence of bony union is evident on X-rays (approximately 6 weeks). If the articular surface of the proximal portion of the lunate is disrupted, a radiolunate fusion is required. Die-punch injuries resulting from impact on the capitate bone also can fracture the articular surface of the distal lunate. To repair this type of injury, a dorsal approach is used to make a drill hole in the dorsal lunate surface. A probe is then inserted, and the distal articular surface is elevated from within the bone. When necessary, the interior of the lunate is bone grafted.

Trapezium Fractures

The trapezium is fractured infrequently. When it is, the injury usually is associated with a fracture of the radius or radial styloid or with fracture or lateral subluxation of the first metacarpal in which the trapezium sustains a split fracture. These injuries frequently result from a fall on a hyperextended hand that was in radial deviation. Fracture of the trapezium alone also can occur and may involve the body or the palmar ridge, as well as avulsion of a bone fragment at a ligamentous insertion. An isolated fracture of the trapezial body typically is produced by a direct blow on an abducted thumb. A trapezial ridge fracture is caused most often by a fall on an outstretched hand.

Diagnosis

A presenting complaint is pain at the fracture site or base of the thumb or thenar eminence. Nonspecific radial-sided swelling and tenderness in the anatomic snuffbox are common. Typically, the pain is reproduced on resisted wrist flexion. Results of the first CMC joint grind test may be negative.

Imaging studies

A standard four-view wrist series should be obtained for suspected trapezium fractures. An oblique view—with the ulnar border of the hand placed on the film cassette and the forearm pronated 20°—is best for illustrating trapezium fractures. Ridge fractures are easy to miss. Thus, if the clinical signs suggest a trapezium fracture but plain films are not diagnostic, ridge fractures are best visualized with a carpal tunnel view or a CT scan.

Treatment

A nondisplaced fracture of the trapezium is treated by immobilization in a short-arm thumb spica cast for 4 to 6 weeks, or until bony union is evident on X-rays. Displaced fractures should be reduced with manipulation and fixated with percutaneous K-wires placed under fluoroscopy or reduced openly with internal K-wire or lag screw fixation. Open reduction and internal fixation are required for displaced vertical fractures accompanied by lateral subluxation of the first metacarpal.

Ridge fractures rarely heal adequately even with open reduction and internal fixation. If the patient remains symptomatic after reduction and immobilization, the nonunited bony fragment should be excised.

Malunion of an old trapezium fracture is treated by an excisional arthroplasty or CMC fusion.

Triquetrum Fractures

Fractures of the volar surface or body of the triquetrum usually are associated with other carpal fractures or injuries, such as perilunate dislocation. Isolated, small avulsion fractures of the dorsal aspect of the triquetrum can result from injuries involving hyperextension of the wrist.

Diagnosis

Patients with triquetrum fractures present with ulnar-sided wrist pain that usually is worse on the dorsum. Nonspecific swelling and point tenderness over the triquetrum are also common.

Imaging studies

Triquetrum fractures are best visualized in lateral or oblique view radiographs. A carpal tunnel view also may be helpful.

Treatment

Nondisplaced fractures are treated by 4 weeks of immobilization in a short-arm spica cast with the thumb free and the wrist in a neutral position. Displaced fractures usually are associated with other injuries, such as perilunate dislocation, and require open reduction and internal fixation. Nonunion of a small avulsion fracture is relatively common, but it rarely produces symptoms and will not affect wrist function. Thus, a small fragment is not clinically significant unless it is painful. If a nonunited avulsion fracture causes chronic pain, the small avulsed fragment should be excised.

Pisiform Fractures

Although uncommon, pisiform fractures can result from direct trauma to the volar and ulnar aspect of the wrist. Pisiform fractures can be longitudinal, transverse, or comminuted. Transverse fractures are chip fractures at the distal end of the bone.

Diagnosis

Patients with pisiform fractures present with pain on the volar ulnar aspect of the wrist. Pain is most pronounced when the wrist is moved in flexion, extension, and ulnar deviation.

Imaging studies

Pisiform fractures are visualized most clearly by a carpal tunnel view or a lateral view in which the wrist is in 30° supination.

Treatment

Healing of pisiform fractures usually occurs after 4 to 6 weeks of immobilization in a short-arm spica cast, with the thumb free and the wrist held in a neutral position. Displaced fractures of the pisiform are rare, but they can occur, especially if an acute fracture involved the articular surface. Displaced fractures or fractures that do not unite after immobilization and remain painful should be treated by excision of the fracture fragment.

LIGAMENTOUS INJURIES, CARPAL INSTABILITIES, AND JOINT DISSOCIATIONS

When the wrist is subjected to excessive loads, its ligaments may lose their ability to maintain stable alignments of the carpal bones with their distal and proximal articulations. Carpal instability, joint dissociation, bone dislocation, or fracture, or any combination of these may result if a ligament is injured in a traumatic event or over a prolonged period of repeated loading. When untreated, ligamentous injuries can cause progressive loss of range of motion, late degenerative arthritis in the intercarpal or radiocarpal joints, and chronic pain and disability.

Injuries to wrist ligaments can occur under a variety of conditions, including a direct blow, distraction forces, and twisting motions. Most patients with ligament injuries report falling on an outstretched hand or describe twisting or jerking movements while the wrist was loaded. There is usually the sudden onset of pain, and a popping or snapping sensation may be heard.

In the most typical injury mechanism, the wrist is forced into a position that rotates the carpal bones and loads an intrinsic ligament to the point where it is torn free from one of the carpal bones. A small bone fragment also may be avulsed as the ligament pulls away from the bone. If loading is limited, only a partial tear of the ligament occurs; when the forces are adequate and persist, the tear can be complete and cause joint dissociation. Under the most extreme conditions, a fracture dislocation, as seen in a transscaphoid perilunate fracture dislocation, may result.

If a ligamentous tear is incomplete or small, there may be no clinical indications of instability until sufficient stress or motion is applied to the wrist, or unless the wrist is regularly exposed to stress or motion before it heals. Partial tears of ligaments, such as the scapholunate and lunotriquetral, can be problematic because they tend to progress into complete tears. Incomplete ligament disruptions cause "dynamic instabilities," which means they are evident on radiographs only when stress views are obtained, including clenched fist, flexion, extension, and radial and ulnar deviation in PA, lateral, or AP positions. Clenched-fist views may be especially helpful for illustrating subtle carpal malalignment. On plain films, angular measurements between the carpal bones usually are normal.

Whenever a patient complains of a painful wrist after a fall on an outstretched hand, but the standard four-view wrist series of X-rays is normal, additional stress views should be obtained. Many injuries that can develop into chronic instabilities are missed because no fracture was evident, and the physician therefore assumed that the injury was not serious.

Complete ligamentous disruptions cause static instabilities and tend to produce clinical symptoms without the application of stress. These injuries usually are visible on the standard four-view wrist series, in part because complete ligamentous disruptions often are associated with joint dissociations, bone dislocations, or carpal fractures.

Although partial or incomplete ligamentous disruptions frequently are limited to only one joint, complete disruptions tend to progress as other carpal ligaments fail in response to the transmission of forces. Complete disruptions cause the most serious carpal instabilities. In most instances, this progression of injury begins in the volar and radial aspects of the wrist and proceeds ulnarly and dorsally as the injuring force continues and disrupts additional carpal ligaments.

As a general rule, the periscaphoid ligaments are injured most often, followed by ligaments around the scapholunate joint, the lunotriquetral joint, and the capitolunate joint. Ultimately, the extrinsic radiocarpal ligaments may be damaged. This scenario produces a progressive pattern of perilunate dislocation (described in greater detail later in this chapter). As the severity of the injury increases, fractures of the scaphoid, radial styloid, capitate, or triquetrum are sometimes associated with this progressive pattern of perilunate disruption and instability.

DISI and VISI Patterns of Injury

Carpal instability results when the restraining effect that intact intrinsic ligaments have on the movement of carpal bones is lost. The most common causes of carpal instability are (1) unstable fracture of the scaphoid, (2) complete disruption of the scapholunate ligament, and (3) complete disruption of the lunotriquetral ligament. Unstable scaphoid fracture and dissociation of the scapholunate joint can produce a pattern of instability called dorsal intercalated segment instability (DISI). Dissociation of the lunotriquetral joint (and sometimes the triquetrohamate joint) produces an instability pattern called volar intercalated segment instability (VISI).

In suspected cases of carpal instability, a true lateral X-ray must be obtained to measure angles between carpal bones. Figure 8-16 illustrates measurement of the scaphoid, lunate, and capitate angles on a lateral radiograph. (Even a slight radial or ulnar deviation can lead to incorrect angular measurements.) The normal angle between the lunate and scaphoid is between 30 and 60° (average = 47°), and the angle between the capitate and lunate is <30°. The capitate, lunate, and radius also appear colinear.

In a DISI pattern of instability, the distal surface of the lunate tilts to an abnormal dorsal position (Fig. 8-17A), and the capitolunate and scapholunate angles increase. In a VISI pattern of instability, the distal surface of the lunate tilts to an abnormal volar position (Fig. 8-17B). In the VISI pattern, the capitolunate angle increases (>30°) but the scapholunate angle decreases (<30°). Both VISI and DISI patterns of

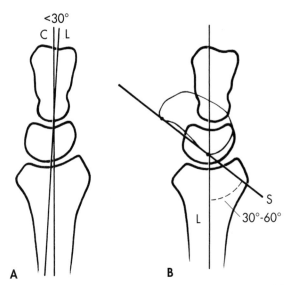

Figure 8-16   Angle measurements in a wrist with normal carpal bone alignments: C = capitate axis; L = lunate axis; and S = scaphoid axis. **(A)** Measurement of the capitolunate angle. Draw the axis of the capitate from the midpoint of its proximal head to the midpoint of its distal articular surface. Draw the axis of the lunate through the midpoint of its distal poles. Both axes should be parallel to the long axis of the radius. In a normal wrist, the capitolunate angle is <30°. **(B)** Measurement of the scapholunate angle. Draw the axis of the scaphoid as a line connecting its proximal and distal volar convexities. In a normal wrist, the scapholunate angle is between 30° and 60°.

instability can result in carpal collapse and degenerative disease if not treated appropriately.

Scapholunate Dissociation and Rotary Subluxation of the Scaphoid Bone

The scaphoid links the motions of the proximal and distal carpal rows of bones. It must therefore have a large range of motion while maintaining stability when stressed or loaded. The scaphoid and its surrounding ligaments are most susceptible to hyperextension injuries of the wrist, particularly when the hand is in radial or ulnar deviation, but severe twisting motions (torque) also can cause injury in this area. The capitate also may be involved in the mechanism of injury because it functions as a "battering ram" against the scapholunate joint in extreme radial deviation.

Partial disruption of the scapholunate ligament alone probably does

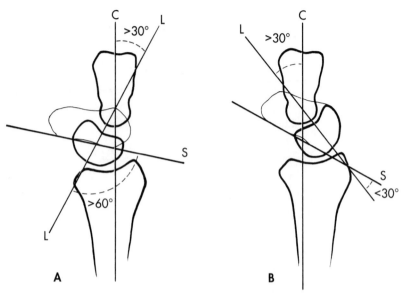

Figure 8-17   Angle measurements in a wrist with malaligned carpal bones: C = capitate axis; L = lunate axis; and S = scaphoid axis. (See Fig. 8-16 for instructions on measuring angles.) **(A)** Angle measurements in a wrist with a DISI pattern of instability. The scaphoid has rotated in a volar direction, and the lunate has tilted in a dorsal direction. The scapholunate angle is >60°, and the capitolunate angle is >30°. The capitolunate angle may be within the normal range in a DISI instability, especially if the capitate has remained in alignment with the radius. **(B)** Angle measurements in a wrist with a VISI pattern of instability. The lunate and scaphoid have both tilted in a volar direction. The scapholunate angle is <30°, and the capitolunate angle is >30°.

not cause instability, and evidence of such an injury is unlikely to appear on standard radiographic studies. If the disruption is complete, scapholunate dissociation develops. This frequent cause of carpal instability occurs when the scapholunate intrinsic ligament is completely torn.

If other periscaphoid ligaments also are disrupted (especially the volar radioscapholunate or radioscaphocapitate) by hyperextension forces, the scaphoid bone is able to flex or rotate volarly more than 70°. This is called complete rotary subluxation of the scaphoid and seems to occur only when at least two of the periscaphoid ligaments are disrupted. In this condition, the radiocarpal joint loses congruity, and the wrist becomes painful when stressed. This injury should be viewed as very serious because it can cause chronic carpal instability or scapholunate advanced collapse (SLAC wrist).

Diagnosis

Patients report dorsal and radial wrist pain that is most pronounced when the wrist is in extension. The injury typically is described by patients as a "sprain" that occurred during a fall on an outstretched hand, with the thenar eminence receiving the brunt of the trauma. The area over the scapholunate joint is usually tender, but swelling may be minimal. The wrist may have a limited range of motion. Extreme tenderness over the anatomic snuffbox should raise the possibility that the scaphoid bone is fractured.

Sometimes patients describe a more chronic history in which the wrist was injured 3 or 4 months earlier, but it did not seem severe enough to warrant medical attention. Then suddenly, they started hearing a loud snapping or clunking noise on the radial side of the wrist when they move a certain way (usually in extension). Pain may have become more severe, crepitus may be evident, and a loss of grip strength frequently is reported.

Late-presenting injuries probably involve a mechanism in which the intrinsic scapholunate ligament and perhaps the dorsal radioscaphoid ligament are disrupted in the initial injury, but the joint remains essentially stable. Because the volar radioscapholunate ligament has to assume more and more loading stress over time, this critical ligament eventually tears and can no longer support the scaphoid and lunate in proper alignment. At this point, the rotary subluxation of the scaphoid becomes complete.

Some patients have radial-sided wrist pain, but their standard four-view X-rays are not diagnostic of scapholunate dissociation. This may be especially true when the scapholunate ligament is only partially disrupted. A positive scaphoid shift test will provide clinical evidence of scaphoid ligamentous injury that is not visible on X-rays (see Fig. 8-6).

Imaging studies

The standard four-view wrist series does not always demonstrate partial disruption of the scapholunate ligament, but stress views or fluoroscopy should reveal evidence of a dynamic instability. A six-view dynamic series can be particularly helpful in diagnosis, with the views consisting of three posteroanterior (PA) views and three lateral views taken in neutral, maximum radial deviation, and maximum ulnar deviation. An anteroposterior (AP) view taken with the forearm in full supination and ulnar deviation while the patient clenches the fist (called a fist-compression view) also may be diagnostic of subtle scapholunate dissociation.

In scapholunate dissociation, the axial length of the scaphoid appears foreshortened on a neutral PA or AP view and a ring sign is apparent over the distal pole (Figs. 8-11 and 8-18). In most cases,

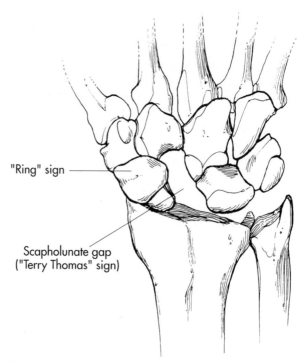

"Ring" sign

Scapholunate gap
("Terry Thomas" sign)

Figure 8-18 Radiographic findings of scapholunate dissociation typically seen on a neutral-position posteroanterior or anteroposterior X-ray.

the normal arc of the proximal carpal row is obviously disrupted, and the scaphoid and lunate are separated by more than 2 to 3 mm of space. This latter finding is called a scapholunate gap (or Terry–Thomas sign). A correctly aligned lunate will have a trapezoidal shape on a PA view; it appears more triangular if it is tilted either dorsally or volarly. If the scapholunate angle is greater than 80°, rotary subluxation of the scaphoid is the probable diagnosis (see Fig. 8-16 for angle measurements). When the space between the lunate and triquetrum is also widened, rupture of the lunotriquetral ligament should be suspected.

Treatment

Treatment of scapholunate dissociation is most successful when the injury is fresh, although successful reduction and ligamentous healing are possible if the correct diagnosis is made even 5 to 6 weeks after an injury.

A conservative treatment approach can be tried in the following situations:

1. Isolated scapholunate ligament injury is suggested by a positive scaphoid shift test, but plain film X-ray findings are nondiagnostic (dynamic instability).
2. There is X-ray evidence of a scapholunate gap, but a negative scaphoid shift test.
3. Plain films are normal, but stress views reveal abnormal alignments of the scaphoid and lunate bones.

In all of these contexts, patients can be placed in a short-arm thumb spica cast with the wrist in a neutral position for 4 to 6 weeks and given nonsteroidal anti-inflammatory drugs. Should pain persist after this period of immobilization, obtain more detailed imaging studies in an attempt to evaluate the severity and exact location of ligamentous injury.

When there is both a positive scaphoid shift test and a scapholunate gap greater than 2 to 3 mm on X-rays, treatment of a scapholunate dissociation should be aggressive. These findings indicate a static instability. With confirmed scapholunate dissociation injuries that are less than a few days old, it may be possible to restore the alignment of the lunate and capitate bones and close the scapholunate gap with closed reduction techniques.

Closed reduction

A local (regional block) or general anesthetic should be administered before the injury is reduced. Then apply fingertrap traction with 10 to 15 pounds of counterweight across the upper arm for approximately 5 minutes. This is followed by manipulation, consisting of dorsiflexion and then gradual volar flexion and pronation of the capitate, to reduce the capitate back into the cup of the lunate. If the lunate is dislocated volarly, use your thumb to stabilize the lunate when bringing the capitate into volar flexion. To eliminate a scapholunate gap, the scapholunate joint is reduced by radially deviating the wrist while holding it in a dorsiflexed position. Traction should be continued while lateral and AP X-rays are obtained to confirm that the reduction is anatomically accurate.

The scapholunate and scaphocapitate joints are then fixed in their reduced positions with percutaneous K-wires inserted under fluoroscopy. Place one wire laterally through the scaphoid into the lunate and the other wire through the scaphoid into the capitate. (A cast alone will not maintain reduction of these joints.) After the wires are inserted, the patient should be put in a bulky dressing for 5 to 7 days or until the swelling subsides enough to apply a cast. If the wrist can be casted, use a short-arm thumb spica cast with the wrist in a neutral position for 6 or 7 weeks. After the wires and cast are removed, the patient is given a removable split to be worn for an additional 4 weeks.

Open reduction

Patients should understand that closed reduction and fixation may not be successful, that instability of the scapholunate joint may persist, and that this type of dissociation can cause progressively serious instability or degenerative changes if the scapholunate gap is not reduced and the surrounding ligaments do not heal. When this is explained, many patients with fresh injuries will choose to have an open reduction rather than a closed one.

If closed reduction is not successful (the scapholunate gap is still evident and/or the scaphoid shift test is still positive), or if a scaphoid subluxation or scapholunate dissociation injury is older than a few days but younger than 6 weeks, open reduction, usually with internal K-wire fixation will be necessary. The torn scapholunate ligament should be reinserted at the same time. When the bulky surgical dressing is removed after the swelling subsides, a short-arm thumb spica cast in a neutral position is used. The cast and wires are removed after approximately 8 weeks, at which time the patient is placed in a removable splint that is worn for an additional 4 weeks.

Late treatment of scapholunate dissociation

When an injury is more than 6 weeks old, treatment for a chronic scapholunate dissociation or complete rotary subluxation of the scaphoid will vary depending on the clinical and X-ray findings. Patients with chronic pain, a positive scaphoid shift test, and an obvious scapholunate gap on X-rays will require surgery. Several options are available, including ligamentous reconstruction or reinsertion, capsulodesis, radioscaphoid arthrodesis, proximal row carpectomy, intercarpal fusions, or total wrist fusion. A specialized hand surgeon will be able to select the most appropriate procedure based on the severity of the injury and factors unique to each patient, such as work demands, recreational activities, and status of the opposite wrist and hand.

The outcome of surgery varies depending on the type. Many patients can expect that after rehabilitative therapy, they will have 70 to 80% range of motion compared with the contralateral wrist by approximately 1 year after surgery. If intercarpal fusion or ligament reconstruction were required, the wrist may not be pain free with all movements. For total wrist fusion, there will be loss of movement but the wrist should be pain free.

Perilunate Dislocations

The lunate is bound with strong ligaments to the radius, scaphoid, and triquetrum, yet these ligaments are damaged more than others in the carpus. Abnormal forces of hyperextension, carpal supination, or ulnar deviation can injure the perilunate ligaments, especially when those forces are concentrated in the area of the thenar eminence.

Most perilunate injuries begin with trauma to the scaphoid on the radial side of the wrist. From there, destabilizing events can progress in an ulnar direction. If the injuring forces are extreme, different combinations of ligament disruptions, bony dislocations, fractures, or a combination of the three can occur. For example, perilunate injuries may be associated with fractures of the scaphoid, capitate, or triquetrum, as well as the connecting intrinsic ligaments; these types of injuries are called transscaphoid, transcapitate, or transtriquetral fracture dislocations. Radial and ulnar styloid processes may also fracture with severe perilunate injuries.

The extent of perilunate injury is categorized by the stages outlined below. Figure 8-19 illustrates the more serious stages of perilunate dislocation.

Stage I: Partial disruption of the scapholunate ligament causes a dynamic instability (see the earlier discussion of scapholunate dissociation).

Stage II: Complete dissociation of the scapholunate joint causes a static instability of the DISI pattern as the distal surface of the lunate tilts in a dorsal direction. The most severe form of Stage II injury is rotary subluxation of the scaphoid.

Stage III: Two or more of the perilunate joints (the scapholunate, capitolunate, or lunotriquetral) are disrupted. The capitate, triquetrum, and/or radial styloid may fracture. All the carpal bones dissociate (usually in a dorsal direction) from the lunate, which may remain in alignment with the radius. In rare cases, spontaneous reduction of the capitolunate and lunotriquetral joints may occur as the wrist recoils from the injuring forces, leaving signs of only a scapholunate injury.

Stage IV: All of the perilunate ligaments are disrupted, along with the dorsal radiocarpal ligaments. In this stage, the lunate tilts in a volar direction and dislocates into the carpal canal (called dorsal perilunate dislocation) to cause a VISI pattern of instability.

Diagnosis

Perilunate dislocation usually causes extreme swelling on the dorsal aspect of the wrist, and the wrist appears obviously deformed. Patients may hold their fingers in a semiflexed position and be unable to fully extend the fingers without pain. In some individuals, there may be

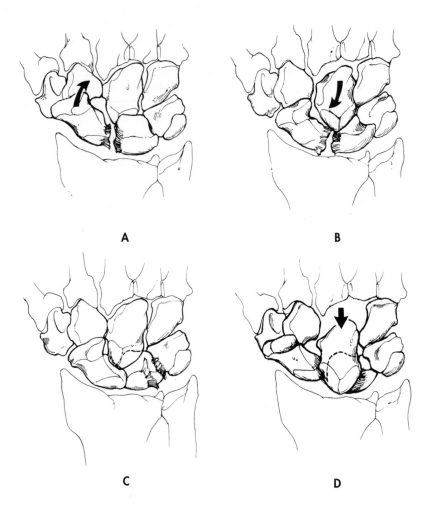

Figure 8-19 Stages II through IV of perilunate dislocation. (A) In advanced Stage II dislocation, there is complete dissociation of the scapholunate joint and rotary subluxation of the scaphoid. In Stage III, additional joints dislocate from the lunate, usually in a dorsal direction. (B) Disruption of the capitolunate and scapholunate joints and dislocation of the capitate and scaphoid (Stage III). (C) The carpal bones may dissociate from the lunate when the lunotriquetral, capitolunate, and scapholunate ligaments are disrupted (Stage III). (D) In Stage IV, the lunate is completely dislocated and tilts volarly into the carpal canal. All the other carpal bones also dislocate.

numbness in the distribution of the median nerve; injury to this nerve should be checked with two-point discrimination.

Imaging studies

Radiographic findings for Stages I and II were discussed in the previous section on scapholunate dissociation. A lateral plain film X-ray should be diagnostic of Stages II, III, and IV perilunate dislocation. In Stage III perilunate dislocation, a true lateral view typically shows the longitudinal axis of the capitate lying dorsal to the longitudinal axis of the radius, while the scaphoid is rotated dorsally (see Fig. 8-17*A*). (In contrast, an isolated lunate dislocation is revealed on X-ray by the fact that the capitate remains in alignment with the radius.) On an AP or PA neutral position radiographic view, the carpus appears foreshortened, and the proximal capitate overlaps the distal margins of the lunate. A scapholunate gap usually is present.

Stage IV dorsal perilunate dislocation is diagnosed easily on a lateral radiograph because of the volar (palmar) dislocation of the lunate (Fig. 8-20). On an AP view, the lunate also will appear to

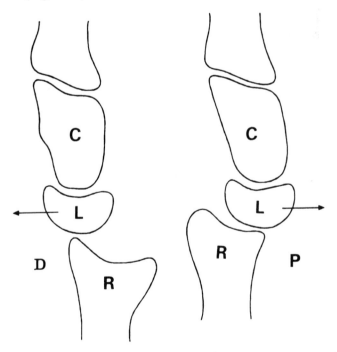

Figure 8-20   Schematic of a lateral radiograph demonstrating severe perilunate dislocation, with palmar (P) and dorsal (D) dislocation of all the carpal bones. C = capitate; L = lunate; and R = radius.

have a triangular shape rather than its normal trapezoidal shape. In severe cases, the lunate can be displaced proximally under the anterior margin of the distal radius. Other radiographic examples of perilunate dislocations are shown in Chapter 3 (Figs. 3-26 and 3-27).

Treatment

Some perilunate dislocations are amenable to closed reduction if the injury is very recent and only a few structures are involved. For example, scapholunate ligament disruption or joint dissociation (Stage I and early Stage II) often can be treated with closed reduction and internal fixation, as was described in the section on treatment of scapholunate dissociation. In some cases, it may be possible to reduce the lunate and other carpal bones with closed techniques, but the scapholunate gap cannot be reduced. Open reduction and internal fixation through a dorsal approach are required for these situations.

Although closed reduction can be attempted, Stage II through Stage IV perilunate dislocations usually require open reduction and internal fixation to reduce dislocations, align the disrupted intrinsic ligaments, and treat the fractures sometimes associated with severe perilunate dislocation. Open reduction is especially important when both ligaments and bones are injured, when fractures are displaced by more than 1 mm, or when a VISI or DISI pattern of instability is present. For Stage IV perilunate dislocation, both dorsal and volar incisions are almost always needed. In addition to reducing and fixating fractures and dislocations, all disrupted intrinsic and extrinsic (radiocarpal) ligaments must be repaired. In many instances of Stage IV dislocation, the carpal tunnel also must be opened and the median nerve decompressed.

At the time of surgery, a bulky dressing is applied. When the swelling subsides after 7 to 10 days, it is replaced with a long-arm spica cast that holds the wrist in a neutral position. A short-arm thumb spica cast is put on 4 weeks later for another 6 to 8 weeks (until there is X-ray evidence of bony healing). Even when healing is complete, a loss of wrist motion frequently follows perilunate dislocation. In a relatively small percentage of patients, perilunate dislocation leads to chronic instability or traumatic arthritis, even after open reduction and ligament repair. In these cases, other surgical options become necessary, including ligament reconstruction, proximal row carpectomy, intercarpal fusion, or total wrist fusion.

Late treatment of perilunate dislocations

Treatment of perilunate dislocations that were not recognized at the time of injury often necessitates sacrifice of a portion of normal wrist motion. Late treatment of perilunate dislocation with open reduction and internal fixation has an above-average rate of success when undertaken as long as 2 months, and maybe even 6 months, after the initial injury is sustained. In some cases, however, it may be impossible to reestablish normal anatomy when scars have formed around the bones and ligaments or the extrinsic radiocarpal ligaments have shortened. If open reduction fails, if treatment is delayed too long, or if the condition of the bones and/or ligaments precludes reduction, a proximal row carpectomy will be required. Carpectomy to treat late perilunate dislocation typically produces pain relief and an adequate range of motion and grip strength. A radiocarpal arthrodesis also may be needed if arthritis has developed as a result of the chronic instability.

Lunotriquetral Dissociation and Instability

Lunotriquetral dissociation, which occurs when the intrinsic lunotriquetral ligament is disrupted, is the injury most often affecting the ulnar side of the wrist and is a common cause of carpal instability. It is characterized by ulnar-sided wrist pain. Even small loads (forces) transmitted across the ulnar side of the wrist when the wrist is flexed can cause fibers of the lunotriquetral ligament to tear. This may be especially true in patients who have an unusually long ulna. Lunotriquetral dissociation also can be caused by injury to the TFCC or ulnocarpal abutment syndrome. Although an isolated disruption of the lunotriquetral ligament should be expected to cause a VISI pattern of instability, some studies have shown that the dorsal radiocarpal ligament also must be torn before the lunate will tilt in a volar direction.

In some patients with diagnoses of lunotriquetral dissociation, a more widespread perilunate injury may have occurred, and the patient actually may have Stage III perilunate dislocation. However, the ligaments around the scapholunate joint may have healed and signs of only lunotriquetral disruption are present when the patient arrives for diagnosis. The mechanism of injury in this context may be excessive loading when the wrist is in maximum extension, in radial deviation, and perhaps in pronation.

Diagnosis

There are two types of lunotriquetral injuries: (1) partial ligament tears (often referred to as a "sprain" by patients) and (2) joint dissociation.

For both types of injuries, the primary symptom is pain and swelling on the ulnar side of the wrist and localized tenderness over the lunotriquetral joint. A clicking sound may or may not be present when the wrist is deviated ulnarly or radially. Some patients also report wrist stiffness or weakness, as well as restricted range of motion and loss of grip strength. Symptom onset usually is associated with a traumatic event, such as a twisting injury or a fall on an outstretched hand when the wrist was in an extended position.

A positive lunotriquetral ballottement test (see Fig. 8-7) is helpful in diagnosing lunotriquetral instability. Because pisotriquetral arthritis can produce a false-positive result on the lunotriquetral ballottement test, this condition should be excluded by stressing the pisiform side to side against the triquetrum bone. If this provocative test causes pain or a grinding sensation is felt, the patient probably has pisotriquetral arthritis. Lunotriquetral instability rarely leads to arthritis because the major force-bearing joints of the wrist remain intact.

Many other disease entities also can affect the ulnar side of the wrist. Thus, the differential diagnosis must include dislocation of the distal radioulnar joint (DRUJ), subluxation of the ulna and extensor carpi ulnaris tendon, TFCC tears, midcarpal instability, ulnocarpal abutment syndrome (DRUJ impingement), and ulnar head chondromalacia.

Imaging studies

Standard four-view radiographs probably will be normal in patients with partial tears of the lunotriquetral ligament. If the ligament is disrupted completely and the lunotriquetral joint is dissociated, plain-film radiographs should show proximal displacement of the triquetrum and discontinuity of the proximal carpal row arc, especially when ulnar deviation produces an overlap of the lunate and triquetrum. A gap between the lunate and triquetrum may be evident.

Stress views may be helpful in establishing the diagnosis, specifically clenched-fist AP and lateral views, a 30° off-lateral oblique that shows the pisotriquetral joint, and lateral views with the wrist in neutral and extremes of flexion and extension. Lateral views often show the triquetrum to be dorsiflexed in relation to the lunate. The average angle between the longitudinal axis of the lunate and the longitudinal axis of the triquetrum is $+14°$. In lunotriquetral dissociation, this angle will be less than $0°$, with an average of $-16°$.

Ulnar variance should be checked with a true neutral-position PA X-ray because disruption of the lunotriquetral ligament frequently is associated with ulnocarpal abutment syndrome, in which a positive ulnar variance of 2 mm or more exists.

If the lunotriquetral ballottement test results are positive but X-rays are negative, arthrography or arthroscopy may be helpful in reaching a diagnosis. When the anatomic relationship between the lunate and triquetrum bones is disrupted, serial arthrograms will show leakage of contrast material between the midcarpal joint and proximal carpal row. However, this finding may be falsely positive in patients who have congenital or degenerative defects that are not clinically significant. Therefore, arthrographic evidence of a lunotriquetral defect must be correlated with the clinical findings and not considered diagnostic in isolation. Bilateral arthrography is recommended for differentiating between an injury and a congenital defect.

Cineradiographs usually are normal with lunotriquetral ligament disruption or joint dissociation but are positive with midcarpal instability. Cine studies can therefore help distinguish between the two.

Treatment

For acute injuries of a lunotriquetral ligament that is not completely torn, conservative treatment with a short-arm spica cast in a neutral position for 4 to 6 weeks and anti-inflammatory medications should be used. Immobilization also may be tried on patients who present with chronic complaints that indicate an old, untreated disruption (either complete or partial) of the lunotriquetral ligament.

If the patient with an acute partial ligament tear still is symptomatic after a trial of immobilization, or if a recent complete ligamentous disruption has occurred, open reduction and internal fixation with K-wires are required. A bulky dressing is applied during surgery and removed after 7 to 10 days, at which point it is replaced with a long-arm spica cast that holds the wrist in a neutral position. A short-arm cast is put on 4 weeks later for another 6 to 8 weeks.

Late treatment of lunotriquetral dissociation

Patients with chronic incomplete tears or complete disruptions of the lunotriquetral ligament require operative management. The best procedure is a four-corner arthrodesis (fusion of the triquetrum, lunate, capitate, and hamate) because it is difficult to fuse only the lunate and triquetrum. This type of arthrodesis is especially preferable for patients who have significant lunotriquetral dissociation or who engage in activities that place greater-than-average stress forces on the wrist. After this surgery, the patient is placed in a short-arm cast for 3 months, or until bony union is evident on X-rays.

Patients who have ulnocarpal abutment syndrome in association with a lunotriquetral injury also will require a joint-leveling procedure to stabilize the lunotriquetral joint.

Other Carpal Bone Dislocations

Isolated dislocations of the trapezium, trapezoid, pisiform, hamate, triquetrum, and capitate bones are rare, but they can occur.

Trapezium Dislocation

Although very unusual, complete dislocation of the trapezium can result from direct trauma to this bone and therefore often is accompanied by open injury. Dorsal dislocation is more common than volar dislocation. Closed reduction should be attempted first, but if normal anatomic alignment cannot be achieved, open reduction will be necessary.

Trapezoid Dislocation

Dislocation of the trapezoid in both volar and dorsal directions has been reported and seems to occur most often in association with dislocations of the second or third metacarpals. Because the volar surface of this triangularly shaped bone is more than twice as large as its dorsal surface, acute as well as old unrecognized volar dislocations should be treated with open reduction. Acute dorsal dislocations of the trapezoid usually can be treated with closed reduction, but open reduction will become necessary if closed manipulation is unsuccessful. Avascular necrosis has been reported as a serious complication of open reductions for both volar and dorsal trapezoid dislocations.

Pisiform Dislocation

Pisiform dislocation is uncommon but has been reported in cases of direct injury and in violent contraction of the flexor carpi ulnaris muscle. The pisiform can dislocate in volar, ulnar, proximal, and distal directions. Closed reduction followed by immobilization has been successful in some cases. However, the pisiform tends to dislocate again after a cast is removed, even with open reductions. Because this bone is expendable, excision of the pisiform may be the best treatment option for both acute and recurrent dislocations.

Hamate Dislocation

Isolated hamate dislocations are extremely rare, but have occurred in both volar and dorsal directions. Successful closed reduction of a volar dislocation has been reported and was achieved by pronating the forearm. In most instances, however, open reduction and K-wire fixation should be the treatment of choice.

Triquetrum Dislocation

Only a few instances of isolated triquetrum dislocation have been reported, in both volar and dorsal directions. Of these, the two volar dislocations were overlooked when the patients were evaluated initially, and late excision of the triquetrum was required to treat the chronic median nerve compression caused by the dislocation. In the one reported case of dorsal dislocation, open reduction of an acute injury was successful.

Capitate Dislocation

Dorsal and volar capitate dislocation has been identified in only three patients. The dorsal dislocation was associated with dislocation of the trapezoid plus the second, third, and fourth metacarpals. In this instance, open reduction plus 10 weeks of immobilization resulted in a return of one third of wrist motion. The two volar dislocations reported were found in association with other carpal injuries. In both cases, open reduction was followed by degenerative changes in the carpometacarpal joints.

Midcarpal Instability

An injured arcuate (deltoid) ligament can cause instability at the midcarpal joint, especially when the triquetrocapitate ligament—the ulnar limb of the arcuate—is damaged. The arcuate is the major supporting structure of the midcarpal area. Although ligaments around the triquetrohamate joint also provide support, injury to these ligaments alone does not seem to cause midcarpal instability. In most patients, it seems that attenuation or congenital laxity of the ulnar aspect of the arcuate ligament causes midcarpal instability rather than an acute tear.

Midcarpal instability is characterized by the following biomechanical picture. The distal carpal row sags volarly and the proximal row assumes a volar flexed position when the wrist is in a neutral or radially deviated position. With ulnar deviation of the wrist, the proximal carpal row suddenly rotates dorsally, and a clunking sound that usually is accompanied by pain can be heard.

Diagnosis

Patients typically present with ulnar-sided wrist pain and tenderness in the area of the triquetrohamate joint. Many mention that an audible clunking accompanies the movements of ulnar deviation and pronation. A slight volar sag of the distal carpal row on the ulnar side often is apparent when the wrist is visibly inspected in a neutral position. Swelling suggestive of localized synovitis may be present in the ulnar aspect of the wrist.

Unlike patients with lunotriquetral instability, most individuals with midcarpal instability do not remember a specific incident of trauma that coincides with the onset of symptoms. Those who do report a traumatic event usually describe a fall on an outstretched hand or a rotatory injury. These patients also may have an injury of the lunotriquetral ligament, which is sometimes found in association with midcarpal instability.

Visual and auditory evidence of the clunk that is characteristic of midcarpal instability can be reproduced easily with this provocative test:

1. Support the patient's hand in a neutral relaxed position with the palm down.
2. Have the patient actively pronate and ulnarly deviate the wrist.

With a positive test result, the clunk can be heard, abnormal movement causing the clunk can be seen, and the volar sagging on the ulnar side of the wrist disappears when the wrist reaches maximum ulnar deviation. This clunk can also be duplicated in most patients if you use passive manipulation and gentle axial compression.

The clunking sound associated with midcarpal instability also may be reproduced when the contralateral wrist is examined; this finding may indicate congenital or degenerative laxity in the arcuate ligament. However, a clunk in the contralateral wrist will not be accompanied by pain, as it is in the symptomatic wrist. With midcarpal instability, the painful clunk will occur spontaneously when the unstable wrist is moved during routine activities.

Imaging studies

When midcarpal instability is present, a lateral plain X-ray obtained with the wrist in a neutral position often shows volar flexion of the lunate. Other plain views probably will appear normal.

Cineradiography is perhaps the best way to diagnose midcarpal instability. Motion in flexion and extension typically is normal, but moving from radial to ulnar deviation will reveal the proximal carpal row snapping from a volar to a dorsal position instead of gliding smoothly. This sudden dorsal rotation of the proximal carpal row produces the clunking sound associated with midcarpal instability.

Arthrograms usually are normal in midcarpal instability. However, a positive arthrogram, in which the contrast material flows into the lunotriquetral area, may indicate that lunotriquetral instability coexists with the midcarpal instability. In most instances, the clinical picture of midcarpal instability is more pronounced than that of the lunotriquetral disruption.

Treatment

A conservative treatment approach for midcarpal instability should be attempted first. In association with anti-inflammatory drugs, including steroid injections into the triquetrohamate joint, immobilization for 4 to 6 weeks in a short-arm spica cast with the wrist in a neutral position may alleviate the pain and clunking.

If symptoms are not relieved by conservative treatment, or they return weeks or months after the cast is removed, a triquetrohamate arthrodesis will be needed. Patients should be informed that this procedure will cause some loss in the range of motion, particularly flexion, but wrist motion should remain within a functional range.

INJURIES TO THE TRIANGULAR FIBROCARTILAGE COMPLEX, THE DISTAL RADIOULNAR JOINT, AND THE DISTAL ULNA

Anatomy

The anatomy of the distal radioulnar joint (DRUJ) consists of several structures that play important roles in the load bearing and mechanical functioning of the wrist (Fig. 8-21).

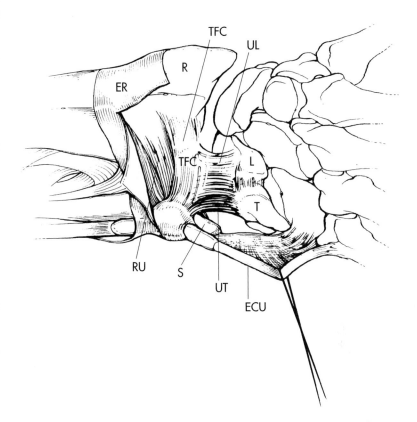

Figure 8-21 Normal anatomy of the distal radioulnar joint (DRUJ) and triangular fibrocartilage complex (TFCC). The articular disk of the TFCC (TFC) is at the center of the complex and is essential to DRUJ stability. Other structures shown are the radioulnar capsular ligaments (RU) and ulnocarpal ligaments (UL = ulnolunate and UT = ulnotriquetral). Distally, the ulnocarpal ligaments merge with the lunotriquetral intrinsic ligament, which is shown adjoining the lunate (L) and triquetrum (T). The extensor carpi ulnaris tendon (ECU) has a thick fibrocartilagenous floor. The extensor retinaculum (ER), the radius (R), and the ulnar styloid (S) also are visible.

The most distal portion of the ulnar head is the ulnar styloid, a post-like structure that serves as an attachment site for stabilizing ligaments. The radius and ulnar head articulate at the sigmoid notch of the radius.

An important component of the DRUJ is the triangular fibrocartilage complex (TFCC). At the center of the TFCC is its triangularly shaped articular disk (also called the triangular fibrocartilage proper or TFC proper) that arises from the sigmoid notch of the radius and inserts into the ulnar styloid. This disk is ~2 mm thick at its radial origin and 5 mm at its ulnar insertion. Covering three quarters of the head of the ulna and the sigmoid notch of the radius, the TFC proper allows simultaneous rotation and sliding of the ulnar head when the forearm is rotated. This articular disk, which serves as a cushion between the ulnar head and carpus, is a major load-bearing component of the DRUJ.

The primary ligaments of the distal radioulnar joint essentially are thickened continuations of the TFC proper that extend from the periphery of the articular disk. They function as the major stabilizing elements of the DRUJ. Several important ligaments that support the ulnar aspect of the carpal bones form the ulnocarpal ligament complex (composed of the ulnolunate, ulnotriquetral, and ulnar collateral ligaments).

The dorsal and volar radioulnar ligaments also are part of the TFCC and function as dynamic stabilizers of the DRUJ. They connect the base of the ulnar styloid and the radius just proximal to the articular disk. These radioulnar ligaments function more as a unit than as independent ligaments to limit rotational and axial migration. The volar radioulnar ligament maintains stability of the distal ulna in pronation. The dorsal radioulnar ligament maintains stability of the distal ulna in supination.

All of these soft tissue structures in the DRUJ are subjected to weight-bearing forces and the transmission of loads across the wrist. The distal ends of the ulna and radius are therefore vulnerable to acute injuries, as well as chronic mechanical degeneration and inflammatory disease.

The articulation between the radius and ulna at the sigmoid notch is encapsulated so that the relationship between the radius and ulna is balanced as the forearm rotates from complete pronation to complete supination. Both bones move together, with the radius rotating about the ulnar head (which remains stationary). The length relationship between the distal ulna and the distal radius is therefore critical for proper mechanical functioning of the DRUJ.

This length relationship, or the ulnar variance, changes with different movements as the ulnar head glides several millimeters within the sigmoid notch of the radius. In supination, the ulnar head moves volarly in the sigmoid notch; in pronation, it moves dorsally. In full pronation and supination, the ulnar head is almost completely uncovered and has little direct contact with the sigmoid notch. If the ulna is longer than the radius (an ulna plus wrist), it can impinge on the proximal row of the carpus, limit wrist rotation, and disrupt the lunotriquetral joint. An ulna that is shorter than the radius (an ulna minus wrist) can cause excess loading on the lunate, which has been associated with an increased frequency of Kienböck's disease.

General Diagnostic Examinations

Identifying the source of pain in and around the area of the ulnar aspect of the wrist can be difficult. The physician must first determine whether the pain originates in the carpus or in the distal radioulnar joint. A simple test can help with localization.
1. Have the patient sit in front of you with elbow flexed and fingers pointed toward the ceiling.
2. Passively move the forearm through a full range of motion.

Pain produced in the wrist when the forearm is moved localizes the site of the problem to the radioulnar joint. If the problem is of carpal origin, forearm motion will not produce wrist pain.

Next have the patient actively rotate the forearm while you observe the extensor carpi ulnaris, the distal ulna, and the ulnar aspect of the wrist for signs of acute dislocation or subluxation. Also apply stress to the DRUJ and note any pain, crepitus, or subluxation.

Imaging Studies

Several radiographic views of the DRUJ are useful for diagnosis, including full supination, midposition supination, neutral, midposition pronation, and full pronation. These views often can identify bone contour defects, malaligned structures, abnormal trabecular patterns, or discrepancies in the length of the radius and ulna.

Because the relationship between the length of the radius and that of the ulna is so important to DRUJ functioning, a plain film X-ray of the radioulnar joint taken with the wrist and arm in a true neutral position is essential. (See the section on the Four-View Wrist Series and Stress View Radiographs.) Figure 8-22 illustrates typical radiographic findings of neutral (normal), positive, and negative ulnar variance.

If plain-film X-rays are not diagnostic, other imaging modalities may be needed, including arthrography, MRI, CT, or arthroscopy.

TFCC Injuries

The TFCC articular disk consists of a central and peripheral portions, and tears or disruptions can occur either centrally or peripherally. The central portion of the disk is thinner than the periphery and is composed of sheets of collagen fibers that are obliquely interwoven and designed to resist multidirectional stress forces. This central articular disk is not well vascularized; consequently, injuries in this area do not heal well. The peripheral areas of the TFCC are more fibrous than the central articular disk and much better vascularized; this superior vascular supply usually leads to prompt healing if peripheral tears are treated promptly.

The TFCC transmits approximately 20% of an axially applied load

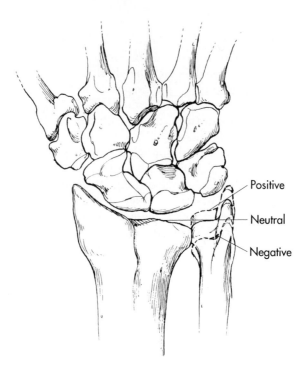

Figure 8-22   Illustration of ulnar variance as might be seen on a true neutral-position posteroanterior radiograph. To evaluate variance, draw a straight line from the distal articular surface of the radius across the ulna. If the line meets the distal articular surface of the ulna, the variance is neutral (or normal). With a positive variance (or ulna plus wrist), the articular surface of the ulna is distal to the articular surface of the radius. With a negative variance (or ulna minus wrist), the distal surface of the ulna lies proximal to the distal surface of the radius.

across the wrist (from the carpus to the distal ulna), with the other 80% being transmitted by the radiocarpal joint. The integrity of the TFCC articular disk is crucial to DRUJ stability, and traumatic disruption of this disk is a frequent cause of ulnar-sided wrist pain. At least 40% of people older than 40 years of age have degenerative defects of the TFCC, but many of these defects are asymptomatic and often bilateral. However, trauma-induced tears are serious injuries and a potential source of wrist instability.

The mechanism of TFCC injury typically is an applied force to an extended and pronated wrist that is axially loaded, or a traction force to the ulnar aspect of the wrist or forearm. Both types of forces can occur when a person falls on an outstretched hand.

There are three types of TFCC disruptions: acute (traumatic),

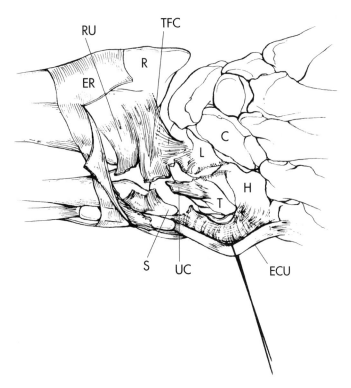

Figure 8-23   Some common injuries to the distal radioulnar joint (DRUJ). This figure shows peripheral detachment of the TFCC articular disk (TFC) from the ulnar styloid (S). Most TFCC injuries seem to begin at the periphery of the TFC proper. The floor of the extensor carpi ulnaris tendon (ECU) and the radioulnar ligaments (RU) also may be torn from the TFC articular disk and ulnar styloid. If the ulnocarpal ligaments (UC) are disrupted, the lunotriquetral intrinsic ligament frequently tears. This injury may ultimately cause midcarpal instability by disrupting the alignments of the triquetrum (T), hamate (H), lunate (L) and capitate (C) bones. Other structures depicted are the extensor retinaculum (ER) and the radius (R).

chronic (degenerative), and congenital. Traumatic TFCC injuries traditionally have been divided into four categories that are defined by the location of damage and the extent to which various DRUJ structures are involved. Several potential injuries are illustrated in Fig. 8-23. The four primary types of injury are:

1. Tear in the central portion of the TFCC articular disk. The tear is most often oriented from dorsal to volar and located several millimeters medial to the origin of the disk in the sigmoid notch of the

radius. The peripheral portions of the TFCC and their attachments remain intact; thus the wrist remains stable.

2. Tear in the periphery of the TFCC at the point of insertion into the ulnar styloid. This type of disruption, which sometimes accompanies an ulnar styloid fracture, causes instability of the DRUJ.

3. Tear of a TFCC distal attachment to ulnocarpal ligaments (ulnolunate and ulnotriquetral ligaments). In this scenario, the ulnar carpus is unstable and may translocate in a volar direction.

4. Tear of the TFCC from its attachment at the sigmoid notch of the radius. This type of injury also causes DRUJ instability.

Disruptions of the peripheral aspect of the TFCC at the ulnar styloid may herald other injuries in the area of the styloid. For example, if the TFCC is torn from its insertion at the ulnar styloid, the extensor carpi ulnaris tendon sheath is also frequently disrupted, causing subluxation of the tendon and ulna. The ulnocarpal ligaments may also be torn, and injury to these structures can propagate distally to disrupt the lunotriquetral, triquetrocapitate, and/or triquetrohamate ligaments. In this instance, perilunate or midcarpal instability may develop. Awareness of the fact that injuries to the TFCC articular disk may involve other structures should be kept in mind when diagnosing ulnocarpal symptoms and planning treatment approaches.

Diagnosis

Patients with disruptions or tears of the TFCC present with ulnar-sided wrist pain that may be exacerbated by ulnar deviation, pronation and supination, or axial loading of the wrist. Swelling over the ulnar aspect of the wrist, as well as point tenderness over the TFCC and distal ulna, are common. A clicking sound heard when the forearm is rotated and/or inflammation of the extensor carpi ulnaris tendon are sometimes present.

A tear in the peripheral aspect of the TFCC at the point of insertion into the ulnar styloid, which causes DRUJ instability, may be indicated by laxity and/or prominence of the distal ulna. Tenderness over the lunotriquetral joint suggests that a tear of the TFCC also involves the lunotriquetral ligament.

Several other problems can cause symptoms similar to those of TFCC injury, including pisotriquetral arthritis, distal radioulnar joint arthritis, lunotriquetral dissociation, ulnocarpal abutment syndrome, or subluxation of the extensor carpi ulnaris tendon. These disorders often are found in association with a disrupted TFCC. Ulnar artery thrombosis can also produce symptoms similar to those seen with TFCC injury. This problem is differentiated by the presence of a positive Allen's test, cold intolerance in the hand (especially the ulnar aspect) and color changes in the ring and little fingers.

Imaging studies

Although plain films often are normal, true lateral and neutral (posteroanterior) position plain film X-rays should reveal fracture, carpal malalignment, abnormal ulnar variance, and a dorsally prominent distal ulna suggestive of subluxation. Plain films can also exclude malalignment of the DRUJ and ulnar styloid abnormalities, including nonunion of a fracture fragment.

Injury to the TFCC occurs more frequently in people who have a positive or neutral ulnar variance, as well as in patients who have sustained a distal radius fracture. Therefore, these radiographic findings should suggest the possibility of a TFCC injury.

Other imaging methods are more accurate for diagnosing TFCC injuries than plain radiographs. For example, arthrography (with injections into the radiocarpal and distal radioulnar joints) can visualize isolated tears of the central articular disk as well as disruptions of the peripheral attachments (Figs. 8-24 and 8-25). Arthroscopy is valuable because it can diagnose and correct isolated central articular disk tears in a single procedure. Computed tomography and MRI (particularly T2-weight images taken in the coronal plane) can be used to obtain information about all structures of the triangular fibrocartilage complex.

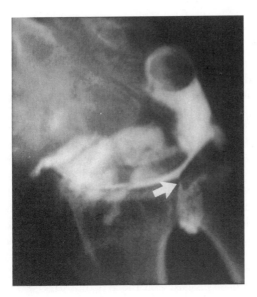

Figure 8-24   Radiocarpal arthrography shows a small communication to the distal radioulnar compartment near the radial attachment of the TFC articular disk (*arrow*).

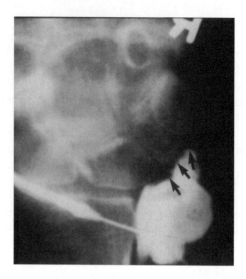

Figure 8-25   Distal radioulnar arthrography shows contrast material surrounding the proximal attachments of the TFCC at the ulnar styloid (*arrows*), which indicates a peripheral detachment of TFCC. Because there is no communication to the radiocarpal compartment, this injury would be overlooked if only radiocarpal arthrography were performed.

Treatment

Acute injury of the TFCC that is not complicated by fracture, subluxation, or instability of the distal radioulnar or radiocarpal joints often can be treated with immobilization. Use of a long-arm spica cast and anti-inflammatory drugs for 4 weeks usually is successful, even when the poorly vascularized central portion of the TFCC articular disk is torn.

Isolated tears of the articular disk, both old untreated tears and large acute tears, often can be treated effectively with arthroscopic debridement.

Old (untreated) and acute injuries that involve ligamentous TFCC structures outside the articular disk, as well as disruptions of the TFCC articular disk that do not heal with immobilization, require open surgical repair. For example, a displaced articular disk can be advanced to its site of detachment at the ulnar styloid and secured with intraosseous sutures. If the ulnar styloid is fractured, the styloid fragment should be excised and the articular disk sutured to the base of the styloid remnant. Ulnocarpal ligament tears can be repaired with direct suturing and/or augmentation with the thick floor of the extensor carpi ulnaris sheath. However, disruptions of the extensor carpi ulnaris sheath itself rarely are suitable for suturing and usually require reconstruction. Triangular fibrocartilage complex tears that also encompass the intrinsic carpal ligaments (such as the lunotriquetral, triquetrocapitate, or triquetrohamate) require the repair methods described in earlier sections of this chapter.

Some extensive TFCC tears that affect the functioning of the distal radioulnar joint may require ulnar resection, hemi-interposition arthroplasty, or carpal/ulnocarpal fusions.

Open repair of TFCC injuries is followed by a bulky surgical dressing for 7 to 10 days (until swelling subsides) and then long-arm cast immobilization for at least 6 weeks. If carpal fusion is required to repair an injury, the period of cast immobilization should be for 8 to 10 weeks or until evidence of bony union is apparent on X-rays. When treated appropriately, the outcome of TFCC injuries usually is quite good, with restoration of DRUJ stability and a pain-free and adequately mobile wrist.

Dislocation/Subluxation of the Ulna

An isolated ulnar dislocation in either a dorsal or volar direction is relatively rare. This type of injury almost always is associated with a disrupted TFCC, which may include the articular disk, the extensor carpi ulnaris tendon, and possibly the ulnocarpal or radioulnar ligaments. Fractures of the distal radius or ulna also contribute to subluxation of the ulna.

Diagnosis

Patients with a dislocated ulna present with a painful and swollen wrist. Any attempt to rotate the forearm and wrist causes extreme pain. Joint deformity is usually obvious. If the dislocation is dorsal, supination is painful and limited, and the ulna is prominent dorsally. With a volar dislocation, pronation is painful and limited, the ulna is prominent volarly, and a sulcus may be evident dorsally. In chronic cases of ulnar subluxation, a grating sensation or audible click also may be present.

Ulnar dislocation is typically caused by a fall on an extended hand, a direct blow to the DRUJ, or excessive rotation (either sustained in acute injury or in response to performance of repetitive tasks). Because ulnar dislocation so often is associated with TFCC injuries, the diagnostic process must consider the possibility that a TFCC disruption exists.

Imaging studies

Exact lateral views of the wrist in a neutral position are useful for identifying ulnar dislocation, but obtaining such radiographs may be difficult if the patient cannot rotate the forearm enough for true lateral views. As little as 10° of rotation can change the radio-carpal relationships and cause an ulnar head subluxation to be over-looked or diagnosed when no subluxation exists (Fig. 8-26). There-fore, CT or MRI images are more accurate for demonstrating subluxation of the ulna. These techniques also will provide informa-tion about the status of the TFCC articular disk and other TFCC structures, as well as the intrinsic carpal ligaments.

A

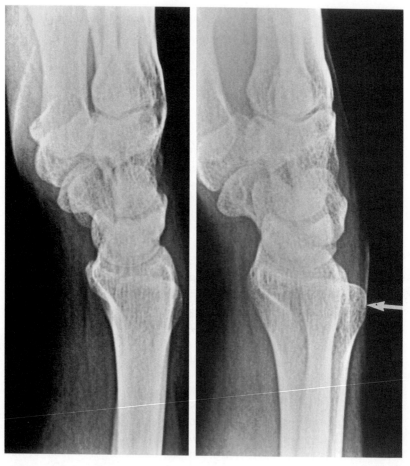

Figure 8-26 Obtaining a true lateral radiograph is important for diagnosing many injuries, including subluxation of the ulna. **(A)** A true lateral view of a healthy wrist and DRUJ, with no evidence of subluxation. **(B)** The same wrist with the radiograph slightly off lateral. Based on this view, a dorsal subluxation of the DRUJ (*arrow*) might be incorrectly diagnosed.

Treatment

Because TFCC disruptions frequently are associated with ulnar dislocation, TFCC injuries should be treated as already described. An appropriate anesthetic should be given before an ulnar subluxation is reduced. Closed reduction of a dorsal dislocation requires forceful supination, and a volar dislocation is reduced by forceful pronation. Reduction is followed by immobilization. For dorsal dislocation of the ulnar head, a long-arm cast with the wrist held in supination for 4 to 6 weeks is the treatment of choice. For volar dislocation of the ulna, use a long-arm cast with the wrist held in pronation.

If the joint cannot be reduced anatomically with closed manipulation, an osteochondral fracture or interposed soft tissue probably is also present. Open reduction will be necessary in these instances.

Fracture of the Ulnar Head

Fractures of the ulnar head and its articular surfaces frequently are associated with radial fractures. The cause is significant direct trauma.

Diagnosis

Patients with a fractured ulnar head have localized pain, swelling, point tenderness, and a history of injury.

Imaging studies

Diagnosis of an ulnar head fracture is made through four-view plain film radiographs. The fracture pattern may be one of comminution of the entire head or an ulnar head that is displaced from the shaft of the ulna.

Treatment

Open reduction and rigid internal fixation are necessary to restore the anatomic alignment of the articular surface or shaft with the ulnar head. If there is extensive comminution, arthroplasty frequently is required.

Distal Radioulnar Joint Impingement/Ulnocarpal Abutment Syndrome

The ulnar head can impinge on, or abut against, the carpus if the head of the ulna lies distal to the head of the radius. Chronic ulnar abutment can lead to degeneration or disruption of the TFCC articular disk, DRUJ instability, and/or tearing of the lunotriquetral ligament. Ulnocarpal abutment occurs most frequently when a radial fracture that was not accurately reduced causes the radius to shorten in relation to the ulna. It also can be a consequence of distal radial epiphyseal growth arrest, wrist fusion in which the radius is shortened, treatments of radial tumors or infections, and occupational repetitive loading in individuals who have a congenital positive ulnar variance.

Diagnosis

Patients present with ulnar wrist pain that is most severe with rotation and ulnar deviation. Clicks and crepitus are common features.

Imaging studies

To determine the relationship between the lengths of the radius and ulna, a true neutral position X-ray must be obtained and the distal ends of the forearm bones evaluated, as illustrated in Fig. 8-22. (Correct positioning was discussed in the section on Four-View Wrist Series and Stress View Radiographs.) Other commonly used radiographic positions can cause radioulnar rotation, which distorts the relationship between the lengths of the ulna and radius. Radiographs of the contralateral, asymptomatic wrist are sometimes necessary for comparison purposes.

Treatment

The treatment of choice for DRUJ impingement is shortening of the ulnar shaft to restore a normal anatomic relationship between the distal ends of the radius and ulna.

KIENBÖCK'S DISEASE

Lunate pain or injury may be caused by the chronic process of avascular necrosis of the lunate bone, leading to collapse of the lunate, carpal instability, and pancarpal arthritis. This is known as Kienböck's disease. The loss of blood supply results from multiple chronic insults produced by repeated compression, ligamentous injury, or multiple or severe fractures. The length relationship between the head of the distal ulna and the articular surface of the radius also is believed to be important in development of this disease.

The lunate receives support from radial and ulnar structures. Some have theorized that the lunate is not as well supported in the ulna minus wrist (in which the ulna is shorter than the radius), and this lack of support leads to an asymmetric stress distribution that produces increased compression at the radial side of the lunate bone. The ultimate cause of avascular necrosis is probably a combination of multiple factors, including compression, synovitis, and anatomic or structural predisposition.

The natural history of Kienböck's disease may be conceptualized as four stages of progressive lunate involvement that is visible on plain radiographs. Treatment of the disease is predicated on the following stages:

Stage I Bony sclerosis of the lunate is evident on X-ray, and a linear or compression fracture may be present, but there is no arthritis.

Stage II In early Stage II disease, the sizes and anatomic relationships of the carpal bones is normal, but there are obvious radiographic density changes in the lunate. In late Stage II, the radial side of the lunate may be shortened as collapse begins. Fracture lines are sometimes evident.

Stage III   The lunate continues to collapse and becomes fragmented. Eventually the capitate migrates proximally and the scaphoid dissociates from the lunate and rotates. The triquetrum may deviate in an ulnar direction.

Stage IV   Extensive lunate fragmentation and collapse leads to pancarpal arthritis and significant carpal instability.

Diagnosis

Patients with Kienböck's disease usually report a gradual onset of pain or acute pain after a seemingly trivial or unrelated injury. There is pain with gripping, decreased grip strength, and a limited range of wrist motion. Symptoms of median nerve compression also may be present. The physical examination reveals localized tenderness over the dorsal aspect of the lunate, nonspecific swelling, and symptoms of synovitis.

Imaging studies

Plain radiographs identify the stage of Kienböck's disease, depending on the common findings evident on X-rays: bony sclerosis, density changes, loss of lunate height, fracture lines, bony fragmentation, and carpal collapse. A true neutral position X-ray (as described in the section on Four-View Wrist Series and Stress View Radiographs) is necessary to determine the relationship between the lengths of the radius and ulna (see Fig. 8-22). When the lunate is collapsed, the capitate moves to a more proximal position, the proximal carpal row appears wider than normal, and the scaphoid may be rotated.

A bone scan usually demonstrates the presence of Kienböck's disease before plain films will show it. A decreased blood supply or marrow edema can be revealed by MRI early in the disease process. Computed tomography is useful in assessing the degree of fragmentation, which is important information when planning treatment.

Treatment

Many hand surgeons currently distinguish between Kienböck's disease occurring in the ulna plus wrist (the articular plane of the ulna lies distal to the articular plane of the radius) and the ulna minus wrist (the articular plane of the ulna lies proximal to the articular plane of the radius). Joint leveling procedures have been advocated for treating Kienböck's disease when there is either a positive or negative ulnar variance, as have other surgical methods designed to diminish stress on or improve the vitality of the lunate bone. Short-arm cast immobilization with and without electrical stimulation can be used to treat Stage I disease in both ulna minus and ulna plus wrists.

The treatment of ulna minus Kienböck's disease generally relies on joint-leveling (radial shortening or ulnar lengthening) procedures to unload the lunate bone. Joint-leveling is an accepted treatment for Stage I, Stage II, and early Stage III ulna minus disease (before development of severe collapse, extensive fragmentation, or arthritis). Radial shortening is preferred to ulnar lengthening because radial healing is more rapid, a bone graft is not required, and corrections in the tilt of the radial articular surface can be achieved. Triscaphe [scaphotrapezium-trapezoid (STT)] fusions have been used to unload the lunate bone in Stages I, II, and III of the disease. In late Stage III or Stage IV, when there is considerable lunate fragmentation and extensive arthritis, partial (radiocarpal or ulnar column) or total wrist fusions commonly are performed.

There is more diversity in the treatment of ulna plus Kienböck's disease. Immobilization with a short-arm cast for periods of 3 to 12 weeks usually is recommended for Stage I disease. Treatment of Stages II and III disease relies on unloading of the lunate by triscaphe (STT) arthrodesis, scaphocapitate arthrodesis, capitate shortening, or joint leveling. Treatment of Stage IV disease is accomplished by partial or total wrist fusion.

The rationale behind triscaphe arthrodesis, joint-leveling procedures, and capitate shortening is that they relieve the load on the avascular lunate and thereby allow revascularization and new bone growth. These procedures are most useful in Stage II and early Stage III disease (in which the lunate is partially collapsed but not extensively fragmented).

Other treatments also are available. Bone grafting of the collapsed or mildly-fragmented lunate bone may be used in Stages II and III. Carved silicone spacers and tendon anchovy grafts have been used as lunate replacements in Stage III, sometimes in combination with a partial (scaphocapitate) carpal fusion. Placement of silicone prostheses has become unpopular because they frequently cause silicone synovitis. As an adjunct to lunate stress-relieving procedures, lunate revascularization also is used in Stages I and II and early Stage III disease.

CARPAL BOSSING

A carpal boss is a normal variant consisting of bony overgrowths from the capitate and the base of the second or third metacarpals. Symptoms occur when degenerative arthritis develops between the opposing bony spurs.

Diagnosis

Patients typically have a history of dorsal wrist pain during extension. Tenderness to palpation at the base of the second and/or third metacarpals usually is present. Impingement of the dorsal capsule and carpal structures by very large carpal bosses can cause a mechanical block that limits full wrist extension.

Imaging studies

A lateral view radiograph of the bases of the second and third metacarpals must be obtained and carefully scrutinized for abnormality. A bone scan demonstrates increased uptake when arthritis or a fracture of the boss is present.

Treatment

Surgical excision of a carpal boss down to normal articular cartilage is the treatment of choice for symptomatic bosses.

DISTAL RADIAL FRACTURES

Fractures of the distal radius represent some of the most challenging injuries encountered by the hand or upper-extremity surgeon. Distal radius fractures frequently occur after a fall on an outstretched arm. The Common mechanisms of injury include athletics, motor vehicle accidents, and falls during inclement weather. Patients typically report falling onto an outstretched arm and developing immediate pain, swelling, and often visible deformity in the distal portion of the forearm or wrist. Radiographs will confirm the distal radial fracture.

Recognize that fractures of the distal radius have a high attendant rate of complications and a potential for poor long-term functional results that have only been appreciated relatively recently. Some physicians have suggested that the biggest potential error in managing a distal radial fracture is to underestimate the functional impairment that may result from such an injury.

Anatomic Considerations

Rational decision making regarding treatment of distal radius fractures mandates an understanding of pertinent normal anatomy of the region. Four anatomic parameters are commonly deranged after distal radius fractures, and their status must specifically be assessed. Any treatment plan must correct major deformities in these areas. The four major parameters include (1) continuity of articular surfaces, including the radiocarpal joint and the distal radioulnar joint, (2) the radial inclination of the radius, (3) the volar tilt of the radius, and (4) the relative lengths of the radius and ulna. First, the congruity of the articular surfaces must be evaluated. Mere fracturing into the articular surface, or more importantly, displacement (step-off) among intraarticular fragments may ultimately result in traumatic radiocarpal arthritis, a potentially devastating condition. Second, radial inclination is important. Radial inclination refers to the normal slope of the radius as

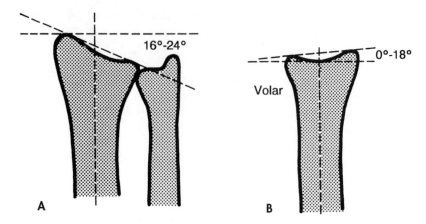

Figure 8-27 **(A)** Radial inclination represents the slope of the radius in a radial to ulnar direction and is normally 16 to 24°. **(B)** Volar tilt represents the slope of the radius in a dorsal to volar direction and is normally from 0 to 18°.

visualized in an AP or PA radiograph, in which the radial (lateral) portion of the radius is relatively longer than the more ulnar (medial) portion of the radius. This degree of inclination varies among individuals, but ranges from 16 to 24° (Fig. 8-27A). Third, the radius is tilted toward the volar surface when viewed from a lateral perspective. This angle commonly measures 0 to 18°, and is termed volar tilt (Fig. 8-27B). Both radial inclination and volar tilt may be affected significantly after impaction, rotation, and displacement of fracture fragments has occurred; failure to correct these deformities predisposes to abnormal wrist biomechanics, altered wrist motion, and the development of traumatic arthritis. The fourth parameter of concern will be the relative lengths of the radius and ulna, or ulnar variance (Fig. 8-28). Among the general population, the ulna normally may be slightly longer than the radius (ulnar positive), the same length as the radius (ulnar neutral), or shorter than the radius (ulnar negative). However, after axial trauma to the wrist, the fractured radius may be impacted and significantly shortened compared with the adjacent ulna. In general, during treatment of distal radius fractures, an ulnar-neutral position should be sought. If the patient's normal anatomy is uncertain, radiographs of the uninvolved hand may be helpful in determining their normal bony anatomy.

The consequences of failing to restore the normal anatomy may be significant. There is a relatively high complication rate with distal radial fractures and a relatively high percentage of poor results. Studies

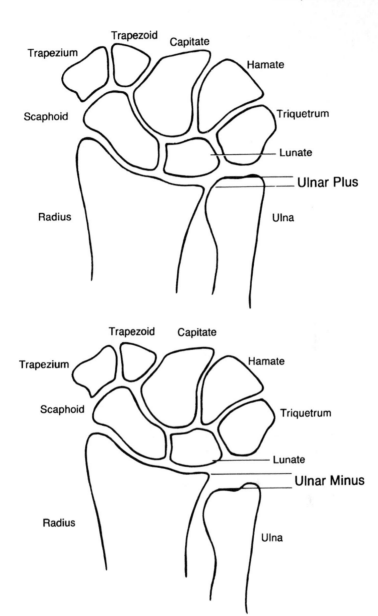

Figure 8-28   (**A** and **B**) Ulnar variance is a measure of the relative lengths of the radius and ulna as evaluated by standard radiographic views. This relationship is termed "ulnar positive," "ulnar neutral," or "ulnar negative."

have indicated that the more abnormal the resultant reduction of the fracture, the greater the chance may be for a poor result. Although unsatisfactory results may be obtained even with anatomic alignment, excessive dorsal angulation following a Colles' fracture, for instance, increases the chances of ultimately developing arthroses or stiffness of the wrist in the future. Similarly, the relative lengths of the radius and ulna, as well as radial inclination also influence outcome. Kopylov et al. provide further insights into the importance of these measurements.

Classification

There are multiple classification systems available for categorizing types of fractures to guide treatment decisions and help estimate prognosis. One of the most common and perhaps the simplest is the Frykman Classification of distal radius fractures (Fig. 8-29). This particular classification scheme relates fracture severity principally to the integrity of the radiocarpal and radioulnar articular surfaces. It assigns fractures to numerical groups, one through eight, based on extensions into the radiocarpal joint, the distal radioulnar joint, or both, and whether the ulnar styloid is also fractured. All odd numbers of classification involve the distal radius only, without fracture of the ulnar styloid, and all even numbers represent corresponding fractures associ-

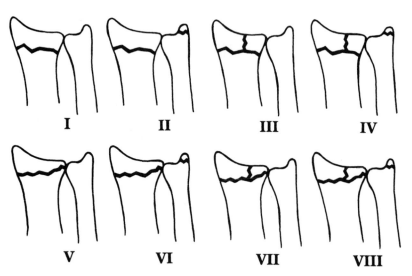

Figure 8-29   Frykman Classification of Distal Radius Fracture Patterns. Higher classification numbers are generally associated with more severe injuries and less acceptable outcomes.

ated with fracture of the ulnar styloid. The more severely involved the articular surface, the higher the classification. Other classifications are stratified by degrees of comminution of the distal radius, as represented by the universal classification schemes. These classifications logically imply that as the amount of energy imparted to create the fracture increases, the extent of bony injury increases. The treating physician can understand readily that the higher the classification, the more severe the fracture pattern and the less stable and more problematic the distal forearm and wrist are likely to be in the future.

Certain common fracture patterns are associated with named fracture types: Colles', Smith's, Barton's, and Chauffeur's fractures. These are classified according to the fracture site and the direction of displacement.

Colles' Fracture

Colles' fracture is the most common of the distal radial fractures and is characterized by dorsal displacement of the distal fragment (Fig. 8-30). The most basic Colles' fracture is a transverse fracture with dorsal displacement or angulation and some dorsal impaction. In the moderately severe Colles' fracture, comminution of the dorsal cortex of the distal radius is encountered. In extensive Colles' fractures, severe comminution of the dorsal cortex and intraarticular extension into the radiocarpal and distal radioulnar joints are common. In addition to simple dorsal angulation, there may be significant dorsal displacement of the fracture (Fig. 8-31).

Smith's Fracture

A Smith's fracture is essentially a reverse Colles' fracture (Fig. 8-32). The distal fragment is angulated toward the palm (volarly/palmerly), and the volar cortex may be impacted and comminuted. Alternatively, an oblique fracture, rather than a transverse fracture, may permit the distal fragment to become displaced volarly rather than angulated volarly. Smith's fractures have been classified further into three types: Type I is a transverse fracture with volar angulation, Type II is an oblique fracture allowing a single distal fragment, including the entire articular surface, to be displaced in a volar direction, and Type 3 occurs when an oblique fracture extends into the radiocarpal surface, thereby allowing a portion of the radiocarpal joint and the carpus itself, to be displaced in a volar direction (Fig. 8-33). Type III is essentially a volar Barton's fracture.

Barton's Fracture

Barton's fractures involve either the volar or dorsal lips of the radius, with the remainder of the radius remaining mostly intact and not involved with the fracture (Fig. 8-34). The carpus itself typically displaces with the fractured fragment.

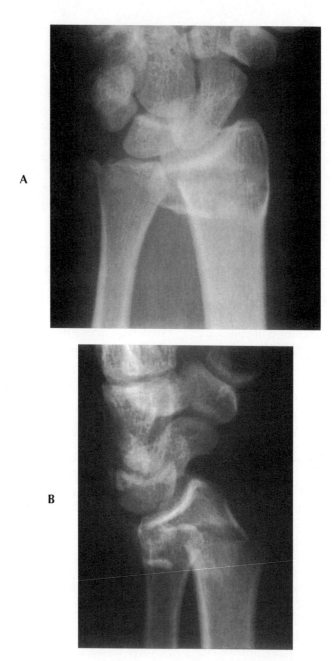

Figure 8-30 (**A** and **B**) Typical Colles' fracture: transverse fracture of the distal radius with dorsal displacement and angulation of the distal fragment.

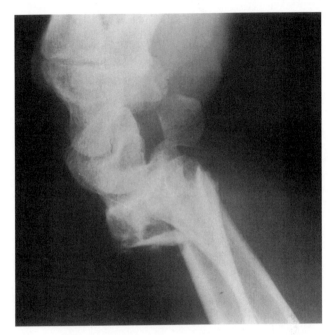

Figure 8-31   Colles' fracture showing significant dorsal angulation and displacement.

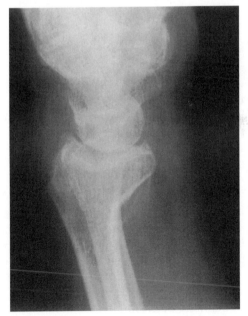

Figure 8-32   Smith's fracture with volar (anterior) displacement and angulation of the distal fracture fragment.

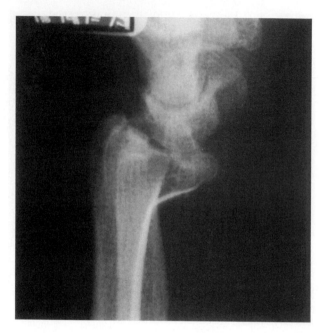

Figure 8-33 Smith Type III fracture or volar Barton's fracture with significant volar displacement of the distal fragment and carpus. The injury is technically a fracture–dislocation.

Chauffeur's Fracture

A Chauffeur's fracture is type of intraarticular fracture in which the radial styloid is fractured from the remainder of the radius. It is an impaction fracture through the radial fossa displacing the radial styloid. A depressed fracture of the radial fossa may accompany the chauffeur's fracture. The carpus usually does not displace with the radial styloid. These are similar in concept to Barton's fractures of the radial aspect of the bone.

Evaluation

First aid for radial fractures consists of splinting the forearm and transporting the patient to a medical facility. Transport can be achieved more comfortably if the patient's wrist is supported with a splint before movement to a hospital or a physician's office. Once in the office or emergency room, evaluation of the patient with a suspected distal radial fracture initially should include a history of the injury. This will facilitate determining the amount of energy that may have been imparted to the wrist. After the history has been obtained,

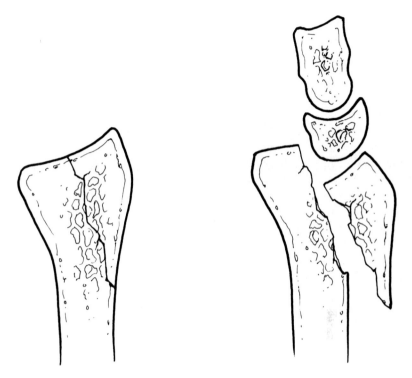

Figure 8-34   Barton's fractures may be volar or dorsal and represent a fracture–dislocation.

the wrist is evaluated carefully for swelling, tenderness, and obvious deformity. The elbow and shoulder should be evaluated for pain, tenderness, or swelling in every patient who has fallen on an outstretched hand or has a wrist injury. Forces that cause injury to the distal radius can be transmitted longitudinally through the radius to the head of the radius at the elbow, and evidence of injury there should be investigated. If the integrity of the elbow is in question, radiographs should be obtained simultaneously with those of the distal radius. Plain radiographs of the distal radius will allow general characterization of the fracture and should include a posteroanterior view, an oblique (semipronation) view, and a lateral view. Plain radiographs are the mainstay in determining whether closed or open methods of treatment will be necessary. In general, nonoperative, or closed, reductions can be expected to produce satisfactory results in the less comminuted, transverse-type fractures, as well as fractures that do not appear initially to be significantly displaced. Fractures that exhibit severe comminution, those with intraarticular involvement with displacement, and most Smith's fractures will require operative reduction and fixation. Additionally, all open fractures of the distal radius should be treated operatively with irrigation, reduction, and appropriate fixation.

Further assessment of the patient always should include evaluation of the neurovascular status of the hand. While a vascular compromise is an extremely rare occurrence after isolated distal radius fractures, a frequent sequelae of distal radial fractures is the development of an acute or traumatic carpal tunnel syndrome. A injury in the vicinity of the median nerve induces edema. The carpal tunnel is an unyielding structure that cannot accommodate the increased nerve soft tissue volume; as a result, progressive ischemia develops within the nerve. Patients who develop paresthesias or anesthesia in the median nerve distribution after wrist injuries should therefore be considered for carpal tunnel decompression to prevent permanent median nerve damage. After thorough evaluation of the involved upper extremity in the distal radial fracture patient, treatment proceeds with initial closed reduction and casting or splinting and organization for operative reduction when indicated. The hand surgeon always should consider concomitant thoracic, abdominal, or other injuries in patients whose distal radius fractures are caused by motor vehicle accidents and other mechanisms likely to induce serious multisystem trauma. Associated injuries must be sought and treated before undertaking treatment of the distal radius when appropriate.

Nonoperative Treatment

Closed reduction and cast immobilization may achieve satisfactory results, especially in the less severe type of Colles' fracture (transverse fracture with dorsal angulation). In general, Smith's fractures do not respond well to conservative treatment and often warrant open reduction and internal fixation.

For the less severe Colles' fractures, closed reduction can be achieved by first administering a hematoma block. The hematoma block is performed using 10 to 20 ml of 1% lidocaine injected directly into the hematoma that will be present at the fracture site. A neurological examination should be performed before injection of the lidocaine. Placement of the needle into the hematoma can first be verified by aspiration of hematoma blood to confirm the location of the needle. Aseptic technique should be utilized. After the hematoma/fracture site has been located, injection of the lidocaine can be undertaken. Allow approximately 10 minutes for the lidocaine to diffuse and anesthetize the fracture site. After the hematoma block, a repeat neurological examination is done before attempting a closed reduction. The treating physician can then better assess any paresthesias that may occur after closed reduction as being either secondary to the development of a carpal tunnel syndrome or secondary to the hematoma block. Sedation is beneficial to alleviate pain and anxiety, and to reduce resting muscle tension.

After adequate local and systemic anesthesia is assured, the patient's involved hand is placed in finger traps and traction of 10 to 15 pounds is applied to the upper extremity (Fig. 8-35). Ten to 15 minutes are then allowed for the ligamentotaxis (passive elongation) to be effective.

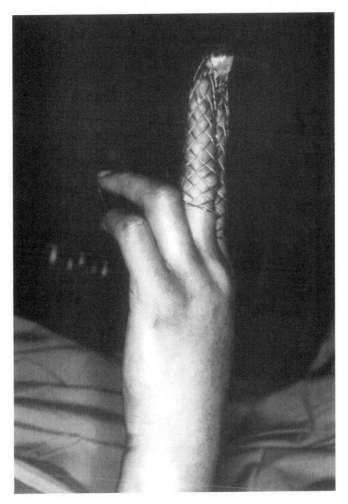

Figure 8-35   Closed reduction of distal radius fractures can be facilitated by use of fingertraps and traction using counterweights.

Simple traction in conjunction with an effective hematoma block and sedation facilitate fracture reduction. The reduction is then accomplished directly. It may be necessary initially to hyperextend the fracture to realign the volar cortex; however, this should be done cautiously to avoid further comminution of the dorsal cortex. After the volar cortex alignment has been achieved, the dorsal forearm is grasped gently with the hands. The physician's thumbs then press on the dorsal distal radius to align the fracture fragments and restore their volar angulation. Ligamentotaxis using traction often will have already restored the radial inclination. In children, manipulation of the fracture should be kept to a minimum and repeated attempts at closed reduction avoided to prevent further injury to the epiphesial plate.

After reduction has been achieved, the patient's forearm is placed in a short-arm cast while the fingertrap traction is maintained. The traction is then removed and a long-arm extension of the cast is added above the elbow. Radiographs are obtained after the reduction to determine the adequacy of bony position and alignment. Once a satisfactory reduction is verified by X-ray, the cast should be split to accommodate postinjury swelling. The importance of avoiding excessive tightness when splinting any acute wrist injury cannot be overemphasized. Arrangements should then be made to reevaluate the patient in a few days. The patient should be counseled emphatically to return to the emergency room or office promptly should sensation change in the hand, the splint feel too tight, or altered circulation to the fingers become evident.

Patients undergoing closed reduction of a wrist fracture should be evaluated in the office within a week. Follow-up radiographs are a crucial aspect in caring for these injuries, which are prone to collapse, angulation, and displacement. These can lead to a devastating outcome if not detected early. Each follow-up X-ray should be scrutinized carefully for the status of the reduction. Deterioration of bone position is an indication of an unstable fracture that would be best treated by operative means. Operative measures may include either an open reduction and internal fixation or percutaneous pin fixation.

If reduction is adequate at the first follow-up visit, patients are advised to return for subsequent X-rays in an additional week as a final check for stability of the fracture and maintenance of the reduction. Patients are treated in a long-arm cast for 4 to 6 weeks; the duration of long-arm casting is dependent on the perceived stability of the distal fragment. More stable fractures may be converted to a short-arm cast earlier than those with involvement of the joint. After 4 to 6 weeks of long-arm casting, the patient is converted to short-arm cast immobilization, which allows pronation and supination of the forearm. Radiographs obtained at 6 weeks will assist in determining the extent of bony healing. Fractures can be expected to unite in 6 to 12 weeks. Some fractures will require longer than 12 weeks to demonstrate radiographic evidence of healing; in such cases, we consider implementation of percutaneous electrical stimulation to stimulate bony union.

After radiographic evidence of healing of the fracture has been obtained, the patient's cast immobilization is discarded and he or she begins aggressive rehabilitation therapy on the wrist itself. During the entire period of cast immobilization, however, the patient must be instructed and actively participate in an aggressive exercise program to maintain mobility of the thumb and fingers. In addition, the exercise program should include manipulation and movement of the shoulder, and at regular intervals during cast changes, the elbow should be flexed and extended in a single plane. Therapy on the wrist after discontinuation of immobilization is conducted for 2 to 4 weeks, depending on the patient's progress. Our typical protocol includes active and passive range of motion exercises and strengthening exercises, which are continued until no further improvement in either range of motion or strength is observed. Total time from injury to discharge from care averages 4 to 6 months, but may be more prolonged in some patients. An individual whose job requires vigorous use of the upper extremity can anticipate a minimum of 4 to 6 months before heavy labor can be resumed comfortably.

Operative Treatment

For patients sustaining Smith's fractures, open fractures, and those with comminuted and/or unstable Colles' fractures, operative treatment is considered essential to maximize the potential for a satisfactory functional recovery. Operative treatment also is indicated for fractures with significantly displaced intraarticular components (see Box) Those patients with dorsal displacement of fractures more than 3 mm

---

Fractures of the Distal Radius

Indications for Surgery:

Unstable Fractures
Badly Comminuted Fractures
Open Fractures
Intraarticular Fractures
Colles' Fractures with: Greater than 3 mm Dorsal Displacement
                          Greater than 15° Dorsal Angulation
Most Smith's Fractures

or dorsal angulation of fractures greater than 15° are considered for open reduction and internal fixation, as are those patients whose fractures cannot be maintained in satisfactory position using closed means. Whether patients with less-pronounced degrees of angulation and displacement will fare better with open or with closed treatment is not clear, and opinions vary among experienced surgeons. Operative treatment of a fracture should be undertaken promptly once a significant deterioration in fracture position has been observed following closed reduction and cast immobilization. If operative intervention is delayed beyond approximately 2 to 3 weeks, it becomes difficult to adequately manipulate the fracture, which necessitates osteotomy of the radius to achieve satisfactory anatomic alignment. Severely comminuted and impacted fractures often remain unstable unless a bone graft is added for dorsal support. The patient awaiting surgery should be counseled that both open reduction and internal fixation, as well as the harvesting of bone graft from the iliac crest, may be required. In addition, patients should be informed that the fixation device (plates, screws, K-wires) can be selected only at the time of surgery, depending on the characteristics of the fracture, and that an external fixation device may be used. These decisions can be finalized only in the operating room when the fracture has been inspected and its inherent stability ascertained after reduction.

Colles' Fracture

The simplest method for fixation of a distal radial fracture is percutaneous pin fixation following closed reduction under an anesthetic. Fractures that can be reduced to an acceptable position manually, but relapse to an unfavorable position with casting, are well suited for this technique. K-wire fixation is performed percutaneously after manual reduction. Portable fluoroscopy and/or intraoperative radiographs confirm alignment. In our experience, fractures amenable to this treatment are the exception rather than the rule. More unstable fractures, those fractures with severe comminution, and those with displaced articular extension will require treatment by open methods. Preferred fixation in patients with Colles' fractures includes application of a dorsal plate, using a bone graft to maintain both the volar tilt after reduction of the distal radius and the radial inclination and radial length when required. Ideally, if rigid plate fixation can be achieved, early motion in the wrist may be considered to minimize the requirements for later therapy and improve the ultimate range of motion obtained.

Colles' fractures are approached through a dorsal incision. Occasionally, it also is necessary to approach the volar aspect of the radius to achieve adequate fracture reduction. In most cases, however, a single dorsal incision provides satisfactory exposure of the fracture site for reduction and fixation.

The surgical approach to the fracture is achieved under tourniquet control. Patients in whom an iliac crest bone graft may be required should receive a general anesthetic. A longitudinal incision is made over the third dorsal compartment of the wrist. A step cut in the extensor retinaculum is designed to facilitate closure of the retinaculum over the third dorsal compartment or beneath the extensor pollicis longus, if necessary, to achieve plate coverage (Fig. 8-36). After the third dorsal compartment is opened, the extensor pollicis longus is retracted either to the radial or ulnar side to aid in visualization. A longitudinal incision is then made in the dorsal periosteum of the distal radius and is extended over and through the dorsal joint capsule. The radiocarpal joint routinely is opened dorsally to permit inspection of the intraarticular surfaces and the carpal ligaments. Then the periosteum is stripped partially from the distal radius to allow direct visualization of the fracture. The patient is placed in finger traction on the operative table to aid in reduction of the fracture and visualization of the radiocarpal joint. If a volar approach is necessary, the initial incision is parallel to and overlies the flexor carpi radialis (FCR) tendon. The volar sheath of the FCR is incised longitudinally toward its radial side and the FCR retracted ulnarly. The dorsal sheath of the FCR is then incised. The interval between the brachioradialis tendonous insertion and the pronator quadratus is then incised. The pronator is elevated off the radius subperiosteally, exposing the fracture site. The periosteal incision is not carried distally into or over the radiocarpal joint to avoid injury to the strong volar ligaments of the wrist. This approach does not provide visualization of the radiocarpal joint, but may assist in fracture reduction and permits easy placement of volar plates if desired.

The fracture is reduced manually under direct vision and the reduction verified intraoperatively using fluoroscopy. The reduction should be evaluated in two planes, and the volar and dorsal cortices should be examined radiographically. Once adequate reduction has been achieved, the fixation type is chosen. Although controversial, patients with adequate bony stock on the distal fragment dorsally are considered candidates for application of a dorsal plate (Fig. 8-37) that will solidly maintain the fixation. Temporary fixation may be achieved using K-wires, which will hold fragments stationary while plate fixation is secured. The intraarticular extensions of the fracture must be examined carefully under direct vision and any discontinuity of the articular surface repaired. The fixation method chosen should maintain the articular surface as anatomically aligned as possible. When severe comminution prohibits satisfactory fixation using plates and screws, several K-wires may be used to immobilize the multiple fracture fragments until healing can occur. In most instances of severe comminution, how-

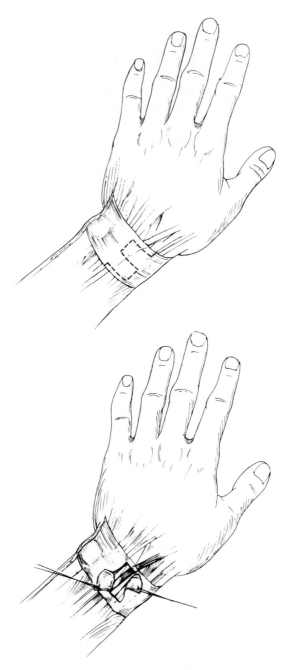

Figure 8-36 The distal radius typically is approached through the third dorsal compartment. The compartment is opened in a "step-cut" fashion that eases closure above or below the flexor pollicis longus.

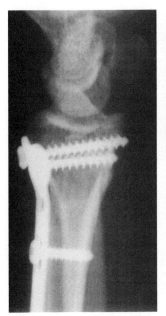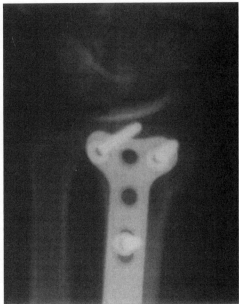

Figure 8-37 Fracture fixation using a dorsal plate. Note restoration of appropriate volar tilt and avoidance of hardware penetration of the radiocarpal joint itself.

ever, it is prudent to apply an external fixator whose purpose is to unload the normal compressive forces exerted at the wrist by the flexor and extensor musculature (Fig. 8-38). Once reduction and fixation have been achieved, the status of the dorsal distal radius is evaluated. In many cases, a small to moderately large bony void may be seen. We routinely bone graft these voids with cancellous bone harvested from the iliac crest in efforts to enhance stability and avoid recurrent dorsal collapse. The surgeon may select plates from a variety of shapes and sizes (Fig. 8-39). Plates are selected depending on the configuration of the fracture segments and the patient's size and anatomy. Fixation may include T-plates, longitudinal plates, and in some instances, a mini-plate applied as a tension band to help maintain joint surface reduction. After application of any fixation method, the fracture reduction and hardware position are assessed radiographically in the operating room where suboptimal pin, plate, or screw placement can be rectified.

External fixation devices are manufactured in a variety of sizes, shapes, and styles. The surgeon will use the device with which he or she is most comfortable and which achieves the best fixation. Additional casting materials are seldom required after application of an

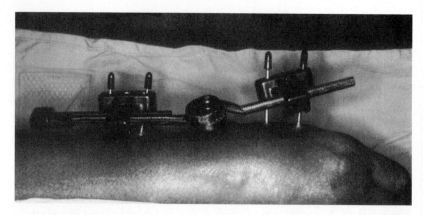

Figure 8-38 An external fixator can be used to counteract the resting muscle forces applied across the wrist, thereby avoiding collapse in more comminuted fractures. Overdistraction should be avoided.

external fixator; a thermoplastic splint may be added on the volar surface if supplemental support is desired. If severe damage of the distal radioulnar joint is present, or if fracture fragments remain unstable, pronation and supination of the forearm can be limited using an articulated long-arm thermoplastic splint that prevents pronation and supination while the elbow is flexed, but allows gentle elbow flexion and extension. During application of an external fixation device, the distal radius should be unloaded, but excessive distraction of the carpus from the distal radius should be avoided. Approximately 5 pounds of traction usually is sufficient to achieve the desired amount of distraction.

Some controversy remains as to whether it is necessary to fix ulnar styloid fractures. In general, we recommend fixation of the ulnar styloid if surgery is undertaken for the distal radius fracture or if more than just the tip of the ulnar styloid is involved. The large fracture fragments imply a more significant potential for detachment of the TFC. Our approach is through an ulnarly placed incision centered over the ulnar styloid. The dorsal sensory branch of the ulnar nerve is identified and protected. The extensor retinaculum is incised volar to the sixth compartment. This should expose the ulnar styloid, which is then reduced under direct vision and pinned with a single longitudinal K-wire. Other alternatives for fixation include wiring the styloid back to the body of the distal ulna. We have found the use of the single K-wire capable of providing adequate fixation.

Once reduction, fixation, and possibly bone grafting have been achieved and confirmed radiographically, the wound is closed in multi-

ple layers. Efforts are made to cover the dorsal hardware with periosteum if possible, although coverage frequently is incomplete. Soft tissue coverage of dorsal plates avoids tendon trauma and adhesion
formation. If coverage cannot be achieved using the periosteum and
the synovial bursal attachments of the dorsal compartments, the step
cut in the extensor retinaculum is brought beneath the extensor pollicis
longus and is used to cover the plates. The tourniquet is released before
final closure of the wound and adequate hemostasis is obtained. A
drain should be left in place if hemostasis cannot be achieved ade-

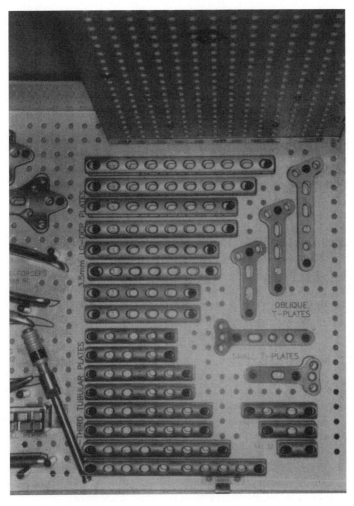

Figure 8-39   Plates of varying sizes and shapes are available for use in fixation.

quately, but it frequently is not necessary. A subcuticular closure of the wound will allow for cast immobilization for a prolonged period of time without necessitating removal of skin sutures. Most patients, particularly those with extensive injuries or those requiring bone grafting, will benefit from at least overnight hospitalization.

Follow-up within 1 week of the operative procedure is arranged; an X-ray is obtained at that time to again verify fracture reduction and to confirm satisfactory position of fixation devices. If these are favorable, further X-rays are performed at 5 or 6 weeks postoperatively as a preliminary evaluation of bony healing. Individuals in whom adequate rigid fixation has been obtained using plates are begun on early, gentle, supervised wrist motion exercises within the first week after surgery. The patients are maintained in a thermoplastic splint between exercise sessions, until radiographic evidence of the healing of the fracture is confirmed. External fixators are left in place for 4 to 6 weeks and then removed. Further immobilization is continued if radiographic evidence of healing has not been achieved. Wire fixation is removed once radiographic evidence of fixation has been demonstrated. Once fracture healing is apparent radiographically, intensive hand rehabilitation therapy is initiated to regain motion and strength in the wrist. As with patients treated with nonoperative means, those undergoing surgical treatment of their fractures may anticipate a 4 to 6 month recovery period until strenuous activity can be resumed.

Volarly Displaced Fractures

Most Smith fractures (volarly displaced fractures) will require open reduction and internal fixation. The approach is volar, as described earlier. An incision is made over the flexor capri radialis. The sheath of the FCR is opened volarly, and the FCR is retracted ulnarly. The dorsal sheath of the FCR is incised, exposing the pronator quadratus and the long adherent insertion of the brachioradialis (BR). An incision through periosteum is made between the BR and FCR. Further subperiosteal dissection will expose the fracture. For most Smith's fractures, the use of a buttress plate is sufficient to maintain reduction of the distal fragment. The fracture is reduced and a volar plate selected and bent to a slightly less volar flare than the reduced radius. Then the plate may be attached to solid proximal bone holding the volar fragment in place (Fig. 8-40). It generally is not necessary to place screws in the distal fragment.

Complications

Distal radial fractures have a relatively high rate of complications, the most common of which are persistent neuropathy, radiocarpal or distal radioulnar joint stiffness or pain, and development of degenera-

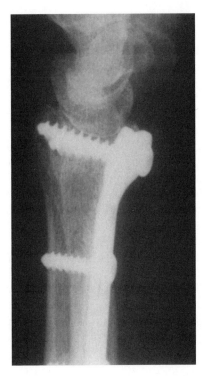

Figure 8-40   Volar buttress plates are particularly useful for maintaining reduction of Smith's fractures.

tive arthritis. Less-frequent complications include late rupture of tendons, most often the extensor pollicis longus; finger stiffness; and the development of Reflex Sympathetic Dystrophy (RSD) or shoulder–hand syndrome. Cooney (1980) reported complication rates of 31% among 565 patients with fractures. An interesting, but unexplained, fact observed by these physicians was a higher complication rate in those individuals who had received local anesthetic or hematoma block during initial treatment. The interpretation of the this fact is difficult. It may represent attempts to treat conservatively fractures that would have been better treated operatively. The treating physician should be aware of the lengthy recovery required and the potential complications that frequently follow them. Patients should be counseled about the seriousness of these injuries to create realistic expectations about recovery. In individuals who have jobs requiring great dexterity, the more severely injured wrist may require a job change or accommodation. Perhaps the higher incidence of complications following closed reduction attempts indicates that the historical acceptance of suboptimal reduction is misguided, and more aggressive attention to restoration of the anatomic features would be beneficial.

Results

Reported long-term results following fractures of the distal radius are inconsistent. Although nonunions are rare, patients sustaining more severe fractures tend to have less satisfactory results than those with simple fractures regardless of treatment modality. Knirk and Jupiter in the *Journal of Bone and Joint Surgery* (1986) reported that 61% of patients had an excellent or good results and 39% of patients had fair or poor results. They noted that 91% of those with residual articular incongruity developed arthritis at the radiocarpal joint. Of those whose joint surfaces were restored, only 11% developed arthritis. These and other studies emphasize the importance of meticulous restoration of anatomic alignment of these fractures, particularly the joint surfaces, regardless of the treatment method used. It is our belief that if nonoperative methods can adequately achieve and maintain reduction, they should be the treatment of choice. For many individuals, however, adequate anatomic alignment is not well maintained by nonsurgical means, and percutaneous fixation, open reduction and internal fixation, bone grafting, and/or external fixation should be considered.

SELECTED REFERENCES

Altissimi M, Antenucci R, Fiacca C, Mancini G: Long-term results of conservative treatment of fractures of the distal radius, *Clin Orthrop* 206:202-210, 1986.

Amadio PC: Scaphoid fractures, *Orthop Clin North Am* 23:7-17, 1992.

Barnaby W: Fractures and dislocations of the wrist, *Emerg Med Clin North Am* 10:133-149, 1992.

Barton NJ: Twenty questions about scaphoid fractures, *J Hand Surg (Br)* 17:289-310, 1992.

Brown JA, Janzen DL, Adler BD, et al: Arthrography of the contralateral, asymptomatic wrist in patients with unilateral wrist pain, *Can Assoc Radiol J* 45:292-296, 1994.

Calandra JJ, Goldner RD, Hardaker WT Jr: Scaphoid fractures: assessment and treatment, *Orthopedics* 15:931-937, 1992.

Carroll RE, Lakin JF: Fracture of the hook of the hamate: acute treatment, *J Trauma* 34:803-805, 1993.

Carroll RE, Lakin JF: Fracture of the hook of the hamate: radiographic visualization, *Iowa Orthop J* 13:178-182, 1993.

Casey PD, Youngberg R: Scapholunate dissociation: a practical approach for the emergency physician, *J Emerg Med* 11:701-707, 1993.

Chidgey LK: Chronic wrist pain, *Orthop Clin North Am* 23:49-64, 1992.

Chin HW, Visotsky J: Wrist fractures, *Emerg Med Clin North Am* 11:703-715, 1993.

Chin HW, Visotsky J: Ligamentous wrist injuries, *Emerg Med Clin North Am* 11:717-737, 1993.

Cooney WP, Dobyns JH, Linscheid RL: Complications of Colles' fractures, *J Bone Joint Surg* 62A:613-619, 1980.

Culp RW, Lemel M, Taras JS: Complications of common carpal injuries, *Hand Clin* 10:139-155, 1994.

De Smet L: Ulnar variance: facts and fiction review article, *Acta Orthop Belg* 60:1-9, 1994.

Golimbu CN, Firooznia H, Rafii M: Avascular necrosis of carpal bones, *Magn Reson Imaging Clin North Am* 3:281-303, 1995.

Hastings H, Leibovic SJ: Indications and techniques of open reduction internal fixation of distal radius fractures, *Orthop Clin North Am* 24:309-326, 1993.

Kauer JM: The distal radioulnar joint: anatomic and functional considerations, *Clin Orthop* 275:37-45, 1992.

Knirk JL, Jupiter JB: Intra-articular fractures of the distal end of the radius in young adults, *J Bone Joint Surg* 68A:647-659, 1986.

Kopylov P, Johnell O, Redlund-Johnell I, Bengner U: Fractures of the distal end of the radius in young adults: a 30-year follow-up, *J Hand Surg* 18B:45-49, 1993.

Kozin SH, Berlet AC: Injuries to the perilunar carpus, *Orthop Rev* 21:435-448, 1992.

Kuschner SH, Lane CS, Brien WW, Gellman H: Scaphoid fractures and scaphoid nonunion: diagnosis and treatment, *Orthop Rev* 23:861-871, 1994.

Lichtman DM, editor: *The wrist and its disorders.* Philadelphia, 1988, WB Saunders.

Markiewitz AD, Andrish JT: Hand and wrist injuries in the preadolescent and adolescent athlete, *Clin Sports Med* 11:203-225, 1992.

Melone CP, Nathan R: Traumatic disruption of the triangular fibrocartilage complex: pathoanatomy, *Clin Orthop* 275:65-73, 1992.

Mirabello SC, Loeb PE, Andrews JR: The wrist: field evaluation and treatment, *Clin Sports Med* 11:1-25, 1992.

Missakian ML, Cooney WP, Amadio PC, Glidewell HL: Open reduction and internal fixation for distal radius fractures, *J Hand Surg* 17A:745-755, 1992.

Palmer AK: *Fractures of the distal radius.* In Green DP (editor): *Operative hand surgery,* New York, 1993, Churchill Livingstone, pp. 929-971.

Posner MA, editor: Ligament injuries in the wrist and hand, *Hand Clin* 8:603-682, 1992.

Prendergast N, Rauschning W: Normal anatomy of the hand and wrist. *Magn Reson Imaging Clin North Am* 3:197-212, 1995.

Smith DK: MR imaging of normal and injured wrist ligaments, *Magn Reson Imaging Clin North Am* 3:229-248, 1995.

Stanley JK, Trail IA: Carpal instability, *J Bone Joint Surg (Br)* 76:691-700, 1994.

Szabo RM, Greenspan A: Diagnosis and clinical findings of Kienbock's disease, *Hand Clin* 9:399-408, 1993.

Timins ME, Jahnke JP, Krab SF, et al: MR imaging of the major carpal stabilizing ligaments: normal anatomy and clinical examples, *RadioGraphics* 15:575-587, 1995.

Tubiana R, Thomine J-M, Mackin E: *Examination of the hand and wrist.* St. Louis, 1996, CV Mosby.

9

Replantation and Microsurgery

David S. Martin, MD
Laurent Lantieri, MD
Roger K. Khouri, MD, FACS

The advent of microsurgical technique has expanded considerably the reconstructive options available to the hand surgeon and may be the most important technical development in hand surgery in the twentieth century. Microvascular technique permits the reattachment or transfer of tissue with restoration of its blood flow, a drastic improvement over archaic attempts at tissue reattachment without reperfusion. Early in the twentieth century, surgeon and Nobel laureate Alexis Carrel developed the principles of vascular anastomoses and tissue transfer, concepts that have been equally applicable using the operating microscope as they had been macroscopically. The first vascularized arm replantation was performed in 1962 by Malt and McKhann, and the first digital replantation by Komatsu and Tamai in 1968. Since these undertakings, replantation and microvascular free tissue transfer have been refined and are now relatively commonplace, particularly in medium-sized and larger medical centers. In the United States the standard of care is to at least consider replantation of any amputated part regardless of its location or size.

As the technical capabilities of hand surgeons have become more extraordinary, restoration of a viable finger or limb after amputation has become more commonplace. It also has become apparent that functional recovery after replantation of badly mutilated parts may not always be satisfactory. Patients may expend valuable resources, including time and money, as well as experience pain, lengthy hospitalizations, multiple operative procedures, and blood transfusions, and still never regain function better than that afforded by simple amputation. It is incumbent on the hand surgeon and emergency room physician to evaluate a patient's injuries carefully and consider not only the likelihood of success in reattaching the amputated part, but also the expectations for ultimate functional recovery.

REPLANTATION

In the upper extremity, replantation is the technique of reattaching a finger, hand, forearm, or entire arm that has been amputated completely. Digital amputations at various levels occur far more frequently than more proximal amputations. Multiple digits may be amputated, and the site of amputation may occur at any level from the tip of the finger to its base.

Prehospital Management

Care of the site of amputated part is of paramount importance and is neglected easily if attention is focused exclusively on the injured patient. Diligent care of the amputated part will enhance chances for successful replantation and avoid further damage to the part. Proper care of the amputated part and the amputation stump must be assured and cannot be assumed to have been conducted satisfactorily. Any amputated part that may be replantable, whether it be an ear, a scalp, a penis, or a portion of the upper extremity, should be placed on a saline-moistened gauze sponge, placed inside a plastic bag, and that bag cooled in an ice water slurry as promptly as possible (Fig. 9-1). Direct contact with ice, the use of dry ice, or immersion in ice water are detrimental. In addition, a pressure dressing should be applied to the site of the amputation and that part elevated to control hemorrhage. These measures should be instituted by the initial care provider. Patients have been transferred to our institution in hemorrhagic shock because no dressing was applied to a major hand wound, and digits have been unreplantable because of extensive soft tissue freezing of the amputated parts. At each level of prehospital and hospital care, it is essential

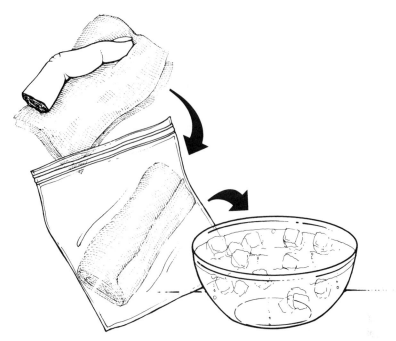

Figure 9-1 Proper care of the amputated part enhances chances for successful reattachment. Prolonged warm ischemia, severe cold exposure, and direct immersion can affect tissues adversely.

that proper attention to the injured extremity and amputated part be confirmed.

Emergency Evaluation

General

Patients who have sustained traumatic amputations at any level have dramatic wounds. Assess both the amputation and any other injuries thoroughly and rapidly, provide proper care to both the amputated part and to the stump, obtain necessary diagnostic tests, such as X-rays, and promptly contact a hand surgeon who can make the ultimate decision regarding efforts at replantation or alternative treatment. The major components of emergency room evaluation of a patient who may be a candidate for replantation surgery are shown in Table 9-1. With the exception of some small fingertip amputations, most patients will require surgery regardless of whether replantation is undertaken, and measures to facilitate their transfer to the operating room should be undertaken. Potential replantation patients should not be allowed

Table 9-1 Components of Emergency Room Evaluation

Proper care of the amputated part	Wrap in saline-moistened gauze, place in plastic bag, and place bag in ice water slurry
Care of amputation stump	Apply pressure dressing
Anesthetic considerations	Nothing by mouth
	Minimal sedation
Obtain history	Mechanism of injury
	Time injury occurred
	Hand dominance
	Usual occupation
	General medical condition
	Smoking history
	Other injuries
	Previous injuries
General physical examination	Evaluate vital signs
	Screening physical for operating room
	Assess other injuries
Examine amputated part	Bony and soft tissue sites of amputation
	Extent of soft tissue damage
Examine amputation stump	Bony and soft tissue sites of amputation
	Extent of soft tissue damage
	Other extremity injuries
Radiographs of the part and stump	Location of amputation
	Degree of comminution
	Joint involvement
	Other injuries
Obtain preoperative testing (as indicated)	
Alert operating room/anesthesia team	
Counsel patient and obtain operative consent	

to eat or drink anything by mouth. The administration of excessive narcotics and sedatives should be avoided, particularly until counseling is complete and a decision about replantation has been made.

History

Mechanism of injury

Obtain a complete history of the injury; it will influence treatment decisions. Patients often are understandably upset and may be reassured with a calm and gentle demeanor. The patient should be queried about the mechanism of injury because this will affect both the likelihood of successful replantation and the likelihood of achieving an acceptable functional result. The most common culprits in digital amputations are the table saw, hand-held circular saw, radial-arm saw, and an array of industrial and nonindustrial heavy equipment. Industrial equipment with moving parts, such as rollers, belts, presses, or hydraulic systems, may "catch" a glove or finger and amputate the digit as it is drawn into the machinery. Home devices, such as leaf shredders or log splitters, also may cause amputation by direct cutting, as may knives, machetes, and hatchets.

The mechanism of injury predicts both the likelihood of successful revascularization and the ultimate functioning of the replanted part. Injuries caused by very sharp amputation with minimal soft tissue and bony injury distally on the amputated part have a much better prognosis for replantation than injuries with concomitant crushing or avulsion of the amputated part. In the latter, revascularization still may be possible, but more frequently is unsuccessful, and the ultimate digital mobility and sensation achieved are diminished. Amputations involving an extensive "burst" injury, burns, and severe abrasions, or those injuries in which the digit has been torn from the limb frequently are unreplantable.

Ischemia time

The tissues of the hand itself are surprisingly tolerant of ischemia, presumably because of the relative paucity of muscle within the hand. There are occasional reports of successful digital replantation after substantially more than 48 hours of cold ischemia, but in general, more than 24 hours of cold ischemia or more than 12 hours of warm ischemia before patient arrival are relative contraindications to replantation. Considerations regarding ischemia times should include the additional time required to prepare the patient for surgery and the process of revascularization itself, which requires between 2 and 6 hours per digit depending on the experience of the surgeon and operating team and the nature of the injury itself. Any patient thought to be even a remote candidate for replantation of any amputated part should have the ischemic part cooled as described previously.

In more proximal amputations, such as at the forearm or arm level, the tolerance of ischemia is reduced. These areas consist of large volumes of skeletal muscle that do not survive ischemia well. More than 6 hours of warm ischemia or 12 hours of cold ischemia would prohibit replantation. Because forearm or arm amputations are relatively rare (often less than one per year even at larger medical centers), conclusive studies using preservation solutions, such as those employed in transplantation surgery, are lacking. Despite these limitations, amputated limbs should be cooled quickly and definitive care assured promptly.

Hand dominance and occupation

The patient's occupational and recreational requirements for the injured extremity affect plans for reconstruction and should be part of the initial evaluation. Patients with jobs that do not require dexterity, patients who are otherwise disabled in using the affected hand, and those who must return to gainful employment quickly may find completion amputation more suitable than efforts at replantation.

General medical condition

Patients who are considered for replantation surgery must be able to withstand the required operative time. This may be prolonged, particularly in multiple digit replantations. A portion of the procedure may be performed under axillary block or other regional anesthetic, but general anesthetic also may be required. A patient's inability to tolerate anesthetic for the duration of these procedures is a contraindication to replantation. The rare replant candidate with preexisting vasculitis or vasospastic disease of the extremity (such as Raynaud's phenomenon) is a poor candidate for replantation.

Smoking history

Although smoking is not a contraindication to replantation, most microvascular surgeons recognize that the vasoactive properties of tobacco may detrimentally affect chances for successful revascularization. Patients should be advised that they will not be permitted to smoke postoperatively during recovery; patients unwilling to comply must be advised that they are jeopardizing their chances for successful reattachment. Some surgeons will not offer replantation to patients who adamantly refuse to cease smoking at least temporarily.

Self-inflicted injuries

Occasionally, amputation of a digit or hand will be the result of a suicide attempt or other self-mutilating behavior. It is imperative that the examiner consider this possibility when interviewing the patient and that, when justified, an appropriate psychiatric consultation be promptly obtained. Replantation surgery is relatively contraindicated in patients who will be unable or unwilling to comply with the extensive postoperative rehabilitation required. However, after consultation with a psychiatrist, attempts at replantation may be considered if the patient's prognosis is more favorable.

Associated injuries

It is unusual for associated injuries to be present in the case of individual digital amputations. However, more proximal amputations frequently are the result of severe high energy trauma. Consequently, other injuries are common. Implications of major limb amputations will be discussed later in this chapter.

Patients should be questioned about other injuries affecting the extremity and other parts of the body. Fractures and dislocations can be overlooked when attention is focused on the site of amputation. Other injuries should be evaluated thoroughly before replantation efforts are undertaken.

Previous injuries

Previous injury to an amputated finger may not be readily visible to the examiner and may not be revealed by the patient. Injuries that affected the finger's function before amputation will persist and may interfere with replantation.

Physical Examination

General

Patients should have their vital signs measured. Patients who have lost a large volume of blood must be resuscitated thoroughly and promptly. Any injuries remote to the site of amputation must be evaluated completely.

Site of amputation

An earlier caregiver or the patient probably will have already placed a pressure dressing over the wound. In examining the injured extremity itself, it often is advisable to encircle the upper arm with a blood pressure cuff in anticipation that a tourniquet may be necessary for inspection of the wound. The tourniquet should not be inflated empirically or injudiciously because it will render all tissue distal to it ischemic. Failure to deflate a proximal tourniquet can lead to disastrous consequences. Except in extraordinary circumstances, tourniquet use should be restricted to the time required for inspection; it should not be used for prolonged control of bleeding. Until operative repair can be undertaken, the vast majority of hemorrhages can be controlled with a pressure dressing and extremity elevation.

It is wise to place a towel or pad under the patient's hand to prevent soiling him/her and to position the hand in an elevated position for inspection. The examiner should wear protective eyewear and gloves in compliance with hospital requirements. The examiner should have several gauze sponges and gauze rolls prepared to cover the wound when the inspection is complete.

With the tourniquet deflated, the dressings should be removed gently. Because transected vessels retract and spasm, it is common to encounter minimal bleeding at the site of amputation and to be able to observe the pulsating transected vessel ends within the wound.

Many patients who have been reported to have amputated a digit will be found to have either deep lacerations of an otherwise intact digit or near-complete amputation of the digit with maintenance of a bridge of skin. These injuries will be addressed in the section on revascularization, but it is worthwhile maintaining any bridges of skin that may offer assistance in providing venous outflow if the digit can be revascularized.

The examiner should note the level of soft tissue transection, as well as the site of bony disruption. In degloving injuries, the soft tissues may be amputated proximally, such as the level of the metacarpophalangeal joint, while a complete bony skeleton remains intact distally.

The degree of contamination must be assessed. Foreign material, whether grease, dirt, grass, or other substance, will influence the amount of soft tissue debridement required, the amount of inflammation and scar expected, and the likelihood of wound infection.

The status of adjacent soft tissue and remaining fingers also must be assessed. The soft tissue injury primarily affects the likelihood of successful revascularization. Fingers or portions of the hand that are white or gray must be scrutinized to determine whether they have been devascularized. The hand should be evaluated for abrasions, contusions, and lacerations. Any soft tissue lacerations proximal to the site of amputation that transect the neurovascular bundles must be detected. In general, amputations in which the primary neurovascular bundles or draining veins have been transected in several places along their course—either on the extremity or on the amputated part—cannot be replanted. The motion of the remaining digits must be examined, as must the sensibility of these tissues. Moving two-point discrimination is the most accurate method for determining sensory nerve function, which typically is 3 to 4 mm for the digital pulp. Flexion and extension of all attached digits should be elicited and any abnormalities of motion noted. After inspection, the gentle pressure dressing should be replaced and the extremity should resume an elevated position.

Amputated part

During other portions of the assessment, the amputated part should be maintained in a saline-moistened gauze sponge that is placed in a plastic bag. The bag should be kept on ice (not dry ice). The amputated part should be inspected for its degree of contamination and for sites of soft tissue and bony amputation. The degree of soft tissue injury distal to the amputation site should be assessed. Digits that have sustained crush injuries during their amputation do not fare as well as clean transections. Fig. 9-2 demonstrates an apparently "clean" multiple digit amputation proximally with muti-

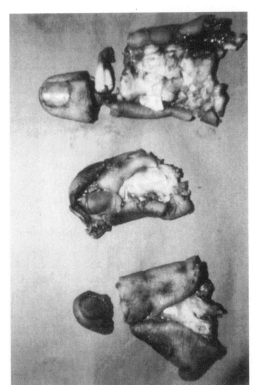

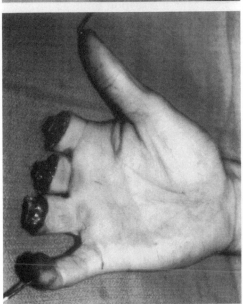

Figure 9-2 Despite the "clean" appearance of the amputation site on the hand itself, extensive mutilation of distal parts from an industrial press renders them wholly unsalvageable.

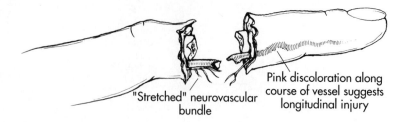

"Stretched" neurovascular bundle

Pink discoloration along course of vessel suggests longitudinal injury

Figure 9-3 Axial neurovascular injury. Avulsion along the neurovascular bundle, rather than direct cutting, is indicative of longitudinal vessel injury. When replantation is attempted, healthy vessel must be repaired to healthy vessel, using vein grafting if necessary.

lated distal parts. These digits are clearly unreplantable. Overall rates of success in replanting digits after crush/avulsion injuries are reportedly as low as 65%, compared with more than 90% for clean transections. Extensive lacerations, particularly "burst" lacerations and other indicators of more diffuse soft tissue crushing injury, may preclude replantation. Any laceration distal to the amputation site must be examined carefully. It is embarrassing to initiate efforts toward replantation only to realize that the neurovascular bundles have been irreparably lacerated distal to the amputation site.

Evidence of axial neurovascular injury should be sought (Fig. 9-3). Unlike the clean cut transection, injuries involving avulsion, or tearing of the tissues, may result in lengthy areas of injury to the neurovascular bundles. Injured portions of vessels are unsuitable for revascularization because they are extremely thrombogenic and therefore incapable of maintaining digital perfusion. Specifically, when lengthy portions of the neurovascular bundles have been torn from the hand, are stretched and dangling from the amputation site, or conversely, are torn from the digit and are hanging from the amputation stump, the likelihood that revascularization will be successful is greatly diminished. The "red line sign," a faint red discoloration seen below the surface of the skin along the path of each neurovascular bundle, indicates longitudinal vessel damage extending well beyond the actual site of amputation. Similarly, the "curly Q" sign, in which the visible neurovascular bundle is coiled, indicates a disruption of the longitudinal structure of the vessel and may suggest that replantation will not be as successful.

Any amputation that has avulsed the tendons of the finger from their musculotendinous junction in the forearm (Fig. 9-4) is more difficult to repair than clean tendon lacerations. These avulsed tendons are almost impossible to reattach satisfactorily to the muscle

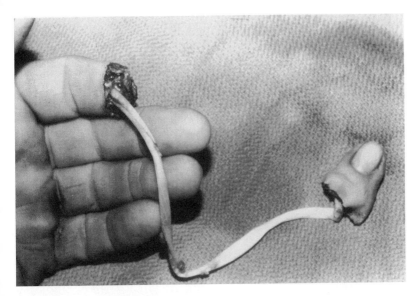

Figure 9-4   Amputation with avulsion of the profundus tendon from its musculotendinous junction in the forearm. The need for tenodesis or tendon transfer makes replantation more difficult.

bellies; tendon transfers or attachment to tendons of adjacent digits often is necessary.

Diagnostic Studies

Radiographs of the hand

It is imperative that radiographs be taken of the involved hand to assess the level of amputation, the involvement of joints, and the structural integrity of both the proximal stump and adjacent bones. The presence of a single digital amputation does not preclude other bony injuries in the hand; they must be sought as attention is often directed exclusively to the site of the amputation. Other fractures frequently require treatment at the time of the operation.

In regard to the actual site of amputation, several factors deserve consideration. First, amputations that do not involve injury to a joint will function better than those that traverse a joint. Fingers without satisfactory motion are more of a liability than an asset; they interfere with the function of the remainder of the hand and do not assist in its activities. Dysfunction of the metacarpophalangeal or proximal interphalangeal joints is particularly devastating for finger function. Amputations with diffuse injuries to either of these joints will not fare well. Figure 9-5 demonstrates extensive bony injury, with significant bone loss and destruction of the meta-

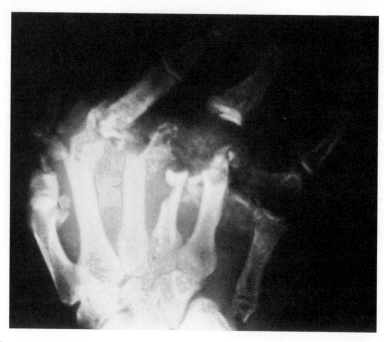

Figure 9-5 Radiograph showing extensive bony injury, including destruction of several metacarpophalangeal joints. These devitalized digits were unsalvageable (leaf shredder injury).

carpophalangeal joints. Significant joint injury was only one of several reasons why these devitalized digits could not be salvaged. The presence of intraarticular injury should be weighed carefully when contemplating replantation, particularly of a single digit. In patients sustaining multiple amputations, where any finger function is desired, salvage of any finger with any expected motion may be desirable. Interestingly, injuries involving the wrist joints, regardless of their severity, may function quite well. Absence of motion at the wrist, such as that observed after total wrist arthrodesis, can be inconvenient but acceptable if finger motion is intact.

Second, badly comminuted fractures tend to fare less well than simple transverse amputations. Early motion for replanted digits is crucial if useful function is to be regained; bony stability is paramount in allowing early motion. Establishing adequate bony fixation and stability frequently is difficult in comminuted fractures. These digits require longer periods of immobilization, which results in increased stiffness. In addition, more severely comminuted fractures indicate a higher magnitude of initial injury to all involved tissues. Badly fractured hands and fingers have prolonged edema, which complicates rehabilitation efforts.

Radiographs of the amputated part

It is worthwhile to evaluate the integrity of the bones in the amputated part. As with the stump, articular involvement and severe comminution lead to problems with bony stability and indicate a higher magnitude of injury sustained. In general, multiple fractures in phalanges distal to the site of amputation suggest that efforts for replantation will not be rewarding.

Angiography

For replantation to be successful, healthy vessels must be repaired to healthy vessels, even if this mandates the use of vein grafts. The best method for assessing the status of the vessels is by direct visualization under high-power magnification and testing of vessel flow after dissection. Angiography, as an indirect method of visualizing vessel continuity and injury, is not indicated in most routine upper-extremity amputations.

Preoperative testing

Hospital policies regarding preoperative testing vary. If laboratory tests, such as an EKG, chest X-ray, or urinalysis are required, these should be initiated at the time of primary evaluation because most patients sustaining amputation will require operative intervention if only to complete and close their amputations.

Most patients should have a complete blood count, including blood typing and an antibody screen, forwarded to the blood bank. Depending on the amount of blood lost before emergency room evaluation, patients may require transfusion, often postoperatively, after equilibration. Many digital replantation patients do not require transfusion, but if anticoagulants are required or if major limb amputation has been performed, transfusion usually is necessary. Unlike most other replantations, patients sustaining major limb transections may require vigorous resuscitation with blood products before the safe administration of an anesthetic and limb reattachment.

Preoperative Preparation and Counselling

Operating room mobilization

Even in centers accustomed to performing replantations, preparations for the procedure may be elaborate and time consuming. Furthermore, replantations may monopolize a dedicated operative team for several hours, depending on the complexity of the procedure. To facilitate preparation, promptly advise the operating room and anesthetic personnel that a patient has arrived in the emergency room who may require replantation. After evaluation by the surgeon who will provide definitive care, the operating room personnel should receive an update. Even if the patient is delayed in the emergency department because of preoperative testing, radiographs, or anesthetic evaluation, a surgeon may be able to make excellent use of precious time by initiating dissection on the amputated part in the operating room as soon as the equipment is available.

The decision to replant

Properly counseling the patient who has sustained an amputation can be extremely difficult. The patient probably has a high degree of anxiety about the injury and the fate of the hand and its missing component(s). Although the patient may be frightened and in pain, the surgeon is responsible for quickly briefing the patient on the nature of the injury, the prognosis, and the options for treatment. Any person unfamiliar with replantation surgery should defer recommendations about replantation to an experienced hand surgeon. Patients may be devastated to have been advised initially that a digit was definitely replantable only to learn later from the hand surgeon that, for whatever reason, replantation cannot even be attempted. It is certainly appropriate for a hand surgeon to be consulted to inform a patient definitively that a mutilated part cannot be replaced even when this conclusion is apparent to everyone involved. Generally, we believe any patient sustaining an amputation in which any portion of the amputated part is available should be advised that replantation may be possible. Efforts should then be made to have the patient promptly evaluated by a hand surgeon, who will assist the patient in making the final decision. The decision to attempt replantation should, therefore, be influenced by the likelihood of success and expectations for functional recovery.

Simply stated, the degree of soft tissue injury determines the likelihood that the part can be replanted successfully, and the level of amputation will determine the functionality of the part if replantation is successful. All patients should be advised that efforts to salvage the amputated part may be futile. The factors influencing success of revascularization are listed in Table 9-2. Relative function by level of amputation are shown in Table 9-3.

SOFT TISSUE INJURY

Reported success rates for digital replantation in clean-cut, transverse amputations exceed 90%, while those for crushed digits, even in experienced medical centers, are closer to 65%. The surgeon's expectations for restoration of tissue viability should be explained to the patient and should be tailored to the individual injury. Patients with multiple fractures within the amputated part, multiple lacerations, extensive abrasions, longitudinal burst injuries, and substantial tissue loss on the amputated part should

Table 9-2   Factors Influencing Success in Replantation

Factor Predicting Survival	Comment
Mechanism of injury	Sharp amputations have a more favorable outcome than more blunt injuries
Soft tissue injury	Extensive soft tissue damage remote to the site of amputation is unfavorable
Axial neurovascular injury	Extensive injury along the transected vessel suggests a poor prognosis
Duration of ischemia	Prolonged warm ischemia reduces the likelihood of a successful restoration of perfusion
Patient age	Replantation attempted in young children or infants is technically challenging Elderly may be less likely to have sufficient inflow to sustain the replanted part
Medical condition	Diabetes, chronic steroid use, connective tissue disorders are less favorable Extensive associated injuries and/or generalized hypoperfusion (shock) fare poorly
Smoking history	Smokers are more prone to thrombosis than nonsmokers

be discouraged from undergoing replantation. Figure 9-6 shows a finger avulsed during an industrial drill accident. The finger is unreplantable.

LEVEL OF AMPUTATION

The level of amputation greatly affects the decision to attempt replantation. The relative prognoses and limitations expected after replantation by level are shown in Table 9-3. Injuries beyond the insertion of the flexor digitorum superficialis (FDS) onto the base of the middle phalanx (Flexor Zone I) tend to function well with replantation because only one tendon traverses the digital sheath distal to the FDS, improving tendon gliding. A Zone I, four-finger replantation is demonstrated in Fig. 9-7. In the event that full distal interphalangeal joint (DIP) motion is not regained, limitation of DIP motion does not preclude otherwise excellent use of the digit. Furthermore, replantation of a Zone I digit restores an almost normal appearance to the hand. Injuries that occur in "no-man's land" (Zone II), between the metacarpophalangeal joint and the insertion of the FDS, are devastating injuries. The prognosis after replantation of these injuries is worse than for any other level of amputation in the hand. Poor

Table 9-3   Function by Level of Amputation

Anatomic Level	Overall Prognosis	Comment
Distal to FDS insertion (Zone I)	Excellent	Technically demanding
Distal palm to FDS insertion (Zone II)	Fair	Limited because of problems with FDS and FDP gliding and frequent MP and PIP joint injury
Midpalm (Zone III)	Good	Favorable with transverse amputations (unusual) compared to oblique amputations with adjacent digits injured at other levels (common)
Carpal tunnel (Zone IV)	Good	Unusual injuries. Outcome determined by success of neural regeneration
Distal forearm (Zone V)	Good	Same as above
Arm/proximal forearm	Fair	Often life-threatening injuries with massive injuries, substantial blood loss, shock, and substantial muscle necrosis following reperfusion

FDS, flexor digitorum superficialis; FDP, flexor digitorum profundus; MP, metacarpal phalangeal; PIP, proximal interphalangeal.

function in Flexor Zone II occurs because two flexor tendons traverse the fibrous digital sheath in this area and must be capable of gliding freely. Adjacent soft tissue and bony injury produce scar tissue that drastically restricts tendon motion. During the recovery after replantation, the digits also may be edematous and require bony fixation, both of which reduce the vigorous motion that would be desirable in isolated flexor tendon injuries in this region. For this reason, single digital amputations in Zone II are not attempted often unless the patient is expected to be highly motivated and/or has special requirements because of his/her occupation (such as being required to fire a weapon as a law enforcement officer) or where cosmesis is a crucial facet. A multiple-digit, Zone II replantation is shown in Fig. 9-8.

Almost any thumb replantation should be attempted. The thumb is the most important digit in the hand. Its primary function is that of a "stable post." As such, it requires relatively little motion and dexterity. In addition, unlike with the adjacent digits,

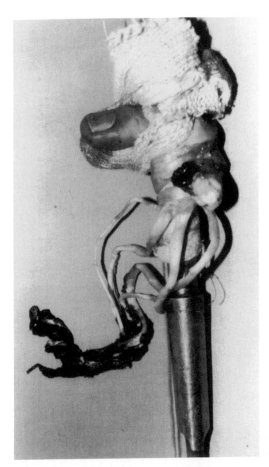

Figure 9-6   Unreplantable digit after industrial drill accident. The magnitude of soft tissue, bone, and tendon injury makes replantation efforts futile.

loss of thumb length by simple closure may greatly impair the function of the hand as a whole. As a result, replantation is preferable (Fig. 9-9). Certainly in instances in which the patient's wounds are so extensive that replant survival is doubtful, other options for either immediate or delayed toe-to-thumb transfer should be considered.

Amputations across the hand proximal to the metacarpophalangeal (MCP) joint are unusual. Tendons at this level do not traverse a digital sheath per se, there is no joint involvement, and bony fixation and microvascular repair is technically easier.

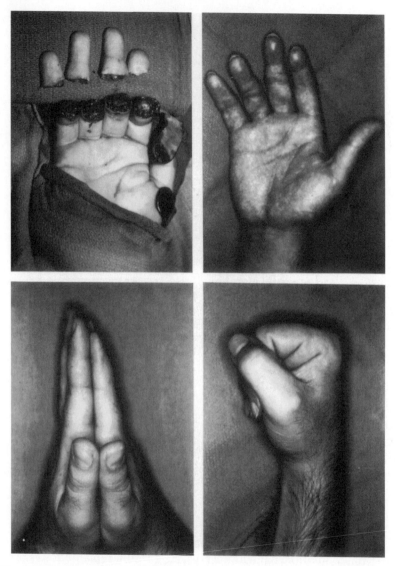

Figure 9-7   Four-finger replantation in Zone I. Function can be quite accept-able, particularly considering that multiple digits are involved.

Therefore, the prognosis after replantation of an entire palm and fingers, or their combination, is good.

Prognosis for replantation after complete amputation at the wrist or distal forearm is in large part determined by the success of neural regeneration. Although multiple tendons traverse this level, their motion is unimpeded by a digital sheath. Overall func-

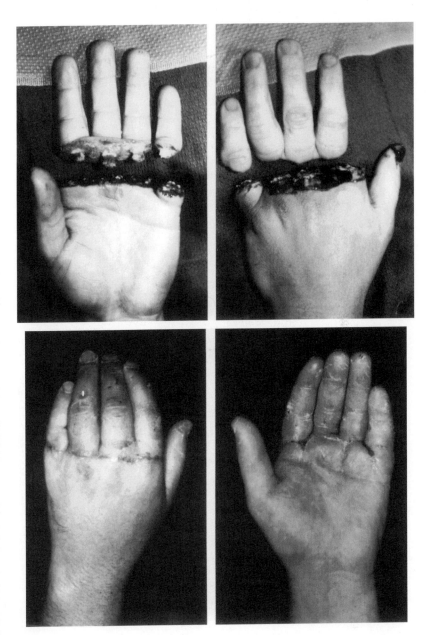

Figure 9-8   Four-finger amputation in Zone II. Accomplishing smooth gliding of the two flexor tendons within the digital sheath at this level is difficult, especially when joint injuries are present. However, for multiple-digit injuries, replantation is preferable to the limitations imposed by closure alone. Alternative reconstruction, such as toe-to-hand transfer, may be a valid option if replantation is unsuccessful.

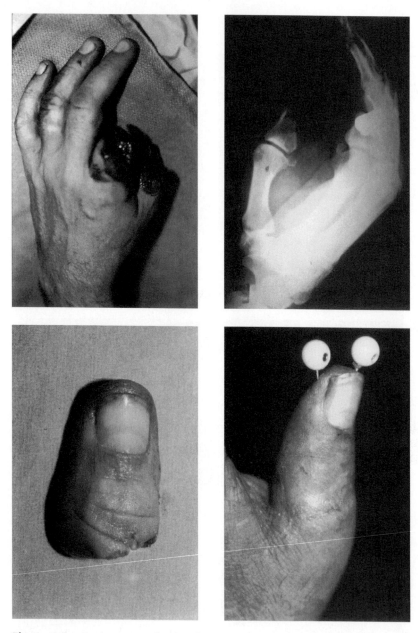

Figure 9-9 Replantation of a thumb amputated between the MP and IP joint. Most thumb amputations should be replanted if feasible; an acceptable contour can be ensured by generous defatting of the subcutaneous tissues at the amputation margins.

tion can be expected to be good, particularly compared with the alternative of simple closure and utilization of a prosthesis (Fig. 9-10).

More proximal amputations, either through the forearm, elbow, or arm, tend to be rare and to have a less encouraging prognosis. First, they occur after the transmission of tremendous force and therefore are commonly associated with multisystem trauma and extensive upper-extremity soft tissue damage. Further, amputations at this level jeopardize large amounts of skeletal muscle, which is relatively intolerant of ischemia and may ultimately undergo extensive necrosis. Finally, neural regeneration over long distances after amputation is less predictable, particularly through a traumatized soft tissue bed. In a stable patient sustaining a clean amputation, we believe all available efforts should be made to salvage the extremity if safely possible.

JOINT INVOLVEMENT

If an amputation injury destroys the metacarpophalangeal or proximal interphalangeal joints, the resulting loss of motion at that joint is a significant liability. A finger that does not flex adequately, particularly if it is a border digit (i.e., the index or little finger), and has altered sensation will be neglected during use of the hand after replantation. This may hinder activities that require the hand to conform to a small size, such as placing a hand in one's pocket. Any traumatic injury to the metacarpophalangeal or proximal interphalangeal joint of an amputated digit will impair the motion of that joint following replantation. The disability resulting from distal interphalangeal joint dysfunction is surprisingly small, however, particularly if the DIP is immobile in a useful position of slight flexion (approximately 15°).

Joint involvement in thumb amputation is less devastating than that observed in finger amputations because the thumb's prominent role is one of stability rather than mobility, and because other thumb joints can often compensate for diminished motion at a single joint.

Wrist joint involvement does not adversely affect efforts to undertake replantation of an entire hand. Because the alternative of simple stump closure at this level leaves the patient with dismal function, and because even total wrist fusion (allowing no wrist motion) is a functional alternative, most hand replantations should be attempted.

PATIENT EXPECTATIONS FOR REPLANTATION SURGERY

Replantation surgery requires a strong commitment both from the patient and the surgeon and should not be undertaken lightly.

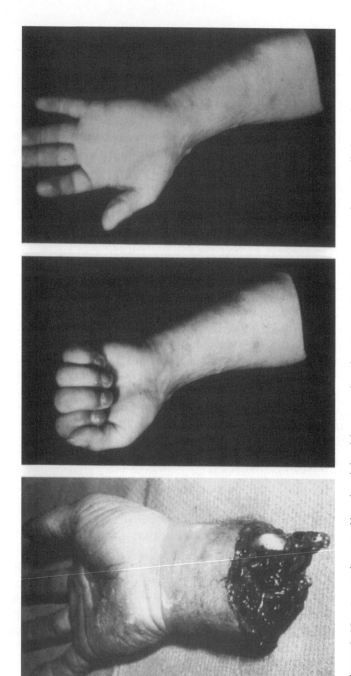

Figure 9-10   Reattachment of hand and distal forearm after clean transection. Prognosis is dramatically better than any alternative reconstruction or currently available prosthesis.

The patient's investment in these efforts should not be understated, and his/her active participation in the process must be assured. Despite the magnitude of the operative endeavor required, the most important factor in the outcome is patient compliance and active involvement in the rehabilitation process.

The patient must be told of the seriousness of the injuries and the prognosis both for initial success and ultimate function. The patient must be told that regardless of the treatment selected, the hand will never function completely normally again. The decision to attempt replantation involves an operation requiring between 2 and 6 hours per digit, depending on the magnitude of the injury and the experience of the surgeons involved. Hospitalization is typically between 5 and 10 days. Further surgery may be required later. The nature of microvascular surgery and the propensity for these tiny vessels to thrombose must be explained to the patient. Based on the surgeon's approach, a rational plan should be made should difficulties be encountered postoperatively. A patient must understand that a vascular thrombosis may unexpectedly and immediately threaten the viability of an otherwise successful replantation, requiring a prompt return to the operating room in an effort to salvage the part. The initial and any subsequent attempts to revascularize the part may fail completely. Between 30 and 50% of patients may require further surgery, frequently for treatment of tendon adhesions, but also for such problems as bony nonunion, painful neuroma formation, or definitive wound coverage. Patients may require anticoagulation, with its attendant risks of bleeding at other sites, and blood transfusions. The possibility of wound bleeding or infection must be explained.

All patients will be expected to participate in hand rehabilitation with an experienced therapist. This may require several trips per week. If patients are located a long distance away from the medical center, arrangements often can be made for therapy closer to home, but the convenience of a local therapist is no substitute for one experienced in rehabilitation following replantation.

Patients will be out of work for between 6 and 12 weeks, depending on their job duties and the status of their wounds. For patients whose injuries were not related to their jobs and are therefore without disability income, the loss of wages for several weeks or months can be a significant hardship. Many choose to have simple completion/closure of their amputation if they can return to work quickly. Patients must be informed that the best motion and sensation in a replanted part will not be achieved for 12 to 18 months after surgery.

Patients will experience discomfort in the replanted part as neural regeneration occurs. They probably will have discomfort on exposure to the cold, particularly in colder climates. This problem may improve, but it may also persist permanently at a diminished level. Patients should be prepared to have a vein graft obtained from the foot or forearm or a nerve graft obtained from the medial or lateral antebrachial cutaneous nerves or a sural nerve. They should understand that these grafts require incisions and that use of a nerve for grafting will lead to an area of permanent anesthesia. Patients must agree to cease smoking immediately and are strongly discouraged from smoking for at least 6 weeks.

PATIENT EXPECTATIONS FOR COMPLETION AMPUTATION

For digital amputations, patients will have a cosmetic deformity, a functional deformity, and grief associated with loss of a body part. Completion digital amputations have the advantages of quick closure (patients can often go home almost immediately), a less painful recovery, and a much less protracted course compared to digital replantation. Patients may resume work perhaps within a week and may expect to achieve an acceptable level of function by 6 weeks. Amputation sites, however, are not immune to problems of pain, neuroma formation, unstable scars, or cold intolerance, any of which can be significant enough to require surgery in the future.

THE ROLE OF THE PATIENT IN THE DECISION

If replantation is an option, patients have the final decision about whether to proceed with replantation efforts or choose completion amputation. The surgeon can explain the alternatives from different perspectives, depending on the specifics of the individual case, but the final decision must come from the patient. In many instances, the degree of mutilation is so great that the surgeon cannot consider replantation, and must advise the patient to have a completion amputation. In the majority of cases, however, patients may choose to proceed with or reject replantation, fully recognizing the consequences of the decision. The surgeon may offer to examine the hand and amputated part in the operating room under magnification to evaluate the extent of vessel injury, with plans to make a final determination there. Overall, we have observed that most patients often will choose to proceed with efforts at replantation even under suboptimal conditions.

MEDICOLEGAL ISSUES

Surgeons are not obliged to perform procedures that are not medically indicated, but because the decision to replant must be made quickly, patients may not have sufficient time to thoroughly consider the options or to independently seek alternative advice from another physician. With some patients in whom replantation could be attempted, the surgeon may feel strongly that the injury, the patient's condition, and the expected level of function do not justify it. Despite these recommendations, a patient may be adamant about trying to salvage the digit. In these cases, it may be appropriate either to consult a second hand surgeon for confirmation or offer to transfer the patient to the care of another physician or to a tertiary medical center where more aggressive replantation efforts may be prevalent.

Operative Planning and Preparation

General

Ideally, a medical center planning to offer replantation services will have thoroughly considered the logistics of undertaking such procedures. The operating room personnel and its equipment, the anesthesia team, and the surgical team should be capable of prompt mobilization. From the time of the decision to attempt replantation, all preoperative testing and X-rays should be completed and the patient and the attendant team should be assembled fully and operational within 1 hour. Larger medical centers, with more extensive operating room capabilities, should be able to expedite these preparations further.

Choice of Anesthetic

The selection of the type of anesthetic is determined largely by the responsible anesthesiologist. In institutions that are comfortable with an axillary block anesthetic, it should be preferred initially for single digit replantations. It can be performed using bupivicaine (Marcaine), with a predictable level of pain relief for more than 6 hours. In addition, the sympathetic block that accompanies it may enhance vasodilation and perfusion. Patients may then be sedated as desired and often will tolerate the procedure well. In cases in which the block resolves before completion of the procedure, a general anesthetic can be administered readily. Alternatively, simply performing the procedure under general anesthetic may be perfectly satisfactory for otherwise healthy patients. The use of IV regional anesthetic or other regional blocks (digital or wrist) usually are unsatisfactory because patients will not remain immobile or will experience tourniquet discomfort during the procedure.

Operating Room Layout

The operating room should accommodate not only the patient, but the operating microscope, other equipment, and a back table where the amputated part can be dissected.

A warming blanket and sufficient padding are required, particularly for multiple amputations that require prolonged operative time. We routinely place a Foley catheter after administration of IV sedation, even in patients who are having surgery under axillary block. This prevents their becoming uncomfortable and moving during more crucial parts of the procedure. A well-coordinated surgical team may be able to reduce replantation time so that bladder catheterization is not required.

The arm should be extended on a broad hand table. Microvascular surgery requires a large flat surface on which the surgeon may position his or her hands. Use of smaller tables, or a regular armboard, will impede the operation. We routinely administer a dose of preoperative antibiotics, such as a first-generation cephalosporin, although its utility has not been established conclusively.

The patient must be well hydrated and resuscitated during the procedure. Patients who are relatively hypovolemic will respond with peripheral vasospasm and decreased perfusion; these are detrimental to replantation salvage. If patients are symptomatic because of blood loss and unresponsive to crystalloid, then packed erythrocytes should be administered. Although controversial, evidence exists to show that once hemodynamic stability is achieved, a lower hematocrit is actually preferable in microvascular surgery—presumably for rheologic reasons.

The anesthesiologist should be asked emphatically not to administer any vasoactive drugs without first consulting the surgeon, unless the patient's life is in imminent jeopardy. It is not unusual for an anesthesiologist to use an alpha stimulant to increase the blood pressure of a patient whose blood pressure has declined during induction; this practice leads to intense peripheral vasospasm that may interfere with replantation efforts.

Plans should be made to update the patient's family periodically as to the progress of the procedure.

Technical Aspects of Replantation Surgery

General Principles of Microvascular Surgery

Microvascular surgery requires the more self-discipline and attention to detail than any area of upper-extremity surgery. Initial experience in microvascular surgery at an animal laboratory should be a prerequisite to participation in patient care. Because microsurgical proficiency depends on experience and reinforcement by repetition, surgeons who perform microvascular procedures infrequently must consider whether they can do so optimally for a specific patient. Any surgeon who is uncomfortable with microsurgical technique should not attempt a replantation, but should refer the patient to a surgeon more experienced with these techniques.

Microvascular surgery must be methodical. Unfortunately, a microvascular anastomosis that is performed flawlessly on a vessel with damaged intima will probably fail, as will an otherwise perfect anastomosis on a twisted or kinked vessel, and a poorly sewn anastomosis. The result of each of these technical errors is the same—microvascular thrombosis with attendant halting of perfusion. The cessation of perfusion will probably be apparent some time after completion of all microvascular repairs; they may not be manifest until the patient is in recovery or is in a patient ward. When it does occur, however, the patient must be returned to the operating room so that the anastomosis can be totally revised. Otherwise, the microvascular effort will be a complete failure. Because technical errors often are not recognizable until after the entire revascularization has been completed, each step of the revascularization procedure must be painstakingly performed. "Cutting corners" in microsurgery will necessitate completely revising an anastomosis and will be regretted.

Although microsurgery must be performed expediently, it cannot be performed awkwardly. The surgeon must be as relaxed as possible and must be sitting in a comfortable position with his or her hands resting comfortable on a well-padded hand table. These tenets are emphasized heavily in most microvascular training programs and should be reinforced.

Initial Dissection of the Amputated Part

Replantation surgery is not fully sterile elective surgery. The amputated part should be cleansed with diluted betadine and placed on the back table for initial dissection. Parts that are contaminated heavily with industrial grease, grass, dirt, or other debris may be scrubbed as an initial step. Copious irrigation is a useful adjunct. If the wound margins are contaminated or traumatized, it is prudent to trim the skin modestly. Efforts should be made to keep the amputated part cool. The part should not be in direct contact with ice or ice water, but may be situated on a piece of plastic that is immersed in ice water. Operating loupe magnification (we recommend at least 3.5×) is used for the majority of the dissection of the amputated part. Use of the operating microscope for initial dissection is unnecessary and tedious.

Most surgeons prefer two longitudinal incisions over the lateral aspects of the amputated part, with the initial dissection on the volar

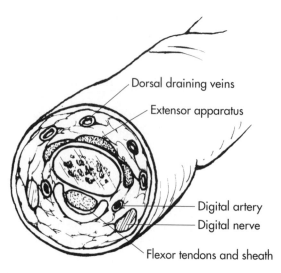

Dorsal draining veins

Extensor apparatus

Digital artery

Digital nerve

Flexor tendons and sheath

Figure 9-11   Cross-section of finger, demonstrating the relationship among volar neurovascular bundles, dorsal veins, and other structures.

aspect. The volar dissection is directed toward locating each neurovascular bundle, or the major arteries and nerves for more proximal amputations (Fig. 9-11). Once each neurovascular bundle is isolated, the end of each identified artery and nerve is tagged with an 8-0 nylon suture for future identification. Precious time can be wasted trying to relocate a previously dissected structure, especially after prolonged concentration. Varying the length of the suture ends may be useful in more specifically identifying structures as nerves, arteries, or veins. Nylon tacking sutures can be inserted in the skin flaps and either placed on traction, or sewed to the digit itself for improved exposure. The surgeon should note the quality of the vessels distal to the site of actual transection. Digital shortening will be used in most replants, but long lengths of discolored artery will require vein grafting and may foretell a poor prognosis overall.

Once the digital nerves have been dissected free, the volar skin flaps and underlying tissues may be defatted. Defatting is an important component of replantation, as it facilitates primary closure of the wounds without exerting excessive pressure on the vascular pedicles and will minimize the persistent swelling that may occur at the site of replantation. Assuming that there will be useful veins on the dorsum of the specimen, there are no other important structures between the flexor tendon sheath and the skin once the neurovascular bundles have been dissected and protected.

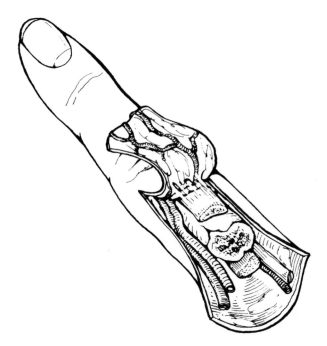

Figure 9-12   Reflection of volar and dorsal flaps allows dissection of volar and dorsal structures and permits preparation of bone and tendon ends. Thin, dorsal-draining veins are located just below the dermis.

The flexor tendons can then be examined. Depending on the level of amputation, preservation of the digital sheath may or may not be an important aspect of the replantation. The anatomy of the flexor tendon system of each finger is illustrated in Fig. 5-4. Briefly, the A-2 and A-4 pulleys, located at the proximal portion of the proximal phalanx and the middle portion of the middle phalanx, respectively, are essential for smooth tendon action. Their disruption, either as a result of the injury or because of surgical technique, will interfere with finger function. They should be preserved, or, if injured, repaired. Other portions of the sheath, however, may be opened to facilitate tendon exposure and repair. If the amputation does not involve these crucial pulleys, then the sheath should be exposed sufficiently to allow primary tendon repair. The more distal joints can be flexed to project the cut end(s) of the flexor tendons in preparation for repair.

Attention should then be directed to the dorsum of the amputated part (Fig. 9-12). Efforts should be made to identify at least two veins for each digit to be replanted. Depending on the level of the amputation, dorsal draining veins can be quite small. Veins can be located immediately under the dermis and are most prevalent on the dorsum. Identified vessels should be tagged with an 8-0 suture after gentle dissection for a few millimeters from the site of transection. The dorsal skin flap should be elevated off these dissected veins, folded backward to enhance exposure, and sutured in place with a 5-0 nylon suture. After several satisfactory veins have been identified, the excess fat on the dorsum of the amputated part can be removed down to the extensor tendon to facilitate closure.

A subperiosteal dissection should then be performed on the bony fragment below the flexor and extensor tendons. A suitable amount of bone should be exposed to allow bony fixation. Although we have been enthusiastic about using plates and screws for more rigid fixation in replantation surgery, the anatomy of most replants, in which bony disruption invariably occurs immediately adjacent to a joint, frequently precludes their satisfactory use. For this reason, we commonly use two parallel cerclage wires with K-wire fixation for most digital replantations (Fig. 9-13). The drill holes can be made in a dorsal to volar direction, the cerclage wires placed, and two crossed K-wires fired from the amputation surface obliquely out of the finger in preparation for fixation to the hand. Additionally, cerclage wiring is more forgiving than plate fixation if the desired bone length or rotation must be adjusted. In more proximal amputations, rigid fixation is attractive when it can be accomplished. In many instances, the amputation is accompanied by a severely comminuted fracture for which no truly satisfactory fixation method can be used. Isolated K-wires for support may be the only valid option in these instances.

After the dissection of the volar neurovascular bundle, the flexor tendon, the dorsal veins, and the extensor tendons, as well as bony preparation and defatting, the part is ready for replantation. It is returned to a cool environment (not directly on ice) until needed.

Initial Dissection of the Hand

The incisions to be performed are marked with a pen. The wounds are debrided of gross contamination and devitalized tissue, and they are irrigated copiously. The arm is then exsanguinated using an Esmarch bandage or sterile ace wrap and an upper arm tourniquet is inflated to a pressure 75 to 100 mmHg greater than the systolic blood pressure. If prolonged dissection is required, the tourniquet is deflated periodically (typically every 2 hours).

The initial skin incisions are then made. They may be best situated on the lateral margins in cases of digital amputation or may use existing lacerations. As in the dissection of the amputated part, the volar dissection is undertaken first. Efforts are made to identify the sites of transection of the neurovascular bundles, which should be tagged with

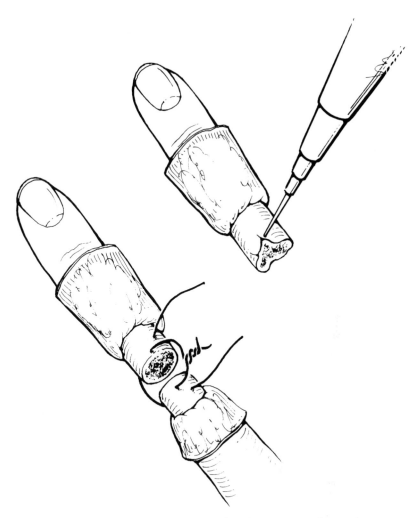

Figure 9-13   Bony fixation using parallel cerclage wires is shown. Attempts at using plate and screw fixation often are hampered by the anatomic proximity of the amputation site to adjacent joints, and by the method's unforgivingness when minor adjustments in bone length or rotation are required.

8-0 nylon suture to facilitate later identification. Attention should be paid to the degree of vessel injury remote to the site of amputation because this may necessitate use of a vein graft. More proximal dissection allows identification of the flexor tendons, which may have retracted considerably. These may be held to length by impaling them on a straight (Keith) needle. The skin flaps may be retracted using 5-0 nylon tacking stitches. Once the volar neurovascular bundles are identified, the skin flaps can be defatted. Attention is turned to the dorsum of the hand, where efforts are made to identify dorsal draining veins suitable for use. These should be tagged with 8-0 suture. The dorsal skin flap should then be defatted to the extensor tendon depth.

A subperiosteal dissection should be performed to allow bony fixation with either cerclage wires or plates. After bony shortening is completed, drill holes can be placed to match those of the amputated part.

The tourniquet can then be deflated and the remainder of the procedure performed with the arm perfused. Any vessel that bleeds uncontrollably can have an Acland (atraumatic microvascular) clamp applied to it until revascularization can be completed.

The vital structures on the stump and on the amputated part should be kept moist with saline. Because typical operating room lighting may cause extensive tissue desiccation that hinders replantation and because microvessels and nerves are particularly susceptible to drying, a saline-soaked gauze should be placed over any area not being dissected.

Sequence of Repair

The amputated part should then be brought to the main operating field and prepared for reattachment. A typical repair sequence is shown in Box. Bony fixation is provided first. Although the foremost goal of most surgeons is to accomplish prompt revascularization, activities requiring gross motor function should be performed before microvascular reconstruction. (Exceptions exist and are discussed below under major limb replantation.) The amputated part is brought into proximity with the amputation stump. In most cases, bony shortening, either by virtue of the mechanism of amputation or in addition to it, facilitates primary repair of all involved structures and avoids the re-

---

Sequence of Repair

Identification, preparation, and suture "tagging" of microvascular structures to be repaired
Preparation of tendon and bone for coaptation
Bony fixation using wires or plates
Repair of flexor and extensor tendons
Repair of arteries and veins
Restoration of perfusion
Repair of nerves
Closure

---

quirements for vein, nerve, and skin grafting. Bony fixation should be obtained so that primary approximation of healthy arteries, veins, and nerves can be accomplished. Bony ends can be shortened or smoothed with a rasp, rongeur, bone cutter, or power saw. Ideal bone fixation includes maximal area of coaptation and appropriate alignment in all planes. The cerclage wires are then placed and tightened. The K-wires are advanced across the amputation site to aid fixation. The use of a C-arm or fluroscan may facilitate optimal placement of these K-wires. Ideally, the bones should exhibit stable fixation, while avoiding transarticular fixation that impedes motion at uninjured joints. Such motion will need to be mobilized vigorously during postoperative rehabilitation. Unfortunately, injuries frequently occur adjacent to the MCP or PIP joints so that bony stability and full joint mobility often are unobtainable. If a finger joint must be immobilized, the MCP should be held in flexion and the PIP joint in full extension as correction of fixed joint contractures in these positions is somewhat easier than for the opposite positions. Efforts should be made to provide proper alignment of the digital axis as malunion with rotation or angulation will influence the patient's long-term satisfaction with the procedure. This is particularly true for thumb amputations, where pulp-to-pulp opposition is crucial.

After bony stabilization, most surgeons advocate repair of the flexor and extensor tendons. This does not add excessively to the ischemia time and avoids the risk of undertaking a tendon repair in the vicinity of a fresh microanastomosis. In the past, successful revascularization of the digit was the primary objective, but more recent observations indicate that tendon and nerve dysfunction ultimately are the limiting aspects of otherwise successful replantation surgery. These tendon repairs should be performed as precisely as possible to facilitate motion in the future. Tendon repairs proceed as described in Chapter 5. All nerve coaptations are performed as precisely as possible, using either loupe magnification or the operating microscope. An epineurial repair is preferable.

For multiple digital replants, arguments abound about the proper sequence for digital revascularization. Some contend that an "ulnar-sided hand" is more functional for grasp and, therefore, those digits should be revascularized first; others conclude that a "radial-sided hand" is better for pinching objects and that consequently those digits should be repaired first. The most logical plan should be to repair first those digits that are likely to contribute the most to overall function of the hand depending on the sites of amputation. We would recommend completing bony fixation and tendon repairs, if possible, before beginning revascularization.

Microvascular Repair

The next step is microvascular repair of the arteries and veins. The operating microscope has been used traditionally, but it is becoming more common for experienced microsurgeons to perform all but the tiniest microanastomoses using high-powered operating loupes (3.5-6.0 ×). The operating microscope is introduced into the operative field or high-powered loupes are worn. It is essential that the surgeon and the assistant be comfortable and at ease behind the microscope. Awkward positioning and posture will impair microvascular technique and lead to fatigue and discomfort for the operator. The hands and forearms of the surgeon must be supported fully with numerous towels for stabilization and to reduce fatigue.

The arteries to be repaired are inspected first. The adventitia of each vessel is trimmed both to facilitate inspection of the vessel and to simplify the anastomosis. The site for vessel repair should appear healthy—without contusion or intimal debris—and should be trimmed to have a smooth end. Paired Acland clamps are applied to each end of the artery to bring them into proximity for anastomosis and to maintain alignment during suture placement. If there is excessive tension on the vessel ends during anastomosis, a vein graft should be used. Care must be taken to ensure that the vessels follow a smooth course, free from kinks and twists. The suture used will be determined by the caliber of the vessels being repaired and consequently by the level of amputation. Digital vessels typically require 9-0 or 10-0 suture, or for the most distal replantations, occasionally an 11-0 suture. Larger caliber vessels in the distal forearm or wrist may require 8-0 suture, and more proximal replantations require vascular sutures as large as 6-0. Use of automatic coupling devices, such as the 3-M microanastamotic coupler, are being used more frequently in replantation and revascularization procedures, particularly for venous anastamoses.

During vessel preparation, the proximal Acland clamp should be released to confirm that the inflow vessel has pulsitile flow that will be sufficient to perfuse the replanted part. If diminished flow is encountered, the surgeon must seek a cause—generalized hypoperfusion, more proximal vessel injury, intimal debris, or vasospasm. Vessels providing inadequate inflow will not perfuse a replanted part.

During the microvascular repair, the lumen of the vessel should be irrigated with heparin 100 U/ml to assist in visualization. Some surgeons also prefer to irrigate the entire amputated part with heparin solution through its digital vessels. During placement of each microvascular suture, the internal lumen must be visualized to ensure that the suture did not penetrate the back wall of the vessel, thereby occluding it. Irrigation of the lumen with dilute heparin near completion of the anastomosis should fill and dilate the vessel symmetrically. Any manipulation of the intima should be avoided because it is extremely thrombogenic when damaged.

The decision to repair one or two arteries depends on the surgeon. The performance of two arterial anastomoses probably does not improve replant survival, but many surgeons, knowing that intolerance to cold is a known complication of digital vessel ligation, prefer to perform two anastomoses if possible. Repair of two vessels also may improve neural regeneration.

The hand may then be turned over and the venous anastomoses performed. Because they have very little structural integrity, venous anastomoses are more technically difficult than arterial repairs. Venous anastomoses are intolerant of excessive tension or other technical errors. A vein graft must be used if the vessels do not approximate easily. No twisting of the vessel can be allowed, and great care must be taken to ensure an even distribution of sutures around the perimeter and to avoid suture placement into the back wall of the vessel. Generally, two venous anastomoses are recommended for digital replantations. However, as in other aspects of replantation surgery, the surgeon may be limited by the anatomy of the injury and the structures available for use. One excellent venous repair is preferable to two average repairs. Once the vascular anastomoses have been completed, remove the venous clamps first, the distal arterial clamp second, and the proximal arterial clamp third. The patient should be warmed during this portion of the operation, and the temperature of the hand should be increased using warm saline to promote vasodilation. Topical lidocaine (up to concentrations of 20%, which is not for intravenous use) and topical papaverine are applied not only to the site of anastomosis, but to the more proximal and distal pedicle.

Confirmation of Revascularization

When the clamps are removed, perfusion should be restored to the involved part. A few moments may be required for the vessels in the replanted part to dilate and for full perfusion to be resumed. Ideally, several signs are encouraging. First, restoration of a pink color to the skin of the part and the nailbed are excellent. The dorsal veins should gently dilate to accommodate increased flow and should dilate on both sides of the microanastomosis (a dilated vein on the amputated part that is flat beyond the anastomosis indicates a nonfunctional anastomosis). The color in the veins should change from a dark blue color of static blood to a lighter color. The arterial pedicle also should dilate and pulsate along its course. Bleeding should be observed at the dermal margins.

The use of the Doppler to evaluate adequacy of revascularization is as an adjunct. Thrombosed arteries may transmit a pulsation that is detected by Doppler, yet not allow any useful flow to the replanted part. Obtaining Doppler signals throughout a replanted part, particularly on the opposite side of the arterial repair, may be reassuring. However, in general, Doppler signals never are interpreted in isolation. The surgeon must be suspicious of any adverse change in appearance of a replanted part. Problems with perfusion of a replanted part should be addressed before leaving the operating room. A digit or other replanted part will not be better perfused after departure; reexploration of the microvascular pedicle is always prudent if perfusion is in jeopardy.

Skin Closure

Once reperfusion has been assured, loose gentle closure of the skin should be completed. The skin closure over a fresh microanastomosis must not be tight. Reapproximated vessels, unlike undisturbed vessels in continuity, are extremely sensitive to external pressure. The site of the microvascular anastomosis is thrombogenic until its intima is reendothelialized, which requires at least several days. When flow is inhibited in the vicinity of the anastomosis, thrombus forms. The thrombosis then persists even if the external pressure is relieved. It is preferable to leave a portion of the wound completely open than to jeopardize the replantation effort by closing the wound tightly. Closure by secondary intention or by later primary closure or skin grafting is far more desirable. Defatting may allow closure that would have been impossible otherwise. In addition, priority should be given to providing coverage for the actual microvascular pedicle to prevent desiccation and disruption. Free-hand split-thickness skin grafts are well tolerated over the anastamoses.

Vascular, Nerve, and Skin Grafts

Surplus vein of appropriate size for digital replantation can be obtained readily from the volar forearm. The wrist and distal forearm often have an abundant supply of suitable veins that can be harvested through a small incision. They should be inserted in their normal direction of flow to avoid any problems related to valves.

Occasionally when a vein graft and overlying skin will be required, it may be possible to design a "venous flow-through flap," which is a patch of skin (from the distal volar forearm/wrist) with its underlying veins that can be inserted as a unit to fulfill both tissue requirements.

In instances where nerve coaptation is impossible, a small segment of medial antebrachial cutaneous nerve (MABC) can be obtained from the medial aspect of the arm in the brachial groove, where its two branches travel adjacent to the cephalic vein. Harvesting of this nerve leaves an area anesthetic along the medial volar forearm. Alternatively, the lateral antebrachial cutaneous nerve (LABC) can be located distal to the elbow at the junction of the lateral third and the medial two thirds of the volar forearm as a continuation of the musculocutaneous nerve. Transection of this nerve for grafting will leave an area of anesthesia along the more distal volar forearm and perhaps across the dorsoradial wrist area. If a small skin graft is needed, it may be taken from the volar wrist, the elbow crease, or the medial arm.

Postoperative Dressing

Caution still must be exercised even after the part is revascularized. Most experienced microsurgeons have seen a replant fail acutely during careless transfer from the operating table to a stretcher, or because a dressing was applied improperly. Many replant surgeons prefer a bulky hand dressing with two essential components. First, it must protect the hand without compromising the inflow or outflow to the part. Apply a petroleum ointment to keep the wound margins moist (such as polysporin), and multiple lightly placed gauze fluffs and pads away from the area replanted, none of which constrict the hand or arm. Second, the dressing must allow immediate inspection of the status of the replanted part by the patient, nursing staff, or surgical team. Dressing pitfalls may be avoided by not using any postoperative dressing whatsoever; this is our preferred method. In tenuous cases, temporary "internal splinting" using K-wires across adjacent joints may provide additional protection of the anastamosis. The injured extremity should be elevated on pillows or other apparatus, and no pressure should be allowed anywhere in the vicinity of the vascular pedicle.

Major Limb Replantation

Traumatic amputations of the forearm or arm are relatively rare. They also imply greater difficulty for several reasons. First, the magnitude of force required to amputate the arm not only is accompanied by extensive destruction of the primary extremity, but also injuries to such other body regions as the head, thorax, and abdomen. Second, transection of large arteries and the accompanying large draining veins in the forearm and arm can lead to exsanguination and a patient who is nearly moribund at the time of initial treatment. Efforts to salvage the patient's life predominate, and the decision to attempt major limb replantation in a patient who is being resuscitated vigorously for profound shock, who has perhaps undergone a thoracotomy, and laparotomy who may have a closed head injury will be difficult. This decision must represent the consensus of the responsible anesthesiologist, the other surgeons involved in the care of the patient, and the upper-extremity surgeon. Major limb replants, because they involve substantial amounts of skeletal muscle that is intolerant of ischemia, may be approached slightly differently from more distal replantations. First, it may be worthwhile to perfuse the amputated limb with a preservation solution such as that used for organ transplantation (University of Wisconsin solution), or at least with a dilute heparin irrigation solution. Second, nondefinitive skeletal immobilization or no immobilization may be used initially to reduce the ischemia time. This can then be converted to plate and screw fixation or use of an external fixator after reperfusion. Third, a shunt may be used briefly to provide arterial inflow until more definitive stabilization or vein grafting can be performed. This will be at the expense of moderate blood loss, which may not be recouped and may interfere with other parts of the surgery. Fourth, given the volume of muscle being reperfused, it may be useful to treat empirically for myoglobinuria primarily with aggressive hydration but also with intravenous mannitol. Dextran also may be used and may benefit both the diuresis and the perfusion to the extremity.

Nonviable muscle must be debrided aggressively to avoid such complications as sepsis and renal failure. Returns to the operating room may be necessary daily until all nonviable muscle has declared itself and been removed.

Although heroic efforts may be undertaken to salvage an amputated extremity, it is prudent to recall that patients can live satisfactorily with an upper limb prosthesis. A patient sustaining a major limb amputation and undergoing replantation may be critically ill as a result of massive blood loss, renal failure, sepsis, and multiple surgeries that jeopardize life. The enthusiasm of the hand surgeon for preservation of limb must be viewed in light of the patient's best interest overall.

Postoperative Care and Monitoring

General

The postoperative care of a replantation patient is almost as important as the technical feat of reattachment itself. The replantation patient must receive diligent postoperative care. There are many pitfalls lurking in the postoperative period that can ruin an otherwise valiant effort at reattachment. The patient should be observed closely in the recovery room because many technical errors in replantation surgery will manifest themselves shortly after completion of the operation. Logistically, it is much easier to return a patient to the operating room from the recovery room than from the hospital ward. The patient should be admitted to a hospital room where close nursing supervision can be assured. It may be necessary to admit the patient to a step down unit or even an intensive care unit if frequent monitoring of the replanted part by the nursing staff (every 1-2 hours) cannot be accomplished on the regular surgical ward.

The patient should be positioned comfortably, with the injured extremity elevated on pillows or other device. The injured extremity never should be allowed to be fully dependent because this may lead to venous engorgement that can threaten the viability of the part. There should be no pressure whatsoever on the replanted part or in the vicinity of the site of vascular repair. Whenever possible, the ambient temperature of the room should be kept warm to encourage vasodilation and increase perfusion, but no external source of warming should be used. Heating pads or warming lights may not only give a false sense of security about the perfusion of the part by elevating its surface temperature, but may cause serious burns in an anesthetic and recently ischemic digit. No external sources of compression are allowed anywhere on the extremity, including blood pressure cuffs, bandages, or tape. Use of the injured extremity for peripheral IV placement should be avoided.

The patient's comfort should be ensured, with ample narcotic medication administered orally or parenterally. Postoperative pain and anxiety lead to peripheral vasospasm and decreased extremity perfusion. These may be devastating to the replanted part.

Patients typically are given ulcer prophylaxis and a first-generation parenteral cephalosporin, an antiemetic is made available. Patients are allowed to resume a regular diet within 24 hours of surgery unless there is evidence that reoperation and a general anesthetic may be required.

Antithrombotic Therapy

The role of anticoagulants and thrombolytic agents in replantation surgery is controversial. The most commonly employed agents are aspirin, subcutaneous heparin, dextran, continuous infusion heparin, and the thrombolytic agents streptokinase and urokinase. Although none of these agents improves patency rates in microvascular repairs performed on undamaged vessels, each enhance patency rates in instances where greater vessel damage has occurred. Our perspective has been that technical errors in microvascular surgery are best corrected by reoperation than by thrombolytic therapy. Patients who have clear evidence of arterial or venous thrombosis should be returned to the operating room where the problem with the anastomosis can be corrected per primum. The thrombolytic agents have been used to salvage flaps under such unusual circumstances as prolonged ischemia or when reoperation is refused, but are used exceedingly rarely at our institution to avoid the systemic risks that such therapy induces. Similarly, the decision to fully anticoagulate a replantation patient must be made carefully. Flaps with marginal perfusion (not those with no perfusion) may survive with systemic heparin, but its use may induce bleeding at other sites or lead to significant blood loss at the operative site. Furthermore, the development of hematoma around the vascular anastomosis induced by systemic heparin may itself lead to vessel compression and thrombosis. Most replantation patients are relatively young and often will tolerate full anticoagulation without sequelae, but the decision to proceed with heparinization or to continue it in the face of serious ongoing hemorrhage at the operative site must be discussed with the patient. Obviously in major limb replants where failure would be particularly devastating, the surgeon will be more likely to recommend full heparinization or a trial of thrombolytic therapy. Any patient receiving any amount of heparin should have his or her coagulation parameters, including the platelet count, measured periodically. Heparin-induced thrombocytopenia, although unusual, can be a cause of major spontaneous bleeding at the operative site or elsewhere. Patients whose replants are salvaged on heparin should be weaned gradually from the heparin over 12 to 24 hours, with careful attention paid to the viability of the replanted part during that time.

Alternatively, aspirin administered daily (80-325 mg), subcutaneous heparin (5000 U two or three times a day administered subcutaneously), or the use of continuous infusion dextran reportedly will not increase the occurrence of spontaneous hemorrhage at other sites. These agents are attractive for use routinely postoperatively, particularly because most replantations occur with varying degrees of vessel damage beyond the site of transection. The dextran infusion is initiated before revascularization, and aspirin is first administered in the recovery room.

Dextran is a high molecular-weight carbohydrate that typically is used as a volume expander. In microvascular surgery, it slightly decreases thrombus formation, perhaps because of its alteration of the rheologic properties of blood. It typically is administered as dextran 40 (40,000 molecular weight), at a continuous infusion of between 20 and 40 ml/hour. Because it is a large complex molecule, it can be antigenic and potentially induce anaphylaxis on administration. For this reason, a 1-mg test dose (Promid) is administered before initiation of the continuous infusion. Other adverse effects of dextran include the development of fluid and electrolyte abnormalities and pulmonary edema. Once initiated, dextran should be maintained until intimal reepithelialization is expected, approximately 5 days. The dextran should be weaned off at that time, with attention given to the replanted part for evidence of altered perfusion.

We routinely prescribe a single aspirin per day to be taken orally by the patient for 4 to 6 weeks after discharge. An aspirin suppository is administered routinely in the recovery room after completion of the operation.

Leeches

Medicinal leeches (*Hirudo medicinalis*) also may have a role in the postoperative management of a replantation patient. In instances in which venous outflow from the replanted part appears sluggish and improved microvascular venous outflow is not thought possible surgically, the application of leeches may improve perfusion by reducing venous engorgement. The leech not only extracts blood from the replanted part, but injects a local thrombolytic agent, hirudin, that promotes bleeding from the leech's puncture site for several hours and may further inhibit thrombus formation. Leeches typically are applied to the congested part approximately every 6 hours. A leech will become engorged and spontaneously fall off the part 20 to 60 minutes after application. For larger replants, more frequent leeching or simultaneous application of several leeches may be necessary. After leech application, one can often see a surrounding area where a less congested color has been restored.

In addition to being unsightly, leeches may induce infection in the replanted part. The saliva of the medicinal leech frequently contains the organism *Aeromonas hydrophilia,* which can infect the replanted part and may lead to systemic complications. All patients subjected to leech therapy should be treated empirically with an agent active against this organism. Several antibiotics have proven effectiveness against *Aeromonas;* we commonly use ceftriaxone, although any second- or third-generation cephalosporin is effective. The same leeches should not be applied repeatedly to a patient or applied among multiple patients.

Monitoring the Replanted Part

The replanted part relies exclusively on its microvascular pedicle to provide satisfactory perfusion. Without that perfusion, the vast majority of the replanted part will undergo necrosis. Microvascular anastomoses are inherently prone to thrombosis. The likelihood of acute arterial or venous thrombosis is affected primarily by the magnitude and extent of soft tissue injury. Even in the sharpest amputations, such as elective free tissue transfer, acute thrombosis can be expected to occur in 2 to 5% of the cases. For more typical replants, thrombosis rates probably average 15%. In crush and avulsion injuries, the rates of vascular occlusion probably approach 35%. Once arterial or venous occlusion occurs, perfusion stops, and the viability of the replanted part is in jeopardy. More than 50% of patients who have acute thromboses that are promptly recognized who are returned to the operating room will have the replanted digits survive completely with exploration and revision of the anastomosis. Therefore, it is imperative that acute changes in perfusion be recognized and that efforts to salvage the part be undertaken quickly. Although relative perfusion may fluctuate, frank occlusion of the artery or, more commonly, the vein, typically leads to a dramatic change in the appearance of the replant.

Arterial thrombosis leads to prompt cessation of inflow to the replanted part. A previously warm and pink digit will now appear cooler and pale. A Doppler signal that was previously detectable throughout the part often cannot be obtained beyond the site of arterial anastomosis. The detection of a Doppler signal within the flap does not imply satisfactory arterial inflow and should be interpreted cautiously. Doppler signals may be obtained distal to a completely thrombosed anastomosis. A replanted part that is pale and cool should be assumed to have a major arterial inflow problem until another cause is isolated.

Venous thrombosis is the most common microvascular catastrophe. Typically, the replanted part becomes engorged, violaceous in color, and cool, implying that perfusion is diminished. Veins are more susceptible to pressure, positioning changes, and to technical error than arteries.

There is no substitute for a trained individual performing sequential examinations of the replanted part to ensure that perfusion is adequate. Although we do not advocate maintaining a physician at the patient's bedside, he or she should be readily available to evaluate the status of a patient with replanted part whose condition is uncertain. As responsibility for the patient is transferred from doctor to doctor or from nurse to nurse, the "receiving" person must feel comfortable about the status of the hand. Has it looked good all day? Has it slowly become cooler and more dark? What is the consensus about how it is doing?

No one parameter is central in monitoring the viability of a replanted part. The examiner should develop a composite picture of the condition of the part. The color, turgor, temperature, and Doppler signal should each be evaluated. A well-perfused digit or hand is pink, warm, and not engorged, with an excellent Doppler signal throughout. Many devices have been used to detect altered perfusion more quickly and objectively. These include laser flow Doppler examination, injection of fluorescein, and various temperature measurements. We often use surface temperature probes as a more reliable measure of the temperature of the replant because these devices are inexpensive, noninvasive, easily used, and not labor intensive. Surface probes are placed on the replanted part and on adjacent normal skin. The difference between the control probe and the replanted part (which often is cooler initially) is noted. As the peripheral perfusion of the patient fluctuates, the control and replant probes both should fluctuate simultaneously.

Therefore, divergence in these measurements often indicates altered replant perfusion before that detectable by gross clinical examination. Previous studies indicate that changes in the difference between the replant and control temperatures of 1.7°C is highly predictive of acute pedicle occlusion.

In our practice, the single most accurate clinical method of assessing the viability of the replanted part is its response to needle stick. At a site remote to the vascular pedicle, a 20-gauge needle is used to puncture the skin. This should result in the protrusion of a small amount of bright red blood. Failure of the replanted part to bleed after puncture or the emergence of a larger volume of dark blood implies an arterial or a venous thrombosis, respectively.

Every time a physician is alerted that a replanted digit appears hypoperfused, a personal examination is warranted. The surgeon should quickly assess the involved part and also consider other reasons for the replanted part to appear threatened. Is the patient perfusing well peripherally elsewhere? The arms and other fingers should be warm, the patient should appear comfortable, and the vital signs should be satisfactory. The patient's urine output should be excellent, and there should be no systemic signs of anemia that would warrant transfusion. Is the hand positioned appropriately? Was it recently dangling beside the bed? The hand should be repositioned promptly to a protected position. Was there any external pressure in the vicinity of the pedicle? Constriction by bandages, identification bands, and tape, as well as rotation of the hand can impair perfusion. Is the wound too tight over the pedicle either because of swelling or hematoma? Removal of sutures at the wound margin may facilitate restoration of perfusion before the development of an actual thrombus. It cannot be understated that veins will not tolerate external pressure. Prompt release of sutures overlying a constricted pedicle may salvage the replantation effort.

Once a significant change has occurred in the perfusion of a replanted part, the surgeon should quickly discuss with the patient the options for treatment. Generally, acute vessel thrombosis in the early postoperative period will result in total loss of the part if the problem is not corrected. Patients should be prepared to return to surgery, in which a vein graft may be required. Some surgeons will prefer to bolus the patient intravenously with heparin either in preparation for surgery or when the halted perfusion is thought to be the result of external compression, pressure, or positioning without thrombus formation.

Early Motion

The microvascular pedicle is susceptible to thrombosis, especially during the earliest days after replantation. However, restoration of motion in the injured part is recognized as one of the most important goals in the rehabilitation process. Decisions about allowing passive motion of the replanted part depends on the adequacy of the vascular anastomoses and perfusion, the stability of bony fixation, and the location of the amputation. Replantations in which the viability of the part was in question, those that require anticoagulation, or those digits that do not look well perfused are not moved at all until optimal perfusion is restored. In replantations that are satisfactorily perfused, we would initiate motion of the involved shoulder and elbow on the first postoperative day under the supervision of a therapist. In finger amputations, the uninjured adjacent fingers are flexed passively and extended gently by a therapist. If the MP joint is not injured in digital replantations, we begin gentle limited passive motion at 2 to 3 days after surgery. It seems apparent that striving for earlier motion is essential if optimal function is to be achieved in finger replantations. In thumb replantations, the importance of early full MP or IP motion may be less because stability of the thumb is more important than its flexibility.

For more proximal replantations, motion will be determined individually by the magnitude of the injury, but, in general, where larger vessels have been repaired and more stable bony fixation accomplished, we would advocate more aggressive and earlier motion of all involved digits.

Rehabilitation

For several weeks to months after replantation, efforts at rehabilitation are intense. Patients are encouraged to perform controlled passive motion exercises of the involved digits. Because of concerns about preserving perfusion to the replanted part, efforts at mobilization often lag behind those used for isolated tendon and nerve repairs. In addition, the presence of a fracture site and the limitations imposed by fixation methods themselves favor more conservative mobilization. For straightforward cases, earlier and more vigorous motion will become the single most important trend in replantation surgery during the next decade. Management of edema, scar optimization, and desensitization efforts are also important. Patients should be reminded to avoid exposure to the cold and additional injury to the part that will be cumbersome and insensate during the recovery process.

Prognosis, Outcome, and Secondary Surgery

Performing replantation surgery in highly compliant and motivated patients can be extremely gratifying. These patients may regain near-normal use of their hands and a return to almost all their preinjury activities without limitation. Patients with more complicated injuries may require prolonged hand rehabilitation for persistent edema, stiffness, and unpleasant sensations in the replanted part. Patience is required because optimal recovery often will not be realized for a year or more after replantation. Secondary procedures frequently are performed after digital replantation. Commonly performed operations include tenolysis, capsulotomy, nerve grafting or neuroma treatment, and bone grafting. Surgeons should not undertake secondary surgery until maximal benefit has been realized from therapy, the patient's wounds are mature, and he or she is prepared emotionally to resume aggressive postoperative therapy requirements.

REVASCULARIZATION

Patients often are seen in the emergency room with sustained injuries that interrupt the blood supply to their arm, forearm, hand, or digits. Most commonly, patients sustain penetrating trauma to the extremity, with complete transection of the brachial, radial, ulnar, or digital arteries. Profuse bleeding may or may not be present because of retraction and spasm of the transected vessels. The perfusion of the hand should be assessed in every patient evaluated for upper-extremity injury. Injuries that appear innocuous externally may have completely interrupted perfusion, which threatens the viability of the extremity distal to the injury. Injuries may range from puncture wounds to near-complete amputations left attached by only a small skin island. Any patient exhibiting a devitalized portion of the hand has a surgical emergency as important as a complete amputation. A hand surgeon should be notified promptly when a finger or hand is cool, pale, and pulseless. Angiography rarely is required because the site of vessel disruption often is clear from the nature of the injury. As with replantation surgery, X-rays should be taken of the injured area and preparations made for surgery.

Revascularization should proceed similarly to replantation. Bony fixation should be provided first. Because bony shortening is rarely an option in these injuries, vein grafts often are required to span the distance between healthy proximal and healthy distal vessels. The tendency to perform a primary microvascular repair under excessive tension is unwise. Each end of a transected vessel should be debrided back to a healthy appearing vessel. If a low-tension primary repair cannot be performed, a vein graft must be inserted.

Whether arterial repair should be performed when the hand is perfused adequately through other routes is controversial. Studies indicate that the long-term patency rates after primary repair of single-transected arteries in the wrist is only approximately 50%. Perhaps the flow characteristics within parallel vessels differs from those of solitary vessels, thereby promoting thrombus formation. Whether these repaired vessels ultimately recanalize or whether use of vein grafts to reduce tension would improve patency figures is unknown. If technically reasonable, we generally repair lacerations of any named upper-extremity arteries in an effort to reduce the chances of long-term intolerance to cold that can occur after disruption of a portion of the arterial inflow to a digit or hand. The repair of lacerations to a single digital vessel is even more controversial; we occasionally perform a repair when the vessel condition is favorable and if the lacerated vessel is the closer of the two to the central axis of the hand (these vessels tend to be the larger ones and presumably provide the majority of digital flow). Again, if there is evidence of impaired perfusion to the part, repair is recommended, using a vein graft when required.

IMMEDIATE FREE TISSUE TRANSFER

Microvascular surgical capability also has allowed the hand surgeon to salvage massively injured extremities by the use of free tissue transfer. Free tissue transfer, or free flap reconstruction, is the process whereby tissue from one part of the body is isolated on its vascular pedicle and transferred to a remote site, where it is revascularized using regional blood vessels. Combinations of skin, subcutaneous tissue, muscle, and bone can be transferred to supplement missing tissue or to provide wound coverage.

Free Flaps for Soft Tissue Coverage

In the acutely injured patient, microvascular free tissue transfer is used most frequently to achieve soft tissue coverage of an open wound in which functionally important tissues are exposed. These wounds are encountered commonly after firearm wounds and as the result of motor vehicle and major industrial accidents. Their hallmark is large amounts of missing and nonviable tissue in the setting of a heavily contaminated wound.

Muscle and fasciocutaneous flaps commonly are employed as free flaps for soft tissue coverage. They can be designed to carry their own overlying skin or be skin grafted if needed. The rectus abdominis, latissimus dorsi, serratus, gracilis, scapular, lateral arm, and temporalis fascia flaps are used commonly. Their vascular pedicle can be anastomosed to the radial or ulnar arteries or to the brachial artery. The upper extremity has an abundance of veins suitable for flap outflow. A critical factor in planning free tissue transfer for upper-extremity reconstruction is timing. A viable, healthy, free flap will assist in sterilizing a wound and can protect bone and other tissues from chronic infection. However, a free flap placed injudiciously into a heavily contaminated wound bed may encounter infection. The presence of gross infection in proximity to a fresh microvascular pedicle is extremely thrombogenic and can lead to total flap loss. Ideally, a free flap would be transferred to the injury site when the remaining tissues are most healthy and most free of contamination. Unfortunately, although daily dressing changes and periodic intraoperative debridement and irrigation may reduce debris and bacteria, additional postponement also allows further wound colonization. In many instances, there is no suitable alternative to undertaking the free tissue transfer. The patient has large areas of exposed bone and tendon, with the vascular supply to the hand floating freely in the wound. An unprotected vein graft traversing a large, open wound is a prerequisite for disaster. In these instances, coverage should be obtained as soon as the patient can safely tolerate the procedure. If the patient already has undergone a prolonged anesthetic, particularly if other major injuries were involved or if there is evidence that the patient is becoming coagulopathic, is extremely cold, or has unstable vital signs, it is prudent to abandon efforts, stabilize the patient in the intensive care unit, and return to the operating room when hemodynamic and clinical parameters are more favorable. Conceptually, however, we recommend the earliest possible reconstructive effort. In patients with heavily contaminated wounds, the anatomic extent of viable and nonviable muscle and other tissue often is difficult to determine acutely. It is unwise to undertake free flap reconstruction without knowing fully the extent of the soft tissue debridement required. These patients should have periodic debridement, often in the operating room, until the tissues appear clean and viable. A few days later, microvascular free tissue transfer is more likely to succeed.

In patients who require immediate coverage but who either have terribly contaminated wounds or a previously failed free flap, liberal debridement of all questionable tissue should be performed. The pedicled groin flap may then be attempted. It is a more reliable salvage form of coverage that will not experience pedicle thrombosis in the event that small areas of infection occur underneath it. In many instances, however, free tissue transfer provides tissue that is better perfused, has improved soft tissue characteristics, and permits earlier mobilization than that afforded by the groin flap.

Toe-to-Hand Transfer

An alternative form of immediate digital reconstruction that is available when the amputated digit is unavailable or unsuitable for reconstruction, is the transfer of a toe to the hand. Transfer of the great toe, or occasionally the second toe, has been used frequently for upper-extremity reconstruction, particularly when a thumb has been amputated. In general, this procedure is undertaken secondarily, when a stable, healed amputation site is present. This offers the advantage of performing the procedure electively under optimal conditions of patient preparation, sterility, and surgeon comfort. Free tissue transfer of a toe or a portion of a toe also may be contemplated as a relatively acute reconstructive effort. Instances in which this may prove useful include ring avulsion type injuries, in which the skeleton of the thumb or another digit has been preserved, but replantation is precluded because the soft tissues have been avulsed and mutilated. Completion amputation would therefore require discarding an intact digital skeleton and, often, the intact flexor and extensor tendons. Because the function of the joints and tendons in a toe transferred later will not equal that expected from the patient's own skeleton, immediate reconstruction using a "toe wrap" or a portion of a toe pulp may be considered. With these techniques, a portion of the soft tissues surrounding the skeletal framework of a toe are transferred to the injured digit using microvascular technique. In experienced hands, the results have been excellent and seem particularly suited to thumb reconstruction. We also have undertaken these efforts for finger ring avulsion injuries, particularly in female patients and others where cosmesis is considered crucial.

Transfer of an entire toe for immediate reconstruction of a thumb or other digit is performed less commonly. It may be considered when simple shortening and closure after amputation would necessitate obliteration of an important joint surface, such as the IP or MCP joints. More typically, however, patients would be advised to undergo initial soft tissue reconstruction of their wound using a groin flap or other coverage, and then undergo a toe-to-hand transfer as a delayed operation under more optimal conditions.

SELECTED REFERENCES

Arakaki A, Tsai TM: Thumb replantation: survival factors and re-exploration in 122 cases, *J Hand Surg* 18B(2):152-156, 1993.

Chow JA, Bilos ZJ, Chunprapaph B: Thirty thumb replantations, *Plast Reconstr Surg* 64(5):626-630, 1979.

Glickman LT, Mackinnon SE: Sensory recovery following digital replantation, *Microsurgery* 11:236-42, 1990.

Johnson PC, Barker JH: Thrombosis and antithrombotic therapy in microvascular surgery, *Clin Plast Surg* 19(4):799-807, 1992.

Jones JM, Schenck RR, Chesney RB: Digital replantation and amputation: comparison of function, *J Hand Surg* 7(2):183-189, 1982.

Khouri RK, Shaw WW: Monitoring of free flaps with surface-temperature recordings: is it reliable? *Plast Reconstr Surg* 89(3): 495-499, 1992.

Kleinert HE, Jabalon M, Tsai TM: An overview of replantation and results of 347 replants in 245 patients, *J Trauma* 20(5):390-397, 1980.

Salesmark L: International survey of current microvascular practices in free tissue transfer and replantation surgery, *Microsurgery* 12:308-311, 1991.

Scott FA, Howar JW, Boswick JA: Recovery of function following replantation and revascularization of amputated hand parts, *J Trauma* 21(3):204-214, 1981.

Urbaniak JR, Roth JH, Nunley JA, Goldner RD, Koman A: The Results of replantation after amputation of a single finger, *J Bone Joint Surg* 67A(4):611-619, 1985.

Wei FC, Chen HC, Chuang CC, Chen SHT: Microsurgical thumb reconstruction with toe transfer: selection of various techniques, *Plast Reconstr Surg* 93(2):345-357, 1994.

Weiland AJ, Villarreal-Rios A, Kleinert HE, Kutz J, Atasoy E, Liser G: Replantation of digits and hands: analysis of surgical techniques and functional results in 71 patients with 86 replantations, *J Hand Surg* 2A(1):1-12, 1977.

10

Management of Mutilating Hand Injuries*

E. Dale Collins, MD
Roger K. Khouri, MD, FACS

INITIAL MANAGEMENT	DIGITAL RECONSTRUCTION
FUNCTIONAL RECONSTRUCTION	Case Examples
THUMB RECONSTRUCTION	SUMMARY
	SELECTED REFERENCES

Industrial accidents involving the hands frequently produce dramatic and severe injuries. The most extreme result is a mangled hand with multiple nonreplantable digits, soft tissue deficiencies, and grossly contaminated open fractures. In the past the functional loss could be devastating to the worker, with potential loss of livelihood. Restoration of function requires multiple procedures to replace the bony framework, soft tissue, motor function, and sensation. Older reconstructive methods produce only marginal improvements in function. More recently, the microsurgical transfer of tissue has revolutionized the management of the severely injured hand. The dramatic losses of tactile soft tissue can now be readily managed through the free transfer of sensate flaps, and vascularized bone grafts can provide a base for functional transfers of toes to replace lost digits. These advances have made it possible to restore a functioning hand with the ability to grasp and pinch discriminatively. As these techniques continue to evolve, the reconstructive surgeon has many more options to solve these difficult problems. Frequently this process entails multiple procedures that must be

---

*Adapted with permission from Collins ED, Khouri RK: *Management of the mangled hand with polydigit loss.* In Pederson WC, editor: *Problems in plastic & reconstructive surgery: reconstruction of the upper extremity,* vol. 3, Philadelphia, 1993, Lippincott, pp. 356-372.

Management of Mutilating Hand Injuries

1. Preserve maximal bony length and joint function at initial debridement.
2. Provide adequate soft tissue coverage to protect preserved vital structures and function.
3. Institute early intensive hand therapy.
4. Provide counseling and emotional support.
5. Secondary reconstruction undertaken after the soft tissue coverage has been restored, a stable skeletal framework is present, and joint function has been maximized.
6. Restore prehension with a functioning thumb or radial reconstruction.
7. A minimum of one, and preferably two digits, should be restored to provide pollicodigital opposition.

---

performed in a carefully orchestrated manner to obtain an optimal result.

This article is an attempt to provide a comprehensive and logical framework to approach the restoration of maximum function for these complicated injuries (see Box). We focus on a specific subset of patients who have suffered significant degloving injuries and multiple nonreplantable amputations. The treatment of these injuries can be divided into two phases: initial management and functional reconstruction. The goal of the first phase is salvage of the injured hand with preservation of maximum digital length, anatomic reduction and fixation of fractures, adequate soft tissue coverage, restoration of sensibility to volar and border surfaces, and optimization of joint mobility. After these goals have been achieved, the second phase of reconstruction can proceed. Sensate three-digit chuck pinch is the ultimate goal of this phase and is achieved through the functional transfer of toes. We present a review of current literature as it relates to toe transfers with algorithms that reflect our preferred management of thumb and digital loss. Two cases are presented to illustrate this approach.

INITIAL MANAGEMENT

The initial management of these injuries must be timely, and the patient should be transferred expeditiously to the nearest microsurgical center where experienced personnel are available. After a standard evaluation in the emergency room, an initial assessment of the injured hand and any amputated parts should be performed, including appropriate radiographic evaluation.

Operative management should follow with minimal delay. Ideally two teams are available: one to clean and debride any amputated tissues and one to manage the injured hand. A jet irrigation system is also required for adequate lavage of the contaminated tissues. After adequate cleansing, vital structures should be dissected back beyond the zone of injury and tagged with appropriate suture. That is, vessels and nerves should be tagged with fine sutures and tendons should be tagged with the suture that will be used in their final repair. This will save time by allowing easy identification of these structures later in the procedure when the field is bloodied. Next, any tissue that is contaminated or devitalized should be meticulously debrided.

At this point, an assessment of what can be salvaged must be made. In polydigit amputations, any amputated part should be replanted in an attempt to preserve maximum function—even digits in which replantation might be questionably indicated in single-digit amputations. Highest priority in replantation should be given to amputated thumb, ring, and long fingers. Fingers that cannot be salvaged may be used as fillet or free flaps to provide needed soft tissue coverage. Composite finger reconstructions may be accomplished using portions of nonreplantable digits to restore partial losses in other fingers. This is particularly true if the replantation to native positions leaves a gap in the palmar grasp.

Whereas bony shortening allows primary repairs of nerves, tendons, veins, and arteries that might otherwise not have been possible in replantable digits, in nonreplantable amputations it is critical to maintain maximal digital length. Therefore great care must be taken to preserve functioning joints and length of the amputation stumps at the initial debridement. To this end, the preoperative radiographs must be carefully evaluated and should be available in the operating theater for reinspection.

The next step is to provide bony fixation of replantable digits and associated fractures. We prefer axial Kirschner wires in many cases because of their ease of placement and the ability for adjustment when necessary. In contrast, rigid fixation requires more time to place and is less easily adjusted, but does allow for earlier mobilization and is appropriate in less severe injuries. Whatever method is chosen, it is critical that the bones be fixed accurately in both longitudinal and rotational alignment. Ultimately, function of the hand depends on the quality of these repairs.

After repairs of fractures, tendons, nerves, and vessels are completed, soft tissue coverage must be provided. In the severely traumatized hand, local flaps or skin grafts alone are rarely sufficient. The alternatives are distant pedicle flaps and free flaps. Pedicle flaps offer several advantages, including their ability to provide a large amount of soft tissue, and, in contrast to free flaps, recipient vessels in the hand may be preserved for subsequent staged reconstructions with functional free transfers. We prefer them for coverage of amputation stumps and dorsal losses. Alternatively, free flaps can provide critical sensation to the volar aspect and borders of the injured hand. Furthermore, earlier motion usually is possible with free flaps, thus preventing the joint contractures that frequently occur with the immobilization required for pedicle flaps.

Whichever coverage is chosen, an intensive program of physical therapy must be instituted as soon in the postoperative course as possible. This should include both exercises for range of motion and passive and dynamic splinting. The therapy program should be supervised by a therapist familiar with the complicated challenges presented by these patients. The therapy must also be closely followed by the hand surgeon, with repeated evaluations of progress. It is essential that during this period of rehabilitation the surgeon and patient develop a relationship, establishing joint goals for the restoration of the mutilated hand, with the ultimate goal being the restoration of pulp-to-pulp, three-digit pinch.

In establishing these goals, it is important that both the surgeon and the patient understand what level of function ultimately can be restored. There are certain prognostic factors that can be of help in this assessment. The first is the severity of digital loss. If the thumb as well as multiple digits are lost, the final outcome is likely to be disappointing. Conversely, if the thumb is preserved, satisfactory function can be achieved even if all four fingers are lost. A second important prognosticator is the level of the digital amputations. Reconstructions of digital loss proximal to the metacarpophalangeal (MP) joints often produce disappointing results because the range of motion obtained with toe transfers at this level is limited. This is particularly true if the web space is also lost. In these cases, combined second and third toes are required to restore the web space and MP joints. If the interdigital web space and MP joint are preserved, the functional outcome after toe transfers is more satisfactory. The best results, however, are achieved when proximal interphalangeal joint function has been salvaged. This is the reason why preservation of length in the amputation stumps is critical, and bony shortening must be judicious at the initial debridement.

A final point to consider is the loss of critical sensibility. A functional but insensate hand is of little value. Not only is the fine prehensile function impaired, but the insensible hand is prone to further injury and neuropathic ulcerations (Fig. 10-1). For this reason, volar and border soft tissue losses are far more debilitating than dorsal deficien-

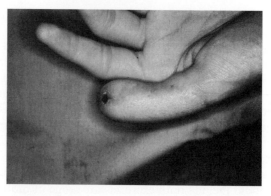

Figure 10-1   Unstable groin flap coverage of thumb degloving injury with recurrent neuropathic ulceration.

cies. In the past, this problem was especially difficult to manage. Skin grafts and local flaps do show reinnervation potential, but the magnitude of loss in the severely traumatized hand often precludes the use of either of these approaches. Pedicle flaps can provide adequate soft tissue coverage, but sensory recovery is protective at best and is inadequate for the volar and border surfaces. The microsurgical transfer of toes to digital amputation stumps and sensate free flap coverage of the volar and border aspects of the hand has provided a better solution to this problem.

Toe transfers can be expected to obtain sensibility that is discriminative (<10 mm two-point discrimination) and is typically better than that of the contralateral toe in its native position if a program of sensory reeducation is instituted postoperatively. This is thought to be because of increased cortical representation after sensory training. In one of the largest reported series, Foucher and Moss reported an average two-point discrimination of 8 mm in a series of 55 patients with second toe-to-hand transfers who received immediate postoperative sensory reeducation.

There are a number of sensate free flaps that been used to restore sensibility to the hand. These have been reviewed by Lee and May, who have also delineated the desirable characteristics for these flaps. First, the flap should have a large number of cutaneous sensory receptors. Second, the skin should be thin and malleable with minimal subcutaneous tissue. Third, the neural supply should be consistent with an axial pattern. Finally, as with any free flap, the vascular pedicle should be reliable and the donor defect must be acceptable. Next to the hands, the feet have the greatest density of sensory receptors; therefore, it is not surprising that donor flaps from the feet provide the best sensibility. The first web-space flap and wrap-around toe flaps provide the best two-point discrimination. These flaps, however, are too small for the magnitude of soft tissue loss seen in severe degloving injuries that typify the patients presented in this paper. In our experience, the lateral arm flap has proven to be a reliable flap that meets all of the above characteristics and is of sufficient size to cover any defect in the hand. All of our patients have achieved at least protective sensibility at the recipient site, and one has 3-mm two-point discrimination.

After establishing realistic goals based on the above prognosticators, the patient and surgeon must then agree on a course of rehabilitation and staged reconstruction that will result in the most functional hand possible. It is often helpful at this stage to have the patient meet with others who have undergone similar procedures. This enables them to visualize both the potential for recovery and the donor defects associated with these procedures.

Finally, it has been our experience that patients with these dramatic injuries typically suffer an intense period of psychological distress and benefit from professional counseling. This impression is supported by Grunert and coworkers, who published the results of their psychological evaluation of 170 patients with severe, work-related hand injuries. They found that these injuries were associated with a number of psychological symptoms, including posttraumatic stress disorder, anxiety, depression, nightmares, and flashbacks. Many of these symptoms appear immediately after the injury and persist for months afterward. Therefore, we also have our patients seen by a psychiatrist early in this rehabilitative process to help them deal with these problems.

FUNCTIONAL RECONSTRUCTION

Functional reconstruction of the severely traumatized hand requires the close cooperation of a skilled microsurgical team, a highly motivated patient, and an experienced hand therapist. The second phase of this process begins only after all wounds are closed, a stable bony base has been established and remaining joint function has been maximized. This sometimes requires that intermediate procedures be performed such as staged tendon reconstruction, tenolysis, capsulotomy, arthroplasty, or bone grafting. Throughout this process the patient and hand therapist must be active participants in the rehabilitation efforts. Once these criteria have been met, functional restoration of the hand can proceed.

The ultimate goal of hand reconstruction is the restoration of prehension and tactile sensation—that is, a hand that is able to grasp and pinch discriminately. This requires a minimum of one stable ray and one mobile ray capable of opposition. In addition, one of these elements must provide sensibility. If it were not for the ability to provide sensation, a myoelectric prosthesis would be in many regards superior to functional hand reconstruction with toe transfers. With experience and training in the use of these prostheses, patients can achieve a strong grasp and precision pinch. Furthermore, they offer superior cosmesis and do not require additional surgery with attendant donor defects. Unfortunately, a prosthesis cannot provide the sensibility critical to hand function. Most experienced reconstructive surgeons believe that function is further optimized by the restoration of two opposable digits in addition to the radial ray to achieve chuck pinch capability. In cases of polydigit loss, the recipient site for toe transfers must be approached in a logical, thoughtful fashion to fulfill these requirements.

THUMB RECONSTRUCTION

Hand function is impaired by 40 to 50% with the loss of the thumb alone; therefore, an absent thumb is clearly the highest priority in restoration of function. Older methods of thumb reconstruction involved creating an immobile radial post. Various methods to accomplish this goal included first metacarpal distraction, pollicization, phalangization (first web-space deepening), and osteoplastic composite reconstructions with bone grafts and flap coverage. Both metacarpal distraction and phalangization require that a portion of the first metacarpal has been salvaged; and even when significant length has been maintained, these methods provide only marginal improvements in opposition. Osteoplastic reconstructions can provide a stable post in the radial position, but the lack of volar sensibility and unstable pad make them poor substitutes for the native thumb. Pollicization remains an acceptable alternative for thumb reconstruction, especially in congenital deficiencies and in pediatric amputations. In the severely traumatized hand with polydigital loss, however, this frequently is not an option for lack of an appropriate donor digit.

Compared to these older methods, microsurgical toe transfer has proved to be a far superior method of obtaining a functional and sensate radial digit to restore opposition. The first toe-to-thumb transfer was performed experimentally on a rhesus monkey by Buncke and colleagues in 1965. The first clinical transfer of a great toe to thumb was done in 1969 by Cobbett. Almost three decades later, toe-to-thumb transfer is still considered the best method of thumb reconstruction, producing superior cosmesis and function to any previous methods. There are now many variations of the toe-to-thumb transfer, including free pulp transfer, wrap-around flap, partial or trimmed toe transfer, second-toe transfer, and great-toe transfer. There is no universal agreement on which is the best method for thumb reconstruction, and each of the options may be the most appropriate choice depending on the level of amputation.

Total great-toe transfers offer the advantage of a broad pad for opposition, which can be an important consideration when the remaining digits have impaired motion. Functionally, the donor defect for great-toe transfers is well tolerated as long as the metatarsal head is preserved. In a detailed analysis of 12 patients who had undergone great-toe-to-thumb transfer, Lipton and associates found 9 had no clinical complaints, 2 had occasional discomfort, and 1 had cold intolerance. The average velocity, cadence, limb stance, and step width did not change significantly, and only a slight reduction in stride length (4.6%) was found. In our experience, patients complain of pain with prolonged standing and ambulation without shoes. Both of these problems improve with time and can be ameliorated with orthotics, and for most patients are an acceptable trade-off for a functional and cosmetic thumb reconstruction. Some patients, however, are unwilling to accept the cosmetic defect associated with great-toe loss.

In these cases, a second-toe transfer may be preferable because the defect is less disfiguring and of minor functional consequence, rarely producing ambulatory disability. For this reason, second-toe transfers should be considered in any patient with a severely mutilated hand in which thumb reconstruction need provide function only, and not cosmesis. Furthermore, in thumb amputations proximal to the proximal third of the first metacarpal, second-toe transfers are indicated because the metatarsophalangeal joint and metatarsal must be taken to provide adequate length. The overall function of the thumb reconstructed from a second toe is acceptable, but the limited contact area for opposition may limit pinch and grip ability in the severely injured hand.

Another relative indication for second-toe transfer is significant size discrepancy between the great toe and the thumb on the uninvolved hand; however, the smaller size, hyperextensibility of the metatarsophalangeal joint, and tendency of the second toe to claw generally result in a less satisfactory appearance. The problem of size discrepancy is better addressed in distal thumb amputations by using various partial great-toe transfers as described by Morrison et al, Upton and Mutimer, Wei et al, and Foucher and Sammut.

The great-toe wrap has been used for first-ray degloving injuries and thumb amputations distal to the MP joint with an iliac bone graft to restore length. This procedure results in a cosmetically acceptable sensate post, but loss of interphalangeal (IP) joint motion, an unstable pulp, and partial resorption of the iliac bone graft limit the functional

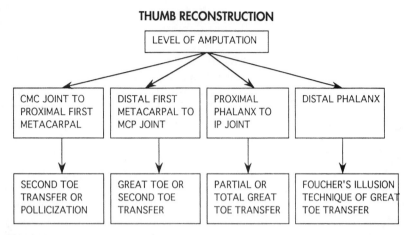

THUMB RECONSTRUCTION

LEVEL OF AMPUTATION

CMC JOINT TO PROXIMAL FIRST METACARPAL	DISTAL FIRST METACARPAL TO MCP JOINT	PROXIMAL PHALANX TO IP JOINT	DISTAL PHALANX
SECOND TOE TRANSFER OR POLLICIZATION	GREAT TOE OR SECOND TOE TRANSFER	PARTIAL OR TOTAL GREAT TOE TRANSFER	FOUCHER'S ILLUSION TECHNIQUE OF GREAT TOE TRANSFER

Figure 10-2   Functional reconstruction of the thumb in cases of isolated thumb amputations. CMC = carpometacarpal; MCP = metacarpophalangeal; IP = interphalangeal joint.

result. Furthermore, although the deep structures of the great toe are not used, completion amputations are often required owing to inadequate soft tissue coverage. Subsequent modifications of this flap incorporate a portion of the distal phalanx to improve support of the nailbed and improve vascularization of the interpositional bone graft. The problems associated with the bone graft and lack of IP mobility remain, however.

In cases of amputations proximal to the IP joint, the trimmed toe technique as described by Wei et al or the modification of the great-toe transfer as presented by Upton and Mutimer present an alternative method of partial toe transfer that incorporates a longitudinal osteotomy through the IP joint of the great toe. This allows both aesthetic tailoring of the transfer and better function in the reconstructed thumb compared to the wrap-around flap. It should be noted, however, that each of these modifications has a potentially diminished range of motion compared to total transfers because the joint is violated. Furthermore, these procedures are contraindicated in pediatric patients because epiphyseal disruption would result in impaired growth.

In thumb amputations distal to the proximal third of the first metacarpal, but proximal to the IP joint, we prefer a total great-toe transfer in cases of isolated thumb loss. The aesthetic benefits derived from the trimmed toe transfers do not compensate for the potential loss of function at the IP joint. This view is shared by other experienced surgeons who also note that atrophy of the great toe transfer in long-term

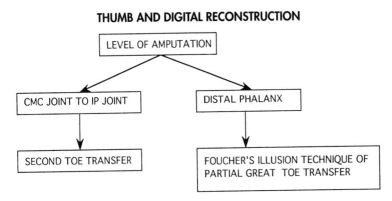

Figure 10-3   Isolated reconstruction of the thumb in cases of thumb and multiple digital losses. CMC = carpometacarpal; IP = interphalangeal joint.

follow-up improves the size match between the native thumb and the reconstruction. This subjective impression is confirmed by Frykman et al in their detailed analysis of toe-to-hand transfer, in which they found great toes shrink an average of 5% in circumference, which is extrapolated to represent a 10% reduction in volume.

In thumb amputations distal to the IP joint, we prefer Foucher and Sammut's "illusion" technique of thumb reconstruction with a partial great toe transfer. Not only does this technique provide a superior cosmetic and functional result to either the wrap-around technique or total great-toe transfer, but the resultant defect in the great toe is quite acceptable. Figures 10-2 and 10-3 summarize our approach to thumb reconstruction in cases of isolated thumb amputation (Fig. 10-2) and combined thumb and polydigit loss (Fig. 10-3).

DIGITAL RECONSTRUCTION

If the thumb is preserved or successfully restored, toe-to-finger transfers are performed as needed to provide functional opposition with the thumb. Much has been written about the optimal placement of transferred toes in four-finger amputations, the so-called metacarpal hand. There is general agreement that at least two toe-to-finger transfers should be performed to provide a three-digit pulp-to-pulp opposition (chuck pinch), which is stronger and greatly improves hand prehension compared to two-digit (key pinch) opposition. Advantages of the tridigital hand include increased lateral stability, grip strength, and pinch.

There is also a general consensus that the placement of transferred toes on contiguous digital stumps is preferable. Adjacent reconstructions provide greater stability, prevent digital drift, and offer a superior cosmetic result. The optimal position of the adjacent reconstructions has been debated. Ulnar, radial, central, and border placement of the transferred toes has been suggested by various groups. Ulnar positioning is believed to give the best power grip and often is given priority in heavy laborers who need a broadbased strong grasp. Radial (second and third ray) reconstructions have the greatest cosmetic appeal and generally provide more precise prehension for fine manipulation. Central (third and fourth ray) reconstructions are an acceptable choice, but should be combined with a second-ray amputation to maximize grasp and prehension. Border (second and fifth) ray transfers have been advocated in situations in which a broad hand span is required, but are the least aesthetic reconstructions, and the transferred digits lack the lateral stability provided by an adjacent digit. Furthermore, the wide gap in the grasp makes it difficult to manipulate small objects, and chuck pinch is less effective. Many advocate the use of a temporary prosthetic post placed in the various positions to determine the ideal location.

It is our belief that the extent and pattern of injury must be analyzed in each case and transfers placed on the most functional contiguous bases regardless of location (Fig. 10-4). Although toe-to-finger transfers that include the MP joint can provide adequate pollico-digital opposition, there is limited palmar digital grasp because of the relative loss of digital length and diminished range of motion. In a detailed functional analysis of nine patients undergoing toe-to-finger transfers (seven proximal to the MP joint), Frykman et al found the total active motion to average 106° or 45% of normal. For this reason, toe transfers are ideally placed on stumps that have a functioning MP joint and a portion of the proximal phalanx. Even better results can be obtained when there is a functioning proximal IP joint. The more distal reconstructions also offer a better aesthetic result.

Having identified the recipient sites, the next decision is which toes should be taken to provide optimum function and the least donor site morbidity. The most common choices include combined second and third toes, and simultaneous versus staged second-toe transfers. Some have also used the third toe. It has been suggested that the defect from third toe transfer is less disfiguring, but its use is limited to situations in which a short donor pedicle is acceptable because it is based on the plantar circulation.

There also are limited case reports of other combinations of toe transfers. In 1990, Pisarek reported the reconstruction of a patient with loss of all digits of both hands from frostbite. The right hand was reconstructed with staged second toe-to-thumb and contralateral second

RECONSTRUCTION OF POLYDIGITAL LOSS

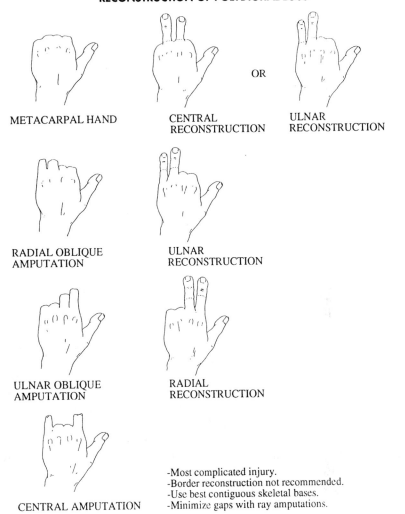

METACARPAL HAND

CENTRAL RECONSTRUCTION

OR

ULNAR RECONSTRUCTION

RADIAL OBLIQUE AMPUTATION

ULNAR RECONSTRUCTION

ULNAR OBLIQUE AMPUTATION

RADIAL RECONSTRUCTION

CENTRAL AMPUTATION

-Most complicated injury.
-Border reconstruction not recommended.
-Use best contiguous skeletal bases.
-Minimize gaps with ray amputations.

Figure 10-4   Approach to reconstruction in relation to pattern of digital loss.

and third toes to the ulnar position. The left hand was then reconstructed with a one-stage transfer of the third, fourth, and fifth toes of the right foot on a single vascular pedicle. The third and fourth toes were placed on the radial stumps and the fifth toe rotated to restore the thumb. Although noting that the cosmetic donor defect is significant, they reported only minor functional impairment in the feet and satisfactory function was achieved in the both the reconstructed hands.

RECONSTRUCTION OF POLYDIGITAL LOSS

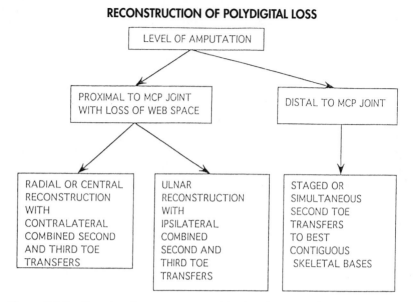

Figure 10-5 Functional reconstruction of the hand in cases of polydigit amputations. MCP = metacarpophalangeal.

Chen and coworkers reported a single case of the simultaneous transfer of the second, third, and fourth toes on a single vascular pedicle to reconstruct a metacarpal hand in a patient who needed three opposable ulnar digits for fine motor function in his work as a calligrapher. Although the reported long-term function was excellent and the functional donor morbidity minimal, the indications for combined three-toe transfers remain limited.

When the recipient site lacks an adequate web space, combined second- and third-toe transfers can provide one. Disadvantages to the combined second- and third-toe transfer are a limited range of motion (typically 25-40°) in the transferred metatarsophalangeal joint and a much more significant donor defect than that of bilateral second-toe transfers. Wei et al suggest using contralateral combined toe transfers for radial reconstructions and ipsilateral transfer of toes for ulnar replacement. This places the longer second toe in a more favorable central position (Fig. 10-5). They also note that the donor defect can be minimized by limiting the dorsal and plantar skin flaps taken from the donor site to allow a tension-free closure of the defect. In particular, the flaps should not extend beyond the midpoint of the web space or scissoring may result in the remaining toes.

When the recipient site has a preserved web space, bilateral second toe transfers are the preferred choice. The decision then becomes whether to perform simultaneous or staged transfers. Simultaneous transfers offer the advantage of more rapid completion of the planned reconstructions with a single surgery and postoperative course. The simultaneous free transfer of tissues has been shown to have no greater rate of complication than those undergoing sequential transfers by Whitney et al in a detailed analysis of 38 patients who underwent simultaneous transfer and 56 patients who underwent sequential transfer of two free flaps. In a follow-up study, they were also able to show that there were shorter hospital stays and lower costs in the subset of patients who were undergoing upper-extremity reconstruction. For these reasons, we believe that simultaneous reconstructions are preferable when technically feasible. Simultaneous transfers generally require two microsurgical teams, however, something not available at all centers. Furthermore, staged reconstructions allow an opportunity for minor adjustments in the initial transfer to realize the maximum functional potential of both transfers.

Case Examples

Case 1

A 23-year-old, left-handed man suffered a crush-amputation of all four fingers of his right hand (Figs. 10-6*A,B*). The amputated parts were flattened and damaged beyond salvage. Except for the small finger that retained a proximal interphalangeal (PIP) joint and a middle phalanx, the skeletal amputation was at the distal proximal phalanx. Because of the degloving effect of the injury, the distal 1 to 2 cm of the proximal phalanges were denuded of skin. To salvage as much as possible of the skeletal remnant, after debridement, the hand was covered with a pedicle groin flap (Fig. 10-6*C*). After division and inset of the flap, an intensive course of hand therapy was required to recover MP range of motion. The amputation level being oblique, he had a useful thumb to small finger pinch; however, it was weak and lacked breadth for stability. We therefore decided to augment the radial side of the hand to restore maximal function.

Four weeks after the injury, we transferred the contralateral second-toe transfer for the index finger reconstruction (Fig. 10-6*D*). Three months later, the ipsilateral second toe was transferred for middle finger reconstruction. After intensive hand therapy, his passive range of motion exceeded his active motion and a flexor tenolysis was performed to help him regain full MP joint motion (Fig. 10-6*E*). He ultimately achieved 15 to 20° of PIP joint motion and 40° of distal interphalangeal (DIP) joint motion. He was satisfied with the reconstruction and returned to his job as a supervisor in his plant 8 months

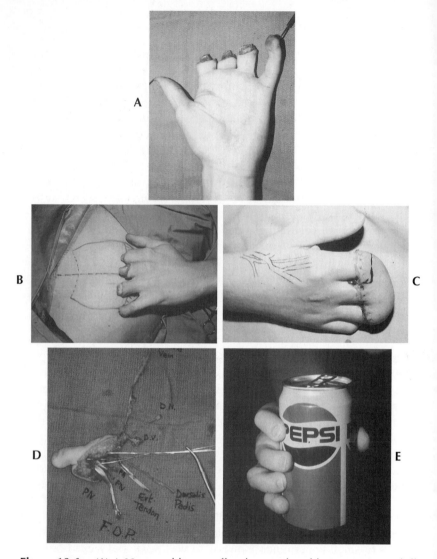

Figure 10-6   **(A)** A 23-year-old man suffered nonreplantable amputations of all four fingers of his right hand. The level of amputation was at or proximal to the PIP joints in the ring, long, and index fingers, and at the level of the DIP joint in the small finger. **(B)** The distal skeletal remnants were degloved. To salvage maximal digital length, the amputation stumps were covered with a pedicle groin flap after debridement. **(C)** After division and inset of the flap, the patient was enrolled in an intensive program of hand therapy to regain MP motion. He then underwent reconstruction of his index and long fingers with staged second toe transfers. **(D)** The second toe before transfer with the pertinent anatomy labeled. **(E)** After a postoperative program of intensive rehabilitation and flexor tenolysis, he achieved useful function. One year after the injury, he complained the that the ring finger stump, still covered with the groin flap, was asensate and had recurrent ulcerations. His right fourth toe was transferred to the ring finger position to provide a stable sensate stump and to restore a more normal digital cascade.

after his injury. He subsequently complained that the ring finger stump, still covered with the groin flap tissue, was asensate, had recurrent ulcerations, and lacked the necessary curve to help him grasp smaller objects. One year after the injury we transferred his right fourth toe to the ring finger position to provide a stable sensate stump and to restore a normal digital cascade. At a 2-year follow-up, he has 6- to 7-mm two-point discrimination in the transferred toes, and a grip strength 60% that of his contralateral dominant hand. He is back to his original employment and has very satisfactory hand function despite limited range of motion of the transferred PIP and DIP joints. He jogs every day and has no morbidity from his feet donor sites except for pain over the toe metatarsal heads on prolonged barefoot walking on hard surfaces.

Case 2

A 25-year-old male sheet metal worker suffered a degloving amputation of the entire right dominant hand except for the thumb, which remained intact. The bony amputation level was at the middle phalanx and all four PIP joints were degloved (Fig. 10-7A,B). He acutely needed both palmar and dorsal coverage. After debridement and reduction of skeletal fractures, we placed his hand in an abdominal skin pocket for 3 weeks (Fig. 10-7C).

This provided dorsal flap tissue for coverage, while the web spaces and palmar defect were covered with split-thickness skin grafts (Fig. 10-7D,E). After intensive hand therapy, he regained full MP range of motion, but the PIP joint remained stiff with only a few degrees of motion. Because the radial side of the hand had a more functional skeletal basis, we proceeded with the staged transfer of both his second toes to the index and middle finger positions (Fig. 10-7F). The dorsal abdominal flap was advanced to reconstruct the second web space.

One year after his injury, he recovered satisfactory three-finger chuck pinch, and good power grip. He returned to light-duty work and was able to type with the two reconstructed digits. Eighteen months after the injury, he complained of recurrent ulcerations over the skingrafted ulnar digital stumps, had inadequate third and fourth web spaces, and a worsening contracture of the skin-grafted palm. We then transferred a trilobed ipsilateral lateral arm fasciocutaneous free flap to cover the ring and small fingers together as a mitt. The flap was neurotized by a sensory branch of the ulnar nerve. Two lobes of the flap were used to reconstruct the third web space and release the palmar contracture. An attempt at flexor tenolysis was unsuccessful in improving range of motion in the toe IP joints.

At 3-year follow-up, he is back to full-time employment. He has

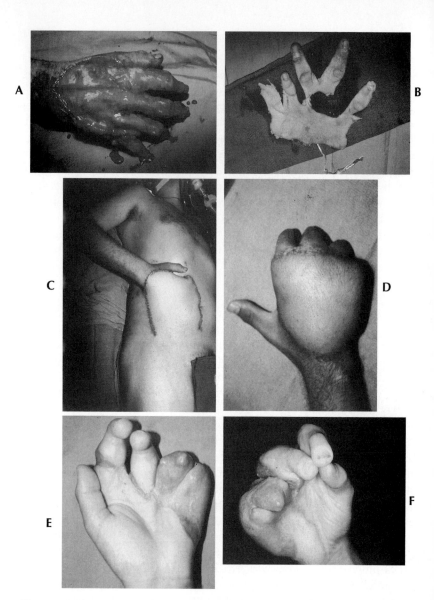

Figure 10-7 **(A)** A 25-year-old male sheet metal worker sustained degloving amputations of his right hand. All four fingers were amputated at the level of the middle phalanx. The degloving injury included his entire dorsum, the amputation stumps, and portions of the palm. **(B)** The amputated parts were severely crushed and could not be salvaged. **(C)** After debridement and reduction of fractures, the hand was placed in an abdominal skin pocket for 3 weeks. **(D)** Division of the abdominal flap provided dorsal coverage. **(E)** The web spaces and palmar defects were skin grafted. **(F)** After an intensive rehabilitation program to maximize joint function, he underwent staged bilateral second toe transfers to the index and long finger positions. One year after his injury he recovered satisfactory tridigital chuck pinch. He is able to write, type, operate light machinery, and pick up a coin from the table.

excellent function in the reconstructed hand and can easily pick up a coin from the table. He uses his hand in writing, typing, and operating light machinery. His two-point discrimination in the toes is 7 to 8 mm and in the flap 10 to 11 mm. The MP joints have full range of motion, but the PIP joints of the ring and small fingers are fused and those of the transferred toes have only 25 to 30° of active motion. He has no residual morbidity from the toes or the lateral arm flap donor sites. Although he required prolonged psychological counseling to overcome situational depression, he is now recovered and volunteers to help patients similarly affected.

SUMMARY

The severely traumatized hand with extensive soft tissue loss and multiple nonreplantable digits is a devastating injury, and presents a formidable challenge to the reconstructive surgeon. Microsurgical reconstruction with sensate free flaps and functional toe transfers has greatly aided our ability to restore function in these cases. As these technical advances continue to evolve, however, the decisions regarding the initial management of the injury, as well as the choice and staging of subsequent procedures, become more complicated. In this paper we have reviewed the literature as it pertains to the functional reconstruction of the mangled hand through microsurgical transfers, and attempted to establish principles for the basic management of these injuries based on our experience and the current literature. We have also presented two cases that illustrate these principles and document the level of functional recovery that can be achieved. Our approach to these problems is summarized in the following:

1. Maintain skeletal base by preservation of maximal bony length and joint function at initial debridement, and by accurate fixation of fractures.
2. Provide adequate soft tissue coverage to protect preserved vital structures and function. Sensate free flaps should be used for volar and border losses, and pedicled flaps for significant dorsal degloving injuries and for coverage of digital skeletal stumps.
3. Intensive hand therapy must be instituted as soon as repairs will tolerate motion.
4. Counseling and emotional support should be a routine feature in the rehabilitative process.
5. Secondary reconstruction to restore sensible opposition should be undertaken only after the soft tissue coverage has been restored, a stable skeletal framework is present, and joint function has been maximized. This may require intermediate procedures such as bone grafts, tendon reconstruction, and capsulotomies.

6. The restoration of prehension must begin with a functioning thumb or radial reconstruction. The best functional results are obtained with partial or total great toe transfers.
7. A minimum of one and preferably two digits should be restored to provide pollicodigital opposition. The reconstructions are best achieved through second-toe transfers to the best two contiguous bases.
8. After completion of hand reconstruction the patient must remain enrolled in an intensive program of hand therapy and sensory re-education to maximize function and sensibility.

SELECTED REFERENCES

Brandt K, Khouri RK: The lateral arm/proximal forearm flap, *Plast Reconstr Surg* 92:1137-1145, 1993.

Buncke HJ, Buncke CM, Schultz WP: Immediate Nicoladoni procedure in the rhesus monkey or hallux-to-hand transplantation utilizing micro-miniature vascular anastomoses, *Br J Plast Surg* 19:332-337, 1966.

Chase RA: Early salvage in acute hand injuries with a primary island flap, *Plast Reconstr Surg* 48:521-527, 1971.

Chen H, Tang Y, Wei F, Noordhoff M: Finger reconstruction with triple toe transfer from the same foot for a patient with a special job and previous foot trauma, *Ann Plast Surg* 27:272-277, 1991.

Chow JA, Bilos ZI, Chunprapaph B: Thirty thumb replantations: Indications and results, *Plast Reconstr Surg* 64:626-630, 1979.

Cobbett JR: Free digital transfer: report of a case of a transfer of a great toe to replace an amputated thumb, *J Bone Joint Surg [Br]* 51:677-679, 1969.

Dellon AL: *Evaluation of sensibility and re-education of sensation in the hand.* Baltimore, 1981, Williams & Wilkins.

Finger and metacarpal hand reconstruction. In O'Brien B, Morrison WA, editors: *Reconstructive microsurgery.* Edinburgh, 1987, Churchill-Livingstone, pp. 370-388.

Foucher G, Moss ALH: Microvascular second toe transfer: a statistical analysis of 55 transfers, *Br J Plast Surg,* 44:87-90, 1991.

Foucher G, Sammut D: Aesthetic improvement of the nail by the "illusion" technique in partial toe transfer for thumb reconstruction, *Ann Plast Surg,* 28:195-199, 1992.

Frykman G, O'Brien BMcC, Morrison W, et al.: Functional evaluation of the hand and foot after one-stage toe-to-hand transfer, *J Hand Surg* 11A:9-17, 1986.

Grunert BK, Devine CA, Matloub HS, et al.: Psychological adjustment following work-related hand injury: 18 month follow-up, *Ann Plast Surg* 29:537-542, 1992.

Hentz VR, Chase RA: *The philosophy of hand salvage and repair.* In Wolfort FG, editor: *Acute hand injuries: a multispeciality approach.* St. Louis, 1980, CV Mosby, pp. 1-26.

Lee A, May JW: Neurosensory free flaps to the hand: indications and donor selection, *Hand Clin* 8:465-478, 1992.

Lipton HA, May JW, Simon SR: Preoperative and postoperative gait analysis of patients undergoing great toe-to-thumb transfer, *J Hand Surg* 12A:66-69, 1987.

Minami A, Masamichi U, Katols H, Ishii S: Thumb reconstruction by free sensory flaps from the foot using microsurgical technique, *J Hand Surg* 9B:239-244, 1984.

Morrison WA, O'Brien BM, MacLeod AM: Thumb reconstruction with free neurovascular wrap-around flap from the big toe, *J Hand Surg* 6A:575-583, 1980.

O'Brien B, Macleod AM, Sykes PJ, et al.: Microvascular second toe transfer for digital reconstruction, *J Hand Surg* 3:123, 1978.

Pisarek W: Transfer of the third, fourth and fifth toes for one-stage reconstruction of the thumb and two fingers, *Br J Plast Surg* 43:244-246, 1990.

Sensory rehabilitation after nerve injury. In Mackinnon SE, Dellon AL, editors: *Surgery of the peripheral nerve.* New York, 1988, Thieme, pp. 530-531.

Smith CB, O'Brien BMcC: Free flap from a nonreplantable digit for microvascular digital reconstruction in a multi-digital hand injury, *Aust N Z J Surg* 61:699-702, 1991.

Strickland JW: *Thumb reconstruction.* In Green DP, editor: *Operative hand surgery,* ed 2, New York, 1988, Churchill Livingstone, pp. 2175-2262.

Terzis JK, Michelow BJ: *Sensory receptors.* In Gelberman RH, editor: *Operative nerve repair and reconstruction,* vol 1, Philadelphia, 1991, Lippincott, pp. 85-105.

Tsai TM, Jupiter JB, Wolff TW, et al: Reconstruction of severe transmetacarpal mutilating hand injuries by combined second and third toe transfer, *J Hand Surg* 6:319-328, 1981.

Tsai T, McCabe S, Beatty ME: Second toe transfer for thumb reconstruction in multiple digit amputations including thumb and basal joint. *Microsurgery* 8:146-153, 1987.

Upton J, Mutimer K: A modification of the great-toe transfer for thumb reconstruction, *Plast Reconstr Surg* 82:535-538, 1988.

Urbaniak JR: *Replantation.* In Green DP, editor: *Operative hand surgery,* ed 2, New York, 1988, Churchill Livingstone, pp. 1105-1126.

Valauri FA, Buncke HJ: Thumb reconstruction: great toe transfer, *Clin Plast Surg* 16:475-489, 1989.

Vitkus K: Aesthetic reconstruction of long fingers with toe-to-hand transfer. *J Reconstr Microsurg* 4:369-378, 1988.

Vitkus K, Vitkus M, Krivulin A: Long-term measurement of innervation density in second toe-to-thumb transfers receiving immediate postoperative sensory reeducation, *Microsurgery* 10:245-247, 1989.

Wei F, Colony LH: Microsurgical reconstruction of opposable digits in mutilating hand injuries, *Clin Plast Surg* 16:491-504, 1989.

Wei F, Chen H, Chuang C, et al.: Simultaneous multiple toe transfers in hand reconstruction, *Plast Reconstr Surg* 81:366-374, 1988.

Wei F, Chen H, Chuang C, et al.: Reconstruction of the thumb with a trimmed-toe transfer technique, *Plast Reconstr Surg* 82:506-513, 1988.

Wei F, Colony LH, Chen H, et al.: Combined second and third toe transfer, *Plast Reconstr Surg* 84:651-661, 1989.

Whitney TM, Buncke HJ, Lineaweaver WC, et al.: Multiple microvascular transplants: a preliminary report of simultaneous versus sequential reconstruction, *Ann Plast Surg* 22:391-404, 1989.

Whitney TM, Buncke HJ, Lineaweaver WC, et al.: Reconstruction of the upper extremity with multiple microvascular transplants: Analysis of methods, cost, and complications, *Ann Plast Surg* 23:396-400, 1989.

Wood M: Finger and hand replantation: surgical technique, *Hand Clin* 8:397-408, 1992.

11

Pediatric Hand Injuries

Greg P. Watchmaker, MD
Peter D. Witt, MD, FACS

PEDIATRIC HAND EXAMINATION

Evaluation of the pediatric hand injury poses special challenges for the physician, who must tailor his or her examination to the child's age and receptiveness without compromising the completion of a detailed examination. The examination of the infant or toddler usually begins with the child in his or her parent's arms. The affected extremity may be observed while obtaining a history of the injury from the parents.

Much information can be gained through this passive observation, including: (1) cascade of the digits; (2) active motion; (3) swelling; and

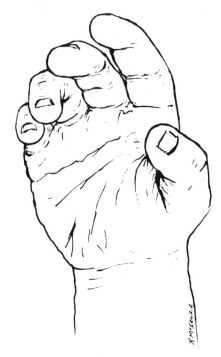

Figure 11-1   Resting posture of the digits.

(4) obvious angulation or deformity. The resting balance between the flexors and extensors holds the digits in a gentle cascade (Fig. 11-1). The index finger is held most extended with the remaining digits held in increasing flexion toward the ulnar side of the hand. Disruption of the cascade can signal injury to the bony support or tendons of the digits. Classically, a laceration of the flexor tendons results in extension of the affected digit out of the normal cascade (Fig. 11-2). Active motion of the hand also may reveal underlying bony or soft tissue injury. The child may be encouraged to hold a pacifier or bottle in the affected hand so the physician can better assess motion. Soft tissue swelling and bruising, whether diffuse or localized, can help direct further studies in the young or uncooperative child. Similarly gross malalignment or angulation should be observed before a more active examination is performed.

The parents should provide a history of the injury. This, along with a passive examination that notes the aforementioned points, often can provide the observant physician with more information than will be gathered by active examination. This passive observation also permits the physician to establish a rapport with the parents and to become a

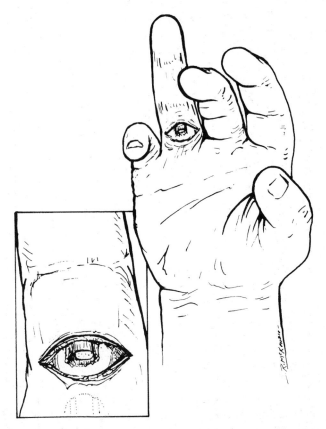

Figure 11-2   Flexor tendon laceration resulting in loss of normal digital cascade.

nonthreatening presence to the child. Formal examination of an older child's hand may proceed as described in Chapters 5, 6, and 7 for the adult. When confronted with an adolescent or toddler, however, the information gathered is significantly limited by the child's inability to describe symptoms and follow instructions. The child often is reluctant to cooperate with the examiner for fear of further injury. Several objective tests may be used to aid the examiner, especially in the difficult diagnosis of suspected nerve injury. The "skin adherence test" is a simple means to assess sweat production in the finger pads. A smooth cylinder (such as the plastic case of a ballpoint pen) is stroked gently across the pad of each digit. Sweat production normally causes a slight adherence or stickiness. The denervated digit that lacks sudomotor innervation will be drier and less adherent. Any suspected nerve injuries require further investigation by a hand surgeon, who is able to perform more sophisticated testing or exploration.

Formal examination of the younger child's phalanges is limited by the abundance of subcutaneous fat. A displaced fracture can be missed easily in the short, thick hand of an infant. The plane of the nailbeds should be examined in both flexion and extension to rule out scissoring because of rotational malalignment (Fig. 11-1). Adjunctive radiographic examination plays an even greater role in the evaluation of suspected fractures in this age group.

Sedation and Anesthesia in the Pediatric Population

The child who will not allow examination or treatment of the injured hand may require sedation or a local anesthetic. On occasion, a screaming toddler may require only a few minutes of quiet time with his or her parents before falling asleep and allowing a gentle examination. When this is not the case, there are several topical, oral, and intravenous agents that can be used.

Two topical anesthetics, TAC and EMLA, may provide sufficient local pain relief and numbness to permit not only examination but also treatment of some uncomplicated lacerations. TAC is a solution composed of tetracaine, adrenaline, and cocaine that is applied to a dental roll and secured with tape over the wound. Good contact with wound edges is important because it will not absorb through the surrounding intact skin. TAC is contraindicated if rapid absorption may occur, such as in burned areas or near mucosal surfaces. Anesthetic action typically requires 15 to 30 minutes and is accompanied by a blanched area secondary to vasoconstriction. In our emergency department, this topical agent is applied after the initial assessment by nursing. Parents are encouraged to take an active role in its application.

EMLA is an emulsified formulation of lidocaine which, even after prolonged contact with intact skin, provides an anesthetic. EMLA is applied generously to the desired area and covered with occlusive dressing (i.e., Tegaderm or Opsite). Typically 30 to 45 minutes are required to achieve satisfactory anesthesia. This new agent in our armamentarium has proven effective, although its long onset of action may delay treatment. If the child's injury could involve a nerve laceration, a sensory examination should be performed before application of EMLA.

A local anesthetic may be administered in a similar manner as with adults. Infiltration using a 27- or 30-gauge needle will not be as painful if the anesthetic is infiltrated slowly with low pressure. Ten milliliters of 2% lidocaine without epinephrine is adequate for an adult, and 3 to

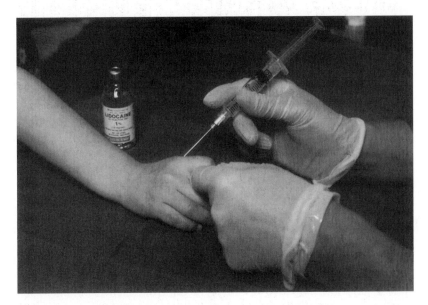

Figure 11-3 Technique for applying digital block anesthetic. Six to 10 ml of anesthetic, without epinephrine, is applied at the base of the digit. Approximately one third is applied to each digital nerve and across the dorsum. The anesthetic is not applied on the volar aspect as a constriction of digital neurovascular structures can result from a true "ring block."

5 ml are sufficient for a child. As with adults, epinephrine is avoided in the digits and palm because of its end-arterial blood supply. If it is anticipated that the procedure may take more than 15 minutes or that the physician may be interrupted, it is prudent to use a mixture of lidocaine plus marcaine 0.5% to prolong the duration of anesthesia.

For digital blocks (Fig. 11-3), begin by infiltrating subcutaneously at the level of the metacarpophalangeal (MCP) joint over the dorsum of the finger to block the sensory twigs of the radial and ulnar nerves. The plane of infiltration should not be so superficial as to raise a bleb (which is not only painful, but ineffective because the nerves are in the subcutaneous plane), or so deep as to infiltrate beneath the extensor hood (which also is ineffective). Next, redirect the needle volarly, without completely removing it, and slowly infiltrate the anesthetic toward the digital nerve. This prevents an additional painful needle stick. The needle is then withdrawn and a second volarly directed needle stick is used to infiltrate near the contralateral digital nerve. Lidocaine (and virtually all local anesthetic agents) is toxic to nerves if injected directly into them. Thus, the older child should be asked if intense pain or a shocking sensation is felt with advancement of the needle. If so, the needle must be withdrawn slightly before injection.

In children 3 years of age and older, it is best to explain that fixing their injury requires two steps. The first step involves making the area feel better with medicine and will involve some pain. We explain that it will take approximately 10 seconds to put the medicine in and encourage the child and parents to count with us during the infiltration. The second step, where we fix the injury, usually does not hurt at all. By explaining this to the calm child before beginning the repair, we are able to maintain their cooperation throughout the procedure. Another maneuver to keep in mind is not to perform the infiltration on the same stretcher that is to be used for the procedure. The child often associates the area where the most discomfort occurred with any future activity. It also is wise to fill the anesthetic syringes before entering the room so the child does not see the large-gauge needle typically used to draw up the local.

Sedatives may be useful to calm the uncooperative or anxious child. It is a safe and effective option in a controlled environment, such as an emergency department, where necessary ventilatory equipment and qualified personnel are available for airway emergencies. Local anesthetic, in conjunction with oral sedation, usually is adequate to perform most procedures. Oral midazolam has several beneficial properties, including rapid onset and short duration. It also produces amnesia, which is comforting to the parents and may prevent future anxiety if the child needs to return to the emergency department. Midazolam typically is mixed with a small amount of fruit juice. An appropriate dose is 0.5 mg/kg of body weight, up to a maximum of 15 mg. After administration of the sedative, the child should be monitored for level of sedation and airway, oxygenation, and hemodynamic status. Sedation usually occurs within 15 minutes. The duration of the sedative is variable, and the child should not be discharged until fully awake. In our institution, we have developed a close working relationship with the pediatric emergency physicians who administer the drugs, including intravenous sedation on occasion, and provide constant monitoring while the laceration closure or fracture reduction is performed. Intravenous midazolam, ketamine, and fentanyl are a few of the agents that may be administered.

On occasion, sedation has a paradoxical effect on the agitated child. In such cases, parental sedation may be appropriate. At times, it is best if the parents are not present because the child does not understand why his or her parents are not intervening in a frightening situation. In these difficult situations, a papoose, such as the one shown in Fig. 11-4, may be helpful. If a papoose is not available, the child can be

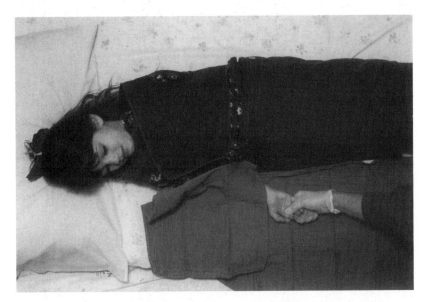

Figure 11-4 Demonstration of "papoose" for immobilizing infants and toddlers.

immobilized with sheets tucked tightly beneath the stretcher. Available support staff also are useful in quieting an agitated child until the procedure is completed.

FRACTURES
Ossification

The evaluation of pediatric hand fractures begins with an understanding of normal hand development and anatomy. The bones of the hand ossify by replacement of a cartilaginous precursor with the bony matrix. The phalanges and metacarpals typically begin ossification by birth, but the carpal bones do not fully ossify for several years. Each of the metacarpals and phalanges lengthen through new production of bone at the growth plate, termed the physis (fi'-sis) or epiphyseal plate. As the growth in each bone is completed, typically in the teen years, the physis closes. Each of the digital bones has only one physis. In the fingers metacarpals and phalanges, the physis is located on the side closest to the MCP joint (Fig. 11-5). An exception to this rule is the thumb metacarpal, which has its growth plate at its proximal end. It is important to know the normal location of each so that a fracture is not overlooked.

The epiphyseal plate is clinically significant for two reasons. First,

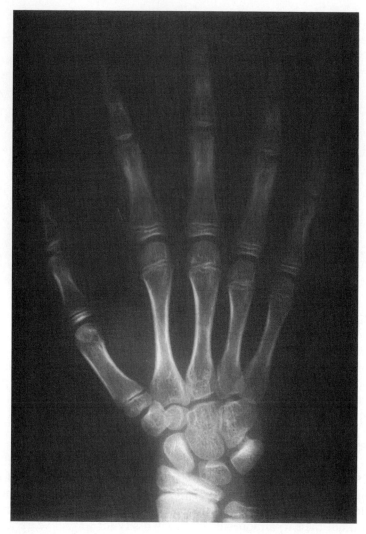

Figure 11-5 Note location of epiphyses. With the exception of the thumb, each metacarpal and phalanx has one growth center located toward the MCP joint. In the thumb, the growth center of the metacarpal is located proximally.

fractures in the young hand typically occur at the physis. Second, future growth and remodeling can be disturbed or prevented if the fracture causes irreparable injury to the growth plate. The Salter–Harris classification system describes fractures that involve the epiphyseal plate. As shown in Fig. 11-6, the severity of the fracture increases from

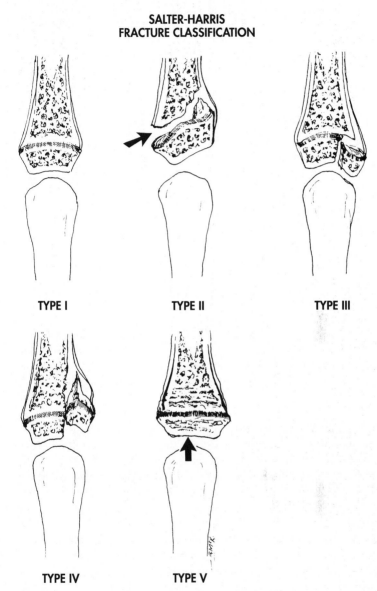

SALTER-HARRIS
FRACTURE CLASSIFICATION

TYPE I   **TYPE II**   **TYPE III**

TYPE IV   **TYPE V**

Figure 11-6   Salter–Harris classification of epiphyseal plate fractures. See text for details.

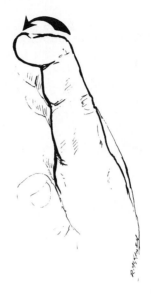

Figure 11-7   Mallet deformity of fingertip.

Type I to Type V. A Type I fracture follows the physis, but remains intact. In contrast, in the Type V fracture, the physis is destroyed. The Type II fracture, which includes a fragment from the adjacent metaphysis, is the most common type of Salter–Harris fracture.

Tuft Fractures

Fractures of the distal phalanx are common; a crush injury is the most common mechanism. The fibrous septae of the finger pad and the nail plate on the dorsum of the fingertip usually prevent significant displacement. Although these fractures rarely require intervention, their associated soft tissue injuries do. The sterile matrix of the nailbed is firmly adherent to the periosteum of the distal phalanx. Subungual hematoma and nailbed laceration must be identified and treated appropriately. If a subungual hematoma occupies more than 25% of the area beneath the nail plate, the nail plate should be removed and the nailbed inspected. If a nailbed injury is not present, the nail plate should be replaced and sutured into position to act as a semirigid splint for the underlying fracture. The treatment of nailbed injuries is discussed in more detail later in this chapter.

Mallet Tip Deformity

Mallet finger deformity results from the loss of active extension at the distal interphalangeal (DIP) joint (Fig. 11-7). In the adult, this

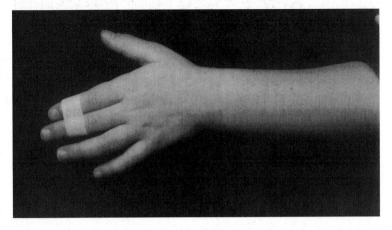

Figure 11-8   An example of "buddy" taping, commonly used to splint digital injuries.

usually is the result of rupture or avulsion of the terminal slip of the extensor tendon. In children, this deformity typically is more the result of a fracture through the physis of the distal phalanx. The extensor tendon, which inserts proximal to the growth plate, pulls the proximal fragment dorsally. The flexor profundus tendon inserts distal to the growth plate and pulls the distal fragment into flexion. Treatment of acute mallet finger injuries usually consists of splinting the distal phalanx in full extension. A padded aluminum splint placed volarly is adequate. If there is a significant intraarticular component, or marked displacement, surgery may be necessary.

Phalangeal Fractures

Most pediatric phalangeal fractures are treated effectively with splinting or buddy taping (Fig. 11-8) the involved digit to the adjacent uninvolved digit after adequate reduction. The majority of pediatric fractures can be reduced with closed manipulation under local anesthesia. Occasionally, more complicated cases may require open reduction in the operating room. The most frequent complication of phalangeal fractures is malrotation, which leads to scissoring, or overlapping, of the fingers in flexion (Fig. 11-9). This is especially true of axial rotation in fractures of the proximal phalanx.

Nondisplaced fractures are best managed by buddy taping and a light dressing in the older and more responsible child. Young children are best cared for by buddy taping and a bulkier dressing to prevent accidental trauma to the involved digit. Children's fractures heal rapidly and, as such, it is uncommon to splint for more than 3 weeks.

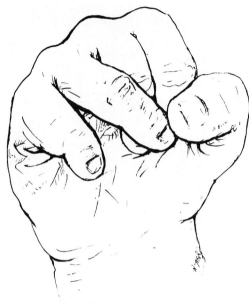

Figure 11-9   Scissoring of ring finger resulting from a proximal phalanx fracture with malrotation.

Displaced or angulated fractures should be reduced after administering a local anesthetic, with or without sedation. As previously described, a digital block provides adequate pain relief for all but the most proximal phalangeal fractures. Several points deserve mention to aid in the reduction of fractures lying close to the MCP joint or proximal phalanx. First, a common fracture in children involves the base of the small finger proximal phalanx. The small finger typically deviates ulnarly, giving rise to the name "extra-octave" fracture (Fig. 11-10). It is difficult to apply sufficient force to restore anatomic alignment through traction and radially movement of the small finger alone. An effective and simple maneuver involves placing a pencil in the fourth web space. The pencil then acts as a fulcrum to aid in reduction of the fracture (Fig. 11-11). This maneuver may be used for nonborder digits as well.

A second maneuver to aid in periarticular fracture reduction takes advantage of the anatomy of the collateral ligaments of the phalanges. This is especially true at the MCP joint. When the joints are in extension, the collateral ligaments are lax (Fig. 11-12). As the joints are brought into a flexed position, the ligaments tighten and become taut in a fully flexed position. This information can be used to advantage when reducing fractures near joints. This is a maneuver commonly

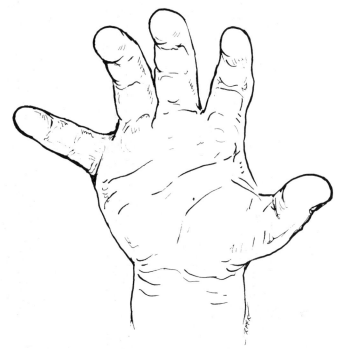

Figure 11-10   Typical appearance of the hand after an "extra-octave" fracture of the small finger proximal phalanx.

performed to reduce a "boxer's" fracture, which is a fracture through the metacarpal neck of the small finger (Fig. 11-13).

It is important to obtain postreduction radiographs to document that adequate alignment has been achieved. The smallest possible dressing that is necessary to stabilize the fracture should be applied without obscuring the details. Previously unidentified fractures or fracture fragments may be identified on the postreduction films. Follow-up films should be obtained 1 to 2 weeks after the injury to ensure that the reduction has been maintained. The postreduction films make a valuable comparison when evaluating the later follow-up films.

Interphalangeal Dislocations

Dislocations of the interphalangeal joints are common and are sometimes reduced by the patient or "coach" before arrival in the emergency department. The terms volar or dorsal refer to the direction in which the distal bone is displaced. Thus, the dislocation illustrated in Fig. 11-14 is a volar dislocation because the distal phalanx is volar to the middle phalanx. Dorsal dislocations are more common at the

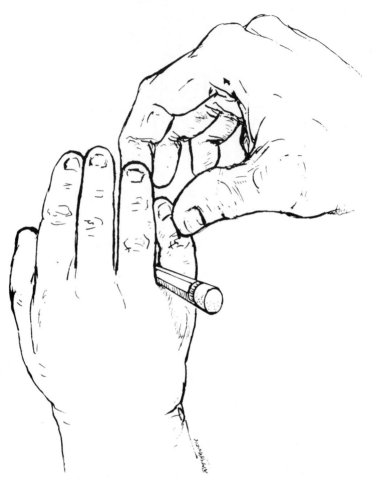

Figure 11-11 Reduction of the extra-octave fracture using a pencil in the web space as a fulcrum.

proximal interphalangeal and distal interphalangeal joints. These dislocations may occur with or without associated fractures.

The management of dislocations includes a history of the causal mechanism, the duration of time since injury (acute, subacute, or chronic), a neurovascular examination, and a radiograph of the involved digit. Dorsal dislocations usually can be reduced after digital block in the emergency department. The digit is distracted gently and hyperextended to regain contact of the articular surfaces. After reduction, it is important to assess stability. The one exception is MCP joint

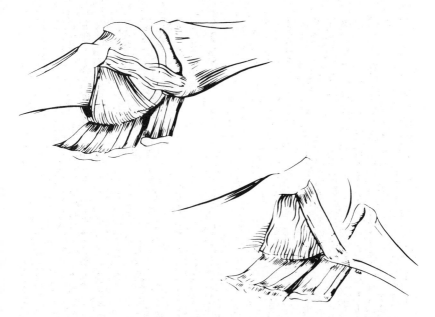

Figure 11-12   Position of the metacarpal collateral ligaments in flexion and extension. Note that the ligaments become taut as the digit is flexed. (From Jupiter, JB: *Flynn's hand surgery,* ed 4, Philadelphia, 1991. Williams & Wilkins.)

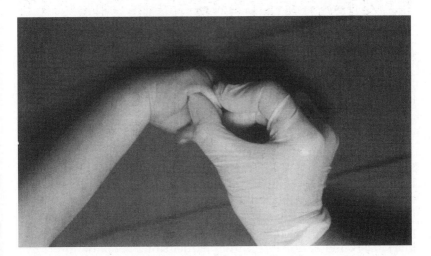

Figure 11-13   Technique for reduction of boxer's fracture. Note that the MP joint is held in flexion. This tightens the collateral ligament and allows better control for fracture reduction.

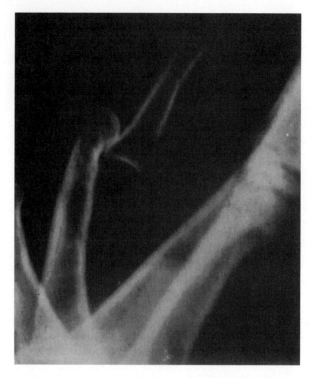

Figure 11-14   Volar dislocation of the distal phalanx.

injuries of the thumb, because the anatomy of this joint differs significantly from the other digital joints. With an injury to the ulnar collateral ligament of the thumb—an injury common among skiers—lateral stressing can change a nonoperative injury into one that requires surgical management. See Chapter 7 for details on the management of this injury.

Often one or both of the collateral ligaments will be disrupted partially following a joint dislocation. This may result in postreduction laxity with radial or ulnar stressing. Buddy taping usually is sufficient to stabilize the joint, and active motion can begin 1 to 3 days after the injury, when the acute discomfort has passed. Formal splinting usually is not necessary unless there is an associated fracture or marked instability. The child is prohibited from participating in sports to prevent recurrent dislocation or further injury. The digit should be reevaluated after 1 to 2 weeks, after which restrictions on activity are liberalized.

Most dislocations are reduced easily. If attempts at reduction fail, there may be several possible causes. First, the dislocation may not be acute. If the surrounding soft tissues are given time to contract, the dislocation may be impossible to correct without surgery. Second, soft tissue, such as the fibrocartilaginous volar plate, may be interposed in the joint space, thereby blocking reduction. Finally, the head of the proximal bone may pierce through the flexor tendon (in dorsal dislocations) or the extensor hood (in volar dislocations). This prevents closed reduction.

Metacarpal Fractures

Metacarpal fractures occur most often in older children; the mechanism of injury is similar to that in adults. The most frequently encountered metacarpal fracture involves the neck or head of the small finger metacarpal. The most frequent mechanism is a closed fist blow directed at another individual or wall; hence the common name of this injury is "boxer's fracture." As the ulnar border of the hand "leads" in the closed fist position, the head of the small finger metacarpal bears the greatest force. Invariably, the distal fragment angles volarly and, occasionally, rotates radially, producing a scissoring deformity.

Physical findings include swelling and pain on the ulnar border of the hand. In addition, because the head of the metacarpal is now pushed volarly, there may be a loss of prominence of the involved knuckle and a corresponding palmar protrusion. This usually is obscured in the acute setting by swelling. The finger may show scissoring or malalignment on flexion. Carefully examine the skin overlying the knuckle for puncture marks, especially if the blow struck involved the face or mouth of another individual. Inoculation of the MCP joint with oral flora can precipitate a florid septic arthritis. In these cases, the wound should be opened and irrigated copiously. Appropriate antibiotics covering typical human oral flora, such as *Eikenella corrodens, Bacteroides,* and *Streptococcus viridans,* should be administered immediately and continued for at least 24 hours. The current recommendation is a 5-day course of a combination of amoxicillin and clavulanate (Augmentin). Patients who are first examined 12 to 24 hours after an injury already may show evidence of infection, with surrounding cellulitis or purulent drainage. In these patients, operative incision and drainage of the joint is required in combination with an intravenous course of antibiotics.

The clinical diagnosis of a boxer's fracture is confirmed by radiographs. Carefully inspect the joint space to exclude the presence gas bubbles produced by anaerobic bacteria. Any chips or indentations of the articular surface are also a clue to direct trauma and bacterial contamination. The lateral radiograph will best reveal the degree of volar angulation. If minimal, the patient may be treated with a closed reduction and an ulnar gutter splint. If angulation is greater than 50°, reduction and pin or plate fixation may be indicated. If this occurs, open reduction and internal fixation are indicated. In cases with intermediate angulation (30-50°), both conservative and operative management have proponents. Scissoring of the digit is unacceptable and must be corrected in all cases.

Fractures of the metacarpal bases are rare, but may be associated with an axial loading injury. These fractures may range from nondisplaced to severely comminuted. Any displaced or intraarticular fractures should receive the attention of a hand surgeon. This topic is covered in more detail in Chapter 7.

Carpal Fractures

Fractures of the carpal bones are both the least common hand fracture and the most often overlooked. If one is not thoroughly familiar with carpal anatomy, it is easy to miss small cortical breaks or dislocations on radiographs. The most frequently fractured carpal bone is the scaphoid. A nondisplaced scaphoid fracture is missed easily and initially may not be visible, even to the trained eye. If a child complains of pain or has tenderness when palpated over the anatomic snuff box (Fig. 11-15), a scaphoid fracture should be suspected. If the clinical examination is consistent with a scaphoid fracture, the child should be treated as though a scaphoid fracture is present, even if the initial radiograph is negative. Opinion differs on whether a short- or long-arm splint is best, but the majority of hand surgeons agree that an ace wrap or Velcro is inadequate. Radiographs which should be repeated in 1 to 2 weeks, often will reveal the injury because of bony resorption

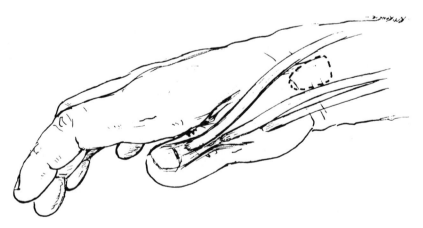

Figure 11-15   Location of anatomic snuff box.

across the fracture site. Most nondisplaced fractures heal uneventfully after appropriate immobilization. However, if the fragments lose their alignment or are immobilized inadequately, surgical intervention will be required. This and other injuries to the carpal bones are covered in more detail in Chapter 8.

SOFT TISSUE INJURIES IN THE PEDIATRIC POPULATION
Fingertip Injuries

The tips of the fingers are the most frequently injured parts of the body. In children, these injuries typically occur when slamming doors and closing folding chairs, or by direct blows to the finger. They often result in lacerations of the nailbed and the surrounding skin, or sometimes in complete or partial amputation of the fingertip. Associated distal phalanx fractures are extremely common.

Anatomy

The fingernail is an important part of the digit. It not only gives character and cosmetic appearance to the fingertip, but also stabilizes the soft tissue and allows it maximal function. The fingernail (Fig. 11-16), or nail plate, lies on top of the nailbed or germinal matrix. It is surrounded by specialized paronychial tissues and overlies the distal phalanx. One full length of nail growth takes about 100 days, and there usually is a 20-day lag from the day of injury to the beginning of nail growth. The germinal matrix contributes 90% of the nail volume, and the sterile matrix the remaining 10%. Most growth occurs proximally at the lunula, a pale, crescent-shaped proximal margin of germinal matrix. As the fingernail grows from the germinal matrix, the more super-

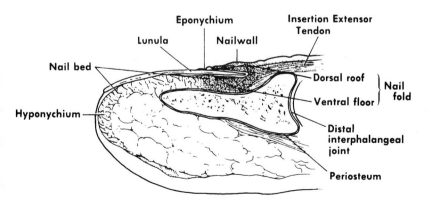

Figure 11-16   Nailbed anatomy. (From Green D: *Operative hand surgery,* ed 3, New York, 1993, Churchill Livingstone, p. 1284.)

ficial cells in the matrix become cornified and the developing nail steadily slides distally into the fingertip. The nail plate is not attached firmly at the lunula, but the nailbed has fibers that anchor its specialized dermis to the periosteum of the distal phalanx. Loss of the lunula, even if the remainder of the nailbed remains, will result in permanent loss of the fingernail. Similarly, if the damaged germinal or sterile matrix is not repaired adequately, the fingernail will be deformed.

Evaluation

When confronted with a fingertip injury in the emergency room, determine whether the fingernail has separated from the underlying nailbed. Separation may indicate an associated nailbed laceration. Radiographs are important in all of these injuries to rule out an underlying distal phalanx fracture and to ascertain the nature of the fracture (simple or comminuted, with or without displacement).

The four types of injuries are as follows:

1. Solitary nailbed injuries. These injuries are fairly unusual. The most frequently encountered is a subungual hematoma, which usually results from a blunt, direct blow to the nailbed. When blood is trapped between the nail plate and the nailbed, the resulting pressure may cause excruciating pain. The hematoma may be drained using a digital block anesthetic by placing a drill hole through the nail plate. A knife with a No. 11 blade can create the drill hole by rotating the point against the nail plate until it enters the hematoma. This must be done carefully to prevent injury to the underlying nailbed. Cautery, or the use of a hot paper clip, generally is discouraged. It may coagulate the blood, which then obturates the opening and curtails egress of blood. Much of the hematoma can thus be drained, and the injured area can then be dressed with absorbent gauze for a short period until the hematoma is resolved completely. With such injuries, one should suspect an underlying nailbed laceration.

2. Lacerations. A stellate laceration to the nailbed can result from a crush injury. There is no advantage in maintaining the nail plate in position. It must be removed by slipping a sharp instrument, such as a fine-curved tenotomy scissors or elevator, under the nail plate and removing the nail plate from the adjacent lacerated nailbed. A finger or arm tourniquet is helpful in aiding visualization of the injury. At this point, the laceration can be cleaned with the edges debrided as needed. A lacerated nailbed must be reapproximated meticulously with 6-0 or 7-0 absorbable sutures using loupe magnification. A single layer of adaptic gauze can

then be placed on top of the repaired nailbed. This, in turn, is incorporated into a finger dressing. It is best to use the removed nail plate as a splint to preserve the contour of the eponychium.
3. Avulsion. Complete nailbed avulsion usually requires a toenail bed graft performed in the operating room. Usually the free nailbed graft can be taken from the small toe or possibly from the great toe. Associated underlying fractures of the distal phalanx involving the tuft, but with minimal displacement of the phalanx, do not require anatomic reduction, although comminuted fractures can be molded manually before repair of the overlying nailbed. Fixation can be accomplished with a battery powered drill or a 25- or 22-gauge needle with a plastic 5 ml syringe. The syringe is used as the driver handle and manually rotated to fix the fracture segments. Fingertip injuries should be splinted for protection and immobilization of the segments. If there is dorsal displacement of the eponychium, replacement may prevent fingernail deformity. The germinal matrix can be slipped back underneath the eponychium and held in place with absorbable mattress sutures.
4. Pulp injuries and partial amputation. Among pediatric patients, maintenance of finger length is of primary importance. Younger patients have an unusual ability to regain sensation and adequate range of motion in the finger, regardless of which procedure is undertaken for reconstruction. In partial amputations without exposed distal bone, relatively simple reconstructive procedures can be employed under most circumstances. Amputated parts can be used for reconstructive purposes. In particular, defatting of an amputated nonreplantable part can be used as a full-thickness graft. Similarly, a composite graft can be used for incomplete amputations, and such treatment meets with success more frequently in children than it does in adults.

Treatment

Management principles include (1) restoration of anatomy; (2) restoration of function; (3) healing of the wound; (4) providing an aesthetically pleasing appearance; (5) maintaining length; (6) avoiding complications that lead to stiff joints; and (7) avoiding residual pain in the fingertip or contour irregularities that may catch on clothing or interfere with the proper fitting of gloves.

If replacement is not possible, the defect is less than 1 cm in diameter, and no bone is exposed, reepithelialization should be considered for treatment. This will require 10 to 21 days of soaks and a fresh daily dressing of nonadhering gauze. The advantage of this method is that reepithelialization and scar contraction decreases the size of the original defect. Subsequent sensory return is often quite satisfactory—even better than if the defect had been covered by a skin graft.

For large partial amputation defects (i.e., greater than 1.5 cm in diameter), application of a free graft may be the preferred procedure. Such primary treatment affords the advantage of early wound closure, thereby obviating numerous dressing changes, which may be logistically difficult in children. Possible donor sites include the hypothenar eminence of the palm, the lateral groin crease, and upper lateral thigh region. The graft can be harvested with a free knife or a battery powered dermatome. Multiple 'fine' absorbable sutures are used for approximation to optimize revascularization. The stint is constructed of moist cotton or foam and gauze, creating pressure on the skin graft for better adherence.

When the amputation creates a concave wound with exposed bone, consideration should be given to shortening the bone with Ronguer forceps and closing the defect primarily. This treatment is less desirable in children than in adults because of the importance of preserving length. In general, when bone is exposed and primary closure cannot be undertaken, formal flap reconstruction of some sort is indicated.

Numerous sophisticated advancement flap reconstructions have been described for management of fingertip injuries. In general, these forms of reconstruction (such as V–Y advancements flaps, cross-finger flaps, and neurovascular island flaps) have fallen out of vogue because of increasingly favorable responses to healing by secondary intention. These procedures are ill advised in an emergency setting. For volar oblique amputations, reconstruction becomes more complex and may necessitate a local pedicle flap from the contralateral digit, or possibly a cross-thenar flap. A detailed discussion of these procedures can be found in Chapter 4.

Conclusion

Injuries in the distal fingertip less than 1 cm in diameter are best managed nonoperatively, providing there is no exposed bone. Wound contraction and epithelialization provide the best results in terms of ultimate form and function (durability, sensory return, and cosmesis) under most circumstances. Larger defects require split-thickness or full-thickness skin grafts, possibly a composite graft, or a neurovascular island flap reconstruction. Transverse and dorsal oblique fingertip amputations can be managed with volar V–Y advancements, which should be performed in the operating room.

BURNS

According to a report issued after a consumer product safety commission survey of 119 hospitals, 38% of all burns involved the upper extremity. The largest number of those injured are children and young adults. Management of upper-extremity burn injuries in children is similar to that in adults, but care must be taken in children to prevent or minimize growth disturbances of injured extremities.

Epidemiology

The causes of burns in children reflect the child's age, sex, cultural background, and economic situation. Eighty-five percent of burns occurring in infants and toddlers younger than 3 years of age are scald injuries. The hand and upper extremity may become involved when the curious child reaches up to the table, counter, or stove, and pulls a cup, dish, or pot of hot liquid onto herself or himself. In underdeveloped countries and among poor families, thermal burns are more commonly caused by exposure to open fires used for cooking and heating or unprotected heating devices.

Children younger than 3 years of age also suffer contact burns involving the palm and volar surface of the fingers from irons, standup room heaters, oven doors, glass fireplace doors, and barbecue covers. These burns can be surprisingly deep. Despite vigorous indoctrination about the dangers of fire, children, particularly boys, are fascinated with it. In the older child, burns from flames are more severe. Deep hand burns can result from playing with matches, adding fuel to a barbecue or gasoline to bonfires, lighting fireworks while holding them in the hand, or experimenting with gunpowder and home-made explosive devices. As such, these children often have burns involving one side of the head, face, neck, chest, arm, or hand. Scald burns of the hand and upper extremity also occur as part of a larger burn when the child crawls into a sink or bathtub of hot water. Typically, these burns have splash marks and an uneven distribution.

Most burns in children are accidental. A small but increasing number are inflicted by adults or other children. The majority of these are scald burns or contact burns (e.g., from cigarettes). Some are caused by chemicals or flames. Physicians must be aware that burns in children may be a manifestation of child abuse and should report suspected cases to the appropriate authorities. Scald burns that are clearly defined and limited anatomically (i.e., in a stocking-glove distribution, or truncal burns associated with extremity burns) insinuate that the patient was forcibly and intentionally held in a hot liquid. If a sharply demarcated stocking-glove distribution is observed (the so-called meniscus sign), the burn may be the result of a purposeful dunking, and child abuse should be suspected. A history of multiple bruises and fractures, and an accident-prone child should raise the question of child abuse.

Classification of Burns

The depth of a burn must be evaluated to properly determine the course of treatment and the prognosis. A cross-section of normal human skin is illustrated in Fig. 11-17. First-degree burns involve only the epidermis. They are dry, do not blister, and generally are painful because of the sensitivity of intact nerve endings. By definition, first-degree burns heal spontaneously in 5 to 10 days. Second-degree burns extend into the dermis and are therefore partial-thickness injuries. They are hyperemic, edematous, painful, and form blisters. They generally heal within 2 weeks, and result in a variable degree of scarring. Third-degree burns indicate destruction of the entire dermis and all of the deep epidermal elements. As such, these wounds are

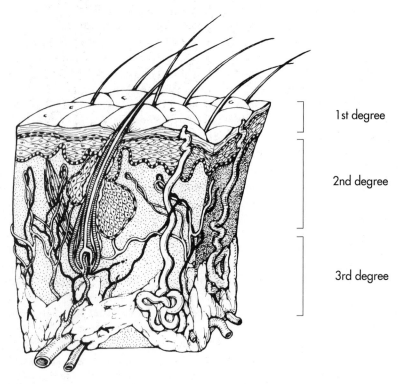

Figure 11-17 Cross-section of normal skin demonstrating depth of burn.

asensate, avascular (because of thrombosed vessels), and leathery. They appear pale to a carbonaceous black, and they do not heal in a timely fashion.

Pathophysiology

Thermal Burns

The extent and depth of injuries relate to the core content of the heat source, the duration and surface area of the contact, the type of tissue and resistance, the age and sex of the patient, the presence of clothing, and the preexisting condition of the tissue. Generally flame burns are more severe than scalds because the temperature of the heat source is maintained. Flame burns to the upper extremities commonly involve the digits, dorsal surface of the hands, and forearms. The burns often are circumferential if the patient was wearing clothing. In young children who are thin skinned and unable to withdraw rapidly, scald burns are often full-thickness injuries.

Chemical Burns

Chemical burns occur less frequently than thermal burns and often involve the upper extremity. Tissue damage by chemicals depends on the type of chemical, as well as its concentration and quantity, the duration of its contact with the tissue, and the mechanism of action. Acid causes coagulation necrosis of the skin, whereas alkali causes liquefaction necrosis. Chemical burns often are deep and severe because the offending substance continues to destroy tissue as long as it is present. Surface contact injuries with acid or alkali should be irrigated copiously with water to wash off and dilute the chemical. Some chemicals, such as hydrofluoric acid, can be neutralized by the injection of small amounts of 10% calcium gluconate solution into the subcutaneous tissue, or alternatively, intraarterially. If an exothermic reaction develops, thermal injury also ensues. Some chemicals, such as picric acid, formic acid, and chromic acid, penetrate the skin and cause minimal skin damage, but injure the subcutaneous tissue. Many of these injuries are caused by industrial chemicals, but quite a few result from every day household and farm chemicals to which children may be exposed.

Electrical Burns

Electrical injuries produce direct tissue coagulation and, in some instances, thermal burns. For example, the classic burn to the corner of the mouth from contact with the male end of an electrical cord is truly a thermal, and not an electrical, injury. The extent of the tissue damage relates to the duration of contact, the voltage and amperage, the tissue resistance at the entry and exit sites, the wave of the current, and the surface of contact. In such injuries, the upper extremity is the most frequently injured part of the body because electrical current passes through tissues that offer the least resistance (i.e., blood vessels) causing thrombosis, ischemia, and delayed hemorrhage. Sometimes the sites are remote from the entry or exit site. Tissues, such as bone, that provide greater resistance, are sites of thermal damage. The development of progressive edema and closed compartment syndrome in the forearm and hand may potentiate tissue necrosis.

Assessment and Diagnosis of the Magnitude of the Injury

The upper extremity represents a large percentage (15-18%) of the total body surface area in a young child. Thus, a burn confined to this area may have significant systemic or regional consequences. Determination of the precise depth of any burn injury can be difficult. Although these judgments are important, they rarely are possible to make in a young, acutely injured, and frightened patent. Fortunately, these determinations are not critical. Equally important in the assessment of burn injuries in children is the fact that their skin is thin and less protected than that of adults. In the adult, the color of burned tissue often is a clue to the depth of injury, but in a child it is less reliable as an indicator. A pink-appearing burn of the upper extremity in an adult may be a partial-thickness burn, but it is likely to be a full-thickness injury in a child. The uncalloused palmar skin of the child's hand is more likely to sustain a deep, full-thickness burn than the thickened keratoid palm of the adult. A waxy white edematous or yellow–brown dehydrated appearance with thrombosed veins corroborates a diagnosis of a full-thickness burn.

Impending or actual vascular insufficiency of an upper extremity is critical. As a result, this condition must be diagnosed and treated expeditiously. Circumferential burns, closed anatomic compartment syndrome, obligatory edema, and significant electric injuries can result in vascular compromise, tissue ischemia, and necrosis. Skin temperature and estimation and capillary refill are notoriously inaccurate signs of diminished vascular perfusion in an acutely burned and edematous upper extremity. Pulses do not guarantee hand perfusion; their absence, of course, is pathognomonic of vascular compromise, and demands immediate action. Measurement of tissue compartment pressures probably is unnecessary in acute management of extremity burns because the development of closed compartment syndrome is uncommon. However, frequent examinations are mandatory during the first 24 to 48 hours after the burn, and along with Doppler evaluation, are the best guides currently available to determine if vascular perfusion to an extremity is satisfactory. If necessary, the hands and fascia of the interosseous muscles are decompressed by dorsal, vertically directed, vein-sparing incisions and the fingers by midlateral incisions if possible. The surgeon should avoid incisions in the radial aspect of the long finger and the ulnar aspect of the thumb and little finger. This procedure can be undertaken at the bedside or in the emergency room.

Minor Burns: Diagnosis and Treatment

In view of the functional importance of the hand to the patient, any burn to the hand is significant. A burn on the distal thumb, although in a small area, may result in hypertrophic sensitive scar with substantial morbidity. It is incumbent on the physician to assess not only the seriousness of the burn, but also the ability of the child's parents to care for the burns properly at home. As a general rule, it is preferable to hospitalize a child with a burned upper extremity if there is any question as to the extent or the depth of the burn or the ability of the family to properly manage the injury on an outpatient basis.

Superficial burns require symptomatic care. Ice-water compresses applied for 12 to 18 hours will decrease edema and provide local analgesia. A small second-degree burn should be cleaned with a physiologic nontoxic solution using sterile technique. Generally, blisters should be left intact and should be protected by nonadherent gauze and fluff dressings to maintain their integrity as biological coverage. Broken blisters, however, or those likely to break, are debrided, and the wounds are covered with fine mesh gauze. More recently, various biologic dressings have been used on debrided wounds, including amnion, biobrane, and pigskin. Application of these materials is the ideal treatment for the uniformly pink, weepy burn wound that is characteristic of a superficial partial thickness burn. In addition to providing protection for the wounds and allowing reepithelialization, these treatments minimize fluid and heat loss, reduce edema, and mechanically prevent or reduce the risk of infection and pain.

Tetanus toxoid and tetanus immunoglobulin are administered as necessary according to the guidelines of the American College of Surgeons (Table 11-1). Frequent follow-up visits, usually every 2 to 3 days, are necessary to confirm the original diagnosis of the depth of the burn injury. It also allows the physician to monitor the patient for possible infection and compliance with the therapeutic regimen. If the pigskin or amnion is adherent, it should be left intact until complete epithelialization occurs. The desiccated amnion will then peel off. If it is not adherent, the wound can be cleaned by removing the amnion or biobrane and replacing it with an antibacterial ointment.

Hand dressings must be applied carefully. A layer of fine mesh gauze is placed next to the wound, which has been covered with a topical antibacterial agent or biologic membrane. A layer of course mesh

Table 11-1   ACS Recommendations on Tetanus*

History of adsorbed tetanus toxoid (doses)	Tetanus-prone wounds		Nontetanus-prone wounds	
	TD	TIG	TD	TIG
Unknown or fewer than 3	Yes	Yes	Yes	Yes
3 or more	No	No	No	No

*Verify a history of tetanus immunization from medical records so that appropriate tetanus prophylaxis can be accomplished.
TD = tetanus and diphtheria toxoids adsorbed (for adult use); TIG = tetanus immune globulin (human)

gauze is then placed about and between each digit, followed by a bulky gauze placed in the palm. Several layers of course mesh gauze are then applied over the remaining areas of the upper extremity, and the entire upper extremity is wrapped with a bandage. The distal finger tips should remain undressed to aid in assessment of vascularity (Fig. 11-18). Topical antibacterial agents, including silver sulfadiazine (Silvadene), are useful during the time that the burn wound is demarcating.

Splints and Splinting

Splints often are necessary for the treatment of upper extremity burns to relieve pain, assist in elevating the injured extremity, diminish tissue edema, provide support for dressings, and promote mobilization. They may be static, maintaining position during the periods of rest, or they may be dynamic. They may be internal or external. Preferably, they are constructed individually for each patient. Some of the newer molding materials, such as Orthoplast, are especially useful in caring for upper-extremity burns, because the splints are easy to make, modify, and clean. Orthoplast can be used for long periods of time and is not damaged by liquids.

External dynamic splints with rubberbands and fingernail bands are excellent adjuncts for mobilization, but they are not substitutes for adequate skin replacement. Splinting should be performed to decrease edema and maintain hand function. This can be accomplished with volar or sandwiched splints in the position of advantage (wrist: 35° extension; MCP: 80-90° of flexion; IP: almost straight); or position of function (wrist: 30° extension; MCP: 70-80° of flexion; PIP: 20-30 degrees of flexion; DIP: almost straight). The former (Fig. 11-19) is preferred for burns of the dorsum of the hand because it maintains the toughness of the dorsal skin and helps decrease edema.

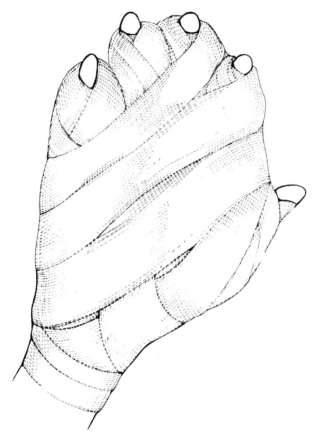

Figure 11-18   Application of a hand dressing. The bulky hand dressing leaves fingertips open for inspection of the circulation and provides comfort.

Occupational Therapy

Physiotherapists and occupational therapists are integral parts of the burn therapy team. Their direct participation is helpful in mobilizing the burned hand and educating others on the burn therapy team to ensure maximal patient benefit. It is essential that all involved joints are placed through range of motion exercises by a member of the treatment team. This must be done without causing undo pain or secondary trauma to injured joints or injured tissues. After the wound has healed, continued guided exercise is necessary to promote the maximal return of functional motion. The ingenuity of the burn therapy team often will be taxed by an uncooperative young child, who is afraid of

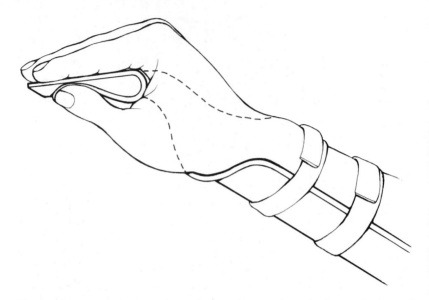

Figure 11-19   External anticlaw splinting. The purpose of splinting the burned hand is to overcome the pathophysiologic forces of burn contractures. This requires keeping the PIP joints straight and the MP joints flexed.

painful manipulations and not yet mature enough to understand the need for stretching scars and mobilizing joints to prevent contractures. Adjunctive techniques include whirlpool baths, ultrasound, pressure garments, and dynamic and static splints to facilitate active and passive motion.

Common late deformities include contractures that result from the persistence of myofibroblasts within the wound. This commonly occurs on the dorsum of the hand. This classical deformity results in hyperextension at the metacarpal phalangeal joints and flexion of the interphalangeal joints (Fig. 11-20). Uncontrolled edema, failure to maintain proper position, full-thickness injury of the dorsal hand, and direct burn injury to the extensor mechanism produce hyperextension at the metacarpal phalangeal joints and allow the strong, unopposed flexor tendons to pull the phalanges into flexion. Secondary scarring and fibrosis produce fixed deformities, thumb adduction contractures, and other dorsal edema-type contracture.

Only very small, deep, partial-thickness or full-thickness burns can be allowed to heal without skin grafting, because these wounds heal by contraction and inevitably lead to functional problems. Initial treatment of these deeper burns, or burns covering a larger surface area, should be in the hospital. The details of surgical treatment of burn

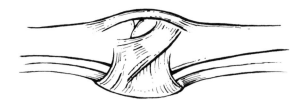

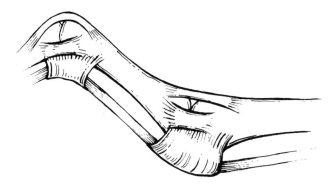

Figure 11-20   Classical dorsal hand burn scar deformity. The MP joints tend to become stiff in extension, in part because contracture of the collateral ligaments.

wounds, including tangential excision, are discussed elsewhere in this book.

SNAKEBITES

Approximately 98% of venomous snakebites are caused by vipers; the remaining 2% are inflicted by coral, as well as captive and foreign venomous snakes. Approximately 21% of such bites involve the digits of the hand. Although surgical management of the patient may be relatively straightforward, the problems that can arise when treating viper bites may require the expertise of numerous medical and surgical professionals, including hematologic, cardiovascular, renal, respiratory, and neurological subspecialists.

The usual culprits of envenomation injuries (rattlesnakes, copperheads, and cottonmouths, which also are known as water moccasins) are pit viper snakes. These snakes are distinguished by the presence of heat sensitive pits located between the eyes and the nostril. With these specialized organs, they can make a direct hit on a warm-blooded animal that they cannot see. Pit vipers can be identified by eyes that have vertical elliptical pupils ("cats eyes") and a single row of subcaudal scutes or scales. The genus Crotalus is further characterized by horny segments on the tail, commonly recognized as rattles.

Envenomation

Envenomation means that a sufficient amount of venom has been introduced into the body to cause either local signs at the site of the bite or systemic signs. The venom apparatus of the Crotalidae consists of a gland, a duct, and one or more fangs on each side of the head. The venom consists of 5 to 15 enzymes, 3 to 12 nonenzymatic proteins and peptides, and at least 6 other unidentified substances. It contains hemotoxin, neurotoxin, venotoxin, cardiotoxin, and necroticin factors. Almost instantly, the venom alters blood vessel permeability, leading to loss of plasma into the tissue and breakdown of blood cells. This results in immediate tissue edema and ecchymosis, and probably is responsible for the signs of local envenomation (severe burning, rapid swelling, ecchymosis, local necrosis, and sloughing about the fang marks). These cardinal signs usually appear within 10 minutes of envenomation, and it is very unusual to have an onset longer than 20 minutes after the bite. If symptoms and signs do not occur within 4 hours, it is almost certain that envenomation has not taken place.

Systemic signs that may occur after the local signs are secondary to toxic effects on the cardiovascular, hematologic, nervous, and respiratory systems. The alterations in bleeding and prothrombin times may result in hematuria, epistaxis, and generalized bleeding diathesis. The hematocrit may fall, along with the platelet count. A rapid fall in blood pressure and a decrease in circulating blood volume may occur along with pulmonary edema.

The systemic signs of envenomation include weakness, sweating, faintness, nausea, and vomiting. Paresthesia and numbness about the scalp, face, lips, fingers, and toes may occur, along with perioral and periorbital muscular fasiculation. The patient bitten by a Mojave rattler may not have the several local signs of edema, but still may be envenomated sufficiently to develop neuromuscular changes causing respiratory dysfunction.

Initial Treatment

No time should be lost in reaching an appropriate medical facility. The following measures should be instituted. (1) The patient should be kept emotionally and physically quiet. The median lethal dose (LD50) of venom can be increased by increasing physical activity. (2) Kill the snake, if possible. Identification of the snake by the treating physician may aid in treatment. For example, the Mojave rattlesnake produces minimal local reactions, yet may require large doses of antitoxin. (3) A small rubber tourniquet should be loosely applied immediately proximal to the bite in such a fashion that it includes lymphatic drainage only. It should not be tight enough to block arterial or venous circulation. The tourniquet should be moved proximally as the swelling advances. (4) An incision 3/4 of an inch linear and 1/4 of an inch deep is made in each fang mark, and cup suction is started. This is effective if it can be undertaken immediately. Little or no benefit from suction avails 30 minutes after the bite; 1 hour after the bite, such treatment should not be considered. Little or no venom can be recovered from the advancing edema. (5) Immobilize the envenomated part to the level of the heart if possible. (6) Icing and/or cooling the wound or extremities should not be used in any form, as cooling potentiates the necrotic effect locally.

Hospital Treatment

First, identify the snake. Then, evaluate the patient's symptoms and signs. Immediately after pit viper envenomation, the following tests should be performed on the patient: CBC, urinalysis, platelet count, prothrombin time, PTT, bleeding time, blood sugar, urea nitrogen, and electrolytes. Be sure to measure and record the circumference of the injured extremity, mark the skin and site selected for measurement wounds for accurate serial comparisons, and document the proximal migration of edema. These measurements should be repeated every 20 minutes because they serve as an index for progression of the poison and a guide for antivenin administration. Severity of envenomation should be documented according to the established recommendations of the Committee on Trauma of the American College of Surgeons (see Box, p. 600).

Almost all authorities agree that antivenin is the single most important therapeutic measure and recommend its use as the initial treatment of all serious envenomations. If antivenin administration is considered, intravenous lines should be started in two separate locations and an adequate amount of polyvalent crotalidae antivenin should be administered. Antivenin should never be injected into a finger or a toe, and probably not locally. Currently, the only commercially available antivenin in the United States is produced by Wyeth Laboratories. In 1981, the following dosage schedule was recommended: minimal envenomation, 0 to 4 vials; moderate envenomation, 5 to 9 vials; severe

---

American College of Surgeons: Recommendations for the Documentation of Envenomation

1. No local or systemic reactions.
2. Minimal envenomation:
   Local symptoms and signs (swelling, pain, or ecchymosis);
   few systemic symptoms and signs (hypotension, nausea, vomiting, sweating;
   weakness symptoms, such as dizziness, perioral paresthesia, and ptosis; and
   minimal laboratory abnormalities.
3. Moderate envenomation:
   Swelling that progresses beyond the area of the bite;
   some systemic symptoms and signs; and
   abnormal laboratory findings (i.e., abnormal clotting factors and a fall in hematocrit and platelet counts).
4. Severe envenomation:
   Marked local systemic symptoms and signs;
   severe systemic symptoms and signs; and
   significant abnormalities and laboratory findings.

Table 11-2   Antivenin Administration

Minimal envenomation	0–4 vials
Moderate envenomation	5–9 vials
Severe envenomation	10–15 vials or more

envenomation 10 to 15 or more vials (Table 11-2). Antivenin is most effective when given within 4 hours of the bite. It is of questionable value if given after 24 hours, but it still should be administered.

Pit viper antivenin is made from horse serum, and anaphylactic reactions can occur even if the skin test results are negative. As such, a skin test for sensitivity to horse serum should be performed. The first vial of antivenin must be given very slowly and with caution. Resuscitation equipment and appropriate drugs, such as diphenhydramine (Benadryl), steroids, and epinephrine, should be immediately available. Serum sickness typically occurs in patients who receive more than 70 ml (7 vials) of antivenin. Although some reports show a 75% instance of serum sickness after treatment with the antiserum, the risk of serum sickness is less serious than the complications of pit viper envenomation. Antibiotics, tetanus prophylactics, and systemic steroids also should be used.

Patient Monitoring

The physiologic status of the patient may change rapidly. Therefore, it is extremely important to monitor the patient in an intensive care unit. Measurement of the circumference of the extremity every 15 to 20 minutes, as well as monitoring of kidney function and respiratory and circulatory status are essential. Coagulation studies also are vital, especially if fasciotomy is contemplated because exuberant bleeding can result from this procedure if coagulation is affected. Access to instruments, equipment, proper lighting, and skilled personnel, including trained intensive care specialists, allows timely intervention (e.g., endotracheal intubation and fluid resuscitation), should it become necessary.

Surgical Management

There is a great deal of disagreement about the role of surgical treatment in the management of snakebites, but most physicians agree that if an incision is made in the depth of each fang mark and suction is performed within 30 minutes, a great deal of venom can be removed. One physician has treated more than 650 cases of snake venom poisoning and has never had to do a fasciotomy. He states that the use of a fasciotomy usually reflects an insufficient dosage of antivenin or no antivenin during the first 12 hours after the bite. The severe pain and acute swelling that occur with snakebites make it difficult to differentiate the acutely swollen limb from a true compartment syndrome. For this reason, intracompartment pressure monitoring (Fig. 11-21) is useful in establishing the correct diagnosis. If a compartment syndrome is diagnosed, a fasciotomy should be performed without delay.

Whitesides' method of measuring intracompartmental pressures is advocated. The advantages of this technique are its simplicity and the ready availability of the required equipment in any hospital seething. The technique requires (1) two plastic extension tubes; (2) two 38-gauge needles; (3) one 20-ml syringe; (4) one three-way stopcock connecting three ports simultaneously; (5) one bottle of normal saline; and (6) one mercury manometer. The technique is performed as follows. A 20-ml syringe with a plunger at the 15-ml mark is attached to the appropriate three-way stopcock with two plastic intravenous extension tubes. One tube is connected to a mercury manometer and one to a sterile 18-gauge needle. The 18-gauge needle is inserted into a bottle of normal saline, and the saline, without bubbles, is aspirated into approximately one half of the length of the plastic tube. The stopcock is turned to close off the tubing so that saline is not lost during the transfer of the needle. The 18-gauge needle is inserted into the muscle, in a compartment of which the tissue pressure is measured. A stopcock is

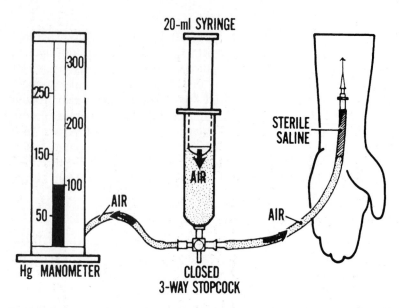

Figure 11-21 Bedside measurement of compartment pressures. Whitesides method of measuring tissue measures is advocated. The advantage of this technique is the simplicity and the ready availability in any hospital setting. See text for details of technique. (From Green, D: *Operative hand surgery,* ed 3, New York, 1993, Churchill Livingstone, p. 666.)

turned so that the syringe is opened to both extension tubes. The pressure and the system is then increased by gradually depressing the plunger of the syringe. When the pressure in this system just surpasses the compartmental tissue pressure, a small amount of saline will be injected into the compartment. The saline column and the plastic tubing will be moved. When the column of saline moves, the operator's pressure on the syringe plunger is immediately stopped and the level of mercury is read on the manometer. This is the tissue pressure of this specific compartment in millimeters of mercury. Common errors in this technique are injecting too much saline into the compartment, which gives an inaccurate reading; placing the needle into a tendon rather than muscle; and aspirating a tissue plug of muscle into the needle before the tissue pressure is measured. A new 18-gauge needle should be used for each measurement. The general range of accuracy with this method is ±3 mmHg. The normal compartmental pressure should be 0 to 8 mmHg. Fasciotomies should be performed when tissue pressure increases to 30 mmHg pressure.

SELECTED REFERENCES

Alexander JW, MacMillan BG, Martel L, et al: Surgical correction of post-burn flexion contractures of the fingers in children, *Plast Reconstr Surg* 68:218, 1981.

Berman W, Goldman AS, Reichelderfer T, et al: Childhood burn injuries and deaths, *Pediatrics* 51:1059, 1973.

Dado D, Angelats J: Management of burns of the hands in children, *Hand Clin* (4):711-722, 1990.

Gold BS, Barish RA: Venomous snakebites. Current concepts in diagnosis, treatment, and management, *Emerg Med Clin North Am* 10:249-267, 1992.

Hueston J: Local flap repair of fingertip injuries, *Plast Reconstr Surg* 37:349, 1966.

Jurkovich GJ, Luterman A, McCullar K, et al: Complications of crotalidae antivenin therapy. *J Trauma* 28:1032-1037, 1988.

Kleinert HE: Fingertip injuries and their management, *Am Surg* 25:41, 1959.

Otten EJ, McKimm D: Venomous snakebite in a patient allergic to horse serum, *Ann Emerg Med* 12:624-627, 1983.

Roberts RS, Csencsitz TA, Heard CW Jr: Upper extremity compartment syndromes following pit viper envenomation, *Clin Orthop* 193:184-188, 1985.

Russell FE, Carlson RW, Wainschel J, Osborne AH: Snake venom poisoning in the United States: experience with 550 cases, *JAMA* 233:341-344, 1975.

Whitesides TE Jr, Haney TC, Morimoto K, Hirada H: Tissue pressure measurements as a determinant for the need of fasciotomy, *Clin Orthop* 113:43-51, 1975.

12

Therapy Considerations Following Acute Hand Injuries

Gail N. Groth, OTR, CHT
Joan Guccione, OTR, CHT
Patty Paynter, OTR, CHT
Erin Casey Phillips, MSOT, OTR/L
Barbara Sopp, MS, OTR/L, CHT
Mary Beth Wulf, OTR/L, CHT
Elizabeth J. Walker, PT
Kathy A. Mantz, BGS
Bruce A. Kraemer, MD

POSTTRAUMATIC HAND THERAPY

To a significant extent, the outcome of a hand injury is determined by the patient's participation in and compliance with a comprehensive program of wound and skin management. It often is stated that a hand surgeon is only as good as the hand therapist who provides the postoperative care. In fact, the therapist–patient relationship is as critical as the doctor–patient relationship because it is the therapist who has more "hands on" interactions with the patient. Scheduling the therapy visits is as important as scheduling the operative procedure. It is essential that the patient and the hand therapist are compatible, and that the surgeon and therapist work closely to formulate an individualized care plan that conforms to certain guidelines and standard therapies.

The surgeon should confer periodically with the patient and the therapist to formulate the care plan and arrange any necessary modifications. The surgeon should give the therapist operative reports and they should meet to review X-rays so that the therapist can offer the patient the best possible care. Confusion and delays in therapy can lead to disastrous results; in many situations, these problems can be avoided through better communication. The surgeon also should evaluate splints to confirm that they are providing proper protection while allowing appropriate therapy to be performed. Such an evaluation also enables the surgeon to assess the patient's ability to understand the therapy instructions and the likelihood that proper therapy will be carried out. When in doubt, more frequent visits (perhaps daily) may be needed to ensure that the patient adheres to the therapy program.

This chapter reviews standard evaluation methods for dexterity, edema, strength, range of motion, and sensory testing. In the treatment section, techniques for edema control, scar management, sensory reeducation, and work-hardening and work-conditioning protocols are discussed. Therapeutic modalities, such as fluid therapy and electrotherapeutic stimulators, also are explained. Finally, options for passive and dynamic splinting are discussed and illustrated. Our treatment of basic hand injuries are summarized in simplified protocols that we follow with some modifications (e.g., immobilization for "take" of a skin graft). In general, the patient's therapy is begun at the earliest possible date, often during the hospitalization or immediately after an outpatient procedure.

EVALUATION PROCEDURES
Tests of Hand Function

Normal hand function depends on adequate range of motion of the upper-extremity joints, muscle strength, normal sensation, and dexterity. Deficits in any of these areas will compromise hand function and need to be addressed in a therapeutic program.

Impairment and compromise of hand function can be evaluated in several ways, depending on the nature of the pathophysiologic condition. Usually, in a comprehensive hand rehabilitation setting, a battery of tests are administered to document the status of a patient's hand function at the time of referral, to guide the therapist in developing an appropriate treatment plan, and to assess the effects of treatment intervention.

Dexterity

Functional tests of dexterity evaluate gross and fine motor control, tool usage, and the manipulation of objects. The commonly used standardized tests include the Nine-Hole Peg Test, the Minnesota Rate of Manipulation Test and the Purdue Pegboard Test.

Nine-hole peg test

This instrument consists of a board having nine evenly spaced holes and a cup that holds nine pegs. The object of the test is for the patient to place the nine pegs in the holes. Instructions are standardized. The obtained value is the time required to complete the task. Normative data are available.

The Minnesota rate of manipulation test (MRMT)

This test instrument consists of a large, rectangular board with a series of holes and a set of large checkerlike disks. The two sides of the disks are of different colors. There are several elements of test performance, including both unilateral and bilateral placing and turning and displacing the disks. Instructions are standardized. The obtained value is the time required to complete each subset of this test. Normative data are available.

The Purdue pegboard test

A standard test board is constructed with two vertically aligned columns of holes. At the top of the board are four recessed cups that hold small metal pegs, washers, and collars. Through a series of five subtests that increase in complexity, patients are instructed to place the test items in specified sequences from top to bottom in the test board. The subtests are designed to evaluate right and left hands separately and in combination. Instructions are standardized. This is a timed test and the obtained values are the number of completed elements within each subtest.

Edema

Reduction in swelling is necessary to permit the patient to have full range of motion in the joints associated with the edematous areas and to restore circulatory support for functional activity. Documentation of the magnitude and location of edema assists the patient and therapist to select the method and duration of techniques that will most effectively manage this problem. Measurement of swelling in the hand and upper extremity can be done by volumetric measurement of the entire distal limb or by simple circumferential measurement of the affected area.

Volumetric measurement

The volume of an entire distal-limb segment can be estimated using a water displacement system, in which the part to be evaluated is submerged in a water tank with an outflow spout from which the water displaced by the limb is collected in a graduated cylinder. The indicator of limb volume is the quantity of displaced water, measured in milliliters. Submersion tanks of clear plexiglass are used most commonly, so that the examiner can observe the position of the limb within the tank.

This method of volumetric measurement is most appropriate when edema is diffuse throughout the distal limb segment. It is not sensitive enough to document very localized swelling, such as the involvement of a single digit or joint or swelling localized to a more proximal site, such as the wrist or elbow. In these circumstances, circumferential measurement is more appropriate.

Circumferential measurement

A circumferential gauge constructed of a centimeter ruler with an adjustable loop affixed to the zero point is used to document digital size. The loop is placed over the area to be measured, and the fixed-length, extended tab of the loop is laid along the ruler. The obtained value is the location of the tab end recorded in centimeters.

Girth measurements using a centimeter tape measure are taken to document edema in more proximal areas, such as at the level of the distal palmar crease, distal wrist crease, or along the forearm.

Strength

Whenever normal functional performance is compromised, the description of the patient's status should identify and document the capability or inability of muscle to generate and sustain force. Muscle strength testing may not be relevant during the acute stage of injury or in the immediate postoperative period, when tissue healing is the primary concern, or during the initial stages of treatment, when pain, edema, and limitation of joint range of motion are important considerations. Under these circumstances, the validity, reliability, and appropriateness of muscle strength testing is questionable. As the rehabilitation phase of treatment progresses, however, strength measures are essential elements in planning programs to restore function.

Many methods are available for measuring muscle strength. The choice of a testing protocol should be relevant to the purpose of testing. For example, if a patient has a suspected peripheral neuropathy, the purpose of testing is to document the level and distribution of involvement by identifying the compromised muscles. The selected approach and instrument will be very different for the individual whose return to work depends on heavy tool use or lifting capabilities.

The most common tests of muscle performance in hand rehabilitation are the Manual Muscle Test and Grip and Pinch Dynamometry.

Manual muscle testing

Manual muscle testing determines "strength" based on the ability of muscle to move its bony level in relationship to gravity and resistance applied manually by the examiner. This procedure is most appropriate in conditions of severe weakness and to screen for specific peripheral nerve pathology. The following table describes the most common grading system (Table 12-1).

Although the manual muscle test can be used to grade performance of the entire musculoskeletal system, a common use of the procedure in hand rehabilitation is to screen for involvement relative to the upper-extremity peripheral nerve distribution. The following is an example of the muscles that would be tested for this purpose.

	Median nerve	*Ulnar nerve*	*Radial nerve*
Intrinsic muscle	Abductor pollicis brevis	1st dorsal interosseous	(none)
Extrinsic muscle	Thumb flexor digitorum profundus	Small finger flexor digitorum profundus	Wrist extensor

Grip and pinch strength measures

The ability to generate force while gripping and pinching requires the integration of the intrinsic muscles of the hand and the extrinsic muscles of the hand and wrist. The Jamar Dynamometer and the B&L pinch gauge are the most common instruments used throughout the United States for measurement of these abilities. The test-retest reliability is acceptable, and normative values are available for both instruments.

The Jamar Dynamometer (Fig. 12-1) consists of a gripping handle and a force gauge that measures the force in pounds generated by the patient. The gripping handle can be set at five different positions to measure forces at five different grip widths in ascending order from Position 1 to Position 5. The normative data are based on forces generated as the mean of three repeated trials in the second handle position, with the patient's arm at the side and forearm

Table 12-1 Key to Muscle Grading

Test Performance	Kendalls Percent	Lovett Word & letter	Abbrev. of percent	Nat. Found. for Inf. Par. & a Study Percent	Alda to Invest. of Per. N. Inj. Numerals	Neurolog. Rating
The ability to hold the test position against gravity and maximum pressure, or the ability to move the part into test position and hold against gravity and maximum pressure.	100	Normal	N	10	100	5	++++
	95	Normal−	N−	—		5−	
Same as above, except holding against moderate pressure.	90	Good+	G+	9		4+	−++
	80	Good	G	8	75	4	
Same as above, except holding against minimum pressure.	70	Good−	G−	7		4−	
	60	Fair+	F+	6		3+	
The ability to hold the test position against gravity, or the ability to move the part into test position and hold against gravity.	50	Fair	F	5	50	3	++
The gradual release from the test position against gravity, or; the ability to move the part toward the test position against gravity almost to completion, or to completion with slight assistance; or, the ability to complete the arc of motion with gravity lessened.	40	Fair−	F−	4		3−	

Continued

Table 12-1   Key to Muscle Grading–cont'd

Test Performance	Kendalls Percent	Lovett Word & letter		Abbrev. of percent	Nat. Found. for Inf. Par. & a Study Percent	Alda to Invest. of Per. N. Inj. Numerals	Neurolog. Rating
The ability to move the part through partial arc of motion with gravity lessened: Moderate arc, 30% or poor +; small arc, 20% or poor.	30	Poor+	P+	3		2+	
To avoid moving a patient into a gravity-lessened position, these grades may be estimated on the basis of the amount of assistance given during antigravity test movements: A 30% or poor + muscle requires moderate assistance, a 20% or poor muscle requires more assistance.	20	Poor	P	2	25	2	+
In muscles that can be seen or palpated, a feeble contraction may be felt in the muscle, or the tendon may become prominent during the muscle contraction, but there is no visible movement of the part.	10 5	Poor– Trace	P– T	— 1		2– 1	
No contraction is felt in the muscle.	0	Zero	0	0	0	0	0

Restriction of range of motion may be denoted by putting the grade in parentheses.
Kendall HO, Kendall FR, Waldsworth GE: *Muscle testing and function.* Baltimore, 1971, Williams & Wilkins, p. 11.

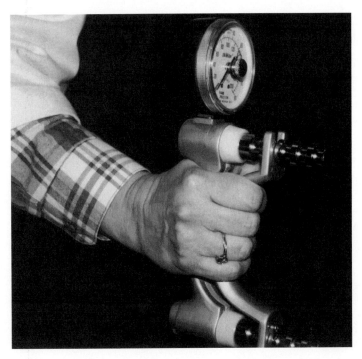

Figure 12-1   Jamar dynamometer for grip strength measurements. The five positions that are possible for the handle correlate with grip width. Normative data are available for measurements of grip at the second position demonstrated in this figure.

parallel to the floor. This has become the standard clinical test position and procedure.

Grip testing in all five positions may be done. Based on the length–tension curve of normal in situ muscle and other biomechanical factors of the hand, maximum force output should be weakest in the first (or smallest width) position, should increase in the second and third positions, and should decline in the fourth and fifth positions. The resultant bell-shaped curve is indicative of normal performance of the patient. Deviations from this pattern may indicate that the patient is not exerting maximum voluntary effort or may indicate deficits in intrinsic muscle function or limitations of joint range of motion.

The pinch gauge (Fig. 12-2) also measures force in pounds generated by the patient. One side of the instrument may be placed on the radial side of the index finger with the thumb on the opposite side to record lateral pinch force. Three-point pinch is tested when

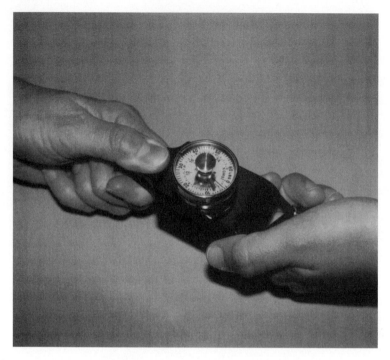

Figure 12-2   Demonstration of lateral pinch measurement using a pinch gauge. Two- and three-point pinch also may be measured with the pinch gauge.

the instrument is placed between the thumb and pads or tips of the index and long fingers. Although many muscles are required to participate in forceful pinch, the lateral pinch test emphasizes the ulnar innervated first dorsal interosseus muscle, and three-point pinch emphasizes the extrinsic finger flexors. Both tests require strong contraction of the median nerve innervated hyperthenar muscles and stabilization by the wrist musculature.

Range of Motion

Range-of-motion (ROM) measurements are integral to the evaluation of a patient's status and progress. Range-of-motion measurements are performed with a goniometer—a protractor with an extended stationary arm and a moveable arm.

Types of Goniometers

These tools are manufactured in a variety of sizes and forms to accommodate joint size and placement preference. We prefer a clear plastic, 360° goniometer, with the moveable arm cut off approximately 2 inches from the fulcrum.

Reliability and Validity

Intratester reliability (within one tester) has been shown to be greater than interrater reliability (between testers). Research shows that when possible, serial measurements of a joint should be performed by the same examiner. The question of the validity of goniometry has not been answered sufficiently to date.

Documentation

All motions are measured from a 0° (neutral) starting position. Flexion measurements are recorded as positive numbers; extension and hyperextension are recorded as negative numbers. This follows the recommendations from the American Academy of Orthopaedic Surgeons and the American Society for Surgery of the Hand. The measurements are recorded most frequently in a table format, but in some cases a graph is used for visual effect.

Goniometer Placement

The goniometer may be placed either dorsal or lateral to the joint being measured. For dorsal placement, the fulcrum should be centered over the joint, with the moveable arm laying dorsally along the long axis of the bone distal to the joint. When a lateral measurement is made, the arms are parallel to the long axis of the bone, and the fulcrum should be as close as possible to the axis of motion. We recommend lateral placement of the goniometer to measure all upper-extremity joints. When measuring the wrist, lateral placement on the radial aspect of the wrist, with the moveable arm parallel to the long metacarpal has been shown to be most reliable.

Active ROM (AROM)

This term indicates the motion achieved by the patient's own muscle power. Joints proximal to the joint being measured should be supported. Digital flexion measurements are assumed to be taken as a composite flexion measurement. Exceptions are noted.

Passive ROM (PROM)

This term refers to the freedom of movement at a joint when an external force is applied. This external force is most typically the examiner's hands, but it also may be the patient's uninvolved hand or a standardized instrument.

Total Active ROM (TAM)

This number represents the sum of the motions of the three finger joints. The three values for flexion are added together. Any extension deficit is subtracted from this value.

Total Passive ROM (TPM)

This number is similar to TAM, but represents the sum of the PROM measurements for the three finger joints. Again, extension deficits are subtracted from the flexion values.

Torque ROM

This term describes PROM measurements taken with an instrument that applies a standardized amount of force to the joint. This primarily has been developed in research laboratories and currently is not used clinically.

Sensory Tests

The following sensory tests can aid in determining the diagnosis, surgical needs, innervation status, and appropriate rehabilitation program. These tests are categorized into threshold, functional, and objective tests.

Threshold Tests

Such tests are helpful in monitoring early return after nerve laceration, as well as in assessing early changes caused by nerve compression.

Pain perception/pinprick

Using a needle, touch the skin until slight blanching. The patient reports if it feels sharp or dull. The uninvolved hand is used as a guide for the amount of needed pressure. There are no normative data, scoring is as follows:

+S	Correct response to sharp
S	No response to sharp
+D	Correct response to dull
D	No response to dull
"S"	Dull stimulus reported as "sharp"
"D"	Sharp stimulus reported as "dull"

This test assesses protective sensation. However, because hypersensitivity can occur during nerve regeneration, a patient's responses are subjective secondary to his or her pain threshold. In addition, the application of force can be variable.

Light touch–deep pressure

The instrument used to assess this area is the Semmes–Weinstein Pressure Aethesiometer Kit (Fig. 12-3). The kit consists of 5 to 20 probes with monofilaments. These probes are marked with numbers ranging from 1.65 to 6.65. Each filament is applied perpendicular to the skin until the filament bends slightly. Filaments 1.65 to 4.08 are applied three times and 4.17 to 6.65 are applied one time. Norms are available and scoring is as follows:

Normal	1.65-2.83
Diminished light touch	3.22-3.61
Diminished protective sensation	3.84-4.31
Loss of protective sensation	4.56-6.65
Untestable	>6.65

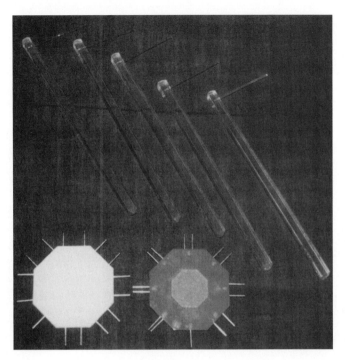

Figure 12-3   Semmes–Weinstein Aethesiometer Kit for measurement of touch threshold and the Mackinnon–Dellon Disk Criminator for two-point discrimination testing.

Vibration

A 30- to 256-cps tuning fork can be used to assess the threshold of touch. The tuning fork can be applied with either the pronged or the stem end. Vibration is scored as more, less, or the same, as compared with the contralateral hand. Norms are not available. The Bio-Thesiometer or the Vibration II (Fig. 12-4) are instruments. In these, the amplitude is variable and the frequency is fixed. The threshold level is recorded in volts or microns of motion.

Functional Tests

Such tests require a higher level of sensory processing and allow the quality of sensation to be assessed.

Static and moving two-point discrimination

Innervation density can be tested by using the Disk Criminator (Fig. 12-3). The test begins with the two ends of the Disk at 5 mm. One or two points are applied randomly until blanching. Seven of 10 responses need to be correct for the distance to be recorded.

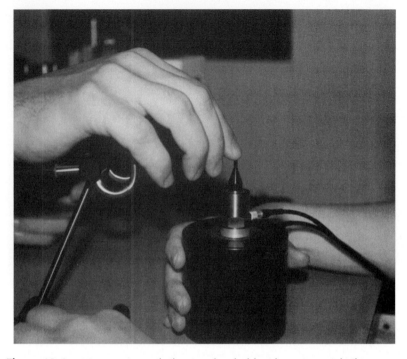

Figure 12-4   Measurement of vibration threshold with commercial vibrometer.

Normative data are available. The normative scale is as follows:

Normal	0-5 mm
Fair	6-10 mm
Poor	11-15 mm
Protective	1 point perceived
Anesthetic	No point perceived

Modified Moberb pick-up test

Standardized items are used and require identification. Vision is occluded and the time required to identify the objects is recorded. No norms have been established. Patients with median or combined median/ulnar nerve involvement are appropriate for this test.

Objective Tests

In objective tests, only passive participation is required; there is no subjective interpretation. Such tests can be helpful in assessing children or possible malingerers. These tests can give "suggestive evidence" of early sensory function or the failure of regeneration.

Ninhydrin sweat test

This test is helpful in assessing sympathetic or sudomotor function. The patients hand is cleaned thoroughly and acetone is applied. The hand is allowed to sweat by placing it under a light for 20 minutes, by it air drying for 30 minutes, or by placing it in a plastic bag during exercise. The hand is then placed on bond paper for 15 seconds. The paper is sprayed with Ninhydrin, which stains the sweat components purple. The grading scale is from 0 to 3 (0 = absent; 3 = normal). Normative data are not available.

Orian wrinkle test

Denervated hands placed in warm water for 30 minutes at 40°C or 104°F do not wrinkle as normal skin would. This test assesses sympathetic function and is graded on a scale from 0 to 3 (0 = absence of wrinkles; 3 = normal wrinkling). Norms are not available.

TREATMENT AND REHABILITATION PROTOCOLS
Edema Reduction

Edema is the accumulation of excessive fluid in tissues. It can result in pain, stiffness, and limited functional movements. Early intervention is essential to prevent soft tissue fibrosis and a chronically stiff, painful extremity.

The primary methods used to reduce edema are active movement, elevation, compression, retrograde massage, and use of contrast baths. Description of these techniques, which can be used individually or in combination, follow.

Active Pumping

Firm active flexion and extension of the digits create a pumping effect that facilitates return circulatory flow. All joints of the involved extremity should be moved through a full range of motion exercises.

Elevation

Elevation is a useful technique in controlling and reducing edema. The edematous part should be positioned higher than the heart. This can be accomplished by propping the extremity on a pillow or a foam wedge when seated or in bed. Excessive elbow flexion should be avoided. The patient should be instructed not to allow the arm to rest in a dependent position and to monitor the extremity for changes in temperature and color.

Compression

Compression to the digit or hand may be accomplished with the use of an elastic wrap, such as Coban (Fig. 12-5*A*). The patient is instructed to snuggly wrap the digit circumferentially, distally to proximally (each digit is wrapped individually) to a point proximal to the area of edema. Depending on the patients tolerance, the wrap can be worn for minutes or for several hours during the day while performing exercises and daily living activities. The patient should be instructed to

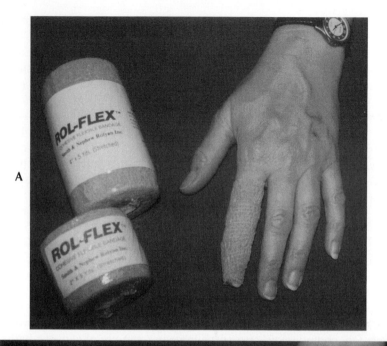

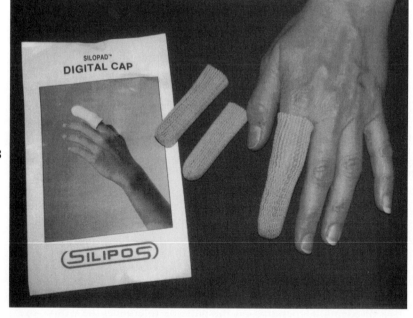

Figure 12-5 Edema control can be accomplished with **(A)** simple elastic bandages or **(B)** prefabricated sheaths.

remove the wrap if signs of ischemia, such as coolness or blanching, occur at the fingertip.

Compressive tubular materials also are available or may be fabricated in a variety of sizes for use on the digits, hand, and forearm (Fig. 12-5*B*).

Use of an intermittent compression pump is a helpful adjunct to facilitate the flow of lymphatic fluid into the venous system. The extremity should be placed in the pneumatic sleeve and elevated during the alternating sleeve inflation and deflation.

The amount of pressure used initially depends on the patients condition. Low pressure is used with acute injuries. The pressure should be greater than 25 mmHg for maximum effectiveness, but should not exceed the patient's diastolic pressure. Depending on the patients response, pressure and time may be increased to 20 to 30 minutes within a treatment session. Use of the intermittent compression pump should be followed by retrograde massage and functional activities when possible.

Retrograde Massage

Another technique for edema control is the use of retrograde massage. This should be performed frequently during the day with the extremity elevated. Massage should be performed with firm strokes moving distally to proximally to facilitate the flow of blood and lymph.

Contrast Baths

Contrast baths can be used to reduce edema and pain. Two basins large enough to accomodate the hand and forearm are needed. One basin is filled with warm water at approximately 96°F; the other basin is filled with water at approximately 66°F. The basins should be situated to allow elevation of the extremity. The extremity is placed in warm water for 3 to 4 minutes, then cold water for 1 minute. This routine can be repeated three to four times depending on the patient's response, beginning and ending with the hand in warm water. The patient should be encouraged to perform digit flexion and extension in the water.

Scar Management

Scar formation is a necessary part of the healing process after injury or surgery. Collagen fibers multiply and are oriented randomly during the initial fibroplasia stage of wound healing. As the scar matures, collagen fibers become organized and aligned in a continuous cycle of production and breakdown.

Intervention at this stage can help the patient achieve a soft, supple scar, thereby enhancing joint motion and limiting subdermal adhesions. Therapeutic interventions include the following.

Mechanical Stress

External stress applied to a scar overlying a joint allows the patient to position the scar on stretch. This process encourages collagen alignment in a lengthened position and prevents scar-joint contractures. Mechanical stress can be applied with PROM exercises or static progressive splinting techniques.

Elastomer/Otoform

External surface moldings over scars enhance collagen alignment with direct pressure. Silicone elastomer (50/50) and Otoform inserts are fabricated to fit directly over the scar. These can be custom made for hypertrophic scarring or difficult-to-reach locations (i.e., interdigital web spaces).

Silastic Gel

Worn in contact with the scar 8 to 10 hours per day, this product helps to soften the external scar to promote joint motion. The gel is manufactured in solid form and is reusable. The effects include flattening and softening of the scar, as well as a decrease in its hypersensitivity.

Massage

Direct pressure and friction gliding massage is the easiest, least expensive way to manage scar. If performed faithfully (a home program of 6 to 8 times daily), massage can demonstrate beneficial results in decreasing scar adherence and sensitivity. Direct pressure is performed with the noninjured hand or a rubber fingertip, with or without lotion. Friction massage is performed along with AROM in the direction opposite the tendon glide to disrupt subdermal scar adhesions.

Vibration

Hand-held vibration units are used to assist with collagen realignment, desensitize scar, and loosen adherent scar bundles. Vibration is used in conjunction with other forms of scar management and small, hand vibration units can be sent home for independent follow-through.

Range of Motion Therapy

Digit

Digital range of motion therapies vary depending on the structures injured and the methods of treatment. Partial ligament injuries of a joint often benefit from protected range of motion therapy, such as with buddy taping, whereas a complete injury may have operative repair with a more graded program of motion that limits maximal ligament strain. With fractures, one needs to provide more careful dynamic splinting for comminuted fractures that are pinned as compared with a plated midshaft fracture.

Continuous range of motion therapy is of benefit to patients with severe and complex injuries, but more often is reserved for secondary reconstruction patients, such as combined flexor and extensor tenolysis patients who need constant motion to limit adhesion formation in any one specific position.

Wrist

Range-of-motion therapy for the wrist often is limited by the degree of swelling and operative intervention. Bony reconstructive procedures often entail a period of immobilization that itself induces stiffness. Therefore, one often is treating a stiff wrist, hopefully in a position of function. Dynamic splinting for both flexion and extension play a major role in wrist management.

As with the digits, continuous passive range of motion devices usually are employed after secondary reconstructive procedures, such as multiple tenolyses of the flexor and extensor tendons crossing the wrist or after wrist capsulotomy following post-Colles' fracture treatment with wrist stiffness.

Guidelines for Sensory Reeducation

Philosophy

Sensory reeducation is a combination of techniques designed to assist patients in interpreting sensory messages that are altered after a nerve injury and repair. These techniques give the patient a new set of matching profiles (cortically) that allow recognition of the altered stimuli. In other words, "sensory reeducation attempts to give an old familiar name to a new unfamiliar sensory image."

Program

Sensory reeducation techniques apply graded stimuli with and without vision. The stimuli is first applied with a patient's eyes closed, then open, and then closed again. Such a sequence allows the patient to absorb the sensory experience and provides reinforcement of what he or she just learned. The program should be performed in a quiet room three to four times a day for short periods (10-15 minutes). This environment and schedule will help improve attention and facilitate learning and memory through repetition. A sensory reeducation program generally consists of two phases: early sensory reeducation (moving and constant touch) and late sensory reeducation (discrimination).

Early Sensory Reeducation

The goal of this phase is to distinguish between moving (quickly adapting fibers) and constant (slowly adapting fibers) touch and to correct mislocalization. Techniques include applying a moving and constant touch stimuli with localization. The stimuli progresses from a pencil eraser to a cotton swab.

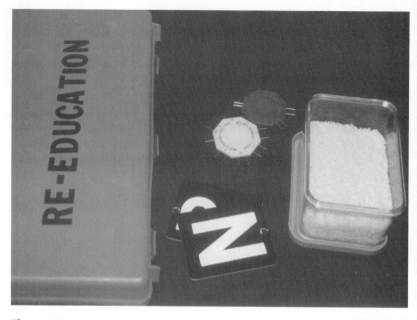

Figure 12-6 Sensory reeducation is a vital component of rehabilitation in patients with nerve injuries. A variety of objects and textures are useful in the reeducation process.

This phase should be initiated when the Semmes–Weinstein test result is 4.31 or lower and when 30 cps and moving touch is perceived to an area. It is critical to initiate reeducation by the time recovery reaches the proximal phalanges. Approximately 4 to 6 months after median and/or ulnar nerve repair at the wrist, early sensory reeducation should be introduced.

During this phase, vibration, Semmes–Weinstein pressure results, moving touch, and constant touch with localization tests should be evaluated. When 256 cps is perceived at the fingertips, this indicates that all touch perception has been recovered. At this point, progress to the next stage of sensory reeducation.

Late Sensory Reeducation

The goal of this phase is to improve a patient's capacity for sensory discrimination. Techniques include identification of large and small objects and textures and numbers, as well as distinguishing between one and two points (Fig. 12-6).

Initiate this phase when moving and constant touch are consistently localized at the fingertips. Approximately 6 to 8 months after a median and/or ulnar nerve repair at the wrist, this phase should be introduced.

At 10 to 12 months after nerve repair at the wrist, patients should be able to perform small-object identification. During this phase, Semmes–Weinstein results moving two-point and static two-point discrimination should be assessed. Continue sensory reeducation until the patients sensory status has reached within normal limits or has plateaued.

Conclusion

The literature shows that the use of sensory reeducation appears to improve a person's level of functional sensation as well as promote a quicker rate of recovery. Research also shows exciting evidence that increased use of an area (i.e., the digits) also increases cortical representation.

Work Conditioning

Work conditioning is a goal-directed therapy for the development or modification of work skills in the actual setting. It is the bridge between acute treatment and return to function. Work conditioning prepares a patient mentally, emotionally, and physically for return to work or activities of daily living. It provides a structured setting to perform extended evaluations and screenings to determine strength and limitation levels. Work conditioning is best for early referrals or referrals with uncomplicated programs or vocational complications.

Work hardening is a therapy for job-specific activities that are simulated for a patient who requires intense conditioning, coordination, and endurance activities to meet the physical demands of their jobs. It prepares an injured worker for return to work by developing a work readiness training program and redeveloping worker's traits.

Work Conditioning	Work Hardening
Acute, focus on specific-injury and exercise program; splinting, ROM, light activities	Chronic, focus on total body conditioning; job simulation and aerobic activities
1-2 disciplines	Interdisciplinary—OT, PT, social work, vocational rehabilitation, psychologist
Patient and therapist share responsibilities of treatment program	High levels of patient responsibility and participation in the direction of the treatment plan
Can be performed in acute clinic area with moderate space allocation	Large space required for job simulation
1-2 hrs/day, 3 times per week	
4+ hrs/day, 5 times per week	
Less costly	More costly

Job analysis is the study of the workers activities and the skills required to perform the job. Analysis may include use of tools, manipulation, body position, and pace required.

Work capacity evaluations measure an individuals total ability to perform a job task. Work tolerance, fatigue level, strength, endurance, flexibility, and performance are evaluated and recorded for determination of a person's abilities.

USE OF THERAPEUTIC MODALITIES IN HAND THERAPY
Therapeutic Heat
Therapeutic Effects
1. To heat those joints of the hand that have little soft-tissue coverage, thereby decreasing joint stiffness.
2. To reduce muscle spasm and increase blood flow through reflex mechanisms.
3. To relieve pain.

Superficial Heating Agents
1. Hot packs: Provide superficial moist heat through conduction. Contraindications: decreased circulation and decreased sensation.
2. Paraffin: Provides conductive heat by coating the hand with a mixture of melted paraffin wax and mineral oil. Because of paraffin's low specific heat, higher temperatures can be tolerated than with water at the same temperature. Contraindications: open wounds and infected skin lesions.
3. Fluidotherapy: Provides dry heat through placement of the hand in a container holding fine cellulose particles through which warm air is circulated. Exercise and dynamic splinting can be carried out during treatment. Contraindications: open wounds should be protected by a plastic bag.
4. Whirlpool: Provides superficial heat through warm water agitation. Excellent aid in debridement and as stimulation for the healing of open wounds. Contraindications: increased edema in the limb receiving treatment.

Deep Heating Agents
1. Ultrasound: Provides increase in tissue temperatures of up to 5 cm through ultrasound high-frequency acoustic energy. Contraindications: Delay use for 8 weeks after tendon repair and 10 to 12 weeks after tendon graft. Avoid use in children with open growth centers in bone. Avoid use in areas of malignancy and lack of sensation, as well as in the presence of impaired circulation.
2. Phonophoresis: Use of ultrasound energy to drive anti-inflammatory drugs and local analgesics through the skin to underlying

tissue. Better-controlled studies on the efficacy of phonophoresis are warranted.

Cryotherapy (Application of Cold)

Therapeutic Effects

1. To decrease blood flow and tissue metabolism, thereby decreasing bleeding and acute inflammation.
2. To diminish muscle-guarding spasms, thereby allowing for greater ease of motion.
3. To elevate the pain threshold.

Application of Cold

1. Ice massages: Effective in treatment of small areas.
2. Cold packs: Effective in coverage of larger areas.
3. Vapocoolant sprays: Lower tissue temperature through evaporation and are used in conjunction with stretch techniques.

Contraindications

1. Avoid use in persons with cold-hypersensitivity syndromes.
2. Impaired circulation.
3. Hypertension.

Clinical Electrotherapy

Therapeutic Effects

1. To electrically stimulate nerves transcutaneously.
2. To decrease pain.
3. To facilitate muscle contraction.
4. To induce ions.

Clinical Electrotherapeutic Stimulators

1. Functional electrical stimulation (FES): Provide pulsating AC current for stimulation of innervated musculature. Used for muscle education or facilitation. Contraindications: Do not apply to tendon repair until 6 weeks postoperative or to tenolysis until 7 to 10 days postoperative.
2. High-voltage galvanic stimulation (HVGS): Indications for use in treating pain, edema, and wound healing. Contraindications: Patients with dysrythmias of the heart.
3. Iontophoresis: Induction of topically applied ions into the tissue by application of a low-voltage direct galvanic current. Indications are for use in acute inflammatory conditions and scar formation. Contraindications: Cannot be used over metal implants, skin abrasions, or open lacerations. Should not be used until at least 6 weeks after tendon repair.
4. TENS: Provides electrical stimulation to peripheral nerves for pain relief.

SPLINTING

There are a large number of splinting devices available for treating patients. They range from over-the-counter splints that a patient might purchase at a local drug store to custom-fabricated splints fashioned by a trained hand therapist. Splints of the latter type usually are required when the patient has a complex injury or requires various attachments to allow focused therapy to support or bend specific joints. Depending on the magnitude and nature of the specific problem, prefabricated splints may suffice. In many cases, however, they are too long, causing unintended rubbing and blocking full flexion, or they are too short, providing inadequate distal forearm and wrist support. Custom-fabricated splints have the advantage of being contoured to a patient's specific anatomy and allowing focused therapy on specific areas. They usually are made of thermoplastic materials that soften when heat is applied. This allows for proper molding and fit and for later readjustment as changes in the hand occur or points of friction are identified. The surgeon should review all splinting devices because improper splinting or patient misunderstandings about the splint can be disastrous. For example, early restrained extension splinting of an isolated finger with a flexor tendon repair, while allowing the other digits unrestricted motion, is likely to result in rupture of the repaired tendon.

Static splinting is used in the early healing process when support to the hand in the "position of function" usually is needed. Such splints have no moving parts. The position of function entails aligning the joints of the hand so that the collateral ligaments of the joints are relatively stretched; if stiffness develops, motion is regained more easily. The wrist should be held in 0 to 30° of dorsal extension with the thumb abducted out of the plane of the palm, the MP joints supported in 60 to 70° of flexion, and the interphalangeal joints flexed from 0-15° (Fig. 12-7). These splints should be comfortable and worn easily at night. They are especially useful in patients with burns to the hand, who should wear them at all times when not performing active therapy. Other examples of static splints are shown in Figs. 12-8 to 12-10.

Dynamic splinting is used as required by the specific injury pattern and joint stiffness. Dynamic splints have moveable parts and are made up of several components, including fingertabs, pulleys, outrigger bars, and tension bands. Stress to the patient that overly aggressive use of the splints can lead to undesirable swelling, redness, or perhaps rubbing. In addition, when there has been an associated vascular injury, the patient needs to assess the part for ischemic changes and avoid focal pressure over the repaired vessel(s). One needs to be sure that splints are not applied too tightly and that they do not cause sensory

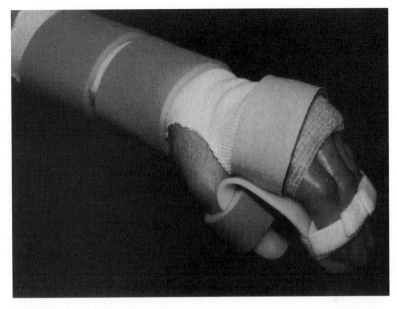

Figure 12-7   Static volarly based orthoplast splint in the position of function.

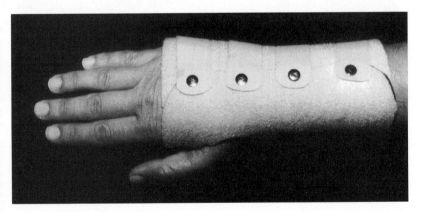

Figure 12-8   Typical prefabricated neoprene static wrist splint.

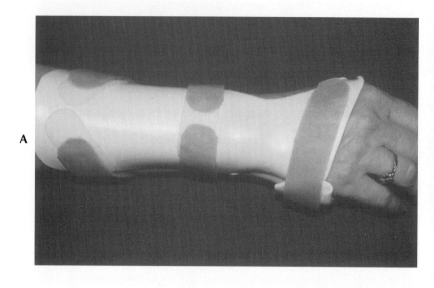

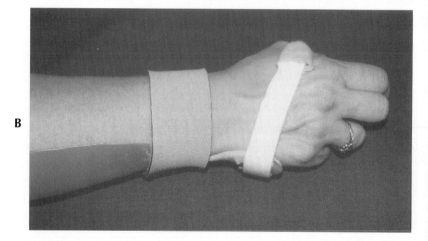

Figure 12-9   Examples of **(A)** dorsally based static orthoplast splint and **(B)** volarly based static orthoplast splint.

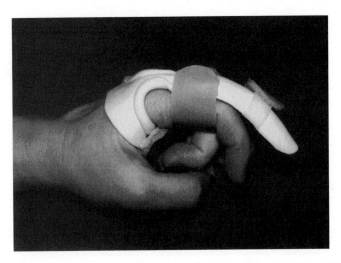

Figure 12-10   Static dorsal extension block splint used frequently for PIP injuries, including limited fractures of the volar lip of the middle phalanx.

nerve compression with continued use. If a splint causes rubbing, the patient should immediately notify the therapist who will adjust the splint to avoid a pressure ulcer. There are many variations of dynamic splints and selected examples are illustrated in Figs. 12-11 to 12-15.

The timing and method of splint discontinuation varies according to the problem being treated, as well as the patient's activities and hand use. Prolonged splinting in an elderly patient can result in an immobile hand, whereas discontinuing a splint prematurely may lead to an incomplete injury, becoming a complete disruption with unprotected use. Providing the patient and family with a full explanation of the purpose of the therapy, the treatment goals, and a list of specific movements and motions to avoid often allows earlier discontinuation of splints and an earlier return to motion.

Buddy Taping

Custom or prefabricated splints (Fig. 12-16) can be fashioned to secure an injured digit to an uninjured digit, thereby providing support to the injured digit. These splints are worn at all times except, when the injured joint is involved in active exercises. They have the advantage of allowing nearly normal digital function while healing is occurring. One should avoid their use in edematous digits. Bands at least 1/2 inch wide are used around the proximal and middle phalanx levels to secure the fingers together. Buddy taping is useful for treating partial collateral ligament injuries of the MP and PIP joints and nondisplaced fractures

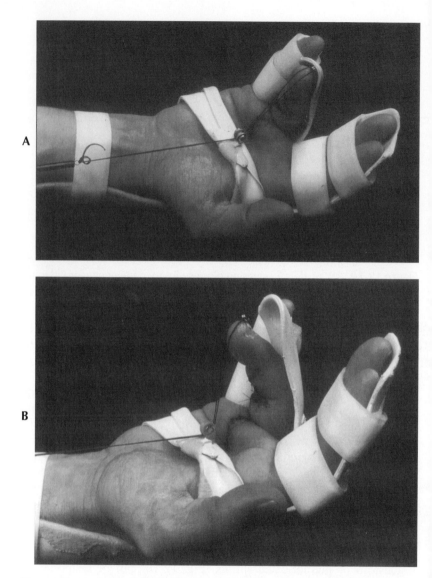

Figure 12-11 (A) and (B) Kleinert splint for flexor tendon repairs. The uninvolved digits also are splinted to prevent rupture of the repaired with forceful flexion. The pulley system provides passive flexion of the involved ring finger.

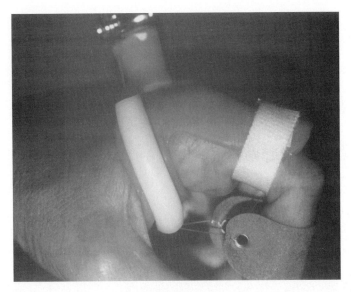

Figure 12-12   Custom hand-based dynamic PIP flexion splint for treatment of stiff PIP joints.

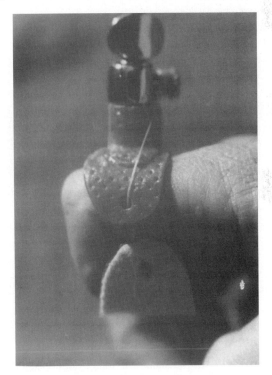

Figure 12-13   Custom hand-based dynamic PIP and DIP flexion splint for treatment of stiff joints.

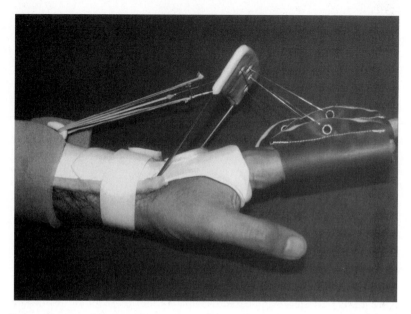

Figure 12-14   Custom dorsal wrist cock-up splint with dynamic extension outrigger for treatment of radial nerve palsy.

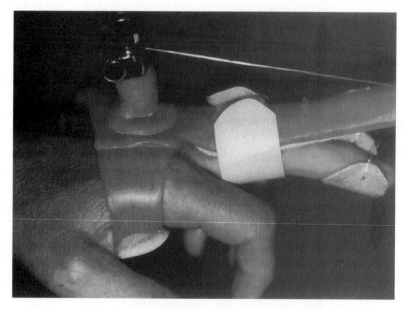

Figure 12-15   Dynamic PIP joint extension splint.

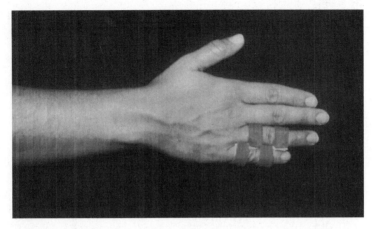

Figure 12-16   An example of buddy taping. See text for details.

of the proximal and middle phalanx as long as there is no displacement in any plane and serial X-rays are used to confirm this. They also are useful in helping a finger regain its normal range of motion by encouraging it to move along with the adjacent finger that has normal motion. Buddy splints also can be worn as protection when allowing the patient to return to sports activities.

Mallet Finger Splinting

After 6 weeks of continuous extension splinting (Fig. 12-17), the finger comes out of the splint to begin 10 to 15° of flexion 5 to 6 times per day. The finger remains in the splint at all other times. The patient is monitored carefully for development of an extensor lag and kept in the splint for an additional 1 to 2 weeks if one develops. The patient gradually increases DIP flexion over 3 to 4 weeks, and the splint is discontinued after 4 additional weeks. The patient is cautioned to carefully avoid forced flexion, which can occur with such seemingly benign tasks as tucking in clothes or sheets or putting on a sweater or a jacket. Patients are cautioned against unsupported use of the finger in contact sports for 3 months. They should use external support to prevent repeated forced flexion.

Ruptured Central Slip Splinting/Boutonniere Splinting

Treatment of a ruptured central slip usually requires immobilization of the PIP joint in extension for a minimum of 6 weeks. If there is an acute boutonniere deformity, the surgeon should consider possible operative treatment of the patient; if so, the splinting program may be

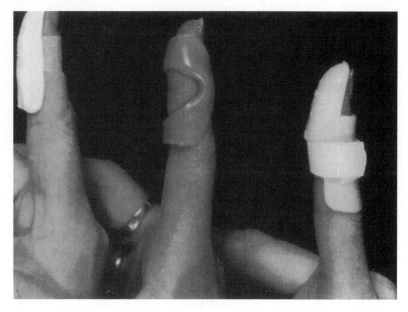

Figure 12-17 A variety of prefabricated and custom splints may be used for the treatment of mallet finger.

modified. While the finger is held in extension, the patient is encouraged to actively flex the DIP joint. This helps to stretch and strengthen the lateral bands that sublux volarly in these injuries. After the 6-week period of immobilization, the patient begins a graded protected program of active PIP flexion 5 to 6 times per day. The finger is kept in the splint at all other times. The patient is monitored carefully for development of an extensor lag and the PIP is totally immobilized for an additional 1 to 2 weeks if a 5 to 10° extensor lag develops. Otherwise, the patient gradually increases active PIP flexion over 3 to 4 weeks, and the splint is discontinued after 4 weeks. The patient is cautioned against unsupported use of the finger in contact sports for 3 months. They should use external support to prevent repeated forced flexion.

SPECIFIC TREATMENT PROTOCOLS

Tables 12-2 to 12-11 describe specific protocols for the treatment of tendon lacerations and hand fractures. Refer to the appropriate chapters in this book for further discussion of the rehabilitation issues related to these injuries.

Table 12-2 DX: Extensor Tendon Laceration: Static Method

	Week 1	Week 2	Week 3	Week 4	Weeks 5–6	Weeks 7–8
Wound Care	Warm water rinse		Remove sutures 10–14 days Begin scar management			
Edema management	Elevation				Continue edema management with retrograde massage as needed postimmobilization	
Static Splinting		Static extension splint: —Wrist: 30–40° extension —MPs: 0° —IPs: 0°			Continue splint at night; as needed to control extensor lags	
Dynamic Splint						As needed to gain full composite fist
Exercise/ROM		AROM of uninvolved digits; elbow; shoulder			Begin AROM; gentle composite fisting	
Strengthening/ Work Conditioning						Resistive exercises to increase grip; facilitate RTW
Activities of Daily Living (ADLs)	One-handed ADLs				Use hand for light ADLs	

ROM, range of motion; AROM, active range of motion.

Table 12-3 DX: Flexor Tendon Laceration

	Week 1	Week 2	Week 3	Week 4	Weeks 5–6	Weeks 7–8
Wound/Scar Management	Warm water soaks performed in clinic only		Silicon gel, scar massage			
Edema Management	Elevation, coban compression					
Static Splinting						At 7 weeks, composite extension splint p.r.n.
Dynamic Splint	Dorsal blocking splint: —Wrist: 20–30° flexion —MPs: 40–70° flexion —PIPs/DIPs: Full extension involved digit held in flexed position by nail hook or suture—rubberband traction through the metacarpal bar in base of splint		At 3–5 weeks, the wrist is splinted in neutral position. All digits remain splinted in protected position with involved digit continued in Kienert traction			At weeks 6–12, discontinue protective splint

Exercise	Duran's PROM exercises hourly, 10 reps. Kienert's active extension exercises hourly, 10 reps. Passive place and hold exercises in clinic only	Active wrist flexion extension; Duran's; Klienert's; Differential tendon gliding	At weeks 4–6 continue previous exercises; add isolated active PIP & DIP flexion/extension	At week 7 begin resistive exercise if warranted by adherent scar; theraputty; hand helper
Strengthening/Work Conditioning				
Activities of Daily Living			At 6 weeks, light functional use progressing to full functional use by 12 weeks	

MP, metacarpal phalangeal; PIP, proximal interphalangeal; DIP, distal interphalangeal; PROM, passive range of motion.

Table 12-4   DX: Mallet Finger

	Week 1	Week 2	Week 3	Week 4	Weeks 5-6	Weeks 7-8
Wound Care	Debridement clinic only					
Edema Management	Elevation					
Static Splinting	DIP joint immobilized. Position: DIP: 0–10° extension	Continue immobilization through 6th week postoperative. Adjust splint as needed				Gradually wean protective splint. Proceed with splint if extensor lag develops
Dynamic Splint Exercise/ROM	Maintain ROM of uninvolved MP–PIP joints	Continue HEP to maintain				Begin AROM upgrade as tolerated with control of extensor lag
Strengthening/Work Conditioning						Hand strengthening at 8 weeks. Resume normal ADLs
Activities of Daily Living (ADLs)	Light activities	Light ADLs as tolerated. Splint at all times				

DIP, distal interphalangeal; ROM, range of motion; MP, metacarpal phalangeal; PIP, proximal interphalangeal; HEP, home exercise plan.

Table 12-5   DX: Distal Phalanx Fracture

	Week 1	Week 2	Week 3	Week 4	Weeks 5–6	Weeks 7–8
Wound Care	Wound care initiated and continued until well healed		Begin desensitization as wound permits and continue until discharge			
Edema Management	Use compression immediately and continue until discharge					
Static Splinting		DIP protective splint is utilized for first 3 weeks of therapy, with removal for hourly AROM		Discharge protective splint if fracture is clinically healed		
Dynamic Splint		May dynamically splint PIP joint with pin or K–wire		providing fracture is stabilized	Initiate DIP dynamic splinting following 1 week of PROM if fracture is well healed	
Exercise/ROM	Perform hourly AROM				Initiate PROM providing fracture is well healed. Continue until discharge	
Strengthening/Work Conditioning	Deferred				Initiate light strengthening, gradually increasing to work conditioning if needed	
Activities of Daily Living	Light functional use			Increase functional use to include all activities		

DIP, distal interphalangeal; AROM, active range of motion; PIP, proximal interphalangeal; ROM, range of motion; PROM, passive range of motion.

Table 12-6   DX: Middle Phalanx Fracture with Rigid Fixation

	Week 1	Week 2	Week 3	Week 4	Weeks 5–6	Weeks 7–8
Wound Care	Light dressing applied and pin care if necessary	Remove sutures and begin scar massage	Initiate silicon gel if needed	Continue scar management techniques as needed until discharge		
Edema Management	Utilize compression as needed and continue until discharge					
Static Splinting	Fabricate protective splint and remove for exercise		Reduce protective splint to only buddy tape	Discharge protective splints when fracture is well healed		
Dynamic Splint			Based on stability of fracture, dynamic splinting may be initiated immediately. Gradually increase the frequency, tension, and duration. Continue until discharge			
Exercise/ROM	Remove splint for A/PROM		Increase frequency of A/PROM and continue until discharge			
Strengthening/Work Conditioning	Deferred			At 4–6 weeks initiate light strengthening progressing to work conditioning if needed. Continue until discharge		
Activities of Daily Living	Light functional use			Gradually increase functional use to include all activities		

ROM, range of motion; A/PROM, active/passive range of motion.

Table 12-7 DX: Middle Phalanx Fracture: Closed Reduction

	Week 1	Week 2	Week 3	Week 4	Weeks 5–6	Weeks 7–8
Wound Care			Initiate scar retraction massage and continue until discharge			
Edema Management	Use of compression initiated immediately and continued until discharge					
Static Splinting	Fabricate PIP and DIP extension splint. For stable fracture, only buddy tape may be indicated	Continue protective splinting with either rigid splint or buddy tape			Protective splinting is discharged when fracture is well healed	
Dynamic Splint	Deferred				Initiate dynamic splinting followed by 1 week of PROM	
Exercise/ROM	Initiate gentle protective AROM when pain subsides (3–5 days for stable fractures and 3 weeks for unstable or oblique fractures) gradually increasing to full AROM				PROM initiated providing fracture is well healed	
Strengthening/Work Conditioning						Initiate strengthening progressing to work conditioning
Activities of Daily Living	Light functional use					Increase functional use to include all activities

PIP, proximal interphalangeal; DIP, distal interphalangeal; ROM, range of motion; AROM, active range of motion; PROM, passive range of motion.

Table 12-8 DX: Proximal Phalanx Fractures with Rigid Fixation

	Week 1	Week 2	Week 3	Week 4	Weeks 5–6	Weeks 7–8
Wound Care	Light dressing applied and pin care if necessary	Remove sutures and begin scar massage	Upgrade to scar retraction and silicon gel	Continue scar management techniques until discharge		
Edema Management	Compression, retrograde massage, elevation, and active puming are initiated immediately and continued until discharge					
Static Splinting	Fabricate protective splint including joints proximal and distal to fracture. Remove for exercises		Reduce protective splint to only buddy tape	At 4–6 weeks may discharge all protective splinting		
Dynamic Splint	Based on stability of fracture, dynamic splinting may be initiated immediately. Gradually increase the frequency, tension and duration and continue until discharge					
Exercise/ROM	Remove splint for full A/PROM	Increased frequency of full A/PROM and continue until discharge				
Strengthening/Work Conditioning	Deferred				At 4–6 weeks initiate light strengthening progressing to work conditioning if needed. Continue until discharge	
Activities of Daily Living	Light functional use				Gradually increase functional use to include all activities	

ROM, range of motion; A/PROM, active/passive range of motion.

Table 12-9   DX: Proximal Phalanx Fracture: Closed Reduction

	Week 1	Week 2	Week 3	Week 4	Weeks 5–6	Weeks 7–8
Wound Care			Initiate scar retraction massage and continue until discharge			
Edema Management	Use of compression, retrograde massage, elevation and active pumping are initiated immediately and continued until discharge					
Static Splinting	Splint including MP and PIP. For stable fracture, only buddy tape may be indicated	Continue protective splinting with either buddy tape or rigid splint			Protective splint is discharged when fracture is well healed	
Dynamic Splint	Deferred				Initiate dynamic splinting following 1 week of full PROM	
Exercise/ROM		Initiate gentle protective AROM when pain and swelling subside (3–5 days for stable fracture and 3 weeks for unstable or oblique fracture) gradually increasing to full AROM			PROM initiated providing fracture is well healed	
Strengthening/Work Conditioning	Deferred				Begin light strengthening at 6–8 weeks progressing to work conditioning	
Activities of Daily Living	Light functional use				Gradually increasing functional use to include all activities	

MP, metacarpal phalangeal; PIP, proximal interphalangeal; ROM, range of motion; AROM, active range of motion; PROM, passive range of motion.

Table 12-10 DX: Metacarpal Fractures: Closed Reduction

	Week 1	Week 2	Week 3	Week 4	Weeks 5–6	Weeks 7–8
Wound Care						
Edema Management	Use of compression, retrograde massage, elevation, and active pumping are initiated immediately and continued until discharge		Begin scar retraction massage and continue until discharge			
Static Splinting	Ulnar gutter or wrist cock-up splint with digits buddy taped—degrees of MP based on fracture location and stability	Continue protective splinting	Continue intermittent protective splinting removing for exercises		Protective splint is discharged when fracture is well healed	
Dynamic Splint	Deferred					
Exercise/ROM	Initiate gentle protective AROM within cast or splint ROM upgrades based on radiographic evidence		Full tendon gliding, wrist AROM, and IP PROM initiated	Continue full AROM program including passive IP motion	Upgrade ROM program to full PROM and continue until discharge	
Strengthening/Work Conditioning	Deferred				Light strengthening initiated progressing to work conditioning Continue until discharge	
Activities of Daily Living	Light functional use				Gradually increased functional use to include all activities	

MP, metacarpal phalangeal; AROM, active range of motion; ROM, range of motion; PROM, passive range of motion; IP, interphalangeal.

Table 12-11   DX: Metacarpal Fractures with Rigid Fixation

	Week 1	Week 2	Week 3	Week 4	Weeks 5–6	Weeks 7–8
Wound Care	Light dressing applied and pin care if necessary	Remove sutures and begin scar massage	Upgrade to scar retraction and silicon gel	Continue all scar management techniques until discharge		
Edema Management	Compression, retrograde massage, elevation and active pumping are initiated immediately and continued until discharge					
Static Splinting	Ulnar gutter or wrist cock-up with digits buddy taped	Continue protective splint	At 3 weeks begin to wean protective splint reducing to only buddy tape		Discharge protective splint if fracture is well healed	
Dynamic Splint	Dynamic MP flexion splint utilized for extremely stable fracture	Continue or initiate dynamic splinting	Increase frequency and duration of dynamic splinting and continue until discharge			
Exercise/ROM	Remove splint for full A/PROM	Increase frequency of full A/PROM and continue until discharge				
Strengthening/Work Conditioning	Deferred			At 4–6 weeks begin light strengthening, progressing to work conditioning if needed. Continue until discharge		
Activities of Daily Living	Light functional use			Gradually increasing functional use to include all activities		

MP, metacarpal phalangeal; ROM, range of motion; A/PROM, active/passive range of motion.

SPECIAL TOPICS
Return to Work

A true measure of successful resolution of a hand injury is having the patient return to his prior employment. Unfortunately, recovering medically from the injury is only a portion of what is needed to have a patient regain employment. Many worker's compensation patients receive partial salary benefits. After prolonged periods of time, the patient has realizes that he/she can "get by" on these reduced payments. As a result, it may become increasingly difficult for that person to reenter the workplace. He or she may even have other sources of income from other types of work so that returning to a previous job might mean a loss of income. However, all injuries reach a point of maximal medical improvement. Determining that point, properly assessing what a patient can do, and conditioning the patient to return to work often is helpful.

One of the best ways to help a patient return to work is keep the time away from work at the absolute minimum. One often can sense if a patient is motivated to return to work before surgery. This should be factored into the decision to operate on a patient. A number of hand problems, such as carpal tunnel syndrome may require patients who perform repetitive tasks to alter their employment after surgery. It often is worthwhile to try a preoperative trial of altered work before surgery in hopes of alleviating the problem by conservative measures. Cooperation of the employer is needed and dealing with an employer who does not recognize that an injury is work related in the first place may prove an obstacle to a smooth return to work.

It often is difficult to truly know if a patient can return to his or her job, especially given the very specific and specialized nature of some work activities. If one cannot visit the workplace or make a careful assessment by a job description, videotapes of the required tasks can help one understand the demands of the job. It is not unusual for the patient's description to be at odds with the real job situation and knowledge of the required tasks entail helps the surgeon make decisions on the advisability of continued work activities. Arranging for the hand therapist or an ergonomic specialist to evaluate the workplace can be useful in difficult situations. At times, small modifications can overcome obstacles that prevent continued work.

In addition, work capacity assessments can be performed to evaluate the patient's ability to perform tasks and to provide initial guidelines as to what can be expected from a patient who returns to work. Work conditioning, as well as work hardening, can be offered to a patient as long as there is a job to return to, but this must be tailored to specific work tasks that increase endurance. Work hardening is helpful for patients who are able to perform tasks and thereby develop the additional body stamina needed to return to work. Work conditioning is tailored more to help the patient regain the capacity to carry out specific tasks than it is related to improvement of the injured hand.

Impairment Ratings and Disabilities

Disability rating is a legal concept and not a real measure of the outcome of a hand injury. Most standard measurement scales of impairment are based on objective measurements of sensibility testing and range of motion, with strength considerations a less quantifiable component. The impairment rating is not the same as a disability rating because based on what a patient does, any given injury or impairment is more or less a real disability (e.g., loss of an index finger of a pianist compared to the same loss in a farmer). The final disability rating is determined by the judicial system because it interprets the patient's impairment in terms of overall lifestyle. It also usually enters in only for work-related injuries, and the way it is reported can vary from state to state (e.g., an impairment rating of each joint of a finger in one state vs. a combined injury rating of each finger or hand in another vs. a single determination of the impairment an injury caused a patient in another). An additional problem arises with a previously injured patient who begins with a disability. One then has to attempt to affix an impairment rating to what the patient has lost as a result of the new injury.

Determination of the final disability rating of a hand-injured patient often is a time of joy for the surgeon, but a time of uncertainty for many patients. Our standard practice is to have the therapist perform the actual measurements of grip strengths, range of motion (with and without appropriate splints and supports), and sensory discrimination. Using the disability rating scales set forth in the *AMA's Guide to the Evaluation of Permanent Disability Impairments,* presently in its fourth edition, one can combine the evaluations into an estimate of the patient's impairment.

One should make the ultimate impairment rating in the context of the patient's overall therapy course and combine it with what one expects the patient to carry out. One can get a feel for the patient's functional capacity by assessing what the patient has been doing recently and then observing the range of motion and attempts at grip strength. Obtaining the patient's previous therapy records can be helpful in deciding the truthfulness of a patient's evaluation. It is not unusual for a patient to demonstrate a poorer function at the time of disability rating, and this should be evaluated carefully. Our practice is to tell the patient that we believe that the initial measurements did not honestly reflect real abilities and to try again. Other signs of a noncompliant patient is seen in grip measurements. Normally one has a bell-curve distribution of Jamar grip strength measurements when tested in the five different positions. In addition, repeated, rapid alternating hand grips of the Jamar grip strength meter should give fairly constant measures in an honest patient. A malingering patient will have widely varied measurements.

There are several computerized disability rating devices currently on the market. Although they still require that the therapist use a variety of tests, including the Semmes–Weinstein measurement, circumference, two-point discrimination, individual muscle strength, fingertip-to-palm measurements, locations of scars, and Tinel's sign, it does rapidly collect the data of joint range of motion as well as pinch and grip strength. These data are all combined for an impairment rating, with a computerized explanation of the rating for medicolegal purposes. This can save the physician the time needed to use the disability scales to derive the impairment rating by hand. Another benefit of the computerized systems is that they can serially display measurements as well as rapidly collect data and determine statistical variances to better detect malingering. These systems can prove a great savings in time for a busy hand therapy unit.

Psychological Issues

The psychological treatment of patients with a major injury needs to begin at the time of injury. The patient often needs a great deal of support, but their acceptance of this and the availability of treatment is unpredictable. Our standard practice is to tell patients from the time of injury that it is not unusual for them to have adjustment problems to the injury and that secondary depressions are common. For major injuries in which it is obvious there will be significant limitations in the use of the hand, we have a psychiatrist meet with the patient before discharge.

Vocational training or retraining is begun early with severely injured patients, so that their lives do not focus on what they have lost, but on future opportunities. The availability of alternative employment opportunities helps patients adjust to new limitations with increased self-pride and allows therapists to focus on new hand needs.

The eventual return to work can be a trying time for a patient who must face the same work environment and perhaps the very machine that caused the injury. This adjustment can be very difficult or even impossible—for some patients, and close monitoring of the patient is needed at this time.

Patients with major injuries who are out of work for a considerable period of time are at a high risk for developing family discord. A previously nonworking spouse may have to seek employment; work additional hours to help cover expenses. A spouse may have to keep a job because it provides medical insurance. The family dynamics often are altered markedly and resentments may develop that can be compounded by the increased stresses that come with child care. One should try to monitor potential home problems and offer assistance as appropriate. Unresolved family problems can significantly affect a patient's attitude toward the injury and its ultimate resolution.

SELECTED REFERENCES

Cannon NM, Foltz RW, Koepfer JM, et al: *Manual of hand splinting,* New York, 1985, Churchill Livingston.

Fess EE, Philips CA: *Hand splinting: principles and methods,* ed 2, St. Louis, 1987, CV Mosby.

Hunter JM, Mackin EJ, Callahan AD: *Rehabilitation of the hand: surgery and therapy,* ed 4, St. Louis, 1995, CV Mosby.

Kendall HO, Kendall FR, Waldsworth GE: *Muscle testing and function.* Baltimore, 1971, Williams & Wilkins.

Mackinon SE, Dellon AL: Sensory rehabilitation after nerve injury. In Mackinon SE, Dellon AL: *Surgery of the peripheral nerve.* New York, 1988, Thieme.

Index

A

Abductor digiti minimi, 58
Abductor pollicis brevis, 58
Abductor pollicis longus, 22
Abscess formation, 86
  dorsal, 86
  palmar, 87
  pyogenic flexor tenosynovitis, 87
  web-space collar-button, 200
Acetylcholinesterase, 295
ACE® wrap, 91
Acid burns, 76-77
Acland clamp, replantation surgery and,
  528
Actin, 2
Acute injury
  anesthesia for, 158
  laceration closure, equipment needs,
    158
  splinting of, 172
  treatment of, 157-168, 172
    lighting requirements, 157
    skin preparation, 158
Acute Trauma Life Support, wound evaluation and, 154
Acyclovir, herpetic Whitlow lesions and,
  204
Adductor aponeurosis, 390
Adductor pollicis, 59
Adhesion formation, *see also* Scar
  formation
  biochemical control of, 28, 29
  filmy, 25
  operative control of, 30-32
  tendon gliding and, 28
  tendon healing and, 26
ADM, *see* Abductor digiti minimi
Adrenaline
  pediatric hand injuries and, 570
  upper extremity injury and, 158
AIN, *see* Anterior interosseous nerve
Alkali burns, 77-78
Allen's test, 43, 44, 421-422
β-Aminopropionitrate, 29

Amputated part
  examination of, 504-507
  initial dissection, 523-526
  prehospital management, 498-499
  radiography of, 509
Amputation
  care of amputated parts, 92-93
  completion, patient expectations for,
    520
  fingertip, coverage options, 209
  replantation and, 498
  site of, 503
  angiography, 509
  associated injuries and, 502
  case examples, 559-563
  diagnostic studies, 507-509
  emergency evaluation, 499-500
  history taking, 500-503
  initial dissection of amputated part,
    523-526
  ischemia time, 501-502
  level of, 511-517
  major limb, 533-534
  mechanism of injury, 500-503
  operating room mobilization, 509-510
  patient expectations for replantation,
    517-520
  patient medical condition, 502
  patient occupation, 502
  physical examination, 503-507
  postoperative care/monitoring, 534-541
  preoperative counseling, 509-521
  preoperative preparation, 509-521
  preoperative testing, 509
  pressure dressing over wound, 503
  rehabilitation after replantation sur-
    gery, 540
  replantation considerations, 510-521
  replantation surgery outcome, 540-541
  secondary surgery, 540-541
  self-inflicted, 502
  smoking history, 502
  surgical considerations, 501-503
  toe-to-hand transfer, 543-544
Anaphylaxis, 156